Pocket CUTANEOUS MEDICINE AND SURGERY

Edited by:

JEFFREY S. DOVER, MD, FRCPC

Chief, Division of Dermatology
New England Deaconess Hospital
Assistant Professor of Dermatology
Harvard Medical School
Boston, Massachusetts

In Collaboration with:

BROOKE A. JACKSON, MD

Instructor, Department of Dermatology
Beth Israel Hospital
Harvard Medical School
Boston, Massachusetts

JACQUELINE M. JUNKINS-HOPKINS, MD

Clinical Associate in Dermatology
University of Pennsylvania Medical
Center
Philadelphia, Pennsylvania

In Consultation with:

KENNETH A. ARNDT, MD

Dermatologist-in-Chief
Beth Israel Hospital
Professor of Dermatology
Harvard Medical School
Boston, Massachusetts

PHILIP E. LeBOIT, MD

Associate Professor of Pathology and
Dermatology
University of California, San Francisco
San Francisco, California

JUNE K. ROBINSON, MD

Professor of Dermatology and Surgery
Departments of Dermatology and Surgery
Northwestern University Medical School
Chicago, Illinois

BRUCE U. WINTROUB, MD

Executive Vice Dean
Professor of Dermatology
School of Medicine
University of California, San Francisco
San Francisco, California

W.B. SAUNDERS COMPANY
A Division of Harcourt Brace & Company
Philadelphia   London   Toronto   Montreal   Sydney   Tokyo

W.B. SAUNDERS COMPANY
A Division of Harcourt Brace & Company

The Curtis Center
Independence Square West
Philadelphia, Pennsylvania 19106

POCKET GUIDE TO
CUTANEOUS MEDICINE
AND SURGERY   ISBN 0–7216–5409–6

Last digit is the print number: 9   8   7   6   5   4   3   2   1

To the Women in My Life

My grandmothers, Bertha and Lillian
My mother, Nina
My daughters, Sophie and Isabel
and especially to my wife, Tania

For their never-ending encouragement,
support, love, friendship,
and patience

PLEASE NOTE

All references to **CM&S** following
headings are to
Cutaneous Medicine and Surgery.

Preface

Cutaneous Medicine and Surgery: An Integrated Program in Dermatology is a new approach to the study of dermatology. It consists of a flagship textbook, *Cutaneous Medicine and Surgery*, and three other texts, the *Atlas of Cutaneous Surgery*, the *Pocket Guide to Cutaneous Medicine and Surgery*, and the *Self-Assessment and Review;* other books and periodicals are to follow. The main text serves as the backbone and outline of the program, while the other publications either complement or supplement it. All of the accompanying books refer back to the main text for discussions in greater depth in order to fully integrate the varied sources of information.

Comprehensive textbooks of dermatology are, by their very nature, encyclopedic and detailed and large, bulky, and impractical as portable sources of ever-ready information. The *Pocket Guide to Cutaneous Medicine and Surgery*, packed with only the most pertinent clinically relevant material, has been written to accompany the main text and has been designed to fit conveniently into a coat pocket or small bag. The *Pocket Guide* serves as an introduction and guide to dermatology for medical students and trainees, and as a quick reference for practicing primary care physicians, internists, and allied health care personnel.

Cutaneous Medicine and Surgery has been condensed into this pocket-sized companion text by incorporating all the essential clinical and therapeutic aspects of the main text. The organization of the *Pocket Guide* is based directly on the outline of *Cutaneous Medicine and Surgery* and is divided into 13 chapters representing our classification of dermatological diseases. These chapters are further subdivided into individual sections that represent a disease or a group of related disorders. The same outline is followed for each topic and includes definition, clinical description, pathogenesis and etiology (where known), pathology, and treatment. Each section is cross-referenced to the appropriate chapter in the main text to make consultation with *Cutaneous Medicine and Surgery* as easy as possible.

The *Pocket Guide* is meant to supplement but not to replace *Cutaneous Medicine and Surgery*. It is comprehensive in its approach to clinical dermatology and sufficient, in many instances, as a single source of information. As a companion to *Cutaneous Medicine and Surgery*, we hope it will assist students and clinicians in delivering optimal care to patients with cutaneous disease.

We would like to thank Drs. Brooke A. Jackson and Jacqueline M. Junkins-Hopkins for their precise, effective, and expeditious condensation and writing of selected chapters in the *Pocket Guide*. We would also like to thank the authors of *Cutaneous Medicine and Surgery*, on whose expertly written work the *Pocket Guide* is based.

JEFFREY S. DOVER, MD, FRCPC
KENNETH A. ARNDT, MD

Contents

chapter **3** _____

What Causes Blistering of the Skin? **227**

chapter 1

What Fundamental Information Is Necessary to Understand Cutaneous Medicine and Surgery?

WHAT IS NORMAL SKIN?

(CM&S Chapter 1)

The skin, a complex organ responsible for numerous physiologic and immunologic functions, is arguably the largest organ in the body. An average human adult's skin weighs 3 to 4 kg, constitutes 6% to 7% body weight, and measures about 2 square meters. The skin's principal duty is to serve as a barrier to harmful exogenous substances, chemicals, and pathogens while retaining water and endogenous proteins. The skin also regulates body temperature, is a sensory organ, protects against physical injury, has psychosocial and aesthetic importance, and is an important component of the immune system. Human skin consists of three layers: epidermis, dermis, and subcutaneous fat.

Epidermis

The major barrier function of skin is provided by the thin stratum corneum. The complex structural and biochemical machinery of the epidermis is, in large part, devoted to production of the cornified layer. Cornification results from a sequence of events including the synthesis and assembly of a series of *keratins,* the addition of *filaggrin,* and, ultimately, the synthesis and assembly of the *cornified envelope.* The major function of keratinocytes is formation of the stratum corneum. Diseases leading to disruption or inadequate formation of the stratum corneum are accompanied by profound defects in the skin's barrier function capability. The skin's protective function is dependent on the integrity of the epidermis (and its attachment to the dermis), which is maintained by elaborate intercellular adhesion structures (desmosomes) and by strong and ordered intracellular intermediate filaments, predominantly keratin, as well as other intracellular structural proteins, actin-containing microfilaments, and tubulin-containing microtubules.

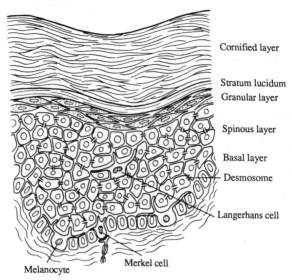

FIGURE 1–1. The epidermis is an integrated epithelium consisting of several zones, or strata, including the basal, spinous, granular, and cornified layers and three "other" cellular components: melanocytes, Merkel cells, and Langerhans cells. (Courtesy of Lynn Kitagawa.)

Although the epidermis is an integrated epithelial layer, four distinct contiguous "layers" or zones are apparent by light microscopic examination extending from the dermis to the skin surface: the basal, squamous, granular, and cornified layers (Fig. 1–1). The *basal layer* consists of cuboidal or columnar cells, one to three layers in thickness, comprising the main proliferative compartment of the epidermis. The undersurface of the epidermis undulates, forming projections called *rete ridges* that separate *dermal papillae* of the upper (papillary) dermis.

The basal layer produces cells that eventually replace terminally differentiated cells that are continuously lost from the epidermal surface. The epidermis replaces itself every 12 to 14 days. One of several distinct populations of basal cells is the stem cell population. They are small in number, divide infrequently, and reside deep within rete ridges. Following division, stem cells give rise to one daughter cell that remains a stem cell and one daughter cell that divides more rapidly but can divide only a limited number of times and can undergo terminal differentiation. The regulation of basal cell growth and division, while not well characterized, is influenced by intrinsic and extrinsic factors, including intracellular and extracellular elements of the dermis, epidermal growth factor, vitamin A, and hormones.

Suprabasal keratinocytes within the spinous layer are polygonal in appearance with numerous delicate "spiny" projections known as *desmosomes* spanning their intercellular spaces to adjacent keratinocytes. Keratinocytes become larger and flatter and have decreased water content as they migrate toward the surface. Langerhans cells—dendritic, immunomodulating cells—are scattered throughout the spinous layer and function in delayed hypersensitivity reactions, allograft rejection, and graft-versus-host disease.

The *granular layer,* composed of keratinocytes replete with *keratohyalin granules,* comprises two or three cell layers between the spinous and cornified layers. Here, cellular proteins and organelles, no longer to be used, are degraded. *Lamellar bodies* (Odland bodies [membrane-coating granules]), found in granular layer keratinocytes, participate in the cornification process by discharging their lipid components into intercellular spaces, enhancing the skin's barrier function, and aiding intercellular cohesion within the stratum corneum. Protein envelopes also develop within the stratum corneum influenced by *filaggrin,* a protein component of the keratohyalin granules, which causes keratin filament aggregation.

Finally, the *cornified layer* (stratum corneum), variable in thickness, is composed of flattened, polyhedral cells (corneocytes) that have lost nuclei and cytoplasmic organelles and are arranged in orderly, but widely overlapping columns in many skin areas. The stratum corneum is thinnest on the eyelids and genitalia and thickest on the palms and soles.

Keratinization

Formation of keratin fibers is one of the major functions of epidermal keratinocytes. The keratins are a family of approximately 20 intermediate-filament proteins that have a molecular mass ranging from 40 to 70. The keratins can be grouped into two classes based on their structure and isoelectric points: acidic and basic keratins. Specific keratin pairs are synthesized in microscopically distinct epidermal cell layers. Each keratin pair assembles to form intermediate filaments that with tubulin and actin form the cytoskeleton of keratinocytes. The major function of keratin appears to be to maintain the three-dimensional architecture of the epidermis by providing an intracellular skeleton for the keratinocyte.

Filaggrin

Filaggrin is a cationic 26- to 48-kd protein present in the stratum corneum. Filaggrin associates with keratin intermediate filaments, resulting in the formation of densely organized aggregates in vitro and aiding in the formation of dense parallel packing of keratin filaments during epidermal differentiation.

The synthesis and assembly of the *cornified envelope* appears to be the other major function of keratinocytes. The precursors of the cornified envelope, such as involucrin, loricrin, and keratolinin, apparently are synthesized first in the outer layers of the spinous layer and in the granular layer. These molecules are translocated to just inside the plasma membrane of keratinocytes in the granular layer and are cross-linked with transglutaminase, forming a durable polymer that is highly insoluble. The 15-nm–thick cornified envelope is stabilized by extensive cross-linking via $\epsilon\gamma$-glutamyl lysine isopeptide bonds.

Skin Pigmentation

Skin color is determined by the amount of melanin present in the skin and the way in which it is distributed. Although the concentration of melanocytes per unit surface area varies markedly in different areas of the body, there are no significant differences among races in the number or distribution of melanocytes in the skin. Black skin is darker than lighter skin because of increased production, distribution, and retention of melanin, not a greater number of melanocytes. Melanin is produced in pigment granules known as *melanosomes*. Melanosomes are synthesized in melanocytes and passed to epidermal cells in the lower layers of the epidermis. Each melanocyte is in contact with about 36 keratinocytes, and each such group of cells is termed an *epidermal melanin unit*.

Melanin synthesis begins with the conversion of tyrosine to *dopa* through the action of tyrosinase. Dopa is hydroxylated and polymerized to melanin in melanosomes. Melanosomes are passed from melanocytes to surrounding keratinocytes, which actively phagocytize them. Melanosomes undergo progressive development from stage I melanosomes, which contain no melanin but have enzymatic activity, to stage IV, or fully developed melanin-laden melanosomes, which lack tyrosinase activity.

Melanosomes in black skin are large, dense, numerous, and distributed singly to epidermal cells. The relative size of the melanosomes correlates with tone in black skin, with darker skin having larger melanosomes. In the skin of white and Asian people, melanosomes are smaller, less dense, fewer in number, and distributed in clusters. Melanin production increases in response to ultraviolet light, resulting in tanning. The ability to increase melanin production in response to ultraviolet light is genetically determined and is greatest for blacks, Asians, and whites of Mediterranean descent.

Dark skin absorbs and disperses ultraviolet irradiation more effectively than lighter skin and thereby prevents much of the damage done by ultraviolet exposure. Black skin has an inherent sun protective factor (SPF) of approximately 5.

Dermoepidermal Junction

The *dermoepidermal junction* (DEJ) is a large, specialized attachment site that forms an extensive interface between the epidermis and papillary dermis. The major function of the DEJ is to keep the epidermis firmly attached to the dermis; other functions include support, regulation of permeability across the dermoepidermal interface, and a role in embryonic differentiation.

Dermis

The dermis consists primarily of connective tissues—collagen, elastic tissue, and ground substance—that protect against trauma and envelop the body in a strong and flexible wrap. Also within the dermis are blood vessels, lymphatics, nerves, and epithelial adnexa—hair follicles and sebaceous, apocrine and eccrine glands.

Collagen fibers measuring from 2 to 15 μm are the major structural components of the dermis. In the adventitial and papillary dermis, collagen forms a finely woven meshwork of fibers, while in the reticular dermis, collagen fibers form thick bundles. The two major types of collagen are types I and III. *Type I collagen,* which accounts for 80% of total collagen in human skin, is present throughout the entire dermis, imparting to it tensile strength. *Type III collagen* constitutes approximately 15% of dermal collagen and is localized mainly in the adventitial dermis, including beneath the epidermal basement membrane where it plays an important role in anchoring the epidermis to the dermis.

Elastic fibers constitute approximately 3% of the dermis by dry weight, measure 1 to 3 μm in diameter, and play a major role in skin elasticity and resilience. Elastic fibers are wavy and appear fragmented when examined by light microscopy, where they cannot be seen with routine stains and for visualization require stains such as silver, orcein, or resorcin-fuchsin.

Ground substance, an amorphous material that fills spaces between the fibrillar and cellular components of the dermis, imparting turgidity and resilience, is composed of water, electrolytes, plasma proteins, and mucopolysaccharides. Mucopolysaccharides are constructed of long chains of aminated sugars (glycosaminoglycans) and uronic acids. Linked covalently to polypeptides, the chains form high-molecular-weight complexes called *proteoglycans.* In the dermis, the most common glycosaminoglycans are hyaluronic acid and dermatan sulfate. Because water is lost during processing of histologic sections, ground substance appears as empty spaces and its demonstration requires special stains, such as colloidal iron or Alcian blue.

Fibronectins, another important component of the ground substance, are high-molecular-weight glycoproteins present on the surfaces of cells, in extracellular fluid, and in connective tissue matrices. Their most important function is to facilitate the attachment of fibroblasts, macrophages, and keratinocytes to cell membranes, basement membranes, collagen, and fibrin.

Vasculature

The blood supply of the dermis originates from a plexus located in the deep reticular dermis that connects via communicating vessels to three more superficial plexuses. The three superficial plexuses are the subpapillary plexus and plexuses around hair follicles and around eccrine glands. From these vascular networks, progressively smaller *arterioles* ascend through the dermis, finally branching into numerous *capillaries* in the adventitial dermis. Capillary loops supplying each subepidermal papilla originate from the subpapillary plexus, each loop consisting of an ascending arterial limb and a descending venous limb. The venous limb drains blood into progressively larger *venules,* which finally empty into small *veins* of the subcutaneous plexus.

Pads and nail beds of the fingers and toes, the central face, and the ears contain specialized vascular structures—*glomus bodies*—concerned with regulation of blood flow and temperature. Glomus bodies are arteriovenous shunts—that is, direct connections between arterioles and venules without interposition of capillaries.

Lymphatics in the skin form a complex network following the distribution of arterioles and venules.

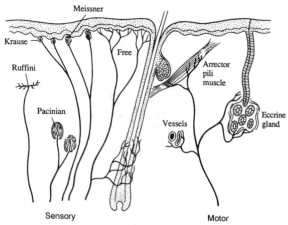

FIGURE 1–2. Both sensory and motor innervation supplies overlapping cutaneous regions. Sensory innervation consists of free nerve endings, some with attachments to epidermal Merkel cells, and some concentrated around follicles, as well as encapsulated receptors (Pacini, Meissner, Ruffini, and Krause end-bulbs [mucocutaneous corpuscles]). Motor innervation to the skin may result in increased sweating, vasoconstriction, or arrector pili muscle contraction causing "goose bumps." (Courtesy of Lynn Kitagawa.)

Nerves and Sensory Receptors

The skin is richly innervated and can be considered a terminus of the peripheral nervous system (Fig. 1–2). Cutaneous nerves, which contain both sensory and motor fibers forming plexuses in the subcutaneous tissue and in the dermis, supply overlapping, contiguous regions of the skin. Innervation of the skin is marked by regional variation—that is, some zones are recipients of more nerve fibers than others. In locations such as palms, soles, glans penis, nipples, and clitoris, the distribution of nerve terminals is more dense than in other regions of the skin. Sensations including touch, pressure, temperature, and pain are perceived in the skin via different receptors, and specific messages are conveyed from the peripheral to the central nervous system.

The autonomic portion of the peripheral system, which serves to ensure internal homeostasis, consists of sympathetic and parasympathetic divisions. Most viscera are supplied by both divisions. Epithelial and nonepithelial structures such as cutaneous adnexa including eccrine and apocrine glands, blood vessels, and muscles of hair erection are innervated by sympathetic fibers only. Autonomic nerve stimulation may result in increased volume of perspiration, blood vessel constriction, and arrector pili muscle contraction, causing "goose bumps" as hairs become elevated.

Sensory Receptors of the Skin

The skin possesses different types of receptors sensitive to different stimuli. Fundamental sensations, including temperature, pressure, pain, and touch, are perceived by the skin and transmitted to the central nervous system, where the information is localized and analyzed. More complex sensations, such as vibration, are combinations of these basic sensations.

Sensory receptors, variable in their degree of complexity, can be classified as *free* or *encapsulated*. Free nerve endings are simple, consisting of single small, unmyelinated or myelinated nerve fibers situated in the epidermis and papillary dermis where they form a network. In human skin, free nerve endings have been detected in eyelids, nasal vestibule, and genital region.

In contrast, the encapsulated type is more elaborate, containing different types of cells, in addition to nerve endings. They include Pacini corpuscles, Meissner corpuscles, Ruffini corpuscles, and mucocutaneous corpuscles, also known as Krause end-bulbs.

Pacini corpuscles are distributed throughout the dermis and subcutaneous tissue, particularly in fingers, external genitalia, and breasts, and function as pressure receptors. They are ovoid or round structures 0.5 to 1 μm in diameter that are formed by a central nerve fiber surrounded by concentric layers of flattened cells, which are in turn surrounded by a subcapsular space and, eventually, a capsule.

Meissner corpuscles, which act as mechanoreceptors, are most numerous in the center of palms and soles, as well as the lips, eyelids, external genitalia, and nipples. Situated high in the papillary dermis, Meissner corpuscles are ovoid structures composed of axons and laminar cells.

Subcutaneous Fat

Subcutaneous fat serves as a shock absorber protecting vital structures, maintaining body heat, and storing energy. The basic unit of the subcutaneous fat is the microlobule, which is composed of collections of adipocytes. Aggregations of primary microlobules form secondary lobules that are separated by connective tissue septa containing nerves, vessels, and lymphatics. Septa connect the reticular dermis to the fascia of the skeletal muscle.

Cutaneous Appendages

Hair Follicles

Longitudinal section of hair follicles reveals three zones (Fig. 1–3): the *infundibulum*, extending from the ostium (opening) of the follicle to the opening of the sebaceous duct; the *isthmus*, extending from the opening of the sebaceous duct to the insertion of the arrector pili muscle; and the *inferior segment*, which extends from the site of insertion of the pili muscle to the base of the hair follicle and is made up of the *stem* and the *bulb*. The inferior segment cycles through growing and resting phases during the life of the hair follicle, while the infundibulum and the isthmus remain constant. The stem cells of the follicle are believed to reside in the bulge that marks the attachment of the arrector pili muscle.

Cross-section of the *inferior segment* (in sequence, from the middle to the outer surface) reveals the following (Fig. 1–4): (1) *medulla* of the hair shaft, present only in terminal hairs; (2) *cortex* of

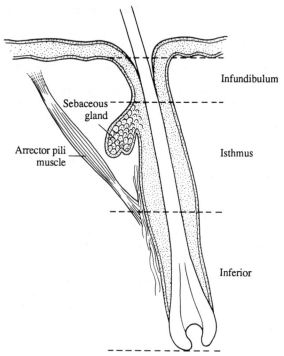

Infundibulum

Sebaceous
gland

Isthmus

Arrector pili
muscle

Inferior

FIGURE 1–3. Traditional division of hair follicles includes the upper fun-
nel-shaped infundibulum, extending from the epidermal surface to the sebaceous duct entrance; the midportion, or isthmus, which is bounded by entry
of the sebaceous duct above to the attachment site of the arrector pili muscle
below; and the inferior segment. (Courtesy of Lynn Kitagawa.)

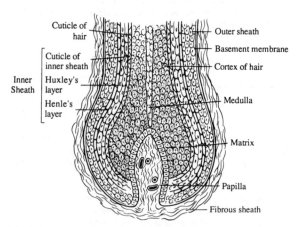

Cuticle of
hair

Cuticle of
inner sheath

Inner
Sheath

Huxley's
layer

Henle's
layer

Outer sheath

Basement membrane

Cortex of hair

Medulla

Matrix

Papilla

Fibrous sheath

FIGURE 1–4. Hair bulbs are complex epithelial-mesenchymal structures.
Matrical cells produced by the germinative basal layer form the medulla, hair
shaft and its cuticle, three layers of the inner hair sheath, and, possibly, the
outer sheath. (Courtesy of Lynn Kitagawa.)

the hair shaft; (3) *cuticle* of the hair shaft, composed of a single cornified layer; (4) *inner root sheath;* and (5) the *outer root sheath. The bulb,* or lowest part of the hair follicle, is composed of germinative cells and numerous melanocytes, some with prominent dendritic processes. The germinative cells have hyperchromic nuclei, little cytoplasm, and numerous mitotic figures, indicating their high rate of proliferation.

Hair growth is cyclical. Most follicles are in growing, or *anagen,* phase, which typically lasts months to years, depending on anatomic site. Through unknown mechanisms, and in apparently random, nonsequential fashion, follicles periodically enter a transitional, involutional, or *catagen,* phase when hair growth stops and the inferior segment begins resorption over a several-week period. The hair bulb assumes a club appearance and completes its upward journey at the level of the erector muscle attachment site, where it remains in nesting, or *telogen* phase, for several weeks to a few months. Following a predetermined period, ill-defined signals result in another growth phase and the cycle begins anew as matrical cells generate a new hair within the regenerating and descending inferior segment.

Sebaceous Glands

Sebaceous glands are present in all cutaneous areas except palms, soles, and the dorsal feet and develop in association with hair follicles, with some exceptions. Free sebaceous glands not associated with follicles are present in modified skin of the nipple and areola of men and women; on the labia minora and inner aspect of the prepuce; and on the vermilion border of the lips and buccal mucosa, where they are known as Fordyce's condition, or spots. The largest and most numerous subaceous glands are on the central face and scalp, particularly the forehead and nose, as well as the upper back.

Sebaceous glands are well developed at birth but atrophy after birth and remain small until puberty, when they respond to gonadal and adrenal androgenic hormones, remaining large through adult life until menopause in women and a slightly later age in men.

Sebaceous glands are made up of lobules, producing centripetally differentiating sebaceous cells that gradually accumulate cytoplasmic lipid, filling and surrounding the centrally placed nucleus. Mature sebaceous cells disintegrate (holocrine secretion) at the entrance to the sebaceous duct, eventually emptying into the follicular infundibulum. The amorphous mass of lipid and cellular debris represents *sebum,* which coats the hair shaft and the epidermal surface with lipid-rich secretions, presumably as a lubricating and protective function. Sebum consists predominantly of triglycerides, wax esters, squalene, cholesterol, and cholesterol esters.

Apocrine Glands

Apocrine glands are found uncommonly except in the skin of the axilla, anogenital region, external auditory canals, and eyelids, and uncommonly on the face and scalp. They do not participate in heat regulation (and therefore are not sweat glands), although they may function in humans as scent glands, their primary function in other mammals. Apocrine glands remain small and nonfunctional until puberty, enlarging under hormonal influences.

Apical portions of apocrine cell cytoplasm protrude irregularly into the lumen of the follicular infundibulum and apparently "pinch off," producing apocrine secretion. Apocrine glands produce a viscous, milky, odorless substance that, in contrast to eccrine secretion, is stored, to be released intermittently with intervening longer refractory periods. Bacterial action on apocrine gland secretion produces short-chain fatty acids and other substances, resulting in characteristic odors.

Eccrine Glands

Eccrine glands, which are the only true sweat glands in humans, are abundant throughout all skin surfaces except the vermilion border of the lips, labia minora, clitoris, glans penis, external auditory canal, and nail beds, with the greatest number of glands located on the palms, soles, and axilla. Eccrine glands are composed of (1) the *secretory gland* and (2) a *coiled duct* that leads from the secretory segment to (3) the straight *intradermal duct* traveling through the dermis and connecting to (4) the spiraled *intraepidermal duct* (*acrosyringium*).

The major function of eccrine glands is to produce the hypotonic solution known as sweat, which facilitates evaporative cooling. Cholinergic nerves of the sympathetic nervous system innervate eccrine glands, producing acetylcholine, which acts on the plasma membrane of pale cells to begin the metabolic process leading to sweat formation. Both thermal and emotional factors prominently stimulate sweating; under severe conditions, adults are capable of producing up to several liters of sweat.

Nails

The nail plate and surrounding tissues form the *nail unit* (Fig. 1–5). The *nail plate* is a translucent, rectangular structure composed of cornified cells that inserts proximally and laterally into continuous skin grooves known as the *proximal* and *lateral nail folds,* respectively.

The cornified layer of the ventral part of the proximal nail fold contributes to the formation of the *cuticle,* which extends over the surface of the nail plate for 1 to 2 mm. Beneath the proximal nail fold, the *matrix* of the nail contains germinative cells, the source of cornified cells for the growing nail. The proximal portion of the matrix supplies cornified cells for the dorsal portion of the nail, while the distal portion of the matrix does so for the ventral portion of the nail. The matrical epithelium, which is composed of a basal, spinous, and cornified layer continuous with the nail plate, lacks a granular layer. The *lunula,* a crescent-shaped zone visible distal to the proximal nail fold, marks the distal margin of the nail matrix. This area is more visible on thumbnails.

The *nail bed,* distal to the matrix, has unique features. The epithelium is devoid of a granular layer with long, thin angulated rete ridges and dermal papillae. The nail bed dermis is highly vascular, with numerous arteriovenous shunts, or glomus bodies, functioning in temperature regulation. The nail plate rests on the nail bed, with both structures firmly attached.

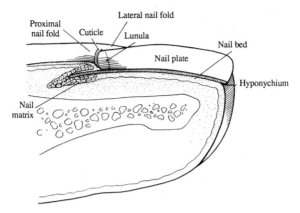

FIGURE 1–5. Nail units are situated on the distal, dorsal aspects of fingers and toes. The nail plate, a product of germinative cells of the nail matrix, including its distal visible portion, or lunula, resides in cutaneous grooves, or folds, proximally and laterally. Cornified cells of the nail bed intercalate with the undersurface of the nail plate, resulting in its strong adherence. (Courtesy of Lynn Kitagawa.)

Skin as a Component of the Immune System

Considerable evidence exists that the skin is an important component of the immune system. Skin contains an organized arrangement of immunocompetent cells that mediate specific and nonspecific immune responses. Key among them are epidermal Langerhans cells: dendritic, bone marrow–derived, antigen-presenting cells distributed among keratinocytes throughout the epidermis in numbers ranging from 350 to 800/mm^2 in different areas of the body. The importance of Langerhans cells in cutaneous immunity is their capacity to take up haptens in the skin and carry them to regional lymph nodes. Application of haptens to skin containing Langerhans cells induced T cell–mediated, delayed-type hypersensitivity.

Langerhans cells express surface antigens characteristic of antigen-presenting cells. They have been shown to take in, process, and present protein, hapten, and allo- and self-antigens and to stimulate naive and primed T lymphocytes. Antigens carried by Langerhans cells to regional lymph nodes are presented to T cells, which proliferate in response to antigen and accessory, co-stimulatory signals. Resultant, activated, antigen-specific T cells are released into the circulation, where they may modulate immune responses in the skin such as the development of allergic contact hypersensitivity and possibly many other cutaneous inflammatory responses. Langerhans cells have been shown to play an important role in skin allograft rejection and in graft-versus-host disease. Depletion of epidermal Langerhans cells has been implicated as playing a causal role in ultraviolet-induced carcinogenesis and in photoaging.

Keratinocytes, the majority epidermal cell population, also may have immune function. Epidermal keratinocytes produce and secrete a wide array of mediators of inflammation. They also can be induced to express HLA class II antigens, antigens normally expressed only by cells belonging to the immune system.

The dermis contains a wide variety of antigen-presenting cells and lymphocytes predominantly distributed around small vessels of the dermal vascular plexus. The T-cell receptor repertoire of normal skin lymphocytes differs significantly from peripheral blood, suggesting that it is shaped by the antigens present within the skin. Papillary dermal venules are surrounded by cuff mast cells that contain many mediators that help control vascular flow and permeability. Lymphocytes and macrophages are found in the dermis in normal skin, while their numbers are increased in many skin disorders. Finally, eosinophils, neutrophils, and basophils infiltrate the skin in many inflammatory skin diseases.

WHAT DOES NORMAL SKIN DO?

(CM&S Chapter 2)

Functions of the Deeper Skin Layers and the Epidermis

External to the muscle fascia is the *subcutaneous fat layer,* the innermost region of the skin. In addition to its critical metabolic functions, this layer acts as an insulator, reducing heat movement into or out of the body and absorbing energy from blunt mechanical trauma. Above the fat layer lies the *dermis,* composed of collagen-glycosaminoglycan complexes, which both protect internal structures from blunt mechanical trauma and provide a conduit for nutrients and metabolites to and from the overlying epidermis. Overlying the dermis is the *epidermis,* which consists of several stratifying layers of *keratinocytes,* characterized by vertical differentiation. The postmitotic, nucleated layers of the epidermis generate the differentiation products, both protein and lipid, which compose the *stratum corneum.* In addition to keratinocytes, the epidermis also contains *melanocytes*, which synthesize UV-absorbing pigments (e.g., melanin), as further protection against UV radiation, and Langerhans cells, which play a role in cutaneous immune surveillance, protecting the organism against antigens that breach the stratum corneum. The epidermis and dermis also contain a variety of cutaneous appendages that have protective functions. The *eccrine sweat glands* and *blood vessels* of the skin aid in the regulation of body temperature; the *sebaceous glands* rapidly transport proteins and lipids to the surface of the skin, where they may function as antimicrobial agents and/or promote cell shedding (desquamation); and finally, afferent and efferent *nerve fibers,* which are chemosensitive, mechanosensitive, and heat-sensitive, act as a rapid warning system to trauma.

Barrier Functions of the Skin

The epidermis, a self-replicating structure that renews itself about every 30 days, is approximately 100 μm thick over most areas of the body. The principal constituent cell of the epidermis is the keratino-cyte, which becomes anucleate at the top, forming the 10-μm-thick stratum corneum. The cells of the stratum corneum, which are orga-nized into geometric stacks and are embedded in a lipid-enriched intercellular matrix, protect not only the host's aqueous interior from excessive water loss to a dry environment, but also against the entrance of microorganisms, as well as against the penetration of natural and man-made toxins. In addition to the stratum corneum, deeper layers of the skin protect from damage by (1) ultraviolet (UV) radiation, (2) mechanical forces, (3) extremes of environmen-tal temperatures, and (4) low-voltage electric current.

Epidermal Differentiation

Differentiation proceeds as mitotically active keratinocytes mi-grate outward from the basal layer, through the *spinous* and *granu-lar* layers, to reach the stratum corneum, where they become flat-tened, devoid of organelles, and progressively dehydrated. The principal cellular events in the process of epidermal differentiation (also termed cornification) are first, *keratinization,* the synthesis of the principal fibrous proteins of the keratinocyte, which impart structural and chemical integrity, filter incident UV light, and ab-sorb water and other small molecules; second, *keratohyalin* deposi-tion, associated with synthesis of ''histidine-rich protein,'' stratum corneum basic protein, or *filaggrin*, which appears to facilitate the assembly of keratin bundles during terminal differentiation and contribute to the water-holding properties of the stratum corneum; third, formation of a highly cross-linked, insoluble *cornified enve-lope,* composed of two or more precursor proteins—*involucrin, loricrin,* and *keratolinin*—which provides a rigid structural ecto-skeleton, a scaffold for the insertion of keratin filaments, a semiper-meable barrier to water, electrolytes, and nonelectrolytes and a highly resistant barrier to external assault; and fourth and finally, the generation of the lipid-enriched intercellular domains of the stratum corneum resulting from the secretion of the lipid-enriched contents of distinctive organelles, termed lamellar bodies (membrane-coat-ing granules, keratinosomes, Odland's bodies, cementosomes), into the intercellular matrix.

Stratum Corneum Formation and Structure

New corneocytes enter the stratum corneum at its base and move apically over approximately 14 days, following which they are shed invisibly (desquamation).

Stratum Corneum Structure

The stratum corneum has a bicompartmental architecture of pro-teinaceous cells embedded within a continuous lipid-enriched but heterogeneous matrix. The protein-enriched components, *corneo-cytes,* interdigitate along their lateral margins and are bound to-gether further by protein- and glycoprotein-enriched bridging molecules termed *desmosomes,* which slowly disintegrate during transit from the inner to the outer layers of the stratum corneum.

Water content of human epidermis remains high and relatively constant at 65% to 70% from the basal through the lower granular cell layer, but falls rapidly from 65% at the outer cells of the granular layer to 40% at the base of the stratum corneum, and to 15% at the outer layer of the stratum corneum. This concentration gradient is responsible for the passive diffusion of water from the internal to the external environments, termed *transepidermal water loss.*

The Epidermal Lamellar Body

The lipid enrichment of the stratum corneum results from the secretion of the contents of the epidermal lamellar body, a 0.2- to 0.3-μm-diameter ovoid, secretory organelle.

Epidermal Lipid Composition

The lipids of the stratum corneum are synthesized de novo within the epidermis. They are a unique mixture of nonpolar lipids that are enriched in cholesterol, adapted to protect the host against excessive water loss.

Langerhans Cells and the Immune System

Lymphocytes are the principal effector cells of the immune system, but they are aided by afferent and efferent accessory cells. The *Langerhans cells* of the epidermis are accessory cells of the afferent immune system, which function to present antigen to T lymphocytes, leading to an immune response. The latter do not recognize these antigens without prior, specific processing by the Langerhans cell.

Protection Against Damage from Extremes in Environmental Temperature

Thermoregulation of the Human Body

Body temperature homeostasis primarily involves maintaining the temperature of the central organs, such as the brain, heart, lungs, and abdominal viscera, within a narrow range of between 36.2° C and 37.8° C. The temperature of these core tissues is therefore generally maintained at or very close to 37° C, which represents the core temperature, and the temperature conducive to optimal organ function. In contrast, temperatures exceeding 39° C can lead to various forms of biologic damage and even to cell death, depending upon the absolute temperature and duration of the insult.

In contrast to central organs, peripheral tissues such as muscles, subcutaneous tissues, and the skin can function over a much wider temperature range. In fact, skin temperature can fall to as low as 20° C and rise to 40° C without cellular damage. However, skin temperatures in excess of 45° C or as low as 18° C usually are associated with pain and injury. Even though there are distinct central and peripheral thermoregulatory tissues, the boundary between the core and the peripheral temperature regions is fluid, expanding or contracting in order to maintain the core temperature region.

Thermoregulatory Responses

The skin participates in thermoregulation in a cold environment with stimulation of the sympathetic nerves, which contracts cutaneous blood vessels so that flow from the core to the skin is decreased. This results not only in a reduction in the transfer of body heat to the surface, but also in the lowering of the temperature gradient between the skin and the environment, which further decreases heat loss.

In contrast, in a relatively hot environment, as sympathetic stimulation decreases, and through direct warming of the skin surface, vasodilatation occurs, allowing blood to accumulate in the skin and heat to be lost rapidly. In addition, there is activation of sweating, panting, and behavioral alterations that enhance heat loss such as skin wetting and movement to a cooler environment.

Skin Structures That Subserve Thermoregulation

The skin provides both the sensory input to thermoregulation and the physical means to allow heat loss or conservation. The *thermoreceptor cells* of the skin are distributed unevenly over the skin in a punctate fashion. Like the neurons in the CNS, both warm-sensitive and cold-sensitive thermoreceptors exist. As the peripheral thermostats, they are thought to be the first component of the thermoregulatory apparatus to experience changes in environmental temperature. Information on changes in their firing rate in response to shifts above or below a threshold temperature is sent to the hypothalamus, triggering either inhibition of sweating or excitation of shivering. However, core temperature first must depart from normal levels before a thermoregulatory response occurs. The net influence of skin temperature is 30 times less than that of the central temperature.

Skin Structure in Relation to Thermoregulation

The skin provides a large surface area (about 2 m^2 for an average adult) for both the absorption of heat from the environment and the loss of heat from the body, and this large surface area facilitates evaporative cooling. The arrangement of the *blood vessels* in the skin is ideally designed to either dissipate or conserve heat. The primary function of the skin vasculature is heat regulation (nutrition is a secondary function). Thermoregulation is achieved by regulating blood flow to the skin surface. Under basal conditions, about 450 ml/minute or 8.5% of total blood flow passes through the skin. However, skin blood flow may increase as much as 10-fold under thermal stress with maximum vasodilation, and during maximum vasoconstriction as a result of cold stress, skin blood flow virtually ceases.

Sweat Gland Responses

Sweat is derived from the secretion of the *eccrine sweat gland*, a simple tubular epithelium consisting of a duct and secretory coil. Sweating is controlled both by thermosensitive neurons in the hypothalamus, which subsequently control the nerves surrounding sweat glands, and by plasma electrolyte concentration reflecting the degree of body hydration. There are from 1.6 to 4 million eccrine sweat glands distributed over the surface of the body. The average density of the glands varies; for example, there are 64 glands/cm^2 on the back, 108/cm^2 on the forearm, 181/cm^2 on the forehead, and 600 to 700/cm^2 on the palms and soles. Under thermal stress, a maximum sweat rate of 3 to 4 L/hour can be attained, and a rate of 1 to 1.5 L/hour can be maintained for extended periods, which corresponds to a heat loss that is 10 times greater than the basal rate.

HOW ARE ABNORMALITIES OF THE SKIN DESCRIBED?

(CM&S Chapter 5)

Dermatology, in contrast to many medical specialties, relies heavily on evaluation of clinical appearances of diseases for diagnosis. When a patient undergoes evaluation of a skin condition, the first contact serves to provide a general sense of the patient's persona. Following the overall assessment, the distribution of lesions over the skin is noted.

Cutaneous diseases may be localized to relatively small portions of the skin, or they may be diffuse and involve large areas. Those that are localized may be confined to specific regions or areas, or they may consist of solitary lesions. Widespread conditions involve large areas of the body in either a symmetrical or an asymmetrical fashion (Fig. 1–6).

Once distribution has been ascertained, the configuration of individual lesions is assessed (Fig. 1–7). Configuration refers to the arrangement of skin lesions with respect to one another. Lesions may be grouped into a characteristic pattern, or they may be arranged randomly. If grouped, they may be very close together, such as in the herpetiform arrangement, or they may be distributed around a central lesion. Lesions may be arranged linearly, either in confluent fashion or separated from one another. Just as a characteristic distribution of a skin disorder may be the most important aspect of the clinical diagnosis, the configuration may be of prime importance. Good examples include the zosteriform configuration characteristically seen in herpes zoster.

After an accurate assessment of configuration has been made, the individual skin lesion itself is examined. Once the fundamental lesion has been characterized, it is important to describe it with respect to whether it involves adnexal structures and whether it is smooth surfaced or dome shaped. Assessment of color, texture, and shape is also essential. The final step is to conceptualize where the pathologic process is ongoing and what might be responsible for it. Skin diseases involve the epidermis, papillary dermis, reticular dermis, subcutaneous fat, adnexal structures, or combinations of the above. Once all of this information has been gathered, the clinician synthesizes it and arrives at a clinical diagnosis.

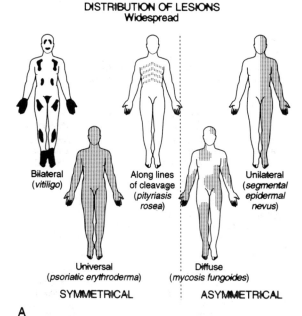

A

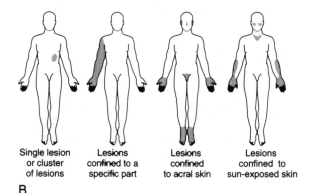

B

FIGURE 1–6.

Fundamental Lesions of the Skin

There are 16 fundamental lesions of the skin. They include the following: (1) macules; (2) patches; (3) papules; (4) plaques; (5) nodules and tumors; (6) vesicles; (7) bullae; (8) pustules; (9) eschars; (10) erosions; (11) ulcers; (12) scales, crusts, and keratoses; (13) atrophy; (14) telangiectases; (15) burrows; and (16) cords.

CONFIGURATION

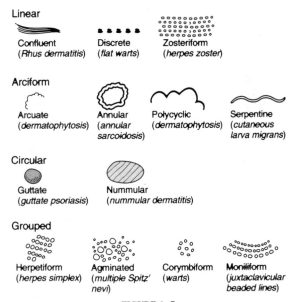

FIGURE 1–7.

These morphologic expressions of skin diseases are the basic entities in the skin on which all diagnoses in dermatology are ultimately founded.

Macules and Patches

A macule is a flat spot on the skin that measures up to 1 cm, whereas a patch measures more than 1 cm at its greatest diameter. Essentially, macules and patches refer to areas of the skin in which the color is different from that of surrounding normal skin (Figs. 1–8 to 1–10). Macules may result from an abnormality in the epidermis alone, such as in vitiligo, or in the dermis alone, such as with petechiae; in some cases, both the epidermis and the dermis are involved, such as in postinflammatory pigmentary alteration.

Papules

A papule is a raised, nonvesicular, nonpustular lesion in the skin that is less than 1 cm at its greatest diameter. Papules may be round, oval, umbilicated, polygonal, flat topped, dome shaped, gently elevated, acuminate, papillated, or digitated (Fig. 1–11). They may have smooth surfaces, or they may be eroded, ulcerated, or covered by keratotic debris. Papules may arise from an abnormality situated mostly in the epidermis, mostly in the dermis, or a combination (Figs. 1–12 to 1–14). They may be associated with hair follicles or eccrine or apocrine structures, or they may be distinctly separate

Text continued on page 24

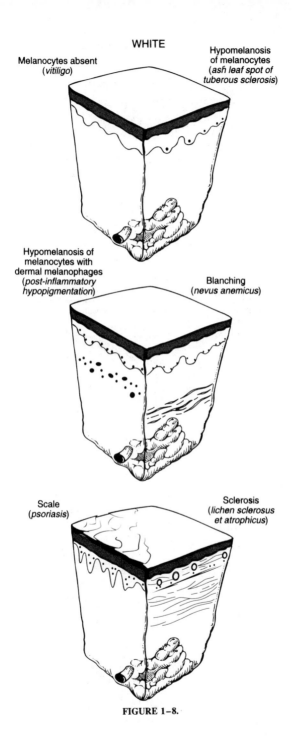

WHITE

Melanocytes absent
(*vitiligo*)

Hypomelanosis
of melanocytes
(*ash leaf spot of
tuberous sclerosis*)

Hypomelanosis of
melanocytes with
dermal melanophages
(*post-inflammatory
hypopigmentation*)

Blanching
(*nevus anemicus*)

Scale
(*psoriasis*)

Sclerosis
(*lichen sclerosus
et atrophicus*)

FIGURE 1–8.

19

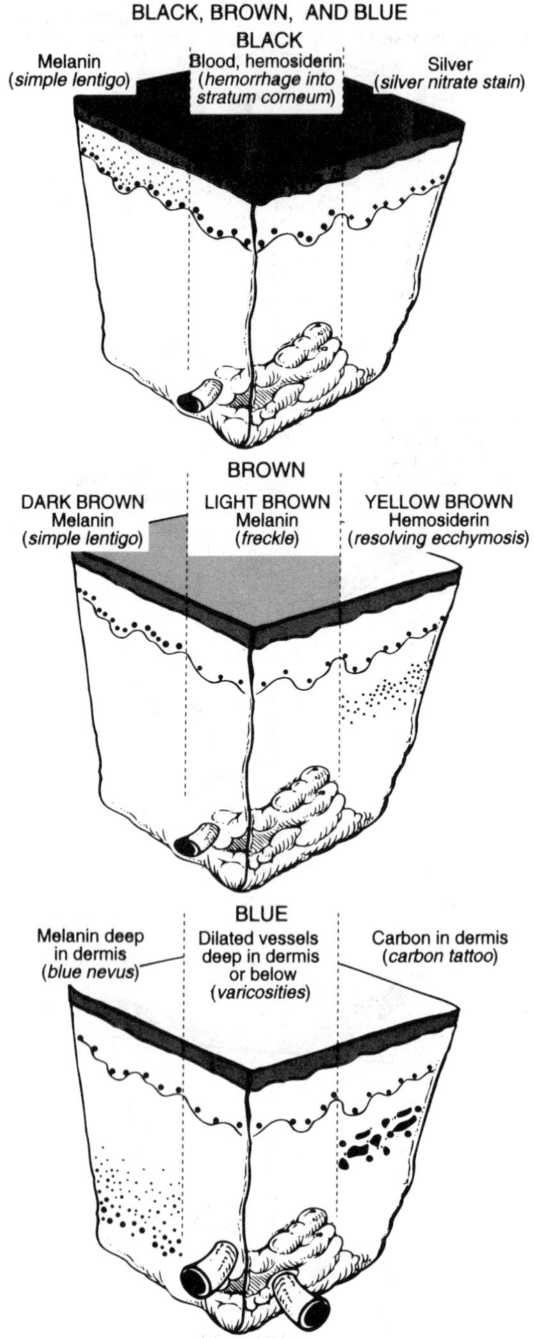

BLACK, BROWN, AND BLUE

BLACK

| Melanin *(simple lentigo)* | Blood, hemosiderin *(hemorrhage into stratum corneum)* | Silver *(silver nitrate stain)* |

BROWN

| DARK BROWN Melanin *(simple lentigo)* | LIGHT BROWN Melanin *(freckle)* | YELLOW BROWN Hemosiderin *(resolving ecchymosis)* |

BLUE

| Melanin deep in dermis *(blue nevus)* | Dilated vessels deep in dermis or below *(varicosities)* | Carbon in dermis *(carbon tattoo)* |

FIGURE 1–9.

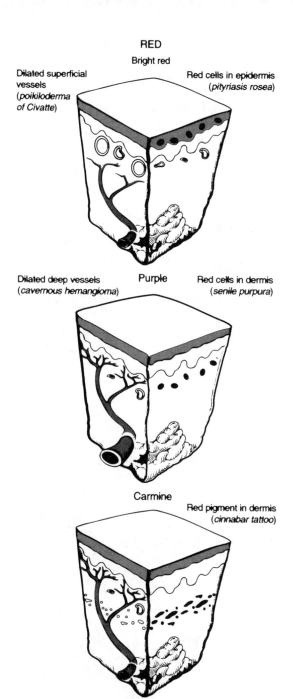

RED

Bright red

Dilated superficial vessels (*poikiloderma of Civatte*)

Red cells in epidermis (*pityriasis rosea*)

Purple

Dilated deep vessels (*cavernous hemangioma*)

Red cells in dermis (*senile purpura*)

Carmine

Red pigment in dermis (*cinnabar tattoo*)

FIGURE 1–10.

21

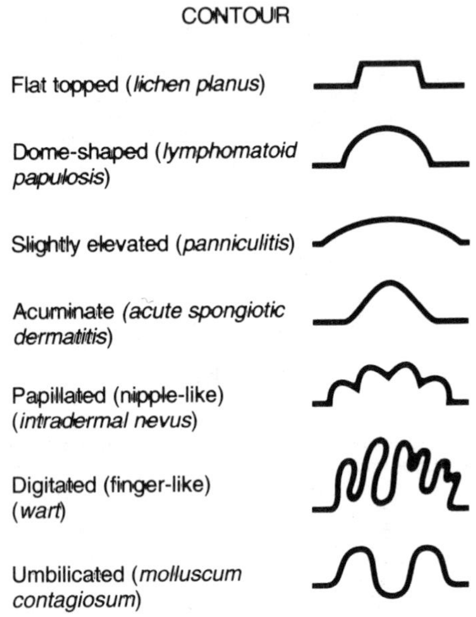

CONTOUR

Flat topped (*lichen planus*)

Dome-shaped (*lymphomatoid papulosis*)

Slightly elevated (*panniculitis*)

Acuminate (*acute spongiotic dermatitis*)

Papillated (nipple-like) (*intradermal nevus*)

Digitated (finger-like) (*wart*)

Umbilicated (*molluscum contagiosum*)

FIGURE 1–11.

MORPHOLOGY OF PAPULES

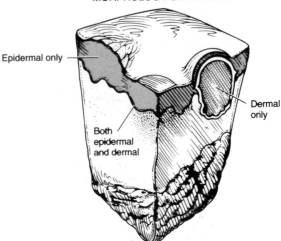

Epidermal only

Dermal only

Both epidermal and dermal

FIGURE 1–12.

PAPULE MORPHOLOGY

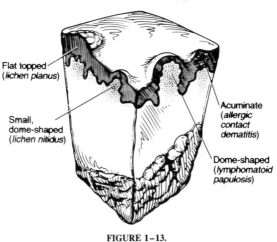

Flat topped
(*lichen planus*)

Small,
dome-shaped
(*lichen nitidus*)

Acuminate
(*allergic
contact
dematitis*)

Dome-shaped
(*lymphomatoid
papulosis*)

FIGURE 1–13.

FOLLICULAR PAPULES

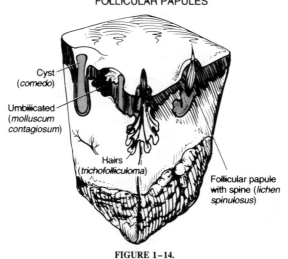

Cyst
(*comedo*)

Umbilicated
(*molluscum
contagiosum*)

Hairs
(*trichofolliculoma*)

Follicular papule
with spine (*lichen
spinulosus*)

FIGURE 1–14.

from any adnexal structure. Papules always have substance and texture.

Plaques

Plaques are broad, elevated flat lesions in the skin that are more than 1 cm at their greatest plane dimension. They may occur as fundamental lesions themselves or arise as a consequence of coalescence of papules. Plaques arise from abnormalities in the epidermis (e.g., seborrheic keratoses), dermis (e.g., xanthelasma), or both (e.g., lichen simplex chronicus).

Nodules and Tumors

A nodule is a dome-shaped or rounded, solid lesion in the skin that is more than 1 cm at its greatest diameter. A tumor is a similar lesion, which, for the sake of convention, measures more than 2 cm in diameter (Figs. 1–15 to 1–17). Nodules and tumors generally result from abnormal augmentations in the dermis and/or subcutaneous fat. As in the case of papules, these may occur as a consequence of infiltrates of inflammatory and/or neoplastic cells, deposits, cysts, or elements of connective tissue.

Vesicles and Bullae

Vesicles are small blisters in the skin that are less than 1 cm in diameter, whereas bullae are blisters that are more than 1 cm in diameter. Vesicles are almost always tense, although bullae may be either tense or flaccid. Both of these lesions may be produced de

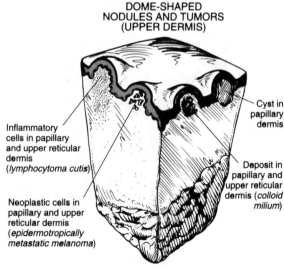

DOME-SHAPED
NODULES AND TUMORS
(UPPER DERMIS)

Inflammatory
cells in papillary
and upper reticular
dermis
(*lymphocytoma cutis*)

Neoplastic cells in
papillary and upper
reticular dermis
(*epidermotropically
metastatic melanoma*)

Cyst in
papillary
dermis

Deposit in
papillary and
upper reticular
dermis (*colloid
milium*)

FIGURE 1–15.

LOW DOMED
NODULES AND TUMORS

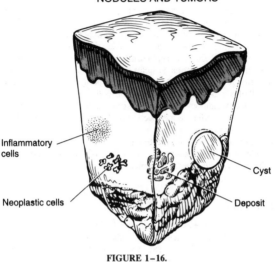

FIGURE 1–16.

SLIGHTLY ELEVATED NODULES
AND TUMORS (SUBCUTANEOUS)

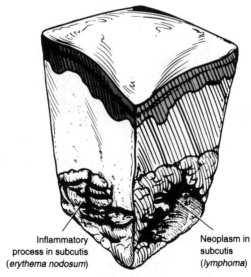

FIGURE 1–17.

novo, or they may arise from other fundamental lesions such as papules that develop into papulovesicles. Either vesicles or bullae may be clear, hemorrhagic, or turbid, depending on whether the content is serum, red blood cells, or white blood cells, respectively.

Vesicles and bullae are classified according to the location of the blister in the skin—namely, whether they lie entirely within the epidermis, beneath the epidermis, or both within and beneath the epidermis. Intraepidermal vesicles and bullae may develop as a consequence of one of three mechanisms: spongiosis, ballooning, or acantholysis. Spongiosis refers to the collection of fluid between individual keratinocytes, typically seen in allergic contact dermatitis; ballooning refers to a collection of fluid within individual keratinocytes, typically seen in viral diseases such as herpes simplex infection; and acantholysis refers to abnormal separation of keratinocytes from one another as a consequence of abnormal desmosome adhesion, typically seen in primary blistering disorders, such as pemphigus.

Pustules

A pustule is an elevated, circumscribed collection of leukocytes in the skin. Pustules in the skin are either follicular or nonfollicular in their orientation (Fig. 1–18). An eruption of follicular pustules is referred to generically as folliculitis, which may be infectious, such as bacterial, or sterile, especially if induced by trauma or exposure to toxins. Examples of nonfollicular pustules include pustular psoriasis and candidiasis.

PUSTULES

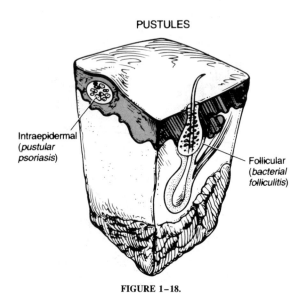

Intraepidermal
(*pustular
psoriasis*)

Follicular
(*bacterial
folliculitis*)

FIGURE 1–18.

Scales, Crusts, and Keratoses

Some cutaneous disorders are characterized by changes primarily at the surface of the epidermis or in the cornified layer. Crusts refer to accumulations of serum containing variable quantities of leukocytes and red blood cells (Fig. 1–19). Eschars are zones of devitalized tissue consisting of coagulated epidermis with variable quantities of dermis in association with dried serum (Fig. 1–20). Disorders that produce abnormalities exclusively in the cornified layer are generally described as keratotic or hyperkeratotic. Although these changes may be the only abnormality of a disease, they usually occur as a consequence of another pathologic process and are associated with papules, plaques, vesicles, or bullae.

Crusts are yellow when they contain neutrophils (e.g., impetigo), red when they contain red blood cells, or black when they contain dried serum (e.g., ulcerative conditions, such as pyoderma gangrenosum).

Erosions and Ulcerations

An erosion is the loss of part or all of the epidermis without involvement of the dermis. Ulcers result when there is loss of all of the epidermis and a portion of the dermis (Fig. 1–21).

Atrophy

Atrophy refers to loss of the dermis and/or the subcutaneous fat (Fig. 1–22). Superficial atrophy is characterized histologically by loss of normal undulating dermal papillae and epidermal retia and clinically by slight depressions of the skin, hypopigmentation, a

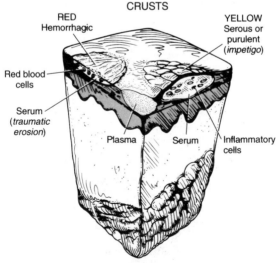

FIGURE 1–19.

ESCHAR

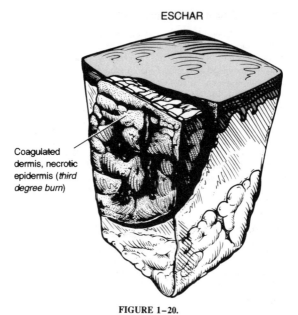

Coagulated dermis, necrotic epidermis (*third degree burn*)

FIGURE 1–20.

shiny appearance, telangiectasia, loss of hairs, and fine wrinkling ("cigarette paper wrinkling"). Deep cutaneous atrophy arises as a consequence of diminution of the reticular dermis, primarily collagen bundles but also elastic fibers. Clinically, deep dermal atrophy manifests as either depressions or as eversions of the skin that are caused by herniations of fat.

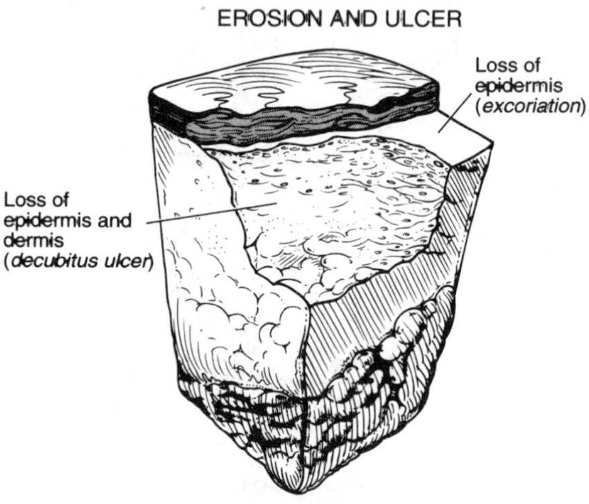

EROSION AND ULCER

Loss of epidermis (*excoriation*)

Loss of epidermis and dermis (*decubitus ulcer*)

FIGURE 1–21.

ATROPHY

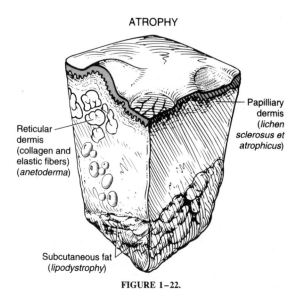

FIGURE 1–22.

Telangiectasia

Telangiectases are visibly dilated blood vessels, usually capillaries, venules, or, rarely, arterioles. Telangiectases may present as other fundamental lesions of the skin, such as papules in nevus araneus (spider nevi), although they may occur alone, such as in telangiectatic acne rosacea.

Burrows

Burrows are linear lesions in the skin, which represent tunnels in the uppermost part of the skin that are produced by the burrowing of a parasite.

Color in Dermatology

Skin diseases may assume many different colors, depending on a number of factors.

Red

Many skin diseases, both inflammatory and neoplastic, cause the skin to be red, to which the term *erythema* is often applied. Red is virtually always a consequence of dilatation of blood vessels in the dermis. The shade of red depends on whether involved vessels are capillaries, venules, or arterioles; whether the blood vessels of the superficial plexus are involved alone or those of both the superficial and deep plexuses are affected; and the degree of hemoglobin oxygenation. The presence of melanin, cornified layer alteration, extravasated erythrocytes, and inflammatory cells and their density and distribution also play a role in the shade of red produced.

Yellow

Yellow is also often compared with natural substances such as apple jelly, buff, cream, copper, fawn, gold, honey, saffron, straw, and wax. Yellow in the skin may result from natural pigments, such as carotene and bile, as well as exogenous pigments, such as cadmium. Lipids also may impart a yellowish color, as in xanthomas, and altered elastic tissues such as solar elastosis commonly result in a yellowish hue. Other sources of yellow include thickening of collagen of the reticular dermis, such as in morphea, and diffuse infiltrates of mast cells, such as those in nodular lesions of urticaria pigmentosa.

Blue

A blue color in the skin can arise from a number of different sources. Melanin within melanophages or melanocytes in the reticular dermis appears bluish-gray when viewed through the whitish skin of light-skinned Caucasians (Fitzpatrick types I to III). Blood in the vascular spaces of hemangiomas or extravasated into the reticular dermis also may impart a bluish color, as may carbon in tattoos. The blue of cyanosis is a manifestation of poorly oxygenated blood, whereas the slate-grayish–blue color of argyria results from the deposition of silver in the dermis.

Brown and Black

Brown lesions may be more precisely described as bronze, buff, café-au-lait, chocolate, or copper colored. Brown is usually due to melanin, and the intensity of brown depends on how much and where the melanin is situated in the skin. If abundant melanin is present in the cornified layer, the color of the lesion is black. Less melanin in the cornified layer leads to a dark-brown color, whereas tan results when there is still less melanin present in lower levels of the epidermis, such as in freckles, café-au-lait spots, and simple lentigines in which most of the pigment is present near the basal cell layer. In general, proliferations of melanocytes lead to darker shades of brown and black in contrast to those in which normal melanocytes produce an increased amount of melanin. Brown may also arise as a consequence of extravasation of erythrocytes with breakdown of heme to hemosiderin. Stains on the skin surface such as those due to nicotine may give rise to a brownish color, whereas pigment produced by dematiaceous fungi causing tinea nigra also results in brownish discoloration.

White

White may assume a number of different shades in the skin. Stark white (dipigmentation) is associated with complete loss of melanin from the epidermis, as in vitiligo. An off-white color (hypopigmentation) results when there is partial loss of melanin from the epidermis, as in postinflammatory hypopigmentation. White also may result from hyperkeratosis, as seen with thick, scaly lesions of psoriasis.

Glossary of Common Terms in Dermatology and Dermatopathology

Acantholysis. Acantholysis refers to dissolution of intercellular bridges so that the keratinocytes separate and become rounded.

Acanthosis. An increase in the number of epithelial spinous cells manifests as a thickening of the epidermis.

Acral Parts of the Skin. Acral portions of the skin refer to the fingers and toes, tip of the nose, and pinnae of the ears.

Anagen. The growing phase of the hair cycle.

Apoptosis. In dermatology, usually applied to necrosis of keratinocytes in which the nuclei of the necrotic cells dissolve and the cytoplasms shrink, round up, and are subsequently phagocytized.

Atopy. A genetic predisposition to the development of hypersensitivity states associated with enhanced mast cell degranulation. Some of the associated disorders include allergic rhinitis, asthma, atopic dermatitis, and urticaria.

Atypia. A cytologic term that refers to cells with large hyperchromatic pleomorphic nuclei that vary in size and shape and often have prominent nucleoli.

Balloon Degeneration. A histologic term that refers to intracellular edema. Recognized in cells with swollen pale cytoplasm, balloon degeneration is commonly associated with viral diseases.

Basal Cell. The basophilic, cuboidal cells at the lowermost level of the epidermis.

Basement Membrane. A histologic term that refers to the pink homogeneous area between the basal cell layer of the epidermis and the papillary dermis.

Basket-weave Cornified Layer. The normal histologic appearance of the cornified layer on most of the body other than the palms and soles.

Blister. A collection of fluid within or beneath the epidermis.

Catagen. The involutional stage of the hair cycle in which the inferior part of the hair follicle undergoes necrosis and involution.

Civatte Bodies. Pink, homogeneous anucleate bodies seen histologically that are the residue of necrotic keratinocytes. Also known as *colloid bodies*, *hyaline bodies*, and *apoptotic bodies*, they are typically seen in lichen planus.

Comedo. A dilated hair follicular infundibulum filled with cornified cells, sebaceous material, and microorganisms.

Cornoid Lamella. A column of parakeratosis that extends above and into the epidermis where there are vacuolated and dyskeratotic cells, typical of porokeratosis.

Cyst. An epithelium-lined space in the skin. The lining of the cyst may be derived from one of a number of different sources, including eccrine ducts, hair follicles, and sebaceous ducts.

Dermatitis. An inflammation of the skin, histologically characterized by an inflammatory cell infiltrate of varying degree in the dermis.

Dermatosis. Any pathologic condition of the skin.

Dyskeratotic Cell. A prematurely cornified cell manifested histologically as having eosinophilic cytoplasm and often a pyknotic nucleus and seen in inflammatory conditions or in neoplasms.

Elastotic Material. Also known as solar or actinic elastosis, this material represents elastin produced by fibroblasts as a consequence of long-standing sun exposure. Histologically manifested as bluish tangled masses in the dermis that stain strongly positive with elastic stains.

Epidermal Hyperplasia. An increased number of cells in the epidermis as a result of a stimulus; the number of cells stabilizes and ultimately diminishes when the stimulus is withdrawn.

Epidermotropism. The growth or movement of neoplastic cells toward and into the epidermis.

Epithelial Structures of Adnexa. Derivatives of embryonal ectoderm such as hair follicles, sebaceous glands, apocrine glands and ducts, and eccrine glands and ducts.

Epithelioid. Histologic term that refers to characteristics of a nonepithelial cell having features similar to those that comprise an epithelium. Many different cells may assume the characteristics of epithelioid cells, such as melanocytes, endothelial cells, and histiocytes.

Epithelioma. Synonym for *carcinoma*.

Eschar. A gray, brown, or black adherent material that overlies an ulcer. Composed of necrotic epidermis, plasma, inflammatory cells, erythrocytes, and, on occasion, degenerated collagen.

Fibrosis. An increased number of fibroblasts in association with an increased amount of collagen in most cases.

Follicular Mucinosis. Collections of acid mucopolysaccharides within the epithelium of hair follicles.

Germinal Centers. Histologic term referring to cortical areas of a lymph node composed of rapidly dividing B lymphocytes.

Giant Cell. Histologic term that refers to a cell that is enlarged and often contains multiple nuclei.

Granulation Tissue. Highly vascular edematous connective tissue that clinically appears pink and glistening and histologically is associated with a proliferation of blood vessels containing a mixed inflammatory cell infiltrate.

Granulomatous. Inflammatory infiltrate in the skin in which macrophages predominate. There are five patterns of granulomatous inflammation that have been described in the skin: tuberculoid, sarcoidal, palisaded, suppurative, and foreign body.

Hamartoma. A malformation that occurs as a consequence of an error in development characterized by an abnormal mixture of tissues indigenous to the organ.

Herpetiform. Designates the arrangement of lesions similar to that seen in herpes simplex and zoster. They are closely approximated and usually touching.

Hyperkeratosis. Increased thickness of the cornified layer of the epidermis.

Hyperplasia. An increase in the number of normal cells in normal arrangement in a tissue.

Hypertrophy. An increase in the size of a cell or organ.

Impetiginization. Secondary infection of the skin with bacteria leading to an appearance similar to that of impetigo.

In Situ. This term is used to denote neoplasms that are confined to their site of origin.

Infiltrate. Any material present in tissue that is not normally present in quantity. May refer to inflammatory or neoplastic cells.

Interface Dermatitis. Histologically, an inflammatory infiltrate that obscures the dermoepidermal junction.

Leukocytoclasis. Fragmentation of leukocytes, usually polymorphonuclear leukocytes and often as a result of antigen-antibody reactions. In histologic sections, appears as "nuclear dust."

Leukoplakia. Clinically manifested as white plaques on a mucous membrane that develop as a consequence of a number of different factors, including hyperkeratosis and maceration. May be seen in association with chronic trauma, neoplasia, or infection.

Lichenification. Thickening of the skin characterized by induration, hyperpigmentation, and accentuation of normal skin markings. Histologically, there is irregular epidermal hyperplasia, hyperkeratosis, and thick coarse collagen bundles arranged vertically in the papillary dermis.

Lichenoid. Clinically, refers to an eruption or a lesion that resembles lichen planus—that is, pink flat-topped polygonal papules. Histologically, refers to an infiltrate of inflammatory cells filling the papillary dermis in band-like fashion that obscures the dermoepidermal junction, usually associated with vacuolar alteration and necrotic keratinocytes.

Lobular Panniculitis. An inflammatory condition of the panniculus in which inflammatory infiltrates are situated primarily within fat lobules.

Lymphoid Follicles. Collections of mononuclear cells that resemble germinal centers of lymph nodes.

Maculopapular. A descriptive term applied to a skin eruption in which there are both macules and papules.

Munro's Microabscess. A small collection of neutrophils within the epidermis found in psoriasis.

Necrosis. Local death of cells or tissue. Histologic features include nuclear fragmentation (karyorrhexis), dissolution of nuclei (karyolysis), and nuclear shrinkage with hyperchromasia (pyknosis). Cytoplasm of necrotic cells is often swollen and eosinophilic.

Nevoid. Hamartomatous; malformative.

Paget's Cell. A large, round cell with an oval nucleus and abundant pale-staining cytoplasm containing mucopolysaccharides found in mammary and extramammary Paget's disease.

Pagetoid Cell. A cell that resembles the cells of mammary and extramammary Paget's disease by virtue of having abundant pale cytoplasm. Often seen in cutaneous melanoma, and contains little, if any, melanin.

Pagetoid Pattern. A description of the scattering of Paget's or pagetoid cells throughout the epithelium in a number of different conditions, such as mammary and extramammary Paget's disease, Bowen's disease, and malignant melanoma.

Papillomatosis. Accentuation of dermal papillae so that they project above the skin surface. The overlying epidermis may or may not be hyperplastic.

Papulosquamous. Refers to skin diseases having papules that are scaly.

Parakeratosis. Retention of nuclei in the cells of the cornified layer.

Pautrier's Microabscess. A collection of atypical mononuclear cells in the epidermis of lesions of mycosis fungoides and related cutaneous T-cell lymphomas.

Pigment Incontinence. Refers to loss of pigment from the epidermis as a result of damage of dermal melanocytes and basal keratinocytes followed by ingestion by macrophages in the dermis.

Pleomorphism. Variability in size and shape of cellular structures, such as nuclei, within an infiltrate or a neoplasm.

Polymorphic Eruption. The presence of more than one type of fundamental lesion within a given eruption, such as a combination of macules, papules, vesicles, etc.

Psoriasiform. Clinically, resembling psoriasis—that is, by having reddish plaques covered by micaceous scale.

Sclerosis. An increased amount of homogenized thickened dermal collagen bundles with decreased numbers of fibroblasts.

Spongiosis. Intercellular edema recognized as a widening of intercellular spaces and stretching of intercellular bridges occurring as a consequence of fluid accumulation.

Superficial Vascular Plexus. Venules and arterioles situated beneath the papillary dermis in the upper part of the reticular dermis.

Systematized. Lesions limited to a well-defined zone, such as a blood vascular, lymphatic, or neural pathway.

Telogen. The resting stage of the hair cycle in which the inferior part of the hair follicle has retracted to the level with the site of attachment of erector muscle.

Umbilicated. Having a central depression, as in an umbilicated papule.

Urticaria (wheal, hive). Evanescent pink papules and plaques that blanch on diascopy and often have pseudopods at their periphery.

Urticarial. Having a hive-like appearance—that is, pink edematous papules and plaques differentiated from true urticaria by the tendency to persist longer.

Vacuolar Alteration. Histologically, tiny clear spaces on either side of the basement membrane at the dermoepidermal junction. Synonymous with liquefaction degeneration.

Vasculitis. Inflammation of blood vessels that results in morphologic evidence of damage to them. In fully developed lesions of small vessel vasculitis, either fibrin is present within the walls of blood vessels and/or thrombi are present within their lumina. In fully developed lesions of large vessel vasculitis, the mere presence of inflammatory cells within the wall of the blood vessel suffices to make the diagnosis. Vasculitis is primary if vessels are the main targets of inflammation and secondary if they are injured incidentally as a result of inflammation directed elsewhere.

Vegetation. A heaped-up collection of scale and crust on the skin surface that may be either hemorrhagic or purulent.

Vellus. Fine, delicate hairs found on much of the body, such as the face, arms, and trunk; in contrast to terminal hairs, which are broader and longer and found on the scalp, axillae, and pubic region.

Verrucous. Like a verruca—that is, a rough, finger-shaped lesion that is characterized histologically by digitated epidermal hyperplasia or neoplasia.

Zosteriform. In the shape of a girdle or, more particularly, the belt-like distribution of lesions along a dermatome such as those seen in herpes zoster.

WHAT BASIC SURGICAL CONCEPTS AND PROCEDURES ARE REQUIRED FOR THE PRACTICE OF CUTANEOUS MEDICINE AND SURGERY?

(CM&S Chapter 6)

Fundamental Anatomy

Knowledge of the underlying anatomic structures of the head and neck is critical to successful cutaneous surgery. Details are beyond the scope of this text but can be found in Chapter 6 of CM&S.

Biopsy Techniques: Description and Proper Use

Selection of Biopsy Site and Type of Biopsy

Biopsies are performed to establish a diagnosis, to remove a neoplasm and check its margins to ensure complete excision, and to assess the effectiveness of a therapeutic procedure on a previously diagnosed condition.

In the case of inflammatory diseases, the biopsy procedure should be planned to encompass a representative portion of the eruption. When the eruption is characterized by lesions in various stages of development, it is usually best to select a well-developed lesion, neither too early nor too late in the state of regression.

An exception to the general rule of selecting a fully developed lesion for biopsy is in the case of vesicular, bullous, or pustular lesions, in which an early intact lesion not older than 24 to 48 hours is preferable.

In the case of pigmented lesions suspected of being malignant, and fungating or nodular processes, an incisional biopsy that extends beneath the deepest part of the lesion and includes as much of the lesion as possible should be obtained, if an excisional biopsy is not practical.

The area that is most representative of the disease process and is uncomplicated by changes unique to the anatomic region should be selected. In general, biopsies of the lower leg, even in young persons, show stasis vascular changes that complicate the interpretation of the histologic presentation and heal very slowly. Similarly, biopsy of the palm and sole should be avoided whenever possible.

The variety of biopsy techniques includes punch biopsy, shave biopsy, scissors removal, curettage, and elliptical excisional or incisional biopsy. Shave biopsy is adequate in superficial disease processes such as a seborrheic keratosis, solar keratosis, or a wart, in which the pathologic changes are largely limited to the epidermis, whereas a deep punch biopsy or, preferably, an incisional biopsy is performed to diagnose deep processes such as panniculitis. Punch biopsies that are 3 or 4 mm in diameter are the usual procedure for obtaining specimens for histopathologic examination. Because it may not be possible to obtain adequate amounts of subcutaneous tissue by punch biopsy, elliptical incisional biopsies often are advisable for the study of subcutaneous lesions or of panniculitis.

When to Delay Biopsy

When the history of the patient indicates a bleeding problem, it is advisable to perform a screening panel of laboratory tests before performing a biopsy. The tests are complete blood count with platelet count, bleeding time, clotting time, partial thromboplastin time, and prothrombin time. If the platelet count is more than 10,000/mm,³ a small punch biopsy may be performed. When the platelet count is less than 10,000/mm,³ the punch biopsy should be deferred.

When problems with blood clotting are present, biopsy must be performed with utmost caution. The physician should make use of all available agents to aid hemostasis, including application of direct pressure, use of suture ligatures to tie bleeding arteries, pinpoint monopolar electrodesiccation in incisional biopsies and use of various chemicals applied to a punch biopsy site, including Monsel's solution (ferric subsulfate), aluminum chloride solution, trichloroacetic acid, and silver nitrate applicator sticks. Oxidized cellulose (Oxycel cotton) and gelatin foam (Gelfoam) sponges provide a matrix to encourage natural coagulation factors, apply pressure to the wound, and may be buried in the wound.

The use of anticoagulants and platelet inhibitors can increase the risk of intraoperative and postoperative hemorrhagic complications. If possible, aspirin should be stopped 9 to 10 days prior to surgery and may be resumed 1 day after surgery. In the interim, acetaminophen may be substituted for aspirin. The routine laboratory evaluations described above do not help predict the clinical antithrombotic effect from aspirin use.

Patients take warfarin for both high-risk indications (e.g., hypercoagulable states and prosthetic heart valves) and low-risk reasons (e.g., deep venous thrombosis, stroke prevention in patients with atrial fibrillation, and after a myocardial infarction or stroke). For the low-risk patient, warfarin is stopped 3 days prior to surgery and resumed 1 day after surgery without the use of a loading dose. In the high-risk patient, warfarin is stopped 1 week prior to surgery, and subcutaneous heparin is initiated. Surgery is performed with the patient receiving either low-dose heparin (5000 units subcutaneously twice a day) or intravenous heparin. After surgery, full-dose heparin resumes, and warfarin is restarted. For smaller biopsy procedures, a patient may continue warfarin with meticulous use of hemostasis and pressure dressings.

Patients who have had joint replacement, heart valve replacement, or valvular disease from rheumatic fever may require a short course (2 hours) of preoperative prophylactic oral antibiotics prior to biopsy of the skin.

Type of Biopsy

Punch Biopsy (Fig. 1–23)

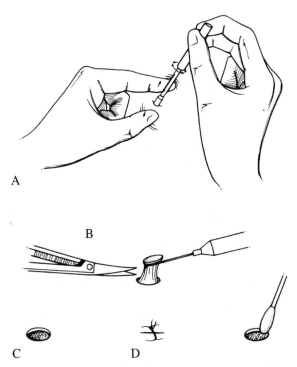

FIGURE 1–23. Punch biopsy. *A,* After the area to be biopsied is anesthetized, the skin around the area infiltrated with anesthesia is drawn taut with the
thumb and forefinger of the physician's free hand.

B, The orifice of the punch is applied firmly to the skin surface with the
handle held perpendicular to the skin. A gentle but firm downward pressure is
exerted at the same time that the handle is rotated between the thumb and
forefinger. This motion will carry the punch through the subcutaneous fat.

Care is required in removing the specimen made with a punch. If a toothed
forceps is used, there is a tendency to crush the tissue as it is being lifted from
its bed. This produces an artifact that may interfere with the pathologist's
ability to make an accurate diagnosis. This artifact may be avoided by a
simple maneuver. Downward pressure on the skin around the cylinder will
cause the skin to pop up. The cylinder can then be lifted with the tip of the
needle that was used to administer the anesthesia.

C, The direction of tension should be along the line of elective incision
(resting skin tension line). This force will cause the eventual defect to be oval
rather than round.

D, It can be closed with a single suture resulting in a closure as close to a
linear one as possible, or a hemostatic agent is applied with a cotton swab and
the area heals by second intention. (*A* to *D* from Robinson JK, LeBoit PE.
Biopsy techniques. *In:* Robinson JK, Arndt KA, LeBoit PE, Wintroub BU,
eds. Atlas of Cutaneous Surgery. Philadelphia: WB Saunders Co., 1995.)

Shave Biopsy and Saucerization Biopsy
(Figs. 1–24 and 1–25)

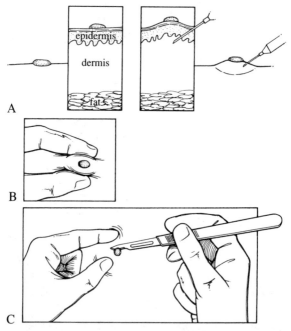

FIGURE 1–24. Shave biopsy. *A*, The epidermal process is elevated above the surrounding tissue by injecting local anesthesia or by (*B*) pinching the skin between the thumb and forefinger. *C*, If the skin is elevated by the bleb of anesthesia and a biopsy at the papillary dermis is required, the skin can be made taut and the blade moves under the lesion in a horizontal plane parallel to the skin surface. (*A* to *C* from Robinson JK, LeBoit PE. Biopsy techniques. *In*: Robinson JK, Arndt KA, LeBoit PE, Wintroub BU, eds. Atlas of Cutaneous Surgery. Philadelphia: WB Saunders Co., 1995.)

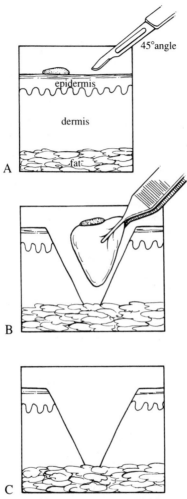

FIGURE 1–25. Saucerization biopsy. *A*, The blade undercuts the lesion at a 45-degree angle to the surface of the skin. *B*, The depth of the incision is carried to the fat. *C*, The resulting defect heals by second intention. (*A* to *C* from Robinson JK, LeBoit PE. Biopsy techniques. *In*: Robinson JK, Arndt KA, LeBoit PE, Wintroub BU, eds. Atlas of Cutaneous Surgery. Philadelphia: WB Saunders Co., 1995.)

Curettage and Scissors Removal

Curettage is a simple technique used for removing benign superficial lesions such as warts, molluscum, milia, and seborrheic keratoses, for scooping out friable tissue, and for demonstrating the size of a basal cell carcinoma prior to its excision. However, curettage is the least satisfactory method of biopsy because the material is usually scanty, is superficial in location, and has lost its architecture with many fragments being present. After the site is anesthetized, the cutting edge of the curette is applied to the lesion, which is removed with a firm, quick, downward scoop. Hemostasis of the biopsy site is obtained by pressure and hemostatic agents or electrodesiccation.

The technique of scissors removal is reserved for benign pedunculated lesions, such as filiform warts, skin tags, and polypoid nevi. The blades of a small scissors such as an iris scissors are slipped under the lesion, and it is snipped off with or without the injection of local anesthetic. The base is transected with a snip of the scissors. Bleeding is controlled by application of 35% aluminum chloride solution. No bandage is required.

Elliptical Incisional and Excisional Biopsy

Use of the elliptical (fusiform) technique is essential when larger or deep specimens must be taken, as in diseases with significant changes in the deep dermis extending to the fascia (e.g., dermatomyositis, scleroderma, eosinophilic fasciitis, panniculitis, or mesenchymal neoplasms). It also is the preferred technique for diagnosis of pigmented lesions that may be melanomas.

Antisepsis, Anesthesia, Hemostasis, and Suture Placement

Antisepsis

Antisepsis consists of the use of antimicrobial solutions to decrease resident and transient cutaneous flora, the adoption of procedures to protect personnel and patients from the transmission of infection, careful handling of all tissue, and the proper use of the surgical suite and instruments to prevent introduction of microorganisms into the environment.

Microorganisms on the skin are generally gram-positive aerobes or anaerobes or fungi. The most common antiseptic solutions, such as chlorhexidine (Hibiclens), isopropyl alcohol, and iodophor (e.g., Betadine) used, either alone or in combination, should provide adequate coverage for cutaneous surgery procedures. However, the solution is only part of the antisepsis. Appropriate application for the recommended time is equally important.

Once an area has been cleaned, a fenestrated drape is used to isolate that site from the surrounding skin and avoid contamination. All skin showing through the opening must be prepared. Instruments, suture, gauze, and hands will be dragged across this skin and, if not antiseptically prepared as well as the surgical site, will increase the probability of an infection.

Prevention of infection in the surgical suite is the responsibility of all personnel. Individuals with active cutaneous infections or dermatitis should not participate in surgery. Hands should be washed before and after each patient contact. Gloves, masks, gowns, and eyeshields are to be worn.

Anesthesia

The most commonly used injectable anesthetic is lidocaine. Lidocaine has an amide linkage, which avoids the problem of allergic reactions from procaine.

The four most frequently used amides are lidocaine (Xylocaine), mepivacaine (Carbocaine), bupivacaine (Marcaine), and etidocaine (Duranest). To prolong the duration as well as for its vasoconstriction effect, epinephrine may be added to the anesthetic. For lidocaine and mepivacaine, the addition of epinephrine more than doubles their average length of duration of 90 minutes. For bupivacaine and etidocaine, epinephrine is not necessary as they have long duration times, averaging 200 minutes without it. These two latter drugs are of use in cases in which epinephrine is contraindicated.

EMLA is a topical cream mixture of prilocaine and lidocaine. It is applied under occlusion for 1 hour to achieve maximal effect. It produces variable degrees of anesthesia, depending on the individual and the site of application. It is helpful in children as a preparation to lessen the discomfort of intracutaneous anesthesia, for some superficial shave procedures, and in some laser treatments.

Adverse Effects

The adverse effects associated with the use of the amide-linked anesthetics (e.g., lidocaine and bupivacaine), which are mainly neural and cardiac, are mostly dose related. The recommended maximal dosages are 7.0 mg/kg, which is about 50 mL of 1% lidocaine with epinephrine for a 70-kg man. The maximum recommended dosage for 1% lidocaine *without* epinephrine is 4.5 mg/kg, or approximately 30 mL for that same 70-kg man. Epinephrine should be avoided in patients who are receiving propranolol, monoamine oxidase inhibitors, triyclic antidepressants, or phenothiazines, and it should be used sparingly in patients with untreated acute angle-glaucoma, vascular disease, hyperthyroidism, or unstable mental status, or who are pregnant.

Neurotoxicity presents as perioral tingling, lightheadedness, and tinnitus before slurred speech, nystagmus and hallucinations, and, ultimately, frank seizures. Cardiac effects include myocardial depression, atrioventricular blockage, ventricular arrhythmia, and hypotension.

Technique

In most situations, a 3- to 10-mL syringe is attached to a 30-gauge needle, $\frac{1}{2}$-inch long. To reduce the discomfort of infiltration, it should be performed slowly. The pain of infection may be reduced further by the use of bicarbonate (nine parts to one part) to alter the acidic pH of xylocaine with epinephrine.

Hemostasis

Control of bleeding is essential during cutaneous surgery. Hemostasis begins with eliciting the patient's medical history. Notation should be made of any bleeding problems, difficulties with previous surgeries, and all medications with a potential effect on clotting, including aspirin, nonsteroidal anti-inflammatory drugs, and anticoagulants. The various techniques available to produce hemostasis include mechanical means (pressure), the use of thermal (electrocautery) devices, and chemical agents, such as silver nitrate, ferric subsulfate (Monsel's solution), aluminum chloride, and absorbable sponges made from gelatin or cellulose.

Suturing Techniques

Sutures are used primarily to close surgical defects. Sutures act as foreign bodies in a wound and thereby increase the risk of infection. Thus, they should be placed under antiseptic conditions and with a minimum of trauma to the tissues. Not every wound needs to be or should be sutured. If infection or bleeding is a major concern, serious consideration should be given to second-intention wound healing.

To begin suturing, the needle should be placed at a 90-degree angle with the surface of the skin (Fig. 1–26). The needle merely punctures the skin surface and then should be rotated through its curvature to the depth desired. The entrance and exit points of the needle should be equidistant from the edge of the wound. As the needle exits the skin, it should be grasped by the forceps and steadied so that the needle holder can get it and pull it through. Always push the needle through far enough to grab it behind the point.

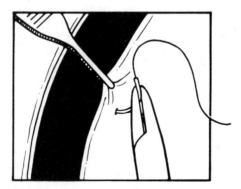

FIGURE 1–26. A 90-degree angle is formed between the needle and the epidermis. (From Robinson JK. Technique of suture placement. *In*: Robinson JK, Arndt KA, LeBoit PE, Wintroub BU, eds. Atlas of Cutaneous Surgery. Philadelphia: WB Saunders Co., 1995.)

Instrument Tie (Fig. 1–27)

When properly done, the edges are apposed. There should be no ischemic (white) areas around the sutures indicating they are tied too tight. There should be no gaping between sutures indicating they are too far apart. The cut ends of the sutures should not stick into the skin. The knots should not lie directly on the suture line, but be to one side of it.

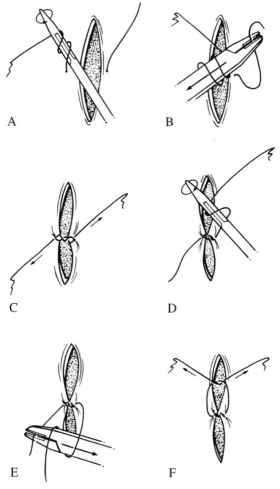

FIGURE 1–27. An instrument tie. (From Robinson JK. Technique of suture placement. *In*: Robinson JK, Arndt KA, LeBoit PE, Wintroub BU, eds. Atlas of Cutaneous Surgery. Philadelphia: WB Saunders Co., 1995.)

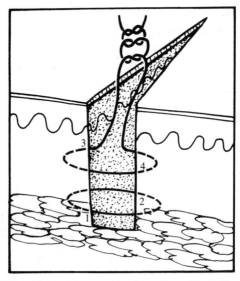

FIGURE 1–28. A buried suture with an inverted knot. (From Robinson JK. Technique of suture placement. In: Robinson JK, Arndt KA, LeBoit PE, Wintroub BU, eds. Atlas of Cutaneous Surgery. Philadelphia: WB Saunders Co., 1995.)

Buried Suture

The workhorse of closures is the buried subcutaneous suture. This stitch is usually done with a slowly resorbing suture material so that it provides stability to the wound after the epidermal sutures have been removed. The level of placement is usually fat and dermis (Fig. 1–28).

chapter 2

What Disorders Present with Inflamed Skin?

A. Mechanisms, Symptoms, and Treatment of Inflammation

MECHANISMS OF PRURITUS

(CM&S Chapter 8)

Definition and Clinical Description

Pruritus (itch, itching) is defined as "that sensation that provokes the desire to scratch or rub." Pruritus is a distinct, unpleasant sensation arising most commonly in the skin, but it can also be experienced in the mucous membranes and upper respiratory tract. In humans, the production of scratching in response to itch demands the functional integrity of at least some part of the cerebrum.

Pruritus may be localized or generalized and has both external and internal causes. External causes can be physical or chemical, whereas internal causes are due either to skin disease or systemic disease and are, with rare exceptions, due to chemicals or to primary neurologic causes.

Excoriations (erythematous or superficially eroded areas in the skin produced by scratching) are the objective sign of pruritus but are by no means universally observed in itchy skin regardless of the cause. Rubbing is less likely to result in excoriations, and rubbing sometimes may be the preferred motor response to try to alleviate the sensation of itch.

Pathology

Although gentle scratching evokes no histologic findings, excoriation causes a range of changes, including necrosis of superficial keratinocytes (seen as brightly eosinophilic cytoplasm and nuclear pallor), erosion of the outermost epidermis, and subepidermal fibrin deposition. Extravasation of erythrocytes and hemorrhagic scale and crusts are also common. In contrast, rubbing induces the

45

TABLE 2-1. Pruritus Due to Skin Disease
Infestations: scabies and other mites, pediculosis
Insect bites
Endogenous eczemas
Lichen planus
Dermatitis herpetiformis
Fungal diseases
Urticaria, symptomatic dermographism
Urticaria pigmentosum
Senile xerosis
Psoriasis
Toxic and drug eruptions

changes of lichen simplex chronicus, namely, psoriasiform epidermal hyperplasia with a thickened granular and compact cornified layer.

Pathogenesis and Etiology

Neurologic Aspects of Pruritus

The many disparate causes of itching resulting in firing of the cutaneous itch ''receptors'' must in humans result in the transmission of a stimulus to the cerebrum that is appreciated there as the sensation that evokes the desire to scratch or rub. It has been established that excitation of unmyelinated and myelinated afferents (C and Aδ fibers) and spinal neurons projecting through the anterolateral quadrant of the cord transmits the itch stimulus to the brain. The mechanism by which this process is achieved is unknown.

Pharmacologic Aspects of Pruritus

Physical stimuli result in itch by firing of C and Aδ fibers capable of responding to altered mechanical and thermal conditions in the skin. In addition, receptors respond to chemical stimuli; that is, they are chemosensitive. Chemosensitivity to naturally occurring as well as exogenously introduced chemical stimuli is attributed to this population of nociceptors. Chemical pruritogens may not produce itch directly but rather result in itch by liberation of histamine by

TABLE 2-2. Systemic Disease Groups Associated with Pruritus
Autoimmune disease
Blood dyscrasias and carcinomas
Endocrine and metabolic disease
Hepatic disease
Neurologic diseases
Pregnancy diseases
Psychological diseases
Renal disease
Tropical and parasitic diseases

degranulation of mast cells in the skin. The ineffectiveness of non-sedative antihistamines against many forms of pruritus indicates that histamine is unlikely to be the only mediator of pruritus in human skin disease. Serotonin, prostaglandin E_1, and prostaglandin E_2 are weak pruritogens on intradermal injection as single agonists but have a stronger pruritogenic effect when injected as a mixture. Aspirin, an inhibitor of prostaglandin synthesis, does not appear to be antipruritic except in polycythemia rubra vera, in which it is conceivable that serotonin released from platelets might have a pruritogenic effect. Substance P induces itch in human skin. It is unclear whether the itch produced by substance P is a result of a direct effect or due to its ability to release histamine from mast cells. In theory, cytokines released from lymphocytes in inflammatory infiltrates in the epidermis or upper dermis in itchy dermatoses might be responsible, at least in part, for the pruritus of these dermatoses. The itching after morphine injection has been attributed to its ability to release histamine from mast cells.

Pruritus in Cutaneous and Systemic Disease

The best understood chemical pruritogen in the pruritic dermatoses is histamine in idiopathic urticaria. The itch of this dermatosis can be attenuated or abolished by nonsedative H_1 receptor–blocking agents, and the effects of intradermal histamine are strikingly similar if not identical to the symptoms and signs of acute and chronic idiopathic urticaria. Evidence is therefore strong for the role of histamine as a pruritogen in urticaria.

The inefficiency of nonsedative compared with sedative antihistamines in the pruritic dermatosis atopic eczema indicates a central attenuation of itch by these drugs and that histamine release in the skin provides an unlikely candidate mechanism for the peripheral initiation of the characteristic itch of this condition. Generalized or localized pruritus is a common complaint among the elderly and leads to substantial morbidity. In the majority of elderly patients, no underlying disorder can be identified; but in many instances, the pruritus is associated with moderately or severely dry skin. As in the case of xerosis, the mechanism of the pruritus is not understood and it is not relieved by nonsedative antihistamines, indicating that histamine is not the pruritogen.

TOPICAL CORTICOSTEROID THERAPY

(CM&S Chapter 9)

Topical corticosteroid preparations vary greatly in potency and are usually categorized into seven groups (Table 2–3). Group I consists of the so-called superpotent agents, and group VII, which includes hydrocortisone acetate, are the least potent. With the exception of the preparations in group I in which Temovate and Ultravate are more potent than Diprolene or Psorcon preparations, there are no significant differences in potency of preparations within a given group and they are listed alphabetically by brand name. Some corticosteroids are found in preparations that are categorized into different groups depending on their concentration in the preparation and the type of vehicle used.

TABLE 2-3. Ranking of Some Commonly Used Topical Steroids by Potency

BRAND NAME	GENERIC NAME
Group I (Super Potent)	
Temovate cream 0.05%	Clobetasol propionate
Temovate ointment 0.05%	Clobetasol propionate
Diprolene cream 0.05%	Betamethasone dipropionate
Diprolene ointment 0.05%	Betamethasone dipropionate
Psorcon ointment 0.05%	Diflorasone diacetate
Ultravate ointment 0.05%	Halobetasol propionate
Group II (High Potency)	
Cyclocort ointment 0.1%	Amcinonide
Elocon ointment 0.1%	Mometasone furoate
Florone ointment 0.05%	Diflorasone diacetate
Halog cream 0.1%	Halcinonide
Lidex cream 0.05%	Fluocinonide
Lidex gel 0.05%	Fluocinonide
Lidex ointment 0.05%	Fluocinonide
Topicort cream 0.25%	Desoximetasone
Topicort ointment 0.25%	Desoximetasone
Group III (High Potency)	
Aristocort cream (HP) 0.05%	Triamcinolone acetonide
Diprosone cream 0.05%	Betamethasone dipropionate
Elocon ointment 0.1%	Mometasone furoate
Florone cream 0.05%	Diflorasone diacetate
Maxiflor cream 0.05%	Diflorasone diacetate
Uticort ointment 0.025%	Betamethasone benzoate
Valisone ointment 0.5	Betamethasone valerate
Group IV (Medium Potency)	
Cutivate cream 0.05%	Fluticasone propionate
Elocon cream 0.1%	Mometasone furoate
Halog ointment 0.025%	Halcinonide
Kenalog cream 0.1%	Triamcinolone acetonide
Synalar cream 0.2%	Fluocinolone acetonide
Synalar ointment 0.025%	Fluocinolone acetonide
Westcort ointment 0.2%	Hydrocortisone valerate
Group V (Medium Potency)	
Aclovate ointment 0.05%	Alclometasone dipropionate
Diprosone lotion 0.05%	Betamethasone dipropionate
Kenalog lotion 0.1%	Triamcinolone acetonide
Locoid cream 0.1%	Hydrocortisone butyrate
Synalar cream 0.025%	Fluocinolone acetonide
Uticort cream 0.025%	Betamethasone benzoate
Valisone cream 0.1%	Betamethasone valerate
Westcort cream 0.2%	Hydrocortisone valerate
Group VI (Medium Potency)	
Aristocort cream 0.1%	Triamcinolone acetonide
Synalar solution 0.05%	Fluocinolone acetonide
Tridesilon cream 0.05%	Desonide
Valisone lotion 0.05%	Betamethasone valerate
Group VII (Low Potency)*	
Nutracort cream 1%	Hydrocortisone
Hytone cream 1%	Hydrocortisone

*Includes other preparations containing dexamethasone, flumetasone, prednisolone, and methylprednisolone. Modified from Flowers FP: Topical coricosteroids use in a dermatologic practice: an algorithm for appropriate use. University of Florida Continuing Education Proceedings, November 1987, pp 4–9.

Types of Formulations. There are five types of topical cortico-steroid formulations: ointments, gels, creams, lotions, and solutions. Ointments are the most efficacious because they provide built-in occlusion, which enhances hydration of the stratum corneum to a greater extent than the other vehicles. Ointments are particularly useful for application to areas of the skin where the cornified layer is thick, such as the palms and the soles. They are also ideal for diseases that produce thick scales such as psoriasis. Their main disadvantage is lack of cosmetic acceptability. Creams have a greater cosmetic appeal and are particularly suited for areas of the skin such as the face, groin, and intertriginous sites. Lotions, gels, and solutions are preferred for hair-bearing areas of the body.

Receptor Binding

Introduction of hydroxy groups into the 11β-, 17α-, and 21-positions, ketone groups into the 3- and 20-positions, and a double bond into the 4-position of pregnane gives hydrocortisone (Fig. 2–1). Each one of these groups, except for the 17α-hydroxy group, enhances the binding of the steroid to the glucocorticoid receptor. The 17α-hydroxy group has the effect of decreasing the mineralocorticoid potency of hydrocortisone.

Introduction of another double bond (in the 1-position), a 6α-fluoro group, or a 9α-fluoro group leads to substantial increases in the binding to the glucocorticoid receptor. The 16β- or 16α- methyl or hydroxy groups are incorporated into the structures of potent anti-inflammatory steroids because of their abilities to decrease mineralocorticoid potency.

The result of the sequential incorporation of the additional functional groups into hydrocortisone is a series of increasingly more potent glucocorticoid steroids. Starting with hydrocortisone, going through prednisolone (double bond in the 1-position), and ending with fluocinolone, flumethasone, and diflorasone (all with 6α- and 9α-fluoro groups and a 16α- or 16β-group) gives the parent steroids of a large number of the more potent commercial products. In gen-

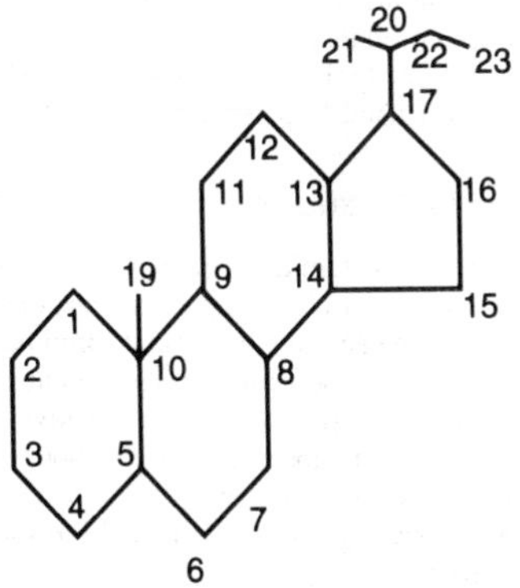

FIGURE 2–1. The pregnane ring system and numbering for substituents.

eral, the most potent steroid in a series is the member that is substituted with a double bond in the 1-position, a 6α- and a 9α-fluoro group and a 16α- or 16β-methyl group. The greatest enhancement of topical potency is derived from the replacement or masking of hydroxy groups in the modified hydrocortisone structure. Such changes have the potential not only for enhancing the solubility of the steroid in the skin but also for enhancing its binding to glucocorticoid receptors. Replacement of the 21-hydroxy group in betamethasone with a chloro group gives clobetasol, which binds much more tightly to glucocorticoid receptors than does betamethasone.

Masking the hydroxy group with ester or ketal derivatives also enhances binding. Representative ketal-type derivatives are the acetonides formed from the 16α-, 17α-dihydroxy groups found in triamcinolone and fluocinolone.

Clinical Considerations

In general, the nonfluorinated steroids are far less potent than their fluorinated counterparts and should be chosen for use on body sites where the skin is very thin (the face, groin, or scrotum) to avoid potential side effects.

Superpotent Topical Corticosteroids

Because all the side effects reported for the less potent topical steroids are more pronounced, it is important to proceed with caution when using a superpotent corticosteroid. Reversible preatrophy can often be observed in the form of vascular changes of the skin during the first 2 weeks of therapy with the superpotent steroids. Sufficient percutaneous absorption can occur with superpotent agents to cause either suppression of the hypothalamic-pituitary-adrenal axis or development of Cushing's syndrome. These effects are particularly prevalent when the corticosteroid is applied to large areas of the skin under occlusion or when it is applied to very thin areas of the skin.

Physicians should follow certain definite guidelines when prescribing superpotent topical corticosteroids. These agents should be used carefully in children and in the elderly. Superpotent steroids should not be used on the face except for severe disease and for no longer than 2 weeks or in flexural areas. Most of the cutaneous side effects are reversible, with the exception of striae. The use of these agents should be restricted to patients with severe dermatoses.

Therapeutic Indications

In general, the corticosteroid is applied twice a day, although daily application and "pulse" therapy have been shown to be as effective, particularly when the more potent formulations are used. Diseases may be classified according to their relative resistance to therapy: resistant, moderately resistant, and sensitive. Resistant dermatoses require the use of superpotent steroids or less potent steroids under occlusion. Moderately resistant diseases respond to mid-strength steroids, whereas sensitive dermatoses respond readily to weak steroid preparations.

Resistant dermatoses include plaque and palmoplantar psoriasis, lichen planus, dyshidrotic eczema, lichen simplex chronicus, granuloma annulare, and sarcoidosis. Moderately resistant dermatoses include adult atopic eczema, nummular eczema, irritant and allergic contact dermatitis, and discoid lupus erythematosus. Sensitive dermatoses include intertriginous psoriasis, infantile atopic eczema, seborrheic dermatitis, pityriasis rosea, and genital pruritus.

Topical corticosteroids are contraindicated in conditions in which a primary infection exists and may actually exacerbate viral, dermatophyte, or yeast infections, as well as scabies infestation. It is always good practice to reduce the potency of the topical corticosteroid when an inflammatory dermatosis has responded to treatment and to consider switching to an emollient nonsteroidal preparation when the inflammation has subsided.

Occlusion with plastic wrapping increases the absorption of hydrocortisone as much as 100 times. Modern occlusion methods make use of plastic gloves, sauna suits, Saran Wrap, Duoderm, and Actiderm patches, depending on the type and amount of surface to be covered.

Tachyphylaxis, development of resistance to previously effective topical steroids with long-term use, can be minimized by short-term or intermittent use of the steroid. Sudden discontinuation of treatment with topical corticosteroids should be avoided to prevent rebound phenomenon.

Side Effects

Thinning of the dermis and epidermis causes atrophy of the skin, probably the most common localized side effect of topical corticosteroids. Atrophy is most frequently on the flexural areas of the skin and results in telangiectasia, striae, purpura, and skin fragility. Perioral dermatitis and steroid rosacea are common side effects of long-term topical corticosteroid application. When topical corticosteroids are used for periods longer than 1 month they may exacerbate preexisting acne, induce steroid acne or cause reversible hypopigmentation.

Chronic use of topical corticosteroids may lead to hypertrichosis. In infants with diaper dermatitis, violaceous red nodules termed *granuloma gluteale infantum* may result when potent topical corticosteroids are applied under plastic diapers. Fungal and bacterial superinfections may occur, particularly when the topical corticosteroid is applied to flexural areas under occlusion. Systemic side effects of long-term use include development of Cushing's syndrome and suppression of the hypothalamic-pituitary-adrenal axis.

B. Inflammatory Diseases That Principally Affect the Epidermis and Dermis

CONTACT DERMATITIS AND OCCUPATIONAL DERMATOLOGY

Definition

Contact dermatitis is an inflammatory process in the skin caused by an exogenous agent or more than one agent, either chemical or chemical plus ultraviolet light (UV). Acute irritant contact dermatitis occurs following direct injurious exposure to an exogenous agent or group of agents that have the inherent ability to produce injury to the skin at the site of contact. Irritant responses are dose-dependent. Occlusion, abrasion, or interruption in the integrity of the stratum corneum (e.g., the result of a eczematous process) augments the absorbed dose of an irritant and enhances its irritancy potential. Contact reactions occur as allergic contact dermatitis, or contact urticaria.

Allergic contact dermatitis is a classic example of a type IV or cell-mediated immune disease. In allergic contact dermatitis, a sensitized person responds to a specific substance or chemically related substance with or without concomitant exposure to UV. In allergic contact dermatitis, an eczematous dermatitis is present at the site of cutaneous contact with a known allergen. In addition, the dermatitis partially or totally resolves with avoidance of allergen exposure. The allergen may be established to have played a causal role on one of two grounds. Exposure to the allergen causes recurrence of the eczematous process after 24 to 72 hours in the patient but not others similarly exposed. A closed patch test using a standard material is positive and confirms the association.

In contrast, contact urticaria is the immediate development of hives or angioedema at the site of skin contact with an urticant. In such sensitized patients, the cutaneous response may be associated with responses in mucosal areas such as the conjunctiva of the eyes and the bronchi. Occasionally, anaphylactic reactions may occur. Contact urticaria occurs on an immunologic or nonimmunologic basis. A limited number of environmental nonimmunologic urticants induce cutaneous mast cell degranulation. Such substances can produce urticarial responses in most humans in a dose-related manner. In allergic contact urticaria, an immediate hypersensitivity response is mediated by a specific IgE that binds to tissue mast cells. A large number of environmental allergens produce contact urticaria, which is frequently seen in small animal handlers, food handlers exposed to raw food protein, pharmaceutical workers, and from rubber latex in surgical gloves.

Clinical Description

Epidemiology

Western industrialized countries have a contact dermatitis prevalence of between 5% and 20%, which appears to be less frequent in the elderly. Contact dermatitis is a common occupational condition constituting a significant proportion of compensated disease in the United States. Irritant contact dermatitis is believed to be five times as common as allergic contact dermatitis in the workplace.

In North America, 20 substances account for most of the positive responses. Although thousands of other contactants have been reported to cause allergic contact dermatitis, the majority of allergens produce a morphologically positive response between 1% and 3% of patients tested. Approximately 70% of persons with allergic contact dermatitis are likely to have a response to one of the 20 contactants. Not included in this list are plant materials, which are a common cause of both irritant and allergic contact dermatitis. The most common plant contact allergen is rhus, the allergen in poison ivy. A few allergens are more likely than others to be work-associated. Younger men without atopic dermatitis have higher odds of having work-related contact dermatitis. Hand dermatitis is common in contact dermatitis in general; hand and arm dermatitis, but not leg dermatitis, are more likely occupational.

Clinical Morphology

Irritant contact dermatitis of the acute type, such as from a chemical burn, is characterized by sharply delineated areas of erythema and vesicobullous changes, which may proceed to erosions and ulcers. The skin may slough when rubbed, yielding a shiny underlying glistening patch with serous discharge. Rarely, such a lesion may be self-inflicted, and in these instances the hallmark of an artifactual process is that the history is often chronic while the morphology is clearly acute with odd location and shape. Large blisters occur with more severe irritant contact dermatitis, and hemorrhage into the blister fluid with deep dermal injury occurs. Such lesions may scar and damage underlying structures. Acid burns (e.g., due to sulfuric acid, phosphoric acid, hydrochloric acid) produce the most damage immediately and resolve quickly. Alkali burns (e.g., due to sodium hydroxide) cause damage over several hours. The initial injury may underestimate the end-results.

For mild or moderately irritating substances, irritant contact dermatitis may occur only at sites of contact under occlusion (e.g., under a rubber glove or a hat band) or in sensitive and/or intertriginous areas of the skin (e.g., eyelids, genitals). Friction, low humidity, or high temperature accentuates irritancy.

Phototoxic contact dermatitis is a specific type of irritant contact dermatitis in which the irritant is capable only of causing a response in association with exposure to UV. After UV exposure, an immediate erythema and edema response occurs. This is often associated with the development of vesicles or bullae. Resolution follows in 48 to 72 hours. Postinflammatory hyperpigmentation may result. Tar products (e.g., creosote, coal tar) and plant oleoresins containing psoralens such as limes, lemons, and celery, psoralens are the most common phototoxins.

Chronic repeated irritant contact dermatitis is the most common type of contact dermatitis. The person complains of itching and fissuring associated with tenderness of the affected area and pain on exposure to irritants, even with simple hand washing. Erythematous scaling patches with indistinct borders, sometimes with microvesiculation, are evident on the exposed areas of the skin, especially on the areas of most sensitive skin (e.g., dorsal hands more than palms). The growth of the nails may be impaired, resulting in ridging of the nails.

In allergic contact dermatitis, erythematous, edematous plaques with vesicles and bullae and distinct borders are typical. Linear lesions with vesicles characterize reactions to plants. Itching is the sine qua non. A widespread macular erythema, and autosensitization (id) reaction, may develop in severe cases. Photoallergic responses occur at sites of contact combined with exposure to light. Airborne contactants like ragweed oleoresin or epoxy resin fumes result in dermatitis on exposed skin surfaces. Photoallergic contact dermatitis differs from airborne contact dermatitis in that the non–exposed skin, such as the upper eyelids, is spared. Following contact sensitization, later oral exposure or inhalation of an allergen can rarely result in a recurrence of the eczematous process at the site of original contact with the allergen.

Pathology

Allergic contact dermatitis, like nummular dermatitis, is a spongiotic dermatitis that begins with slight spongiosis, edema that separates keratinocytes from one another, stretching their intercellular bridges with mononuclear and eosinophilic perivascular dermal infiltrate, and can develop intraepidermal vesiculation, but often evolves into a psoriasiform dermatitis prior to its resolution.

Somewhat different changes occur in irritant contact dermatitis. The changes of irritant contact dermatitis are largely due to necrosis of the outermost portion of the epidermis often accompanied by infiltrates of lymphocytes and neutrophils. Eosinophils are not present in number unless the contactant is an allergen as well as an irritant, or an allergen diffuses into the dermis as a result of diminished barrier function.

Contact urticaria is histologically similar to other forms of urticaria, with infiltrates of lymphocytes, mast cells, neutrophils, and eosinophils, edema of the reticular dermis, and no epidermal changes.

Diagnosis and Differential Diagnosis

Careful clinical evaluation will in most instances of irritant contact dermatitis make the diagnosis. Skin disorders that may pose a problem in the differential diagnosis are listed in Table 2–4.

The identification of the irritant cause depends on careful history taking and a knowledge of irritancy of commercial products. Usage tests or work exposure trials to detect irritant contact dermatitis are occasionally used with a mild irritant, but when acute irritant

TABLE 2-4. Differential Diagnosis of Contact Dermatitis
Dyshydrotic Dermatitis
Atopic Dermatitis
Seborrheic Dermatitis
Neurodermatitis
Psoriasis
Tinea

contact dermatitis is due to a potent irritant, re-exposure is never justified.

Diagnosis of allergic contact dermatitis may require that the patient be re-exposed to a suspect allergen. In plant dermatitis, this is not commonly done, as the history and the morphology is usually diagnostic. In cases of eczematous dermatitis due to cosmetic or work exposure, a long list of possible allergens may be presented. While one may perform usage trials with each suspect formulation, this is time consuming and may cause re-exacerbation of skin disease.

In patch testing, a suspected allergen is applied to the skin and left in contact for 48 hours. Once the patch is removed, the site is examined for morphologic evidence of an eczematous response. If the person develops such a response at a concentration below the irritant threshold concentration, the response is taken to signify that the individual may be allergic to the test substance. Standard patch test kits are available that provide allergens in the appropriate concentrations for testing. The sensitivity and specificity of the collection of test substances that make up the standard patch test tray for the United States approved by the Food and Drug Administration for sale in the U.S. are 77% and 71%, respectively.

Treatment

Treatment of irritant contact dermatitis requires limiting exposure to the irritant. In the case of severe irritants, this is best accomplished by assiduous use of personal protective devices (gloves, aprons, gauntlets, etc.) and in some instances through engineering controls such as enclosures or automated methods of handling the material. For mild irritants causing repeated-insult irritant contact dermatitis, the use of gloves to protect the skin from exposure and the use of emollients to offset desiccation of the skin are of some value. Once the irritant contact dermatitis has become chronic, it is often persistent, and unless such patients significantly modify their cutaneous habits, both at work and at home, they may not improve. In spite of diligent chemical avoidance and aggressive therapy, complete clearing of their skin is unusual. Skillful use of emollients, low-potency intermittent topical corticosteroid use, and avoidance of irritant exposure are the mainstays of management (Table 2-5).

Allergic contact dermatitis offers the possibility of eliminating exposure to the contact allergen and eliminating the component of the patient's dermatitis that is due to allergen exposure. Not infre-

TABLE 2-5. Treatment of Irritant Contact Dermatitis

Avoidance of irritants
Personal protective equipment
Emollients (e.g., Eucerin, Moisturel)
Mild topical steroids (e.g., hydrocortisone 1%, triamcinolone 0.1%)

quently, allergic contact dermatitis and irritant contact dermatitis coincide, as, for instance, rubber gloves may be donned to protect the skin from irritant exposure only to result in an allergy to rubber accelerators. Identification of an allergen and avoidance of further exposure are associated with improvement, but not complete resolution of dermatitis. In acute severe allergic contact dermatitis, oral corticosteroid therapy with prednisone at 1 mg/kg body weight tapered over a 3-week period coupled with topical care and avoidance of further exposure will result in rapid clearing of contact dermatitis (Table 2-6). In less severe disease, topical steroid medication of mid potency such as betamethasone-17-valerate 0.1% or fluocinolone 0.25% three times per day in a lotion, cream, or ointment base depending on the site of application, is often effective. If vesiculation and weeping are present, open wet compresses with saline or Burow's solution should be added to help dry, cleanse, and debride the area.

In instances of phototoxic and photoallergic contact dermatitis, the contactant should be removed and sun exposure should be limited until the dermatitis improves. In work situations, contact dermatitis may require an alteration of workplace conditions.

DIAPER DERMATITIS

(CM&S Chapter 11)

Definition and Background

The term *diaper dermatitis* is a description rather than a diagnosis, referring to an eruption occurring in the area of skin covered by the diaper. Diaper dermatitis is very common, occurring in 16% of children with a primary or a secondary skin complaint visiting a pediatric clinic. Seven to 35% of the infant population is affected at

TABLE 2-6. Treatment of Allergic Contact Dermatitis

Avoidance of allergen(s) indentified
Avoidance of irritants
Personal protective equipment
Emollients (e.g., Eucerin, Moisturel)
Moderate to potent topical steroids (e.g., betamethasone 0.1%, clobetasol dipropionate 0.05%)

a given time, with the highest incidence occurring in infants from 9 to 12 months of age.

Clinical Description and Differential Diagnosis

Diaper dermatitis can be classified by both appearance and etiology, with morphologic changes varying from diffuse erythema to vesicular, pustular, bullous, or nodular infiltrative lesions. Although many dermatologic conditions can occur in this region, the term *diaper dermatitis* should be reserved for those conditions caused, either directly or indirectly, by wearing diapers. Four clinical forms of diaper dermatitis are believed to be related to diaper wear: (1) *chafing dermatitis* with mild redness and scaliness in areas of diaper contact; (2) *sharply demarcated confluent erythema* with involvement of the skin folds; (3) *discrete shallow ulcerations* scattered throughout the diaper area including the genitalia; and (4) *beefy red confluent erythema* of the entire perineum with satellite lesions, seen when secondarily infected with *Candida albicans*. Large nodular lesions without *Candida* superinfection are termed *granuloma gluteale infantum*. The two major categories of diaper dermatitis most frequently diagnosed are primary irritant contact dermatitis and microbial (primarily candidal) infection. Primary irritant contact diaper dermatitis presents as parchment-like, poorly marginated erythema, papules, vesicles, and small superficial erosions. The inguinal folds are usually spared. Candidal diaper dermatitis presents as clusters of erythematous papules and pustules that later coalesce into a beefy red confluent rash with well-marginated borders with satellite lesions. Folds are commonly involved as well. The differential diagnosis includes allergic contact dermatitis, atopic dermatitis, child abuse, congenital syphilis, herpes simplex, histiocytosis X, psoriasis, scabies, seborrheic dermatitis, and tinea cruris.

Pathogenesis and Etiology

Diaper dermatitis is not a single entity but can result from multiple causative factors. The factors most commonly associated with the pathogenesis of diaper dermatitis are skin wetness, elevated pH, fecal enzymes, and infectious agents.

Treatment

Parents should be counseled to change the infant's diaper as soon as it is wet or at least every 2 to 4 hours, and to cleanse after bowel movements with warm water. If severe inflammation is present, 1% hydrocortisone cream may be used, but topical use of fluorinated glucocorticosteroids should be avoided. In ulcerative dermatitis, a protective ointment such as petrolatum or zinc oxide is added. Seborrheic and atopic dermatitis in the diaper area respond well to low-potency topical steroids. Impetigo and folliculitis should be treated with systemic antibiotics such as erythromycin or penicillinase-resistant penicillin. Infection with *C. albicans* should be treated with a topical antifungal agent such as nystatin or an azole cream. If severe inflammation is also present, 1% hydrocortisone can be used in addition to the antifungal agent. Combination fluorinated steroid–anticandidal agents should not be used in diaper dermatitis since their steroid component is potent and may contribute to skin atrophy, scarring, or adrenal suppression. The addition of oral anti-fungal therapy to decrease gastrointestinal colonization by the yeast has not been demonstrated to be more effective than topical therapy alone.

Several compounds that have been recommended in the past should be avoided in the treatment of diaper dermatitis: boric acid, camphor, phenol, methyl salicylate, tincture of benzoin, mercury-containing preparations, and talc.

HAND AND FOOT DERMATITIS

(CM&S Chapter 12)

Dermatitis of the hands and feet is a common clinical problem whose cause is often unknown. Both endogenous and exogenous factors can adversely affect treatment, response, and prognosis. The focus here is on the endogenous dermatoses affecting the hands and feet. Endogenous disorders that can manifest as a hand or foot der-matitis include atopic dermatitis, nummular dermatitis, pompholyx, hyperkeratotic dermatitis of the palms, psoriasis, palmoplantar pus-tulosis, and acrodermatitis continua. Because many of these disor-ders can overlap, these diseases are considered in two major groups: dermatitis of the hands and feet and psoriasis and pustular syn-dromes.

Definition and Clinical Description

Dermatitis of the Hands and Feet

Atopic dermatitis is the major endogenous or constitutional cause of hand dermatitis. Atopic hand dermatitis is common in children, and the hand is the most frequent site of atopic dermatitis in adults, with the fingers being the most common site of involvement.

A history of dermatitis affecting the hands in childhood is of predominant importance in the development of atopic hand derma-titis in later life. Other factors are severe widespread dermatitis in childhood, persistent dermatitis on other parts of the body, and dry, itchy skin. Atopic hand dermatitis may occur alone or with disease elsewhere, particularly in a flexural distribution. It commonly presents as a patchy vesicular rash that mainly affects the dorsa of the hands and fingers. Fissures may be present and are often in-fected. The skin is dry, and lichenification is typically present with chronic disease. The fingernails may be pitted and ridged, and other features of atopic dermatitis may be present.

Nummular or discoid dermatitis consists of sharply demarcated, coin-shaped lesions that may be exudative and crusted. It is a chronic endogenous condition that affects adults between the ages of 50 and 70 years. It is more common in males. Lesions commonly affect the trunk and limbs but typically begin on the hands and forearms in younger individuals. The eruption consists of discrete vesicular or crusted, discoid lesions. These typically occur over the dorsal surfaces of the hands and the backs or sides of fingers. Lesions may be single or multiple.

Pompholyx (dyshidrotic eczema), a vesiculobullous dermatitis affecting the hands and feet, accounts for 1% to 6% of all cases of hand dermatitis. The condition is characterized by recurrent eruptions of clear vesicles or bullae that occur symmetrically on the palms and soles. The volar aspects and sides of the digits are also affected. A sensation of burning and itching preceding an attack is common. The attacks tend to be more common in spring and summer. Secondary infection is a common complication, and fissures, hyperkeratosis, and nail dystrophy may eventually develop.

Hyperkeratotic dermatitis of the palms commonly presents as hyperkeratotic, fissure-prone, infiltrated lesions over the palms of the hands. It may also be located on the soles of the feet. The disease mainly occurs in adults and tends to be chronic. The lesions characteristically occur proximally or in the middle of the palms with only slight clinical inflammation and without vesicles.

Psoriasis and Pustular Syndromes of the Hands and Feet

Psoriasis affecting the palms and soles may present as typical discrete scaly plaques, as diffuse hyperkeratotic scaling mainly distributed over the pressure points, or as a pustulosis. Psoriasis affecting the palms and soles may be difficult to distinguish from a chronic dermatitis. Psoriasis typically has a sharply defined margin at the wrist or forearm. Nail involvement may be present, including pitting, subungual hyperkeratosis, and onycholysis.

Palmoplantar pustulosis is a chronic dermatosis characterized by recurrent sterile pustules affecting the palms and soles. It is a disease of adults with a slight predominance in females. It typically affects persons 40 to 60 years of age. Crops of discrete pustules measuring 2 to 4 mm in diameter typically develop on palmar and plantar skin. The thenar eminence is most often affected, followed by involvement of the hypothenar eminence and central palm. Occasionally, the pustules spread to the volar wrists and the dorsa of the digits. The instep and medial and lateral borders of the foot and heel are characteristically involved. The pustules subsequently change from yellow to brown, followed by shedding of scale.

Acrodermatitis continua is a sterile pustular eruption that affects the distal fingers and toes with severe nail involvement. It is more common in females. A preceding history of trauma or paronychia is common. Usually a thumb or finger is affected first, followed by slow proximal extension and severe nail dystrophy. The condition is characteristically painful and may be associated with soft tissue sclerosis and osteoporosis.

Acute palmoplantar pustular psoriasis is an acute pustular eruption affecting palmar and plantar surfaces and extends onto the dorsa of the fingers, hands, and feet. Lesions can also be seen scattered sparsely on the trunk and limbs. It is frequently preceded by an upper respiratory tract infection, and it characteristically resolves over 2 to 3 weeks. It may also present with leukocytoclastic vasculitis.

Infantile acropustulosis is a condition that mainly affects black male infants between the ages of 2 and 10 months and typically resolves by 2 to 3 years of age. Intensely pruritic 1- to 2-mm pustules occur on the palms, soles, and dorsa of hands and feet. The condition is refractory to treatment with topical corticosteroids but responds to dapsone.

Juvenile plantar dermatosis largely affects young children. It causes scaly erythematous plaques on the weight-bearing areas of the soles and often results in fissuring. The fingertips can also be involved. The wearing of shoes made from nonabsorbent materials, overgrowth of aerobic cocci, and an atopic diathesis are proposed causes.

Pathology

The typical finding in the dermatitides is a spongiotic dermatitis, while that in psoriasis and that in pustular syndromes range from changes typical of psoriasis to intraepidermal neutrophilic pustules without other psoriatic changes.

Diagnosis and Differential Diagnosis

The diagnosis of hand and foot dermatitis is usually not problematic, although the possibility of allergic contact dermatitis or dermatophytoses must always be considered.

Treatment

Dermatitis of the Hands and Feet

The mainstay of treatment of atopic dermatitis and nummular dermatitis is the avoidance of irritants and therapy with emollients and topical corticosteroids. Usually a mid- to high-potency topical corticosteroid is required for a short period of time. Recalcitrant disease may require treatment with superpotent topical corticosteroids under occlusion for 3 to 7 days. Antihistamines can be of benefit but usually the sedating type is required. Infection is common in exudative cases and should be treated with antibiotics. Resistant cases may require phototherapy or cyclosporine. The management of these disorders is discussed on pages 55 and 56.

Psoriasis and Pustular Syndromes of the Hands and Feet

Localized psoriasis vulgaris is treated similarly to psoriasis elsewhere on the body, starting with topical treatment before phototherapy or systemic therapy is considered. It may respond to topical therapy with tar or potent topical corticosteroids with or without occlusion. Topical vitamin D or calcipotriol (calcipotriene in the U.S.) has been shown to be as efficacious as a potent topical corticosteroid without the adverse side effects. UVB phototherapy and photochemotherapy are of proven benefit for psoriasis and can be conveniently used for localized disease. Retinoids, cytotoxic drugs, and cyclosporine are reserved for severe refractory disease, particularly when functional impairment of these sites is present.

Treatment of palmoplantar pustulosis is often difficult, and this disorder is usually refractory to topical therapy such as corticosteroids, tar, and anthralin. A wide variety of other therapeutic modalities have been used. These include intralesional corticosteroids, methotrexate, colchicine, etretinate, and PUVA therapy (systemic or topical). The combination of etretinate and PUVA is more effective than when these treatment modalities are used alone. Cyclosporine has been used successfully to treat palmoplantar pustulosis at doses as low as 1.25 mg/kg per day.

ATOPIC DERMATITIS

(CM&S Chapter 13)

Atopic dermatitis is a common chronic or relapsing eczematous dermatitis characterized by intense pruritus and occurring primarily in infants and children with a personal or family history of atopy.

Clinical Description

Epidemiology

Estimates are that approximately 10% of children suffer from atopic dermatitis. The incidence of atopic dermatitis has been increasing significantly over the past 3 decades. The onset of the disease occurs before the age of 7 years in over 80% of patients, with a female-to-male ratio of 1.4:1.

The pairwise concordance rate of atopic dermatitis is about 0.75 in monozygotic twins and 0.25 in dizygotic twins and nontwin siblings. In up to 80% of patients with atopic dermatitis there is a personal or family history of allergic disease. The incidence of atopic dermatitis in patients with a family history of atopy is as high as 80% when both parents have atopic dermatitis.

Studies have shown that 70% of patients with severe dermatitis will be affected into adult life while 60% of patients with milder disease have persistence into adult life.

Clinical Findings

Atopic dermatitis is characterized by acute, subacute, and chronic lesions. In the acute phase, the involved areas present as intensely pruritic, erythematous papules and vesicles that become excoriated and exudative. These areas commonly become secondarily infected. In the subacute phase, the involved skin has excoriated, erythematous, scaling papules and plaques. Chronic eczema is characterized by changes secondary to repeated rubbing and scratching called lichenification, in which the skin is thickened with increased skin markings.

The distribution of the rash in atopic dermatitis varies with the age of the patient. In infancy the rash usually presents after 2 to 3 months of age and is most characteristically an acute dermatitis. It is at this time that infants begin to develop coordinated scratching. During this period the disease tends to most frequently involve the scalp and face, as well as the extensor surfaces of the extremities. These areas are most prone to being scratched and rubbed as the infant begins to crawl and then walk. Infants and young children commonly develop periauricular fissures with weeping and crusting that are reasonably diagnostic for atopic dermatitis. The groin area is usually spared during infancy, probably because of increased hydration secondary to the occlusion of the area with diapers. At the age of 2 years the infants begin to develop flexural involvement. By the age of 5, the face is less frequently involved and the rash takes on a more subacute appearance. Also, between the ages of 2 and 4 the child develops involvement of the posterior thighs and buttocks. The chest, back, and abdomen are also commonly involved sites in infants and children. During childhood, cheilitis, characterized by dryness, scaling, and fissuring especially of the upper lip, is common.

Atopic dermatitis in adults tends to occur in the same distribution as in late childhood, mainly in the neck, antecubital and popliteal fossae, wrists, and ankles. The groin and axillae are unusual areas of involvement in atopic dermatitis. If eczema is found in these areas, another cause should be sought. Perifollicular accentuation is common in patients with dark skin. Nipple dermatitis, an uncommon although specific finding for atopic dermatitis, may be present in young women.

Pruritus is a major symptom of atopic dermatitis, leading many to believe that the dermatitis is a result of scratching and rubbing. In contrast to this, lesions of atopic dermatitis have been noted earlier than 2 months of age, when scratching is not coordinated. Also, in some atopic infants dry skin has been noted shortly after birth.

Associated Clinical Findings

Xerosis and Ichthyosis Vulgaris

Dry skin or xerosis occurs with a frequency from 48% to 98% in patients with atopic dermatitis and appears as fine-scaled, noninflammatory areas of skin that have a rough texture, often with perifollicular accentuation. The dry skin of atopic dermatitis has reduced water-binding capacity, increased transepidermal water loss, and decreased water content.

Ichthyosis vulgaris has been found to affect up to one third of patients with atopic dermatitis, and features of atopic dermatitis are found in approximately 50% of patients with ichthyosis vulgaris. Keratosis pilaris, a frequent manifestation of ichthyosis vulgaris, is commonly found in atopic dermatitis as hyperkeratotic follicular papules located on the extensor aspect of the arms, thighs, and buttocks. In addition, hyperlinearity of the palms and soles, another manifestation of ichthyosis vulgaris, is commonly found in atopic dermatitis.

Pigmentary Changes

Patients with atopic dermatitis, especially with chronic skin changes, can develop postinflammatory hyperpigmentation and hypopigmentation. These changes resolve months after the dermatitis is brought under control. Pityriasis alba, a condition characterized by hypopigmented, scaly patches located most commonly on the cheeks, upper arms, or shoulders and surrounded by pigmented skin, is commonly seen in atopic dermatitis, although it can be seen in patients without atopic dermatitis. Reticulate hyperpigmentation of the neck, the so-called dirty neck sign, is occasionally present.

Eye and Periorbital Changes

The eyelids may show changes of mild dryness and scaling to severe lichenification and ectropion. Loss of the lateral eyebrow may occur secondary to chronic rubbing. Chronic rubbing of the eyes may be secondary to allergic conjunctivitis. The Dennie-Morgan fold, a single or double fold in the lower eyelid, which may be secondary to eyelid edema caused by eyelid dermatitis. The Dennie-Morgan fold appears to be of no diagnostic significance. Orbital darkening may be caused by chronic edema, lichenification, and postinflammatory hyperpigmentation. Cataracts have been noted in patients with atopic dermatitis with a frequency in the past as high as 20%, although recently the incidence has been found to be much lower. Anterior subcapsular cataracts usually present in young patients with severe disease, while the posterior cataracts may have developed secondary to the use of systemic steroids and topical steroid use around the eyes. Keratoconus, which can cause serious visual impairment and can sometimes lead to a detached retina, is seen with increased frequency in patients with atopic dermatitis.

Hand and Foot Dermatitis

Approximately 70% of patients with atopic dermatitis have had hand dermatitis at some time, while as many as three fourths of patients with hand eczema before age 15 years also experienced hand eczema after that age. Foot dermatitis is especially common in winter.

Complications

Bacterial Infection

The most common bacterial pathogen in atopic dermatitis is *Staphylococcus aureus*, which colonizes the skin in over 95% of patients with atopic dermatitis, with increased numbers in areas of active dermatitis. Acute flares in atopic dermatitis may be driven by *S. aureus* infections and can be recognized clinically by small superficial pustules, new crusted and weeping skin lesions, and poor control by the use of previously effective treatment. There is an excellent clinical response to antistaphylococcal antibiotics.

Viral Infection

Patients with atopic dermatitis are susceptible to viral infections caused by herpes simplex, vaccinia, warts, and molluscum contagiosum. Herpes simplex infection can spread rapidly to become generalized, a condition known as eczema herpeticum. Clinically this is a vesiculopustular eruption in which the lesions are umbilicated and often become hemorrhagic.

Fungal Infection

Patients with atopic dermatitis are susceptible to chronic infections of the hands and feet caused by *Trichophyton rubrum*. Chronic dermatophytosis may contribute to a flare of atopic dermatitis on areas of skin not involved with fungus.

Exfoliative Erythroderma

In some patients, atopic dermatitis may progress to an exfoliative erythroderma. This may occur secondary to widespread infection or after the withdrawal of systemic corticosteroids.

Mental and Emotional Dysfunction and Growth Retardation

Patients with atopic dermatitis commonly experience anger, frustration, and anxiety. Psychic stress is a major aggravating factor. Children with chronic, generalized, severe atopic dermatitis can develop growth retardation secondary to being placed into a catabolic state.

Pathology

The earliest pathologic change is likely spongiosis, papillary dermal edema, and a sparse perivascular and interstitial lymphoeosinophilic infiltrate. As lesions progress, vesicles appear, and the features approximate those of lichen simplex chronicus.

Pathogenesis

The cause of atopic dermatitis is unknown. Food allergens in some patients with atopic dermatitis have been found to be an exacerbating factor. Up to one third of atopic individuals have food hypersensitivity that contributes to skin symptoms. Withholding foods that give positive challenges can result in remarkable improvement. Aeroallergens, such as trees and grass pollens, may also play an important role in the exacerbation of atopic dermatitis. Both immediate hypersensitivity skin tests and delayed-type hypersensitivity patch tests to aeroallergens are often positive in patients with atopic dermatitis. Flares of atopic dermatitis in some patients have been precipitated by environmental contact with known aeroallergens that had elicited eczematous patch test reactions. The house dust mite may also be an exacerbating factor in atopic dermatitis.

Differential Diagnosis

The differential diagnosis includes allergic contact dermatitis, seborrheic dermatitis, nummular dermatitis, tinea, scabies, and mycosis fungoides.

Treatment

The goal of treatment in atopic dermatitis is to restore hydration to the skin, to identify and eliminate triggering factors, and to decrease pruritus and inflammation.

Hydration

Hydration is a key element in the treatment of both the acute and the chronic stages of atopic dermatitis. During acute flares this can be accomplished by soaking the affected area for 15 to 20 minutes in tepid water two to three times per day. In addition to skin hydration, the soaks help to remove crusts and reduce exudation. Burow's solution at a dilution of 1:40 for a brief period of time provides astringent and antibacterial effects for localized weeping lesions. The addition of sodium bicarbonate or colloid substances such as oatmeal (Aveeno) or starch to the bath water may be soothing to some patients. Upon leaving the bath, patients should remove excess water with a soft towel, followed by the application of the appropriate topical medication. The skin should be occluded within 3 to 5 minutes to prevent evaporation that could lead to further drying of the skin. Uninvolved areas of the skin should be treated with a bland ointment such as white petrolatum or a moisturizing cream. The use of moisturizers is recommended at least three times a day other than when applied after bathing. When the skin disease is under control, bathing can be reduced to once a day.

Trigger Factors

Irritants

The dry, sensitive skin of patients with atopic dermatitis is easily irritated by soaps, solvents, and fabrics made of wool and nylon. Minimally defatting soaps with a neutral pH such as Dove, Basis, or Purpose should be used. Residual laundry detergent should be eliminated by a second rinse cycle if necessary. Patients with hand dermatitis should avoid jobs that require frequent exposure to the irritants or frequent hand washing. Patients should also modify their activities and surroundings to minimize sweating, which may also cause itching. They should work and sleep in surroundings where a constant temperature and humidity is maintained.

Allergens

Aeroallergens and foods are two known possible exacerbating factors in atopic dermatitis. Patients in whom positive skin testing correlates with their history of exacerbations by environmental allergens should carefully avoid exposure to those allergens. In patients who are found to be mite sensitive, benefit may be obtained from the encasement of pillows and mattresses in plastic. Electrostatic air purifiers may also be helpful. In patients who are found to have food sensitivities that flare their dermatitis, the avoidance of those foods can be beneficial. One must be careful to avoid restrictive diets, especially in children, which can lead to malnutrition.

Infection

It is important to recognize bacterial, viral, and fungal infections can cause recurrent flares of the dermatitis. *S. aureus* is usually resistant to penicillin, and bacterial culture for antibiotic sensitivity can facilitate choosing the proper antibiotic. Erythromycin is the initial drug of choice for acute flares, and dicloxacillin or an oral cephalosporin is indicated in cases of erythromycin resistance.

Extensive local or widespread infection with herpes simplex requires systemic therapy with acyclovir. Dermatophyte infections require topical or systemic antifungal treatment.

Antipruritic Agents

Antihistamines have been the mainstay of therapy for the treatment of pruritus in atopic dermatitis; however, little effect has been demonstrated in most studies. Children seem to respond to sedating night-time doses of antihistamines. Modifying the environment to maintain a constant temperature and wearing loose-fitting cotton clothing are beneficial.

Anti-inflammatory Agents

Corticosteroids

Corticosteroids are effective when used topically in decreasing inflammation and pruritus. As a general rule, the lowest potency topical corticosteroid that is effective should be used. The agent should be applied immediately after bathing to maximize penetration through hydrated skin. The choice of drug varies according to the location and extent of lesions, and the drug should be applied no more than twice daily. In the acute flare of atopic dermatitis, a mid-potency corticosteroid such as triamcinolone ointment 0.025% to 0.1% may be applied after bathing to all affected areas except the face, groin, and axillae, on which a low-potency preparation such as hydrocortisone 1% may be used. As the dermatitis improves, the frequency of application as well as the strength of the corticosteroid should be decreased. When the dermatitis becomes well controlled, a tar preparation or moisturizer may be substituted.

The use of systemic corticosteroids is highly discouraged in the care of atopic dermatitis. Although these agents provide dramatic relief when used, they often promote flares when they are discontinued and are associated with serious side effects when used chronically.

Ultraviolet Therapy

Both psoralens plus ultraviolet A (PUVA) and ultraviolet B (UVB) have been found to be effective in the treatment of atopic dermatitis by modulating the immune response in the skin. Some patients, however, experience flares when exposed to ultraviolet irradiation; thus, obtaining a thorough history before considering phototherapy is important. Carefully monitoring treatment is essential, because patients frequently have partial relapses during a phototherapy treatment course. The acute side effect of phototherapy is phototoxicity, while in the longer term these patients are at a greater risk for skin cancers.

Other Therapies

Patients with atopic dermatitis seem to have decreased secretion of IFN-γ. Recombinant IFN-γ injected subcutaneously has been associated with significant improvement in patients with dermatitis while they are receiving the medication, but relapse occurs once the IFN-γ is discontinued.

Cyclosporine has a dramatic clinical effect, although there is a rapid relapse shortly after the discontinuance of the drug. In addition, the drug is associated with serious side effects, including hypertension, elevations in serum creatinine, and paresthesias.

Thymopentin is a polypeptide that mimics thymopoietin, a thymic hormone that influences the differentiation of thymocytes and the function of mature T cells. Studies utilizing thymopentin have shown that patients have moderate improvement in their dermatitis, responding at the sixth week of treatment but with relapses in some cases after the seventh week of treatment.

The future promises to bring forth new anti-inflammatory and immunomodulatory agents as the pathogenesis of atopic dermatitis is elucidated. Investigators are looking at new phosphodiesterase inhibitors as well as traditional Chinese herbal mixtures, which have yielded initial positive results in trials with children and adults.

LICHEN SIMPLEX CHRONICUS, PRURIGO NODULARIS, AND NOTALGIA PARESTHETICA

(CM&S Chapter 14)

Lichen Simplex Chronicus

Definition and Clinical Description

Lichen simplex chronicus is a common, extremely pruritic disorder characterized by well-circumscribed, erythematous, thickened plaques with accentuated skin markings. It may be idiopathic but more frequently it is secondary to atopic dermatitis or other conditions in which pruritus is especially intense. The plaques are dry, and scaling and scratch marks are sometimes present. Intense itching is the predominant symptom but not necessarily a complaint, in that some patients describe a pleasurable sensation from rubbing and scratching. The most common sites of involvement include the lower legs, wrists, ankles, posterior and lateral neck, extensor forearms, upper eyelids, retroauricular area, and the opening of the external auditory canal.

Pathogenesis and Etiology

Lichen simplex chronicus is produced by repetitive rubbing and/or scratching and is maintained because persistent underlying pruritus and ''itch hyperexcitability'' in affected areas perpetuate these behaviors.

Differential Diagnosis

The differential diagnosis includes psoriasis, atopic eczema, contact dermatitis, and tinea.

Treatment

A careful explanation of the traumatic perpetuation of lesions is essential. Local treatment includes the use of potent topical corticosteroids, sometimes under overnight or more prolonged occlusion. Simple occlusion is sometimes sufficient. Intralesional injection of corticosteroids may be effective in instances in which topical therapy has not been beneficial. Relapses are common.

Prurigo and Prurigo Nodularis

Definition

Prurigo nodularis is an intensely pruritic disorder in which persistent rubbing and scratching in particular areas lead to the formation of distinctive skin nodules. Excoriated lesions of prurigo nodularis are termed *picker's nodules*. These occur as an idiopathic form or as a manifestation of itching caused by an underlying cutaneous or systemic disease.

Clinical Description

The lesions of prurigo nodularis are excruciatingly pruritic, 1- to 2-cm, dome-shaped, hemispherical nodules, often eroded, scaling, or crusted, and most often distributed predominantly on the extremities. The intervening skin is usually normal.

Diagnosis and Differential Diagnosis

The differential diagnosis includes hypertrophic lichen planus, persistent bite reaction, and any cutaneous or underlying systemic cause of generalized pruritus.

Treatment

Unless elimination of an underlying provocative factor or disease can be achieved, therapy is symptomatic and there is no uniformly effective treatment. Treatment principles are similar to those involved in management of lichen simplex chronicus except that nodular prurigo is usually even more resistant to treatment.

Notalgia Paresthetica

Definition and Clinical Description

Notalgia paresthetica is a localized itch that usually occurs just to one side or the other of the midscapular area. In most cases it probably arises as the consequence of an isolated peripheral sensory neuropathy.

The patient complains of itching in a single focus on one side of the upper back. In most cases there is no visible cutaneous change, but secondary changes include hyperpigmentation and lichenification as rubbing or scratching persists.

Treatment

Notalgia paresthetica has been successfully treated with topical application of capsaicin and of anesthetic creams.

NUMMULAR DERMATITIS

(CM&S Chapter 15)

Definition

Nummular dermatitis is characterized by coin-shaped (discoid) patches that may vary from papulovesicular and exudative to red and scaly and that preferentially affect the extensor extremities, but may be seen on the trunk.

Clinical Description

Idiopathic nummular dermatitis occurs in both men and women and seems ti be most common in persons older the 50 years of age. The eruption characteristically begins with bright red, often edematous papules or tiny vesicles. Individual lesions coalesce into small, round patches that vary from 1 to several centimeters, and the surface may become exudative and crusted. The extent of cutaneous involvement varies from a few to many such lesions, which are usually symmetrically distributed. With time, the acute papular and vesicular plaques may develop into drier, less red, scaling plaques. The favored sites are the extensor surfaces of lower legs and the dorsa of the feet. However, the upper extremities, dorsal hands, trunk, and thighs may be involved as well. Pruritus is most often moderate to severe, leading to excoriation, while persistent rubbing and scratching of the lesions may lead to hyperpigmentation and lichenification. As the eruption resolves, the erythematous component disappears first, leaving dry, scaling patches that ultimately clear.

Differential Diagnosis

Discoid atopic dermatitis, allergic contact dermatitis, irritant dermatitis of the hands, psoriasis, tinea corporis, and autoeczematization—an acute, sometimes discoid eruption that is secondary to a preexisting localized severe dermatitis, most commonly stasis dermatitis—are the most frequent differential diagnoses.

Treatment

See Table 2–7.

Marked improvement or total clearing of the eruption may be expected in 3 to 4 weeks. However, recurrences are common, especially if the patient does not continue to adhere to an emollient regimen.

TABLE 2-7. Treatment of Nummular Dermatitis

GENERAL MEASURES

Short (5-7 minutes), lukewarm bath or shower every 1-2 days
Mild cleansing agent
Emollient over entire body
Avoidance of irritants
Avoidance of low humidity if possible

SPECIFIC THERAPY

Milder cases: midpotency steroid ointment twice daily
Severe or unresponsive cases: high-potency steroid ointment
  twice daily; occlusive dressings may be necessary
Extensive involvement, unresponsive to topicals: systemic
  corticosteroid
Oral prednisone, 40 mg per day, tapered over 3 weeks
Triamcinolone
H_1 antihistamine (hydroxyzine, diphenhydramine), 25-50 mg
  bid to qid
Secondary infection: Dicloxacillin, erythromycin, cephalexin

SEBORRHEIC DERMATITIS

(CM&S Chapter 16)

Definition and Clinical Description

Seborrheic dermatitis is a common, subacute or chronic inflammatory disorder of unknown cause typically confined to the sebaceous gland-rich skin of the head and trunk and occasionally involving intertriginous areas. It is seen in early infancy and in adulthood but rarely in children older than 6 months of age. Seborrheic dermatitis is found in 3% to 5% of adults and is more common in men than women. It is more common in persons with human immunodeficiency virus (HIV) infection and those with Parkinson's disease, in whom the severity of disease is often greater.

Infantile seborrheic dermatitis, which appears to be asymptomatic, typically involves the scalp, the flexural creases, and the diaper area. Erythematous plaques with sharply defined borders and a glazed, or shiny, surface are characteristic. Small erythematous papules with fine scale may be scattered around and between larger plaques. While scales may be absent in flexural areas, seborrheic plaques on the scalp often develop thick, yellowish white plates of scale colloquially termed *cradle cap*.

Adults with seborrheic dermatitis usually have diffuse erythema and scaling of the hair-bearing portions of the scalp. Typical lesions are well-defined pink plaques with powdery scale that form in the eyebrows, nasolabial creases, and the postauricular sulci. Seborrheic blepharoconjunctivitis is seen in persons with severe facial involvement. Patients with a moustache or a beard commonly have involvement of those sites as well. Occasionally the presternal, interscapular, or genital skin will also exhibit seborrheic changes.

Pruritus of the scalp is nearly universal in adult seborrheic dermatitis, while patients with facial seborrheic dermatitis may complain of an "irritated" or "burning" discomfort, rather than true pruritus.

Secondary infection of seborrheic dermatitis with *Staphylococcus aureus* or *Streptococcus* is common and manifests as crusting, pustule formation, or frank cellulitis.

Pathology

The histopathology of both the adult and the infantile forms of seborrheic dermatitis is that of a spongiotic dermatitis, with perifollicular accentuation. Despite the suspicion that *Pityrosporum* plays an etiologic role, sections through follicular infundibula do not show a discernible increase in their numbers.

Diagnosis and Differential Diagnosis

Infantile seborrheic dermatitis is readily recognized by its nearly universal tendency toward prominent scalp involvement, as well as facial and diaper dermatitis. The most common skin disorders of infancy to be considered in the differential diagnosis of seborrheic dermatitis are atopic dermatitis and psoriasis, while the Letterer-Siwe type of Langerhans' cell histiocytosis must also be considered.

In adults, the diagnosis and differential diagnosis of seborrheic dermatitis are most easily approached from a regional point of view. The differential diagnosis of scalp disease includes psoriasis, atopic dermatitis, pediculosis, and dandruff. The differential diagnosis of facial disease includes perioral dermatitis and rosacea. Truncal and intertriginous seborrheic dermatitis may resemble tinea corporis or tinea cruris, candidiasis, psoriasis, Reiter's syndrome, atopic dermatitis, or various forms of contact dermatitis. Darier's disease has the identical distribution of seborrheic dermatitis, but is morphologically different.

Treatment

In general, therapy is directed toward loosening and removal of scales with keratolytics and shampoos, inhibition of yeast colonization with antifungal medication, control of secondary infection, and reduction of erythema and itching by judicious use of topical steroids (Table 2–8). Patients should be educated about the chronic nature of seborrheic dermatitis and must understand that all presently available treatments work by controlling this chronic condition rather than by curing it.

PITYRIASIS ROSEA

(CM&S Chapter 17)

Definition

Pityriasis rosea is a common acute inflammatory dermatosis of unknown etiology. It is characterized by a self-limited course that

TABLE 2-8. Treatment of Seborrheic Dermatitis

INFANTS

1. Daily shampoo of scalp and face with baby shampoo. Keratolytic shampoos (containing salicylic acid) used for thick scales on the scalp. Avoid general use because of the potential salicylic acid toxicity.
2. Mild topical corticosteroids (e.g., 1% hydrocortisone cream) for short courses when dermatitis unresponsive to shampooing alone.

ADULTS

1. Daily shampoo of scalp, face, and other involved sites with shampoo containing
   a. Zinc pyrithione
   b. Selenium sulfide, 1% to 2.5%
   c. Sulfur-salicylic acid (for heavy scale)
   d. Ketoconazole 2%
   e. Coal tar, juniper tar
   Shampoo must be left in contact with skin for at least 5 minutes to be effective.
2. Thick scalp scales may be loosened with overnight application of salicylic acid 6% gel or solution under occlusion.
3. Systemic antibiotics may be required to control secondary bacterial infection.
4. Ketoconazole 2% cream is effective maintenance therapy of sites prone to steroid-induced side effects (e.g., face and groin).
5. Topical corticosteroids:
   a. For scalp: solutions of hydrocortisone 1%, mometasone furoate 0.1%, fluocinolone acetonide 0.01% daily after shampooing.
   b. For face, groin, and axilla: hydrocortisone 0.5% to 1% cream or ointment once or twice daily initially; tapered once controlled. Steroids should not be used regularly on the face.
   c. For trunk: higher-potency topical steroids are relatively safe.

often starts with a primary isolated scaly plaque followed by a secondary, generalized, symmetrical, papulosquamous eruption typically distributed on the trunk and proximal extremities.

Clinical Description

Three fourths of patients are between 10 and 35 years of age. The disease is more prevalent in the cooler months of the year in temperate zones.

Typical cases of pityriasis rosea can be easily recognized morphologically; the primary lesion, seen in up to 95% of patients, referred to as the "herald patch," is an asymptomatic solitary papule that enlarges rapidly in 1 to 2 days to form an annular or oval lesion that can measure between 2 and 10 cm in diameter with an erythematous, salmon-colored border with fine scaling. The trunk, primarily the anterior chest, is the most common location.

The secondary eruption is more generalized and symmetrical. The lesions are smaller but retain morphologic features similar to those of the primary lesion. The eruption can have lesions at different stages of development from early erythematous, nonscaly papules to annular or oval, salmon-colored, erythematous lesions with fine, peripheral, cigarette–paper thin scales. Pityriasis rosea usually follows the lines of cleavage of the skin in a distribution that resembles a "Christmas tree" pattern on the trunk. The eruption is most often limited to the trunk, neck, and proximal areas of the arms and legs. The interval of time between the herald patch and the more generalized eruption is between 2 and 21 days. The latter eruption will peak in 10 days and will involute in 2 to 10 weeks, leaving no permanent sequelae. Pruritus is often absent, but when present it may be severe.

Atypical cases of pityriasis rosea account for approximately 20% of cases. At variance with the typical features are the distribution and the morphology of the primary and secondary lesions as well as the chronology of events between the two. The primary lesion may be absent or overlooked, may be multiple, may appear on unusual locations, may have an atypical morphologic appearance, and may not be succeeded by the secondary eruption. The secondary eruption may be asymmetrical or have an atypical distribution with involvement of the face, palms, and soles near sun-exposed skin, or even mucosal surfaces. The individual lesions can look eczematous, psoriasiform, and, in blacks and Latinos, lichenoid.

Recurrence of pityriasis rosea is infrequent, occurring in less than 3% of cases.

Pathology

Pityriasis rosea is a spongiotic dermatitis whose distinctive findings include extravasated erythrocytes in the papillary dermis, scattered dyskeratotic cells, and stubby mounds of parakeratosis.

Diagnosis and Differential Diagnosis

Classic pityriasis rosea in patients with white skin is easy to diagnose. Atypical presentations can be challenging. The herald patch can be confused with tinea corporis, figurate erythemas such as erythema annulare centrifugum, as well as nummular eczema or psoriasis. The secondary eruption can mimic secondary syphilis, nummular eczema, guttate psoriasis, tinea versicolor, pityriasis lichenoides chronica, lichen planus, or lichenoid eruptions as well as drug eruptions.

Pityriasis rosea–like drug eruptions occur, particularly to captopril, but also from barbiturates, clonidine, gold, isotretinoin, metronidazole, and penicillamine.

Treatment

Treatment is usually not indicated in typical cases of pityriasis rosea. In those instances in which pruritus or inflammation is severe or long lasting, antipruritics or anti-inflammatory agents such as oral antihistaminics or topical steroids are recommended. Phototherapy with either ultraviolet B light or psoralens and ultraviolet A light has also been shown to be effective in controlling the symptoms as well as in inducing a faster remission.

SMALL PLAQUE PARAPSORIASIS

(CM&S Chapter 18)

Definition

The term *small plaque parapsoriasis* refers to a benign, chronic, persistent, asymptomatic cutaneous disease of unknown etiology.

Clinical Description

Small plaque parapsoriasis is characterized by well-defined, uniform, round to ovoid, asymptomatic brown or yellowish macules and patches with fine adherent scales. The lesions usually measure less than 5 cm, with a few larger lesions sometimes seen. They are devoid of either substance or atrophy. Sites of predilection are the trunk, proximal extremities, and buttocks, with sparing of the face, anterior surfaces, palms, and soles. One variant of small plaque parapsoriasis, digitate dermatosis, consists of ellipsoid, tan macules and patches that favor the trunk, where lesions assume the shape of fingers pressed against the skin.

Men are affected three times more than women, the peak incidence being between the fourth and fifth decades. Some cases involute without treatment, and others persist for years to decades with no progression to malignancy.

Pathology

Histopathologic examination of a typical lesion of small plaque parapsoriasis shows elongated mounds of parakeratosis, slightly hyperplastic epidermis with varying degrees of focal or diffuse spongiosis, with occasional small lymphocytes scattered within the epidermis. There is a sparse to dense inflammatory infiltrate of lymphocytes around the vessels of the superficial vascular plexus.

Pathogenesis and Etiology

There are two major subgroups within the parapsoriasis group, namely, small plaque parapsoriasis and large plaque parapsoriasis. Large plaque parapsoriasis and its variants have come to be recognized as the patch stage of mycosis fungoides. Although the cause of small plaque parapsoriasis is obscure, the clinical appearance, histopathologic features, and course distinguish it as a separate, benign inflammatory disease that is apparently unrelated to mycosis fungoides.

Diagnosis and Differential Diagnosis

The differential diagnosis includes pityriasis lichenoids, pityriasis rosea, nummular dermatitis, and, most importantly, large plaque parapsoriasis. Large plaque parapsoriasis presents as broad, irregularly shaped, slightly scaly, elevated patches or plaques that are usually greater than 5 cm and often measure more than 10 cm in diameter on the buttocks, thighs, flexural surfaces, and, in women, over the breasts.

Treatment

Small plaque parapsoriasis tends to be resistant to treatment. Topical corticosteroids, ultraviolet B phototherapy, and oral psoralens and ultraviolet A light (PUVA) are occasionally effective.

GRAFT-VERSUS-HOST DISEASE

(CM&S Chapter 19)

Graft-versus-host (GVH) disease refers to the spectrum of organ dysfunction that occurs when immunocompetent leukocytes attack specific tissues in a relatively immunocompromised host. A GVH reaction refers to the expression of GVH disease in a specific organ, for example, the acute cutaneous GVH reaction. The most common clinical setting for GVH disease is after bone marrow transplantation, but GVH disease may develop after liver transplantation, after blood transfusions, and in fetuses after maternal-fetal passage of lymphocytes. GVH disease occurs in distinct acute and chronic phases. Epithelial damage in the skin, gastrointestinal tract, and liver mediated by lymphocytes and cytokines causes the constellation of findings recognized as GVH disease.

Acute Cutaneous GVH Reaction After Allogeneic Bone Marrow Transplantation

Clinical Description

An acute cutaneous GVH reaction develops in 50% to 80% of allogeneic bone marrow transplants. The earliest clinical manifestations of the acute cutaneous GVH reaction may develop with the appearance of donor leukocytes in the peripheral circulation by 10 to 14 days after bone marrow infusion as late as several months later. Erythematous macules typically appear on acral sites, usually the palms, soles, and ears. As the eruption evolves, the trunk and extremities may become involved, occasionally leading to erythroderma. Established sites of the acute cutaneous GVH reaction often become edematous, causing patients to complain of tenderness, especially of the palms and soles. Patients may complain of pruritus with or before the development of the eruption. The most serious clinical manifestation of GVH disease in the skin is the progression from erythematous macules to edematous plaques and then to subepidermal bulla formation, which bears a striking resemblance to toxic epidermal necrolysis.

As the eruption subsides, desquamation is apparent similar to that observed after a sunburn. The erythema slowly becomes fainter and edema resolves concomitantly.

Pathology

The combination of vacuolar alteration of the basilar epidermis and the presence of dyskeratotic epithelial cells in the epidermis or hair follicle serves to establish the diagnosis of GVH disease.

Differential Diagnosis

The differential diagnosis of the acute cutaneous GVH reaction includes viral exanthem and drug hypersensitivity reactions.

Treatment

The emphasis in the treatment of GVH disease is on prophylaxis. To avoid fully evolved expression of GVH disease, current practice is to place patients on cyclosporine, methotrexate, or both on the day of marrow infusion or to partially remove donor T lymphocytes from the marrow graft by counterflow centrifugal elutriation or treatment with lymphocyte-specific monoclonal antibodies. Subsequent development of signs of GVH disease prompts the administration of systemic corticosteroids. The skin is not directly treated in GVH disease, beyond application of emollients. If however, a bullous GVH reaction develops, treatment is similar to that of toxic epidermal necrolysis.

Chronic Cutaneous GVH Reaction After Allogeneic Bone Marrow Transplantation

Clinical Description

Clinical signs of chronic GVH disease appear months to years after bone marrow transplantation and primarily involve the skin and liver. The evolution of chronic GVH disease may be, but is not always, preceded by acute GVH disease. The chronic cutaneous GVH reaction is divided according to the type of skin lesions into lichenoid and sclerodermoid variants.

The more common lichenoid GVH reaction bears striking resemblance to idiopathic lichen planus with the primary lesion a violaceous or erythematous papule without scale, which progresses from an initial oral distribution to become more widespread. Oral lesions are also similar to lichen planus. Resolution of the inflammatory phase of the disease often leaves hyperpigmentation and hypopigmentation.

Sclerodermoid GVH reaction bears a striking resemblance to the cutaneous findings in progressive systemic sclerosis. This GVH reaction usually evolves from the lichenoid GVH reation and occurs later after bone marrow transplantation. Limited patches of progressively thickening skin may appear in any location. Commonly, there is extension of involved areas, sometimes resulting in generalized sclerosis of the skin with associated widespread alopecia.

Pathology

Tissue from the lichenoid GVH reaction, resembles lichen planus. In skin biopsy specimens from a sclerodermoid GVH reaction, the progression of sclerosis is from upper dermis toward the subcutis, in contrast to the pathologic change occurring in morphea and progressive systemic sclerosis.

Prognosis

Survival of patients with chronic GVH disease is approximately equal to that for patients without chronic GVH disease regardless of treatment. Death from chronic immunodeficiency and infection in patients with chronic GVH disease is offset by a lower incidence of relapse of the malignant neoplasm. Spontaneous resolution of sclerodermoid chronic cutaneous GVH disease may occur.

Treatment

Immunosuppressive therapy including systemic corticosteroids, cyclosporine, and azathioprine is the mainstay of treatment of the chronic cutaneous GVH reaction. Newer treatments include psoralens plus ultraviolet A light and thalidomide.

Acute Cutaneous GVH Reaction After Autologous and Syngeneic Bone Marrow Transplantation

Autologous bone marrow transplants are performed by harvesting and storing a patient's marrow followed by intensive, high-dose antineoplastic therapy and subsequent marrow rescue. Disease following autologous bone marrow transplantation is usually mild and confined to the skin.

Clinical Description and Treatment

A cutaneous eruption is the primary clinical manifestation of autologous GVH disease. Hepatic and gastrointestinal disease is exceedingly rare. The rash is characterized by erythematous, variably edematous macules and papules, initially acrally located. The eruption is clinically similar to a mild allogeneic GVH reaction. Chronic cutaneous manifestations are rare. Morbidity due to autologous GVH disease is mild, and the prognosis is excellent. Treatment of autologous GVH reaction is generally not required.

LICHENOID DERMATITIDES (LICHEN PLANUS, LICHEN NITIDUS, AND ERYTHEMA DYSCHROMICUM PERSTANS)

(CM&S Chapter 20)

Lichen Planus

Definition

Lichen planus is an inflammatory disease that has characteristic clinical and pathologic features and affects the skin, mucous membranes, nails, and hair. Several clinical types have been described, including typical, hypertrophic, vesiculobullous, and actinic. The etiology of lichen planus is unknown, and in many cases therapy is unsatisfactory.

Clinical Description

Typical cutaneous lesions of lichen planus are small, flat-topped, polygonal, violaceous papules that have a predilection for the wrists, ankles, and genitalia. Lesions typically have a scant, often translucent scale. White lacy lines called Wickham's striae are often visible within lesions. Lesions may occur at sites of injured or traumatized skin (Koebner phenomenon). Papular lesions may coalesce to form plaques. Residual hyperpigmentation is often observed after clearance of the lesions.

Oral involvement of lichen planus is common and variable. Reticular, white patches or plaques on the buccal mucosa are most common. Atrophic, violaceous patches and ulcerations also occur. Mucosal ulcerative lichen planus is generally painful and is notoriously difficult to treat.

Typical nail involvement is manifested by longitudinal ridging, thinning, and distal splitting. In its most severe form, lichen planus of the nails leads to destruction of the nail matrix, scarring of the proximal nail fold, and loss of the nail plate.

A form of lichen planus that involves hair follicle epithelium is known as lichen planopilaris. Early involvement in lichen planopilaris is characterized by dusky erythema surrounding involved hair follicles. Older areas of involvement contain acuminate papules and keratotic debris in follicular orifices. Chronic, untreated lichen planopilaris leads to irreversible destruction of hair follicles and permanent scarring alopecia that may resemble pseudopelade of Brocq.

Hypertrophic and vesiculobullous variants are less common. Typical hypertrophic lesions are large, hyperkeratotic, thick, violaceous, pruritic plaques with surrounding hyperpigmentation occurring most commonly on the anterior lower legs.

The vesiculobullous variants include bullous lichen planus and lichen planus pemphigoides. Bullous lichen planus is characterized by blisters that arise within lesions of lichen planus as a consequence of the intense lymphocytic infiltrate in lesions and extensive basal cell hydropic degeneration. In contrast, lichen planus pemphigoides is characterized by generalized blisters involving both lesional and nonlesional skin. It may represent an independent autoimmune disease precipitated by lichen planus or could also be the coexistence of lichen planus and bullous pemphigoid.

Actinic lichen planus is observed primarily in Middle Eastern countries, affects mostly young persons, and is confined to sun-exposed areas. The lesions are dark, blue-brown macules, papules, and plaques, which are often annular and can sometimes resemble melasma.

Natural History

The prognosis of cutaneous lichen planus is generally favorable. The duration of the rash was less than a year in 68% of cases in a long-term follow-up study of patients with cutaneous disease. Spontaneous clearance occurs most frequently between 12 and 15 months. Up to 50% of affected individuals have recurrences, but multiple recurrences are rare. The oral and hypertrophic forms of lichen planus are more chronic.

Risk of Malignancy

Malignant transformation of lesions of lichen planus is controversial. In a large study of patients with lichen planus there was no increased risk of malignant transformation of the skin lesions or development of internal malignancies. There was, however, an increased risk of developing squamous cell carcinoma of the oral cavity. The risk of oral squamous cell carcinoma developing in a patient with oral lichen planus is probably only twice that of the general population. Close monitoring of patients with chronic oral lichen planus to detect the development of malignancy is generally advised, as is avoidance of smoking and alcohol abuse.

Pathology

Lichen planus is the prototype of lichenoid interface dermatitis. Typically there is a dense band-like lymphocytic infiltrate in the papillary dermis, associated with vacuolar change and necrotic keratinocytes to the basal layer of the epidermis. Necrotic keratinocytes are incorporated into the papillary dermis, where their anucleate remnants are termed *colloid bodies* or *Civatte bodies.*

Pathogenesis and Etiology

Some cases of lichen planus or lichen planus–like (lichenoid) eruptions have been linked to exposure to contact allergens or to ingestion of certain drugs. Parasubstituted phenylenediamines present in color film developer are the contact sensitizers most closely linked to the development of lichenoid eruptions. The drugs most closely linked to lichenoid drug eruptions are the antimalarials, gold, and penicillamine.

There appears to be an association between lichen planus and chronic liver disease. Lichen planus has developed in association with positive serology for viral hepatitis, including hepatitis C.

Diagnosis and Differential Diagnosis

Typical lichen planus has characteristic clinical features that make it relatively easy to recognize and distinguish from other skin diseases. However, some cases, particularly those with atypical cutaneous lesions, may be difficult to differentiate from lichenoid drug eruptions, lupus erythematosus, psoriasis, and secondary syphilis. The differential diagnosis of oral lichen planus includes leukoplakia, candidiasis, erythema multiforme, secondary syphilis, and the blistering disorders.

Treatment

Therapies designed to suppress immune responses are commonly effective in treating lichen planus (Table 2–9).

TABLE 2-9. Treatment of Lichen Planus	
TYPE OF TREATMENT	**COMMENT**
Topical corticosteroids	Superpotent and potent (class I and II) topical corticosteroid ointments applied to hydrated skin are effective in most patients. Topical corticosteroids in dental paste are available to treat oral lesions.
Intralesional corticosteroids	Intralesional triamcinolone acetonide is used for recalcitrant or hypertrophic lesions and to treat nail involvement.
Cyclosporine mouthwash	In most studies, mucosal lesions of lichen planus respond to cyclosporine solution (100 mg/mL) used as a mouthwash.
Systemic corticosteroids	Esophageal erosive lichen planus, widespread and recalcitrant lichen planus, lichen planopilaris, and nail involvement may be treated with oral prednisone (1 mg/kg/day × 6 weeks, then tapered over 4 to 6 weeks).
PUVA	8-Methoxypsoraien and ultraviolet A photochemotherapy has led to clearing in patients with widespread cutaneous lichen planus.
Retinoids	Systemic isotretinoin (0.25 to 0.5 mg/kg), etretinate (0.3 to 0.6 mg/kg), and acitretin (0.25 to 0.75 mg/kg) have been used to treat widespread or recalcitrant lichen planus. The retinoids are teratogenic, and risks and benefits should be carefully considered in women of childbearing potential.
Systemic cyclosporine	Systemic cyclosporine (3 to 6 mg/kg) has been used successfully to control oral and widespread cutaneous lichen planus. Because of drug toxicity, the use of cyclosporine should be limited to the patients with the most severe and recalcitrant disease.

Lichen Nitidus

Definition

Lichen nitidus is an uncommon cutaneous disease of unknown etiology that affects children and young adults. It has no racial or sex predilection; however, there may be a predilection of the disease for blacks and males. The skin disease is chronic and may last many years, sometimes for a lifetime.

Clinical Description

Lesions characteristically consist of 1- to 2-mm, flat-topped, flesh-colored papules that typically involve the forearms, genitalia, and trunk. The lesions are usually asymptomatic, but mild burning on sun exposure has been reported.

Treatment

Although treatments that have been used include topical steroids, antihistamines, systemic steroids, and PUVA, their efficacy has not been established.

Erythema Dyschromicum Perstans

Definition and Clinical Description

Erythema dyschromicum perstans is a rare, difficult to treat, asymptomatic, slowly progressive dermatosis characterized by annular blue-gray macules. The initial lesions may be erythematous patches or plaques, sometimes with an elevated border, which later in the disease become ashy gray. The macules are usually well demarcated and may coalesce to form extensive patches. The dermatosis is localized on the trunk, arms, and face with sparing of palms, soles, scalp, nails, and mucous membranes. Most cases of the disease have been observed in Latin America and India. Erythema dyschromicum perstans may represent the end stage of lichen planus in darkly pigmented individuals.

Pathology

The histopathologic findings, which are similar to those of lichen planus, include vacuolar degeneration of basal layer keratinocytes and a perivascular mononuclear cell infiltrate. Civatte bodies and melanophages are often observed.

Treatment

There is no effective treatment.

LICHEN STRIATUS

(CM&S Chapter 21)

Definition and Clinical Description

Lichen striatus is a fairly common, self-limited, linear dermatosis of unknown origin that is seen primarily in children. In its classic form, lichen striatus begins suddenly with the eruption of 1- to 3-mm flat-topped skin-colored to pink papules on a proximal extremity. Over a few weeks the papules coalesce into small plaques in a continuous or interrupted linear band that progresses toward the distal extremity. Usually one, but occasionally two or more linear lesions may develop. This band ranges in length from a few centimeters to the full length of an extremity and is usually 1 to 3 cm wide. After months to 1 year, the lesions spontaneously resolve, often in the same proximal to distal manner in which they appeared. Hypopigmentation is a common temporary sequela especially in darkly pigmented persons.

Diagnosis and Differential Diagnosis

Early linear epidermal nevus or inflammatory linear verrucous epidermal nevus (ILVEN) is often the main source of confusion. The clinical course is usually more helpful than the morphologic features in distinguishing lichen striatus from epidermal nevi. Epidermal nevi will persist forever. Other disorders that may take on a linear configuration are lichen planus, psoriasis, porokeratosis, and verruca plana.

Treatment

Because the process resolves spontaneously, treatment is usually not necessary.

ERYTHEMA MULTIFORME

(CM&S Chapter 22)

Definition

Erythema multiforme is an acute, self-limited, inflammatory cutaneous or mucocutaneous disorder with distinctive skin lesions and characteristic histopathology. Until recently this broad definition was used to denote a heterogeneous spectrum of disease manifestations associated with a multitude of causes, encompassing the classic form, the severe febrile mucocutaneous form of Stevens and Johnson, and a severe form with widespread blistering that overlaps with toxic epidermal necrolysis.

The clinical classification of the erythema multiforme spectrum is undergoing evolution and clarification as distinct clinical and etiologic subsets are identified and delineated and diagnostic criteria are established. Erythema multiforme minor is primarily an acral eruption with characteristic target lesions variably accompanied by oral mucosal involvement, without systemic symptoms; and erythema multiforme major (Stevens-Johnson syndrome) is a severe form with involvement of at least two mucosal surfaces, associated with systemic toxicity. Toxic epidermal necrolysis is now viewed by many as a distinct disease entity precipitated by drugs and characterized by the abrupt, rapid development of large areas of confluent erythema and blistering with sheet-like, full-thickness epidermal necrosis, without target lesions.

Clinical Description

Erythema Multiforme Minor

Erythema multiforme minor, comprising the majority of cases of erythema multiforme, is a relatively mild, self-limited cutaneous illness that is frequently recurrent. The typical clinical picture is of a symmetrically distributed erythematous eruption with a predilection for the extensor aspects of the extremities and the presence of target lesions, a clinical hallmark. Mucosal involvement, when present, is usually limited to the oral cavity. Prodromal symptoms, particularly mild malaise, are rarely seen.

Morphology

The primary skin lesion is a round, erythematous papule that, over hours to days, may enlarge and develop a central vesicle or bulla. At least some of the lesions evolve with concentric zones of color change to form characteristic target or iris lesions. A classic target lesion has a well-defined border and at least three different zones of color: typically, a central dusky erythematous area is surrounded by a pale edematous ring with a peripheral erythematous margin. Individual skin lesions are usually symptomless but may be associated with burning or itching.

Distribution

The eruption appears in successive crops with a centripetal mode of spread, initially appearing on the extensor surfaces of the extremities and later involving, to a lesser degree, the trunk and face. In cases of recurrent erythema multiforme minor, the most prevalent site of involvement was the dorsum of the hand.

Course and Epidemiology

Erythema multiforme minor is self-limited and resolves within 2 to 4 weeks, typically leaving residual postinflammatory hyperpigmentation as the sole sequela.

Erythema Multiforme Major

The term *erythema multiforme major* is used by some synonymously with Stevens-Johnson syndrome and by others to indicate a disease spectrum that encompasses bullous erythema multiforme, Stevens-Johnson syndrome, and overlap between Stevens-Johnson syndrome and toxic epidermal necrolysis. The disease is a severe, self-limited, extremely variable mucocutaneous illness characterized by an extensive eruption with areas of epidermal detachment and systemic symptoms. Significant involvement of multiple mucosal surfaces occurs typically. A prodrome with constitutional symptoms, such as fever, cough, sore throat, myalgias, and malaise usually heralds the onset of the eruption and may be indistinguishable from symptoms of an illness that leads to the episode of erythema multiforme major.

Morphology and Distribution

The cutaneous morphology and distribution of erythema multiforme major are variable. Skin lesions begin as erythematous macules or papules and frequently evolve with central vesiculation and bulla formation. Some may undergo concentric color change, forming typical but more commonly raised or flat atypical target lesions. In some cases, bulla formation may result in limited areas of epidermal necrosis and detachment, involving less than 10% of the cutaneous surface. The eruption is typically more generalized than that of erythema multiforme minor and may be quite prominent on the trunk.

Mucosal involvement is frequently severe and associated with significant morbidity. Painful, extensive oral mucosal bullae, erosions, and stomatitis result in a foul-smelling mouth and decreased oral intake, which may cause dehydration. Involvement of the lips produces characteristic erosion and hemorrhagic crusting.

Ocular involvement produces erythematous, edematous, and crusted eyelids and hyperemic, painful conjunctivae with associated photophobia. Late complications include scarring of the lids and conjunctivae and lacrimal abnormalities with tear film deficiencies. Permanent visual loss and ultimately blindness may ensue.

Balanitis and vulvovaginitis with ulceration may cause difficulty with micturition and may result in scarring and stenosis. Bronchitis and pneumonia may occur in up to 30% of cases.

Course and Epidemiology

The duration of erythema multiforme major, reflecting more severe mucocutaneous damage, is typically 4 to 6 weeks. Erythema multiforme major primarily occurs in children and young adults.

Pathology

Erythema multiforme is the prototype of a vacuolar or acute cytotoxic interface dermatitis in which there is a superficial perivascular infiltrates of lymphocytes, intracellular edema of keratinocytes and vacuoles at the dermoepidermal junction that can coalesce to form clefts, leading to subepidermal vesiculation.

The histopathologic picture in erythema multiforme minor and major and in toxic epidermal necrolysis can be identical, a fact cited in support of the unitary nature of these conditions.

Pathogenesis and Etiology

Erythema multiforme has been considered to be a hypersensitivity reaction in a host manifesting an immune response to one of a variety of etiologic factors capable of generating foreign antigens, primarily infectious agents or drugs. Of etiologic associations suggested, the three best documented and described are recurrent HSV infection, *Mycoplasma pneumoniae* infection, and drugs.

Recurrent erythema multiforme minor occurs after recurrent HSV infection (type 1 or 2). The eruption of erythema multiforme minor typically occurs 7 to 14 days after the appearance of a recurrent herpes lesion (oral, genital, or other location), with an initial frequency of up to 10 attacks per year. Nevertheless, in a given patient, not all recurrences of HSV infection are followed by an episode of erythema multiforme and not all episodes of erythema multiforme are preceded by a clinically apparent recurrence of infection with HSV, suggesting a potential role for subclinical herpes infections. HSV antigens and DNA have been localized to skin lesions of erythema multiforme.

Erythema multiforme major may also be triggered by *M. pneumoniae*. *Mycoplasma*-associated Stevens-Johnson syndrome usually follows symptoms of an upper respiratory tract infection, occurs in children and young adults, and is rarely recurrent.

Erythema multiforme major is most commonly associated with exposure to certain drugs. The major offenders include sulfonamides — systemic (including trimethoprim-sulfamethoxazole) and topical; anti-convulsants (phenytoin and barbiturates); penicillins; allopurinol; and nonsteroidal anti-inflammatory agents. Many other drugs have also been implicated. Determining the causative agent is often difficult because of the frequency of multiple drug therapy and the coexistence of either an infectious disease or prodromal symptoms of erythema multiforme major.

Diagnosis and Differential Diagnosis

Diagnostic criteria have been proposed for erythema multiforme minor and major. For erythema multiforme minor, these include acute, self-limited or episodic disease of less than 4 weeks' duration; symmetrically distributed, fixed, discrete, round erythematous skin lesions, some of which evolve with concentric color changes to form classic target lesions; mucosal involvement absent or limited to one mucosal surface (usually the mouth); and compatible histopathology on skin biopsy. In cases of recurrent erythema multiforme minor, a careful evaluation for evidence of associated HSV infection is essential. The differential diagnosis includes urticaria, insect bites, drug eruptions, viral exanthema, Kawasaki disease, bullous pemphigoid, and erythema annulare centrifugum.

Erythema multiforme major is characterized by an acute, self-limited course of less than 6 weeks' duration; presence of symmetrically distributed, fixed, discrete erythematous skin lesions; concentric color changes in some lesions causing target lesions or raised or flat atypical target lesions; evolution of some lesions to form bullae, with subsequent areas of epidermal detachment; common prodrome of fever, cough, sore throat, and malaise; severe mucosal involvement (usually of at least two mucosal surfaces); and compatible histopathology on skin biopsy. When sheet-like loss of the epidermis involves more than 10% of the body surface, a diagnosis of Stevens-Johnson syndrome – toxic epidermal necrolysis overlap or toxic epidermal necrolysis is appropriate. Differential diagnosis includes bullous pemphigoid, cicatricial pemphigoid, dermatitis herpetiformis, pemphigus vulgaris, lupus erythematosus, vasculitis, Behçet's disease, Sweet's syndrome, staphylococcal scalded skin syndrome, and acute graft-versus-host disease.

Treatment

General Therapeutic Approach

Optimal therapeutic strategies for erythema multiforme are controversial because specific pathogenic mechanisms of tissue injury have not yet been defined and no controlled studies have yet been performed to evaluate the effectiveness of various treatment modalities. A rational approach to therapy should encompass a diligent search for possible etiologic factors, careful consideration of clinical characteristics (including extent and severity of mucocutaneous lesions and patient discomfort), and assessment of potential complications.

Frequently, erythema multiforme minor requires only symptomatic care. However, because of the degree and extent of epidermal and mucosal involvement that can occur in erythema multiforme major, careful monitoring is critical, opthalmologic consultation and hospitalization are often required, and supportive care is usually necessary.

Specific Therapeutic Modalities

Identification and Elimination of Etiologic Factors

Measures taken to attempt to prevent recurrences of HSV including sun avoidance in ultraviolet light–induced cases and the use of prophylactic acyclovir should lessen or abort subsequent episodes of erythema multiforme minor. Immediate withdrawal and future avoidance of any incriminated, suspected, or unnecessary drug is imperative. *M. pneumoniae* infection, if diagnosed or strongly suspected, should be treated with a course of appropriate systemic antibiotic therapy.

Skin Care

For pruritic or painful skin lesions, use systemic antihistamines or analgesics. For oozing and crusted erosive skin lesions frequently apply open, wet-to-damp compresses of tepid water or a dilute solution of aluminum acetate, and with frequent bathing in lukewarm to cool water. Topical corticosteroid therapy has not been shown to be beneficial. Open lesions should be cultured and, if there are signs of infection, treatment initiated with the appropriate systemic antibiotic. If extensive epidermal detachment occurs, involving as much as 20% to 30% total body surface area, surgical intervention and transfer to a burn unit are advisable.

Mouth Care

Good oral hygiene consisting of mouthwashes, irrigations, and toothbrushing, as tolerated, is essential. Topical anesthetics such as dyclonine, viscous lidocaine, or a mixture of Kaopectate and elixir of diphenhydramine (1 : 1) may be used as a mouthwash. Systemic antibiotic therapy may be required for secondary infection. A liquid or soft diet is usually better tolerated, but with extensive involvement administration of fluids and electrolytes and parenteral nutrition may be required.

Reduction of Morbidity and Mortality

The use of systemic glucocorticosteroid therapy in herpes-associated erythema multiforme minor is not recommended. Since no controlled studies have been conducted to document efficacy, the use of systemic glucocorticosteroids in erythema multiforme major is still highly controversial. Reports have suggested that patients treated with systemic steroids have an increased incidence of complications and morbidity and prolonged hospitalization times. In an attempt to minimize the extent of tissue damage, early use of a short (less then 1 week) course of high-dose systemic steroid (prednisone, 1 to 2 mg/kg per day or an equivalent drug) in the severe, progressive phase of the disease process may at times be justified.

Current recommendations for therapeutic strategies in a burn unit include withdrawal of systemic steroid therapy because of increased risk of sepsis, complications, and adverse effects on wound healing; avoidance of indwelling lines whenever possible; monitoring for secondary infection and aggressive treatment if sepsis or localized infection occurs; supportive care with pain relief, correction of fluid loss, parenteral nutrition, and respiratory therapy; and early gentle debridement of appropriate skin lesions followed by application of silver nitrate dressings, biologic dressings, allografts, or porcine xenografts to facilitate rapid reepithelialization.

Prognosis

Resolution should occur within 4 to 6 weeks since both major and minor forms of erythema multiforme are self-limited disorders.

PITYRIASIS LICHENOIDES

(CM&S Chapter 23)

Definition and Clinical Description

Pityriasis lichenoides is an idiopathic dermatosis consisting of recurrent crops of spontaneously regressing papules that affects patients in all age groups but is more common in the first few decades. It consists of a spectrum of disease with a variable clinical presentation ranging from mostly acute lesions to mainly chronic lesions, with many patients showing intermediate features or a mixture of acute and chronic lesions either concurrently or sequentially.

The acute form is known as pityriasis lichenoides et varioliformis acuta. Patients with this variant exhibit recurrent crops of erythematous, variably purpuric papules that develop crusts, ulcers, vesicles, or pustules before spontaneously regressing over the course of a few weeks. The chronic form is known as pityriasis lichenoides chronica. Patients with this more indolent variant exhibit recurrent crops of erythematous, scaly papules that gradually arise and regress over the course of weeks or months. Many patients develop lesions with intermediate clinical features or a mixture of lesional types. Lesions are usually asymptomatic, but occasionally they may be pruritic or burning. The disease may resolve spontaneously after several weeks or months or may persist indefinitely. Acute lesions may result in smallpox-like (varioliform) scars and chronic lesions can resolve leaving hypopigmented macules that are sometimes the presenting complaint, especially in dark-skinned patients. Systemic findings are uncommon.

Pathology

The histopathologic features of pityriasis lichenoides include an interface dermatitis, often with necrotic keratinocytes, and a perivascular lymphocytic infiltrate. In acute lesions, extravasation of erythrocytes is a common feature. In chronic lesions the epidermis exhibits a parakeratotic scale, lymphocytic infiltration, and fewer extravasated erythrocytes, often accompanied by vacuolar degeneration along the dermoepidermal junction and scattered necrotic keratinocytes.

Diagnosis and Differential Diagnosis

The diagnosis of pityriasis lichenoides is based on the correlation of clinical features with lesional skin biopsy histopathology. The clinical differential diagnosis of pityriasis lichenoides includes dermatitis herpetiformis, folliculitis, drug eruptions, guttate psoriasis, bites, vasculitis, varicella, and secondary syphilis.

Treatment

A variety of treatments have been described (Table 2–10), including the systemic antibiotics erythromycin and tetracycline, ultraviolet phototherapy, methotrexate, and other immunosuppressive agents. None has proven ideal. Topical preparations and antihistamines are used mainly if lesions are symptomatic. Topical or systemic antibiotics may be needed in cases with ulcerated or secondarily infected lesions.

LUPUS ERYTHEMATOSUS

(CM&S Chapter 24)

Definition

Lupus erythematosus (LE) is an autoimmune disease of unknown etiology defined by characteristic clinical features in association with autoantibody production. LE exists across a spectrum from mild, localized, cutaneous disease at one extreme to severe, life-threatening systemic disease at the other. Different LE subsets are

TABLE 2-10.   Treatment of Pityriasis Lichenoides

ANTIBIOTICS

Erythromycin
Tetracycline

ANTIHISTAMINES

Wide variety

ANTIMETABOLIC AGENTS

Methotrexate

IMMUNOSUPPRESSIVE AGENTS

Cyclosporine
Prednisone

PHOTOTHERAPY

Helarium (ultraviolet A and B light)
Natural sunlight
Psoralens and ultraviolet A light
Ultraviolet B light

TOPICAL AGENTS

Antibiotics
Coal tar preparations
Corticosteroids

---

defined by shared clinical features together with distinct autoantibody profiles (Table 2-11).

Clinical Description

Discoid Lupus Erythematosus

Discoid lupus erythematosus (DLE) may occur either as a cutaneous eruption without systemic disease, sometimes referred to as chronic cutaneous LE (CCLE), or as part of systemic lupus erythematosus (SLE). Approximately one fourth of all patients with SLE have lesions of DLE. Approximately 5% of cutaneous DLE patients evolve to SLE. The more severe the skin lesions and the more widespread their distribution, the more likely they are to signify systemic disease.

Discoid lesions are distinctive because of their round, disc-like shape and their tendency to scar. They occur most commonly on the head, face, ears, and scalp. Generalized lesions typically involve the upper chest, back, and arms. The earliest lesion may be an erythematous papule. Subsequently, lesions expand to become annular with indurated erythematous borders and central clearing with hypopigmentation and atrophy. Follicular plugging appears as punctate hyperkeratoses. More mature lesions are characterized by marked pigmentary changes. On the scalp, a scarring alopecia is seen. DLE can affect the lips, tongue, and oral mucosa, where in-

TABLE 2-11. Lupus Erythematosus: Different Types
CHRONIC
Discoid lupus erythematosus (DLE)
Lupus panniculitis
ACUTE
Systemic lupus erythematosus
LUPUS SUBSETS
Subacute cutaneous lupus erythematosus (SCLE)
Neonatal lupus erythematosus (NLE)
Drug-induced lupus erythematosus (DIL)
Hereditary complement deficiencies
Overlap syndromes

volved areas appear as plaques. The natural history of DLE lesions is chronic and slowly progressive.

Variants of DLE include hypertrophic (verrucous) LE, acral (palmoplantar) LE, and tumid LE (edematous plaques without epidermal changes).

Lupus Panniculitis

Lupus panniculitis (lupus profundus) is a rare manifestation of LE and may occur either with SLE, DLE, or independently. These lesions affect the subcutaneous fat and cause tender nodules that give rise to disfiguring saucer-like atrophic lesions. The overlying skin may be normal, have partially or fully developed changes of DLE, or be hyperpigmented. Ulceration is common. The areas most commonly involved are the upper arms, trunk, and face.

Systemic Lupus Erythematosus

SLE is a multisystem autoimmune disease that typically affects women of childbearing age, although it may be seen at any age. All ethnic groups are affected, with a higher prevalence among non-Caucasian races. Eighty per cent to ninety per cent of all SLE patients will have cutaneous manifestations at some point.

Cutaneous Manifestations of SLE

Cutaneous manifestations of SLE can be divided into two categories (Table 2-12). Those that are specific to the disease can be used in establishing the diagnosis and are also histologically specific.

Specific Lesions. The *malar rash* (butterfly rash) occurs across the malar eminences, sparing the nasolabial folds, and may be the presenting sign in 40%. The morphology of the lesions varies, presenting as a very "rosy complexion," indurated confluent plaques of erythema with distinct borders, or in certain patients, the lesions are papular or vesicular. Discoid lesions can also occur in a malar distribution. The nose, forehead, chin, and upper chest may

TABLE 2-12. Cutaneous Lesions of Systemic Lupus Erythematosus (SLE)

SPECIFIC	NONSPECIFIC
Malar rash	Alopecia
Photosensitivity	Vascular
Oral lesions	Vasculopathy
Discoid lesions	Raynaud's
	Livedo reticularis
	Chilblain
	Vasculitis
	Palpable purpura
	Urticarial vasculitis
	Angioedema
	Rheumatoid nodules
	Calcinosis cutis

also be affected. The malar rash is often precipitated by sun exposure.

Photosensitivity (usually to ultraviolet A [UVA] or ultraviolet B light) occurs in approximately 50% of SLE patients. It can present as a "bad sunburn" that can last for weeks to months. The rash begins as a macular erythema and then usually becomes more maculopapular and indurated with irregular borders. Sometimes the rash extends to involve non–sun-exposed skin. Sun exposure also can precipitate a generalized flare of disease activity.

Oral lesions occur in about 20% to 25% of SLE patients and include petechia, gingivitis, cheilitis, and shallow, painful ulcers. Other mucosal surfaces may rarely be involved.

Nonspecific Lesions. See Table 2–12. Thirty percent of SLE patients get a reversible, generalized *alopecia* often associated with disease flares. "Lupus hairs" are broken hairs that occur along the frontal hair line. Raynaud's phenomenon, periungual erythema, palmar erythema, and nail fold capillary changes are seen in lupus and are indicative of underlying vascular disorders.

Livedo reticularis appears as a reticulated net of violaceous discoloration over the skin of the extremities. It can be exacerbated by cold exposure. In some cases, it is associated with fibrin deposition in vessel walls. In severe cases, it may cause ulcerations that heal with an atrophic scar known as atrophie blanche. When livedo reticularis occurs in association with thrombotic events, fetal loss, and/or thrombocytopenia, it may reflect an underlying antiphospholipid syndrome (see Chapter 63, CM&S).

Chilblain or perniosis is an uncommon type of cold-induced injury that results in tender, erythematous to violaceous plaques and nodules over the toes and fingers and is reported to occur in lupus patients.

Cutaneous vasculitis occurs in lupus patients and may affect either small or medium-sized vessels. The most common (20% of SLE patients) is small vessel leukocytoclastic vasculitis, also referred to as a hypersensitivity vasculitis, which affects the postcapillary venules and is most commonly clinically appreciated as *palpable purpura*, but sometimes results in necrosis and ulceration.

The hands and feet are common sites. Urticarial-like lesions that are <2 cm, last longer than 24 hours, and on biopsy show a leukocytoclastic vasculitis are called *urticarial vasculitis* and may be associated with hypocomplementemia. Medium-sized vessel vasculitis gives rise to tender nodules, ulcers, and gangrene of the extremities. Other organs, such as the kidney or brain, may be affected.

Rheumatoid nodules are painless subcutaneous nodules that typically occur on the hands or over the extensor surface of the elbows. Smaller, more superficially located papules have been referred to as "rheumatoid papules." These papules occur in SLE and rheumatoid arthritis, and histologic examination shows both vasculitis and palisaded granulomas.

Bullous SLE. Bullous lesions may be seen in three different settings. First, some primary bullous disorders have been described in association with SLE, including bullous pemphigoid, dermatitis herpetiformis, pemphigus vulgaris, epidermolysis bullosa acquisita, and porphyria cutanea tarda. The second instance in which blistering occurs is a severe lupus reaction. The blisters are typically small and are confined to sites of cutaneous LE involvement. There is also a nonscarring blistering reaction that is unique to SLE. Clinically, these blisters are of variable appearance. They are typically tense, appearing on the sun-exposed areas on either lesional or normal skin, and may be pruritic. Oral lesions occur in approximately one third of patients.

Systemic Manifestations of SLE

The most commonly affected systems affected by SLE include joints (90%), kidneys (50%), lungs (40%), and the central nervous system (30%). In addition, SLE patients frequently experience constitutional symptoms such as fatigue, fever, weight loss, and malaise.

Joint pain affects over 90% of patients. Most commonly involved are the small joints of the hands, feet, wrists, ankles, and knees. Although swelling with inflammation of the synovium (arthritis) may be appreciated, most patients complain of pain without evidence of swelling (arthralgia). The arthritis does not tend to be deforming or erosive.

Avascular necrosis of bone typically affects the femoral heads bilaterally, where it presents as hip or groin pain. It is much more common in patients who have been on steroids.

Renal disease, which affects 50% of patients with SLE, carries the worst prognosis. Early kidney disease may be asymptomatic; therefore, it is essential that all SLE patients be monitored with routine urinalyses, serum creatinine, and blood urea nitrogen. In addition, monitoring of blood pressure is critical because hypertension is a risk factor for renal disease. Elevated anti–double-stranded DNA antibodies along with decreased complement levels are predictive of renal disease and may be used to follow the course of lupus nephritis.

Serositis, or inflammation of a serosal surface, can present as pleural, pericardial, or peritoneal effusions, causing pain at the affected site. *Pleurisy*, acute pleuritic chest pain, occurs in about 50% of SLE patients. A transient friction rub (a small pleural effusion) may be appreciated. Chest pain relieved by sitting forward may indicate a pericardial effusion, and abdominal pain without apparent cause may indicate peritonitis.

Central nervous system (CNS) involvement occurs in as many as one third of all SLE patients. Symptoms as subtle as attention deficit, depression, and headache may reflect CNS lupus activity. Events as catastrophic as seizure, psychosis, and stroke may result from CNS lupus. There are no specific laboratory tests or imaging studies that consistently predict or document CNS disease.

Additional organs are affected in SLE, including the cardiovascular, pulmonary, gastrointestinal, ophthalmologic, peripheral nervous, and hematologic systems, as well as others.

Lupus Subsets

Subacute Cutaneous Lupus Erythematosus

Subacute cutaneous lupus erythematosus (SCLE) accounts for approximately 10% of lupus cases. These patients are somewhat older than the typical SLE patient (mean age, 43 years versus 31 years for SLE), present with a characteristic nonscarring skin rash, prominent photosensitivity, milder systemic disease, and a higher incidence of the anti-Ro/SSA autoantibody.

There are two characteristic cutaneous photodistributed eruptions in SCLE patients. One is an erythematous annular, polycyclic eruption with central clearing. The second consists of scaly pink to red papules. These nonscarring eruptions may spare the face.

Neonatal Lupus Erythematosus

In the syndrome of neonatal lupus erythematosus (NLE), infants born to mothers with SLE or anti-Ro/SSA with or without anti-La/SSB antibodies develop heart block or DLE or SCLE lesions, usually on the face and scalp. The rash is typically not present at birth, although it may be present. It usually appears a few weeks post partum and is transient, lasting for a few weeks to months. It is an annular erythema with mild scale and central clearing. It can be photosensitive and is generally nonscarring, although residual hypopigmention and atrophy have been described. These cutaneous features of NLE bear a striking resemblance to the rash of SCLE. The rash disappears at about 6 months of age, presumably at the time when the maternal IgG autoantibodies disappear from the infant's system.

Drug-Induced Lupus

Drug-induced lupus (DIL) can be precipitated by hydralazine (Apresoline), procainamide (Pronestyl), isoniazid, chlorpromazine, quinidine, methyldopa, D-penicillamine, and others. Some drugs have been reported to exacerbate existing SLE, including estrogens in SLE and thiazides in SCLE.

A typical DIL patient develops pleuritic chest pain, pleural effusions, fevers, and arthralgias; an ANA test is positive, and antihistone antibodies may be positive. The offending drug is stopped and the patient's symptoms gradually resolve. Cutaneous manifestions of DIL are uncommon.

Hereditary Complement Deficiencies

The most common cause of complement deficiency is the excessive consumption of complement by the formation of immune complexes. Complement levels usually correlate inversely with disease activity. In addition, lupus-like syndromes and other immune complex–mediated disorders such as glomerulonephritis, Henoch-Schönlein purpura, vasculitis, and Sjögren's syndrome have also been described in complement-deficient individuals. C2 deficiency is the most common homozygous complement deficiency.

Overlap Syndromes

Overlap syndromes occur when two or more connective tissue diseases are diagnosed in a single patient. Combinations of SLE, scleroderma, dermatomyositis-polymyositis, and rheumatoid arthritis may occur in a single patient. Mixed connective tissue disease (MCTD) is an overlap between SLE, scleroderma, polymyositis, and rheumatoid arthritis. The MCTD patient typically has arthralgias-arthritis, Raynaud's phenomenon, swollen hands, esophageal dysmotility, pulmonary disease, and myositis, but not renal disease. Cutaneous manifestations are not as prominent as they are in SLE. Cutaneous lesions that have been described in MCTD include malar erythema (SLE-like), periorbital heliotrope (dermatomyositis-like), squared-off telangiectasia (scleroderma-like, typically on the face and hands), as well as periungual erythema (nonspecific) and alopecia (nonspecific). The autoantibody profile of MCTD patients is unique in that they have positive ANAs with high-titer anti-U_1RNP antibodies in the absence of other serologies such as anti-Sm or anti-Ro/SSA.

Undifferentiated connective tissue disease (UCTD) designates a patient with one or two symptoms and/or one or two laboratory abnormalities that are suggestive but not diagnostic of a connective tissue disease. UCTD is considered a temporary designation. Sjögren's syndrome is an ''autoimmune exocrinopathy'' in which lymphocytes invade lacrimal and salivary glands resulting in dry eyes (xerophthalmia, keratoconjunctiva sicca) and dry mouth (xerostomia). It can occur in a primary form (without an associated connective tissue disease) or in a secondary form (with an associated connective tissue disease, most commonly rheumatoid arthritis but also SLE and SCLE). It is associated with positive rheumatoid factor and positive anti-Ro/SSA and/or anti-La/SSB autoantibodies in many cases.

Pathology

Histology

The histologic features of LE (DLE, SCLE, and SLE) include (1) hyperkeratosis and follicular plugging, (2) epidermal atrophy, (3) thickening of the basement membrane zone, (4) vacuolar degeneration of the dermoepidermal junction, (5) superficial and deep perivascular and periappendageal lymphocytic infiltrate, and (6) mucin deposition.

Lupus panniculitis is a lobular panniculitis. A prominent and distinct feature of lupus panniculitis is hyaline necrosis of the adipocytes.

Bullous SLE shows a subepidermal blister with a neutrophil infiltrate clustered in microabscesses in the papillary dermis, or lined up along the dermoepidermal junction.

Immunopathology

In general, immunoreactants (immunoglobulins and complement components) are seen in a linear pattern at the dermoepidermal junction in a variety of LE lesions. Direct immunofluorescence may be helpful in distinguishing SLE from other interface dermatitides; however, in general, it does not offer much over serologic testing and light microscopy in the diagnosis of LE. Positive immunoreactivity at the dermoepidermal junction of nonlesional, non–sun-exposed skin (the lupus band test) may, along with anti–double-stranded DNA antibodies, correlate with systemic disease.

Diagnosis and Differential Diagnosis

Discoid Lupus Erythematosus

The diagnosis of DLE is based on clinical appearance and can be confirmed by biopsy. The differential diagnoses for some of the individual cutaneous manifestations of LE include lichen planus, lupus vulgaris, polymorphous light eruption (PMLE), psoriasis, tinea, and sarcoid lesions. A similar approach is appropriate for lupus panniculitis and SCLE.

Systemic Lupus Erythematosus

The diagnosis of SLE depends on a combination of clinical and laboratory abnormalities. Criteria for the diagnosis of SLE are listed in Table 2–13. If 4 of the 11 listed criteria are present, the patient

TABLE 2-13. Criteria for the Diagnosis of SLE	
CLINICAL FEATURES	**LABORATORY FEATURES**
1. **Malar rash**	9. **Hematologic disorders**
2. **Discoid rash**	a. Hemolytic anemia *or*
3. **Photosensitivity**	b. Leukopenia
4. **Oral ulcers**	($<$4000/mm³ $\times$ 2) *or*
5. **Arthritis**	c. Lymphopenia
6. **Serositis**	($<$1500/mm³ $\times$ 2)
7. **Renal disorder**	d. Thrombocytopenia
a. Proteinuria ($>$0.5 g/day) *or*	($<$100,000/mm³)
b. Cellular casts	10. **Immunologic disorders**
8. **Neurologic disorder**	a. Positive LE prep *or*
a. Seizures *or*	b. Anti-dsDNA *or*
b. Psychosis	c. Anti-Sm *or*
	d. False-positive test for syphilis
	(with negative FTA)
	11. **Positive antinuclear antibody**

Adapted from Schumacher HR (ed): Primer on the Rheumatic Diseases, 9th edition. Arthritis Foundation, 1988, p 319.

has a 95% chance of having SLE. These criteria were devised for research purposes and may be somewhat restrictive. They provide a reasonable framework when evaluating a patient for SLE.

Bullous SLE

The following five criteria have been proposed for the diagnosis of bullous SLE: (1) diagnosis of SLE (based on the criteria listed above), (2) chronic and widespread blistering eruption, (3) subepidermal blister with acute neutrophilic infiltrate on skin biopsy, (4) immunoglobulin and complement at the basement membrane zone on direct immunofluorescence, and (5) immune deposits on or beneath the lamina densa by immuno-electron microscopy. The differential diagnosis of bullous SLE includes bullous pemphigoid, dermatitis herpetiformis, and epidermolysis bullosa acquisita.

Treatment

Discoid Lupus Erythematosus

Local Therapy

In general, the treatment of DLE should reflect the severity of the lesions. Small, localized lesions should be managed topically, while more extensive, disfiguring lesions require systemic therapy. Emphasis should be on prevention. The daily use of a broad-spectrum sunscreen with an SPF of 15 or greater, hats, protective clothing, and avoidance of direct sunlight is recommended. The objective of therapy is to prevent or minimize scarring. Once scarring is present, it will not respond to therapy. Camouflage make-up and hair pieces (even in male patients) are effective interventions.

Treatment of limited, localized DLE should start with local therapy. The strength of the topical steroid should be adjusted according to the severity of the lesions and their response. On the face, steroids should be limited. For particularly recalcitrant limited lesions (and verrucous lesions), moderate to potent topical steroids under occlusion (e.g., Duoderm) may be helpful. Intralesional triamcinolone acetonide suspension (Kenalog) injections, 3 to 5 mg/mL for the face and 5 to 10 mg/mL for the scalp every 4 to 6 weeks, can provide good control.

Systemic Therapy

Antimalarials. If a DLE patient has advancing disease despite local treatment, systemic antimalarial therapy should be considered (Table 2–14). Therapy should begin with hydroxychloroquine (because it is effective, safe, and available) 400 mg daily for the first 6 weeks, then decreasing to 200 mg daily thereafter. A full 6-month to 1-year trial may be needed before deciding whether there has been a therapeutic response.

After 6 to 12 months, if there has not been an adequate response, or if the patient has developed intolerable side effects, switching to another antimalarial or "combination therapy" may be considered. Chloroquine is somewhat more effective than hydroxychloroquine,

TABLE 2-14. Guidelines for the Use of Antimalarials in Lupus

DRUG	DOSAGE	MONITOR
Hydroxychloroquine (Plaquenil)	200–400 mg per day (≤6.5 mg/kg per day)	*Baseline:* G6PD, CBC, platelets, LFTs, creatinine, BUN, ophthalmologic exam *Follow-up:* CBC, platelets, and ophthalmologic exam every *6 months*
Chloroquine (Aralen)	250 mg per day (5 mg/kg per day)	*Baseline:* Same as above *Follow-up:* CBC, platelets, and ophthalmologic exam every *3 months*
Quinacrine (Atabrine)	100 mg per day	*Baseline:* G6PD, CBC, platelets, LFTs, creatinine, BUN *Follow-up:* CBC, platelets every *6 months*

but it is more toxic. Finally, if therapy with either of the prior two antimalarials has not been successful, or if side effects limit their usefulness, adding quinacrine (Atabrine), 100 mg daily, can be tried. Synergy between antimalarials justifies their use in combinations.

Miscellaneous Agents in the Treatment of DLE include isotretinoin (Accutane) in doses from 0.5 to 1.0 mg/kg per day, dapsone (25 to 100 mg daily), clofazimine (Lamprene), and thalidomide. Azathioprine (Imuran, 1 to 2 mg/kg daily) may be considered a drug of last resort in extensive, severe, refractory, debilitating DLE, or in cases in which severe cutaneous vasculitis complicates DLE.

Lupus Panniculitis

Lupus panniculitis is difficult to treat. In general, antimalarials are used in the same manner as described for DLE. Intralesional steroids are contraindicated in lupus panniculitis because they can exacerbate the atrophy. Systemic corticosteriods may have a temporary beneficial effect. Plastic or reconstructive surgery should be approached with caution. Reactivation of lesions that have been quiescent can occur with surgery.

Systemic Lupus Erythematosus

From the outset, it should be stressed that there is no definitive treatment or cure for SLE. The management of the SLE patient often requires a team of specialists. A rheumatologist is best trained to handle the overall complexity and complications of this disease and its therapies. Patient education is a starting point for patients and their families (Table 2–15).

Bullous SLE

Bullous SLE has been reported to respond dramatically to dapsone (50 to 150 mg per day), usually within 12 to 48 hours. Prednisone (0.5 to 2 mg/kg per day) may be effective.

TABLE 2–15.   Treatment of SLE

MILD DISEASE

Rest (for fatigue and malaise)
Sun avoidance/protection (for photosensitivity, DLE)
Physical therapy (for range of motion and strength)
NSAIDs (for joint/body pain)
Antimalarials (for skin involvement, joint pain, malaise, fatigue, and fever) as outlined for DLE
Prednisone (low-dose: 2.5–10 mg per day for joint pain)

SEVERE DISEASE WITH END-ORGAN DAMAGE

Prednisone (high-dose: 60 mg per day)
Addition of steroid-sparing agent
   Azathioprine, cyclophosphamide
   (methotrexate, chlorambucil, cyclosporine)

Lupus Subsets

Subacute Cutaneous Lupus Erythematosus

SCLE is best managed with sun avoidance and antimalarials. Sometimes topical steroids are beneficial. Typically, high-potency topical steroids for a 2-week course may be required. Often, however, the patient will have extensive cutaneous lesions, and systemic therapy with antimalarials (either single-agent or combination therapy) will be required. The use of systemic corticosteriods is discouraged. In cases of refractory cutaneous SCLE, the treatments described for refractory DLE are applicable.

Neonatal Lupus Erythematosus

In women with SLE or Sjögren's syndrome who are considering pregnancy, it is reasonable to test for the SSA/Ro and the SSB/La antibodies. It would be important to test for the antibodies in an asymptomatic woman who gave birth to a child with congenital heart block or a rash consistent with neonatal lupus. If the antibodies are present, it is important to counsel these women regarding the increased risk of having additional children with neonatal lupus. Cardiac monitoring beginning at the second trimester of pregnancy is recommended. Cutaneous neonatal lupus is a self-limited condition that does not require specific interventions. Sun avoidance is recommended. One percent hydrocortisone cream may also be of benefit.

DERMATOMYOSITIS AND POLYMYOSITIS

(CM&S Chapter 25)

Definition

Dermatomyositis and polymyositis constitute similar idiopathic acute and chronic nonsuppurative inflammatory disorders of striated muscles. In contrast to polymyositis, which presents as a myopathy, characteristic and distinctive cutaneous changes usually allow an immediate suspicion or clinical diagnosis of dermatomyositis. Both dermatomyositis and polymyositis often represent serious systemic disease beyond skin and muscle.

Five criteria define these disorders. A definite diagnosis consists of three or four criteria plus the cutaneous changes for dermatomyositis and four criteria without the rash for polymyositis.

1. Proximal muscle weakness
2. Elevation of levels of skeletal muscle enzymes
3. Electromyography consistent with a myopathy
4. Muscle biopsy evidence of myositis
5. Cutaneous disease (dermatomyositis but not in polymyositis)

Clinical Description

A bimodal pattern is seen with an initial peak in children and a second larger peak in adults in the 40- to 60-year age range. Polymyositis occurs more commonly than dermatomyositis in adults, while dermatomyositis is more common in children (20 : 1).

Adult Polymyositis and Dermatomyositis

Polymyositis and dermatomyositis may affect several organ systems, including skin, muscle, lungs, heart, gastrointestinal tract, blood vessels, and joints; 41% to 93% present with cutaneous changes.

In amyopathic dermatomyositis, cutaneous changes precede any muscle symptoms by 2 to 13 years; however, asymptomatic histologic myositis may be documented early. Skin disease may persist after the myositis has resolved.

Cutaneous manifestations of dermatomyositis include a variable color change that ranges from an intense erythema to a violaceous hue with mottled hypopigmentation, often associated with scaling and edema. This is often most prominent on the face and upper trunk, possibly reflecting exacerbation by ultraviolet B (UVB) light. Gottron's papules, which occur in 70% to 80% of patients, and heliotrope changes, which are seen in 30% to 60%, are considered to be pathognomonic of dermatomyositis. Features considered pathognomonic include *Gottron's papules*, erythematous to violaceous papules, nodules, or plaques over the metacarpophalangeal or interphalangeal joints or over other extensor joints; and *heliotrope*, the violaceous edema of the eyelids and periorbital area. *Poikiloderma*, a violaceous erythema with hyperpigmentation, hypopigmentation, atrophy, and telangiectases, is seen in the heliotrope and facial distribution and also over extensor prominences in the areas of Gottron's papules, or more widespread over the "V" of the neck, upper extremities, upper chest, and back in a "shawl" pattern. Dermatomyositis can present as generalized erythroderma distinct from both poikiloderma and the heliotrope changes.

Nail fold and cuticular changes can be prominent. The cuticles have an unkempt, picked appearance characterized by irregular overgrowth and thickening. Periungual areas are erythematous with telangiectases, seen better with capillary microscopy. These changes occur in juvenile dermatomyositis, adult dermatomyositis, and in some cases of adult polymyositis. Capillary changes can parallel the clinical course, normalizing during remission. Pruritus is a significant symptom in dermatomyositis, especially affecting the scalp, it may be associated with a gritty or sandy feel to the skin. Vasculitis may be manifested by digital ulcerations, periungual infarcts, oral ulcerations, and dermal nodules. Cutaneous vasculitis may be a marker for malignancy. "Mechanic's hands" resemble the calluses of manual laborers with changes of hyperkeratosis, scaling, fissuring, and hyperpigmentation on the ulnar aspect of the thumbs and radial aspect of the fingers extending onto the palms.

Myopathy can be painful or painless and most commonly involves pelvic, shoulder, neck flexors, cricopharyngeal, and esophageal muscles. The initial sign of lower extremity muscle involvement may be an abnormal gait or difficulty climbing steps or arising from a seated position. Chewing impairment and dysphagia secondary to cricopharyngeal and upper esophageal myositis or lower esophageal dysfunction may be seen. Asymptomatic cardiac manifestations, and pulmonary complications related to dysphagia (aspiration pneumonia), medication toxicity, or interstitial lung disease are also seen.

Overlap syndromes can appear most commonly with scleroderma, systemic lupus erythematosus, and Sjögren's syndrome. Fever, weight loss, fatigue, Raynaud's phenomenon, and a nonerosive, usually nondeforming arthritis occur frequently in the overlap group.

Juvenile Dermatomyositis

Both childhood and adult forms of dermatomyositis and polymyositis adhere to the same diagnostic criteria, but childhood disease has the unique features of vasculitis and calcinosis. Juvenile dermatomyositis has two presentations. Approximately one half of the patients have rapidly progressive disease with a high mortality rate characterized by fever and anorexia and vasculitis which can result in gastrointestinal hemorrhage and perforation. Therapeutic response and prognosis are poor. The remainder of children have a more subacute, gradual presentation with subsequent calcinosis. Calcinosis can be superficial, subcutaneous near joints (knees, elbows, fingers), or in the fascial planes.

Malignancy Association

Malignancy is associated with dermatomyositis, with estimates of risk varying from 6% to 60%. Malignancies in association with dermatomyositis parallel the types identified in the general population. Cost-effective malignancy screening should include a thorough history and physical examination with special focus on the pelvic examination, routine laboratory studies, chest radiography, mammography, stool guaiac testing, and computed tomography of the abdomen and pelvis at least at the time of diagnosis. Abnormal test results, poor response to therapy, and unexplained flares of myositis require further investigation for malignancy. Juvenile dermatomyositis is not associated with malignancy.

Pathology

The histopathologic findings in dermatomyositis are those of a cell-poor vacuolar interface dermatitis resembling lupus erythematosus. Immunofluorescent studies are not key in making the diagnosis of dermatomyositis and include a variety of abnormalities.

The preferred site for muscle biopsy is the quadriceps or biceps muscle, avoiding sites of recent electromyographic needles and extremely weak or strong muscles. Magnetic resonance imaging can assist in selecting the site. Histopathologic features include inflammatory cell infiltrate, vascular damage, fiber necrosis and phagocytosis, and a greater percentage of B cells. Perifascicular atrophy is considered diagnostic of dermatomyositis.

Diagnosis and Differential Diagnosis

Polymyositis or dermatomyositis can usually be diagnosed by a complete history and physical examination, laboratory studies (complete blood cell count, biochemical screen, creatine kinase), electromyography, and muscle biopsy, based on the above-outlined criteria. Antinuclear antibodies occur in more than 90% of patients with polymyositis and dermatomyositis, and myositis-specific auto-antibodies such as anti-JO–1, occur in 35% to 45%.

Several diseases cause lesions on the fingers that can simulate Gottron's papules. In lichen planus, lupus erythematosus, and psoriasis, red scaly lesions do not occur only on the skin overlying knuckles as do Gottron's papules. Edematous erythematous facial skin can be distinguished from cellulitis and acute allergic contact dermatitis by the presence of closely spaced telangiectases. Other causes of muscle weakness should be included, such as certain

---

TABLE 2–16. Treatment of Dermatomyositis and Polymyositis

GENERAL RULES

Accurate diagnosis essential
Avoid active exercise
Guide to treatment effectiveness: improvement in muscle strength (not creatine kinase)
Physical therapy: passive then active range of motion; graded exercise program after inflammation controlled

TREATMENT OF THE SKIN DISEASE

Sun protection
Topical corticosteroids
Hydroxychloroquine
  Juvenile dermatomyositis: up to 7 mg/kg per day
  Adult dermatomyositis: 400 mg per day
Systemic corticosteroids (see below)

TREATMENT OF THE MUSCLE DISEASE

Initial Therapy

Corticosteroids
  1–1.5 mg/kg per day in adults, up to 2 mg/kg per day in children, until stabilized; reduce dose by 10 mg per month until 20 mg per day, then slowly taper; alternate-day regimen may be used; maintenance dose is often required for extended period.

Refractory Disease, Severe Disease, Corticosteroid Side Effects

Methotrexate
  Adults: 7.5–15 mg per week
  Children: up to 20 mg/m^2 per week
Azathioprine
  1.5–3.0 mg/kg per day
Intravenous gammaglobulin
  2 g/kg per month in divided doses over 2–5 days

Additional Therapies of Possible Value

Cyclophosphamide
Chlorambucil
Cyclosporine
Plasmapheresis/leukapheresis
Combination treatment (chlorambucil/methotrexate, methotrexate/azathioprine, and others)
Total-body irradiation

drugs (corticosteroids, penicillamine, zidovudine), human immuno-deficiency virus (HIV) infection, neurologic diseases, polymyalgia rheumatica, and thyroid disease.

Treatment

See Table 2–16.

Prognosis

Remission is observed in 30%, and a course complicated by contractures, persistent or intermittent weakness, and/or calcinosis is seen in 62% of juvenile dermatomyositis. In adults, poor prognostic indicators include cardiac or pulmonary involvement, dysphagia, severe muscle weakness, older age, delay of therapy, and associated malignancy. Mortality approaches 30% at 8 years. Relapse is common.

PIGMENTED PURPURIC DERMATOSES

(CM&S Chapter 26)

Definition

The pigmented purpuric dermatoses, are a group of diseases that are likely variants of each other resulting from lymphocyte-mediated leakage of erythrocytes. They include Schamberg's disease, purpura annularis telangiectodes of Majocchi, the lichenoid purpura of Gougerot and Blum, and the itching purpuras or the eczematid-like purpura of Doucas and Kapetanakis. These diseases have similar clinical and histologic features. The eruptions usually present in middle-aged adults as asymptomatic, purpuric macules on the lower extremities; there is usually no significant venous or arterial insufficiency, and hematologic parameters are normal. The common shared clinical feature is the appearance of multiple, pinpoint, non-blanching red or purple macules that resemble cayenne pepper spots.

Clinical Description

In Schamberg's disease, or progressive pigmentary purpura, symmetrical hyperpigmented patches develop on the lower extremities, especially the pretibial area, most frequently in men. Purpura annularis telangiectodes occurs more frequently in women in the same distribution as Schamberg's disease, but expands in an annular configuration, leaving brown, sometimes atrophic, pigmentation in the center. In lichenoid purpura of Gougerot and Blum, purpuric plaques are typically flat-topped with predominant scaling and erythema, whereas the eczematid-like purpura of Doucas and Kapetanalcis shares some features of Schamberg's disease, but differs by its extensive nature, shorter course, and the system of pruritus.

Lichen aureus is much less common than the classic pigmented purpuras; this disorder is notable for its golden, copper-colored, flat-topped papules that spontaneously appear and persist indefinitely.

Pathology

Common to all of the forms of pigmented purpuric dermatoses are superficial perivascular infiltrates of lymphocytes, extravasated erythrocytes, and macrophages laden with hemosiderin.

Differential Diagnosis

The differential diagnosis of the pigmented purpuric dermatoses includes vasculitis, Kaposi's sarcoma, lichen planus, fixed drug eruption, purpuric mycosis fungoides and purpura secondary to impaired hemostasis.

Treatment

Treatment of the classic pigmented purpuras is usually unsatisfactory. Improvement demonstrated with a variety of topical agents, such as ascorbic acid, antihistamines, and topical corticosteroids, has not been routinely reproduced. Systemic use of steroids has the most reliable and beneficial results, but the lesions recur on discontinuation of the drug, the risks of this therapy outweigh its benefits.

PSORIASIS

(CM&S Chapter 27)

Definition

Psoriasis is a chronic, inflammatory scaling disorder of the skin that affects 0.5 to 1.5% of the U.S. population, which is punctuated by exacerbations and remissions. The pathogenesis of psoriasis involves a complex interaction of genetic and environmental factors. An autosomal dominant mode of inheritance with variable penetrance has been postulated.

Clinical Description and Pathology

Different patterns of psoriasis exist; and, in an individual patient, more than one pattern of psoriasis may be present concurrently, which may change over time.

Plaque Psoriasis

The classic clinical appearance is a well-demarcated, erythematous scaly plaque. A pale ring (Woronoff's ring) may be seen immediately surrounding the lesion. Overlying the erythematous base is a loosely adherent, silvery-white scale. Resolving and newly eruptive lesions are often erythematous but may lack scale. If scale is scraped away, a moist tissue composed of the lowest layers of the epidermis remains. When this last epidermal layer is removed, the capillaries lying closely beneath the scales are disrupted, resulting in pinpoint bleeding (Auspitz sign).

Initially, plaques of psoriasis may be localized or appear in clusters. The primary lesions may enlarge and coalesce into sharply bordered plaques as the disease progresses. This produces lesions of various shapes and patterns: nummular (coin-like), serpiginous, and geographic. As plaques regress (either in response to therapy or spontaneously), they often begin to clear in the center while the disease persists at the edges; this leads to an annular pattern.

Koebner Phenomenon

The production of new lesions in previously normal-appearing skin after local injury is referred to as the Koebner (isomorphic) response. Many types of skin injury, including burns, excoriations, skin infections, contact dermatitis, chemical irritation, and photosensitivity, may elicit this response. The occurrence of the Koebner response does not appear to be associated with the type or duration of psoriasis, extent of skin surface involved, or worsening disease.

Distribution of Lesions

Lesions of plaque psoriasis may occur anywhere on the body and are usually relatively symmetrical. The most commonly involved sites are the elbows and knees, lumbosacral area, intergluteal cleft, and scalp. These areas are frequently subject to friction and other mechanical trauma.

Plaques vary in size and number or enlarge to cover an extensive area of the body. Localized plaque-type psoriasis may be confined to the palms and soles. Such palmoplantar lesions are sharply demarcated, are erythematous, and have overlying scale, which is often very thick. Painful fissures may occur.

Systemic symptoms are generally absent with stable plaque psoriasis but commonly occur with pustular or erythrodermic forms of the disease.

Usually, plaque psoriasis has a gradual onset and chronic course. The lesions persist for months to years. Periodic pustular or erythrodermic flares may punctuate otherwise relatively stable plaque psoriasis. Complete, spontaneous remission is unusual. Factors believed to trigger the onset or exacerbation of psoriasis include oral medications (beta-blockers, lithium, systemic corticosteroid withdrawal, NSAIDs, oral contraceptives), pregnancy, and infection (streptococcal pharyngitis).

Histopathology

The epidermis is thickened (acanthotic) with narrow, elongated, club-shaped rete ridges. The granular layer is absent and the epidermis overlying the dermal papillae is thinned. Collections of neutrophils that migrate from dermal vessels can be found in the epidermis. A subcorneal microabscess is formed when these cells reach the subcorneal layer. The papillary dermis contains an increased number of tortuous, dilated capillaries, which spiral upward and almost to the epidermis. In the upper dermis, perivascular infiltrate composed chiefly of lymphocytes and macrophages is present.

Differential Diagnosis

The differential diagnosis of plaque psoriasis includes seborrheic dermatitis, eczematous dermatitis, lichen planus, pityriasis rubra pilaris, and mycosis fungoides.

Pustular Psoriasis

Pustular psoriasis is subtyped according to the extent of involvement and localization.

Generalized Pustular Psoriasis (GPP)

Acute (von Zumbusch) GPP. The prototype of GPP is characterized by the acute onset of sheets of sterile pustules on a background of erythema. The pustules arise in existing plaques or on previously uninvolved skin and rapidly become widespread. Palms, soles, and the oral cavity may be affected. The pustules often become confluent, forming lakes of pus. The skin is painful and tender. The pustules are accompanied by fever, malaise, arthralgia, and diarrhea. A polymorphonuclear leukocytosis is a common laboratory finding. Typically, pustules erupt in repeated waves, which may recur every few days for weeks.

Localized Pustular Psoriasis

Pustular psoriasis may be localized to the palms and/or soles and is often termed *palmoplantar pustulosis*. The disease typically presents in the fifth or sixth decade with erythematous plaques studded with pustules. Lesions may be painful and develop fissures. The thenar and hypothenar eminences, the instep, and the sides of the heels are most often involved. Systemic symptoms do not occur. The condition is often persistent and resistant to therapy. An acute, self-limiting variant of palmoplantar pustulosis precipitated by infection is also described.

Acrodermatitis continua of Hallopeau is a chronic, treatment-resistant form of localized pustular psoriasis. Scaling and pustules are found on the distal fingers and sometimes toes. Nail deformities are common (onychodystrophy). Underlying bone changes are sometimes seen in affected digits.

Differential Diagnosis

The differential diagnosis of pustular psoriasis includes subcorneal pustular dermatosis, pustular drug eruptions, dyshidrotic eczema, acute generalized exanthematous pustular dermatitis, and the keratoderma blenorrhagicum of Reiter's disease.

Guttate Psoriasis

This pattern is most commonly found in children and young adults. Acute onset is usual, with varying degrees of chronic preexisting plaque psoriasis. Acute onset of a generalized eruption of numerous erythematous, scaling, rain drop–like papules is typical of guttate consistent psoriasis. The findings on biopsy differ from those seen in fully developed plaques in that the rete ridges are only slightly elongated, there may be slight spongiosis, and suprapapillary plates are not yet thinned. Mounds of parakeratosis with neutrophils are present. Streptococcal infection is a frequent trigger factor. The trunk is the most heavily affected. Palms and soles are often spared. The eruption is sometimes pruritic. Spontaneous remission may occur, and it responds rapidly to therapy; especially with ultraviolet light.

Differential Diagnosis

The differential diagnosis of guttate psorasis includes secondary syphilis and pityriasis rosea.

Inverse Psoriasis

Psoriasis may affect intertriginous areas including the axilla, groin, submammary region, navel, and intergluteal fold. Patches of inverse psoriasis are erythematous and may be fissured. Due to friction and maceration, the usual fine scale of psoriasis is often absent in these sites. These moist macerated areas are subject to colonization with yeast and bacteria, which may elicit a Koebner response. Inverse psoriasis is often difficult to treat. Obesity and diabetes may be predisposing factors.

Differential Diagnosis

The differential diagnosis of inverse psoriasis includes candidal infections, tinea corporis, and erythrasma.

Erythrodermic Psoriasis

Erythrodermic psoriasis is a severe, life-threatening eruption characterized by intense generalized erythema and scaling. Erythroderma may complicate plaque or pustular psoriasis or may be the initial manifestation of psoriasis. Systemic symptoms including fever, chills, pruritus, malaise, and fatigue may occur. Generalized exfoliation produces hypoalbuminemia. Lower-extremity edema and hypothermia due to excessive heat dissipation from dilated capillary beds may occur. Those with underlying heart disease are at high risk of "high output" cardiac failure.

Differential Diagnosis

The differential diagnosis of erythrodermic psoriasis includes drug eruptions, and other skin conditions that may evolve into erythroderma such as eczematous dermatitis, pityriasis rubra pilaris, and mycosis fungoides. Reactions to a variety of drugs and withdrawal of topical and systemic steroids in patients with psoriasis and eczema may trigger erythroderma.

Nail Involvement

Psoriasis may affect the nail matrix, nail bed, and nail fold, causing faster than normal nail growth. The matrix lies beneath the proximal nail fold and is responsible for the manufacture and development of the nail plate. Tiny areas of psoriasis in the nail matrix produce focal parakeratosis on the portion of the matrix that forms the superficial layers of the nail plate. When the nail plate emerges, these bits of keratin separate from the surface of the nail, leaving characteristic pits. Nail pits are nonspecific and occur in other dermatoses, such as alopecia areata. With more severe involvement of the nail matrix, the nail may become discolored, deformed, and detached from the nail bed. This is termed *onychodystrophy*. Involvement of the nail fold and paronychium can also lead to onychodystrophy.

The nail bed lies directly underneath the nail plate. With psoriasis of the nail bed, collections of neutrophils and parakeratotic material accumulate underneath the nail plate, resulting in yellowish brown discolorations that are several millimeters in diameter called "oil spots." When oil spots reach the free edge of the nail, the parakeratotic material crumbles and the nail plate is lifted from the hyponychium, producing onycholysis. Involvement of the nail bed also produces subungual hyperkeratosis and splinter hemorrhages. Psoriatic nail disease produces proximal onycholysis.

Mucous Membrane Involvement

Oral and ocular involvement occasionally occur with psoriasis. The typical pattern of psoriasis occurring on the tongue is: benign migratory glossitis otherwise known as geographic tongue, which consists of erythematous patches with a raised, advancing yellow-white border. There is atrophy of filiform papillae, while fungiform papillae are unaffected. This atrophy is usually limited to the dorsal aspect of the tongue. The occurrence of oral lesions does not appear to be correlated with severity of psoriasis or with one type of psoriasis.

Genital lesions, especially on the penis, are frequent. Plaques may arise on the scrotum but are more frequent on the glans penis. In circumcised patients, balanitis circinata of Reiter's syndrome appears hyperkeratotic and may mimic psoriasis. In uncircumcised patients, the moist erosions of balanitis circinata on the glans penis resemble those of geographic tongue. Blepharitis and keratitis are the most common ocular manifestations of psoriasis. Scaling occurs most often on the upper eyelids. It is often impossible to distinguish psoriatic blepharitis from seborrheic blepharitis. Conjunctivitis, keratitis, photophobia, and disturbed lacrimation may also occur.

Scalp Involvement

Despite frequent involvement of the scalp, permanent hair loss appears to be uncommon.

Psoriatic Arthritis

Psoriatic arthritis is a seronegative spondyloarthropathy. The hallmark of this group, which includes ankylosing spondylitis,

Reiter's disease, and arthritis associated with gastrointestinal disease, is the absence of serum rheumatoid factor. Many seronegative arthropathies are associated with HLA-B27. It is unclear whether psoriatic arthritis is a unique entity or whether arthritis and psoriasis occur coincidentally. In most instances, skin lesions precede the onset of arthritis. Nail involvement is common. Patients with psoriatic arthritis appear to have more severe skin disease, but the severity of skin disease does not appear to correlate with the severity of arthritis.

Oligoarticular involvement often affects knees, ankles, and metatarsophalangeal and proximal interphalangeal joints. Polyarticular involvement often affects wrist, metacarpophalangeal, metatarsophalangeal, and distal interphalangeal joints. Spondyloarthropathy includes spondylitis and sacroiliitis. It may be symmetrical or asymmetrical and may occur with or without peripheral arthritis. Arthritis mutilans is least common. The first episode of psoriatic arthritis most frequently involves the knees, metatarsophalangeal joints, or wrist. An elevated erythrocyte sedimentation rate, leukocytosis, or a polyclonal gammopathy often occurs.

Radiologic findings, which are often indistinguishable from those of rheumatoid arthritis, include erosion of terminal tips, "pencil in cup" deformity, ankylosis, sacroiliitis, joint space narrowing, and syndesmophytes. Psoriatic arthritis is progressive. Treatment may reduce the rate of progression but does not halt the disease.

Treatment

The chronic nature of psoriasis should be emphasized to all patients. Although treatment may reduce or even clear signs of the disease, the underlying disease persists and exacerbations are common. Topical steroids, phototherapy, photochemotherapy, topical anthralin, and methotrexate are the most established treatments. The choice of therapy depends on the pattern of psoriasis and evaluation of risks and benefits for each patient. Topical therapies are often sufficient to control localized plaques. Systemic therapies are usually reserved for more severe cases, such as erythrodermic and pustular psoriasis or recalcitrant, widespread plaque psoriasis. Individual treatment regimens vary according to the response to therapy, and treatment needs vary greatly over time.

Topical Therapy

Emollients are an important adjunctive measure to both topical and systemic therapies. They help hydrate, soften, and loosen hyperkeratotic scale, especially in areas where plaques are thick, hyperkeratotic, or fissured. They are safe and relatively inexpensive.

Pharmacologically active topical therapies include mid-strength corticosteroids, tars, anthralin, and vitamin D analogues. Topical therapies are most useful as adjunctive agents in the treatment of plaque psoriasis.

Topical Corticosteroids

Topical corticosteroids have vasoconstrictive, antiinflammatory, antimitotic, and antiproliferative properties. The precise mechanism(s) of action in psoriasis is, however, unknown. For general concepts regarding topical corticosteroids, see "Principles of Therapy" (Chapter 9 in CS&M).

Use of milder steroids, such as hydrocortisone, on the face and intertriginous areas will help reduce the risk of steroid side effects such as striae, telangiectasia, and atrophy, which most often occur on these sites that allow greatest penetration of these agents. Ultrapotent fluorinated steroids such as halobetasol propionate (Ultravate) and clobetasol propionate (Temovate) are especially likely to induce these changes on sensitive areas. Although the advantages of multiple applications are not well quantified, topical steroids are generally applied twice a day. Use of ultra high-potency steroids is generally limited to 2-week courses.

Occlusive dressings enhance the delivery of steroids and increase the efficacy of topical corticosteroids. Except in very hyperkeratotic areas and for short periods of time they should not be used with high-potency preparations. Hydration of the stratum corneum, decreased mitotic activity, and protection from trauma may explain the improved efficacy of steroids under occlusion. Occlusive dressings may be applied to local areas (steroid-impregnated tape, hydrocolloid dressings, plastic wrap, shower cap) or the entire body (plastic jogging suit).

Plaques that fail to respond to topical agents may improve with intralesional therapy. Suspensions of a relatively insoluble steroid such as triamcinolone are injected directly into the dermis of small, persistent plaques. The dose of the steroid is gradually released over 3 to 4 weeks. Side effects include local atrophy and systemic absorption. This method is painful and not practical for treating large areas.

Anthralin

Anthralin (1,8,dihydroxy-9-anthrone) is a synthetic hydroxy anthrone that is concentrated in the mitochondria, undergoes oxidation and produces oxygen radicals and insoluble brown oxidation products, which produce local irritation and staining. Anthralin has been reported to inhibit in vitro and in vivo keratinocyte proliferation.

Anthralin should only be used to treat stable plaque psoriasis. The irritation it produces may aggravate erythrodermic and pustular psoriasis on mucous membranes or intertriginous areas. Anthralin-induced staining of skin resolves in a few weeks after therapy is stopped. Light-colored hair may also be stained purple or green. Anthralin penetrates lesional skin more rapidly and readily than normal skin. This facilitates "short contact therapy," with anthralin cream or paste applied to lesions for only 10 to 30 minutes.

Topical Tar Preparations

Tars are the products of distillation of oil and have been used for many years as adjunctive therapy with ultraviolet-B as part of the Goeckerman regimen. Tars are messy and smelly, greatly limiting their acceptability to patients.

Vitamin D

Vitamin D and some of its derivatives stimulate differentiation and inhibit DNA synthesis and cell proliferation in cultured keratinocytes and in vivo from normal and psoriatic epidermis. Vitamin D may also have immunomodulatory effects. Calcipotriol, a synthetic analog of vitamin D_3, binds with high affinity to skin receptors.

Unlike topical therapy, which has been extensively evaluated, lack of data from controlled studies supporting substantial efficacy and safety of oral Vitamin D therapy makes it unlikely that this treatment is highly effective. Comparison studies of calcipotriol ointment (50 μg/g) with betamethasone valerate ointment (0.1%) have confirmed the efficacy of calcipotriol to be comparable to that of topical steroid.

Side Effects. A potential side effect of therapy with vitamin D and its analogues is disruption of calcium metabolism. The use of oral calcitriol is limited by its potent effects on calcium metabolism. Application of 1 topical calcipotriol (100 g of ointment containing 50 μg/g of calcipotriol) has no effect on calcium metabolism in terms of serum calcium and phosphate, urinary calcium, serum calcitriol, or parathyroid hormone. The most common side effect of the use of topical calcipotriol is facial irritation.

Systemic Therapy

Patients who fail to improve with topical therapy may respond to systemic therapy. Many systemic therapies produce substantial complete clearance of lesions. The more effective treatments carry a higher risk of side effects. Relative and absolute contraindications must be carefully considered before prescribing a systemic therapy.

Methotrexate

Mechanism. Methotrexate (MTX) is a folic acid antagonist that competitively binds to the active catalytic site of dihydrofolate reductase and interferes with the production of methyl donors that are essential for nucleotide and amino acid synthesis. The drug selectively affects rapidly dividing cells, decreasing DNA synthesis and inhibiting mitosis. MTX has an antiproliferative effect as well as an immunomodulatory effect on psoriasis, and blocks chemotaxis of neutrophils.

Principles of Therapy. MTX is reserved for patients with severe disease in whom other modalities have failed or are contraindicated. Indications include patients with extensive plaque psoriasis, erythrodermic psoriasis, localized and generalized pustular psoriasis, psoriatic arthritis, and physically and emotionally disabling disease.

Baseline laboratory tests including complete blood cell count, liver function tests, and creatinine clearance should be performed prior to initiating therapy. Pregnancy and nursing are absolute contraindications to the use of MTX. Relative contraindications include active or recent hepatitis, cirrhosis, excessive alcohol consumption, moderate to severe renal dysfunction (creatinine clearance less than 50 mL/min), severe anemia, leukopenia or thrombocytopenia, active infectious disease or evidence of immunodeficiency, and inability or unwillingness to use contraception during treatment. During MTX therapy, liver function studies should be monitored, especially in the first months of treatment. Patients should not use alcohol while taking MTX.

Dosage. MTX is given as a single weekly oral, intravenous, or intramuscular dose or as a weekly divided dose over 24 hours. The single oral dose is 7.5 mg to 25 mg per week; the single parenteral dose is 7.5 mg to 50 mg per week given intramuscularly or intravenously. Improvement in symptoms is usually seen within 6 weeks.

Drug Interactions. Salicylates and NSAIDS interact with MTX to increase toxicity. Trimethoprim-sulfamethoxazole (Bactrim) also blocks dihydrofolate reductase, and should be avoided while on MTX. Retinoids have an independent hepatotoxic risk and should generally be avoided while on MTX therapy.

Side Effects. The most frequent acute side effects are malaise, headache, nausea, and anorexia. These commonly occur shortly after drug administration. Stomatitis, diarrhea, and myelosuppression reflect acute toxicity to the rapidly proliferating cells of the gastrointestinal mucosa and bone marrow. Alopecia occurs infrequently and is usually mild and reversible. MTX sometimes causes reactivation of ultraviolet light–induced erythema or increases the erythema response to ultraviolet-B radiation. In case of profound pancytopenia or other signs of acute overdose, leucovorin calcium, the physiologically active form of folic acid, should be administered immediately.

Hepatotoxicity. The most serious complication of long-term MTX therapy for psoriasis is chronic hepatotoxicity, which is dose related. Biochemical tests of liver function are a poor indicator of MTX-induced chronic liver damage. The standard means of monitoring MTX therapy of psoriasis is by liver biopsy performed after each cumulative dose of 1.5 g of MTX. Cirrhosis appears to become substantial with cumulative doses over 4.0 g. Other side effects of MTX therapy include myelosuppression, teratogenicity, pneumonitis, and increased risk of malignancy.

Retinoids

The retinoids are a group of vitamin A–derived compounds. Etretinate, a synthetic retinoid and its carboxylic acid derivative, acitretin, has been proven effective in the treatment of psoriasis. Isotretinoin (Accutane), is primarily used to treat acne and has only modest antipsoriatic activity.

Mechanism. The precise mechanism of retinoid action is unknown but may act through suppression of DNA synthesis and modulation of epidermal keratins and differentiation. Retinoids also have anti-inflammatory effects. Etretinate reduces PMN chemotaxis, as well as the chemotaxis-stimulating activity of psoriatic serum.

Principles of Therapy. Retinoids are effective first-line agents for pustular and erythrodermic forms of psoriasis and respond more rapidly to etretinate than to MTX. Response and toxicity of retinoids are dose related. Usual starting doses of etretinate are 0.5 to 1 mg/kg per day. Erythrodermic and plaque psoriasis tend to require relatively higher doses (about 1.0 mg/kg per day), but pustular psoriasis often responds to lower doses (0.5 to .75 mg/kg per day).

Patients should be evaluated with regard to severity of disease, baseline lipid profile, and hepatic function and for a woman's desire to conceive. Severe hyperlipidemia, active or recent hepatitis, pregnancy, and inability or unwillingness to use long-term contraception are contraindications to retinoid therapy. Relative contraindications include history of liver disease, osteophyte formation, and excessive alcohol consumption. A serum pregnancy test, lipid levels, and liver function tests should be obtained before beginning therapy and monitored throughout therapy.

Side Effects. Side effects are dose related and may be related to duration of treatment. The most serious side effects of retinoids include teratogenicity, hyperlipidema, hepatotoxicity, and musculoskeletal changes. Diffuse idiopathic skeletal hyperostosis (DISH Syndrome) is associated with both etretinate and acitretin therapy. Dryness of the skin and mucous membranes is the most frequent side effect. Ocular effects of etretinate include conjunctivitis, keratitis, corneal opacities, and impaired color perception. Pruritus, scaling, and alopecia may occur. Nails may become thin and fragile and shed. Xerosis and cheilitis may be alleviated with emollients. Ophthalmologic ointments or artificial tears help to relieve ocular dryness and irritation. Mucocutaneous side effects, including alopecia, are rapidly reversible on decreased dosage or withdrawal of the retinoid.

Hydroxyurea

Hydroxyurea is an analogue of urea that is used primarily in cancer chemotherapy for chronic myelogenous leukemia. It inactivates the enzyme ribonucleotide reductase, thereby inhibiting DNA synthesis and selectively killing cells in S phase. It may specifically inhibit epidermal proliferation.

Hydroxyurea produces best results when used in combination with PUVA or UVB therapy. It may be useful in patients who are unresponsive to these treatments alone. Bone marrow depression is a constant hazard. Hydroxyurea is probably teratogenic and may be carcinogenic in long-term use.

Cyclosporine

Cyclosporine a powerful immunosuppressant agent produced by certain species of fungus, was initially used to prevent rejection in transplant recipients and it has since been shown to be beneficial in the treatment of psoriasis. The use of cyclosporine should be limited to the short-term treatment of patients with extremely disabling plaque psoriasis who are resistant or intolerant of other systemic therapies.

Mechanism. The precise antipsoriatic mechanism of cyclosporine is unknown. Possible mechanisms of action include suppression of T lymphocytes, inhibition of IL-2 synthesis, and inhibition of keratinocyte proliferation.

Principles of Therapy. Daily doses of 3 to 5 mg/kg per day are usually sufficient to clear lesions within 8 weeks with minimal acute toxicity. Cyclosporine should be avoided in patients with hypertension, hyperlipidemia, renal or hepatic disease, malignancy, or current therapy with immunosuppressants or radiation. During therapy, blood pressure, serum lipids, and renal function should be closely and regularly monitored. Glomerular filtration rate is a more reliable indicator of renal function than is serum creatinine.

After therapy is stopped, most severely affected patients relapse within a few months. The cumulative toxicity of cyclosporine maintenance therapy greatly limits its long-term use for this chronic disease.

Drug Interactions. Cyclosporine, which is metabolized through the hepatic P-450 enzyme system, has numerous drug interactions. Drugs which increase cyclosporine blood levels through inhibition of the P-450 system include erythromycin, oral contraceptives, and calcium channel blockers. Rifampin, phenytoin, and trimethoprim-sulfamethoxazole decrease the blood concentration of cyclosporine through induction of the system.

Side Effects. Cyclosporine is associated with numerous serious side effects, such as nephrotoxicity, carcinogenicity, neurologic symptoms (headaches, tremors, paresthesias), gastrointestinal symptoms (nausea, vomiting, diarrhea), hyperlipidemia, gingival hyperplasia, and hypertrichosis.

Other Immune Modulators

Azathioprine. Azathioprine is a powerful immunosuppressant and antimetabolite derived from 6-mercaptopurine, which interferes with DNA synthesis and thus cell proliferation. It suppresses cell-mediated immunity, inhibits PMN and monocyte activity, and blocks production of prostaglandins. Although it may have modest beneficial effects on psoriasis, its potential side effects include hepatotoxicity and bone marrow suppression.

FK 506. Like cyclosporine, FK 506 (tacrolimus) is a fungal metabolite with potent immunosuppressant activities. Initial results with FK 506 in small numbers of patients with psoriasis have been promising. Whether it is safer than cyclosporine is not established.

Systemic Corticosteroids

Systemic steroids may reduce inflammation in the absence of alternative therapies for severe erythrodermic or pustular psoriasis. Unfortunately, withdrawal of oral steroid treatment may precipitate a worsening of disease. Hazards of long-term treatment with systemic steroids include osteoporosis, cataracts, glucose intolerance, and hypertension.

Phototherapy and Photochemotherapy

Phototherapy is the use of ultraviolet radiation to treat skin diseases. Light is absorbed by molecules in the skin (chromophores) that trigger a sequence of photochemical events that may alter the structure and function of skin or the immune system. Different wavelengths of light produce different effects on the skin. Exposure to sunlight has long been known to improve the symptoms of psoriasis. Both ultraviolet B (UVB) (wavelength 290 to 320 nm) and ultraviolet A (UVA) (320 to 400 nm) light are useful in psoriasis therapy. UVB may be used as monotherapy or in combination with other agents. UVA is used with topical or systemic photosensitizers, most notably the psoralens (PUVA therapy). The use of exogenous photosensitizing agents to enhance the therapeutic effect of ultraviolet radiation is termed *photochemotherapy*.

Phototherapy

Mechanism. The precise mechanism of UVB therapeutic effect in psoriasis is unknown. UVB may have antiproliferative effects. UVB induces DNA pyrimidine dimers and inhibits epidermal DNA synthesis, mitosis, and proliferation. UVB also has immunomodulatory actions.

UVB Phototherapy. Erythemogenic doses of UVB administered at least three times per week appear most effective. Optimal treatment is based on a patient's minimal erythema dose, i.e., the dose of ultraviolet radiation (in millijoules per square centimeter) that produces a barely perceptible erythema.

A hydrophobic emollient should be applied before each treatment to maximize UVB penetration. Initial doses of 0.8 to 1.0 minimal erythema dose are typically used. Subsequent increases are governed by the patient's response to the prior dose. Patients generally required three to five treatments per week for a complete response. Treatments are continued until the lesions are cleared. Typically 25 or more treatments are required. Maintenance therapy with UVB appears to prolong remission after clearing.

UVB phototherapy usually clears acute guttate psoriasis rapidly. Generalized plaque psoriasis will often respond, but more treatments are usually required and some exposed areas including the lower legs, buttocks, and elbows are often especially difficult to clear.

Goeckerman Regimen. Topical agents may slightly enhance the beneficial effect of UVB. In the Goeckerman regimen, tar is applied to the skin several hours before exposure to UVB irradiation. Tar may have an antiproliferative effect.

UVB and Anthralin. The Ingram technique uses a combination of tar, UVB, and anthralin. It is effective but messy and time consuming and not much more effective than anthralin alone.

The modified Ingram method, which is more convenient, uses a combination of short-contact coal tar, phototherapy usually from metal halide lamps emitting UVA and UVB, and short-contact high-potency anthralin therapy in a psoriasis day-care center. Both the traditional and modified Ingram methods require use of costly facilities and are unlikely to be cost effective.

Side Effects. The acute side effects of phototherapy are identical to those of sunburn, redness, pain, and pruritus. Phototoxic reactions may also exacerbate psoriasis. Patients with diseases exacerbated by ultraviolet light, such as lupus erythematosus or porphyria, should be treated with great caution. Use of sensitizing medications such as tetracycline, sulfa drugs, and phenothiazines might increase the risk of erythema, but the peak action spectrum of most of these drugs is in the UVA range. Chronic actinic degeneration (photoaging) and increased risk of nonmelanoma cancer are long-term side effects of phototherapy. Increased risk of nonmelanoma skin cancer is the most serious long-term risk of UVB, but the magnitude of increase is probably modest for most patients. Males exposed to high doses of UVB have been shown to have a greater than fourfold risk of genital tumors compared with patients with less UVB exposure. Ocular damage, especially keratitis and conjunctivitis, may occur if eyes are not protected during ultraviolet light exposure.

PUVA Therapy. Psoralens are photosensitizing compounds that naturally occur in certain plant species, including lime, lemon, parsley, celery, fig, and clove. PUVA therapy, which combines oral synthetic psoralens followed by exposure to UVA (320–400 nm), is widely used to treat severe psoriasis. The most widely used psoralen is 8-methoxypsoralen (8-MOP).

Mechanism. The mechanism of action of PUVA is unknown. Psoralens intercalate with DNA and, after exposure to UVA, form photoadducts, which may inhibit mitosis and reduce the rate of epidermal proliferation.

Acute Toxicity to PUVA. The most frequent acute side effects of oral PUVA are erythema, pruritis, nausea, headaches, and dizziness. These effects are usually mild and reversible. The onset of erythema (24 hours after exposure) and the time to peak erythema (48 to 72 hours) are delayed compared with that produced by UVB therapy (onset 2 to 6 hours with peak at 12 to 24 hours). The erythema induced by UVA may last longer (up to a week compared with 24 to 48 hours for UVB).

Treatment of Psoriasis. Although different treatment schedules have been used in the United States and Europe, certain aspects of the treatment protocols are fairly standard. Between 0.4 (liquid form) to 0.6 (crystalline form) mg/kg of 8-MOP is given, followed in 1½ (liquid) to 2 hours (crystalline) by UVA exposure. Treatment is given two to four times per week until clearing is achieved. PUVA is then continued less frequently on varying schedules to "maintain" the cleared state. Patients are frequently "maintained" on one PUVA treatment every two weeks.

Treatment of Psoriasis Variants. Erythrodermic psoriasis responded less favorably than guttate and plaque psoriasis.

Side Effects. The long-term side effects of PUVA therapy include a cumulative dose-dependent association between PUVA exposure and increased risk of cutaneous squamous cell carcinoma. A small and barely significant dose-dependent risk of basal cell carcinoma is seen. The risk of male genital squamous cell carcinoma, a rare tumor in the general population, is greatly increased in male patients exposed to PUVA. These observations indicate the importance of shielding unaffected parts of the male genitalia and minimizing exposure of affected areas.

Other sequelae of PUVA therapy include development of pigmented macules ("PUVA lentigines"). Unlike solar lentigines, which consist of collections of normal melanocytes, ultrastructural studies of PUVA lentigines show features including nuclear atypia and melanosomal pleomorphism and degenerative changes.

Accumulation of photoproducts may potentially lead to cataract formation. Patients are advised to wear UVA blocking glasses immediately after ingestion of the drug and for the remainder of the day of treatment.

Combination Therapies

The goal of combination therapy is to maximize efficacy and minimize toxicity. These qualities are particularly desirable when treating psoriasis, which often requires long-term maintenance therapy.

Re-PUVA. Combination therapy with retinoids and PUVA may be an effective alternative in patients who are resistant to monotherapy. In addition to their direct therapeutic effects, retinoids probably also enhance the response to UVA by decreasing the thickness of psoriatic plaques and epidermis. Patients are treated with 0.4 to 0.8 mg/kg of etretinate or acitretin for 2 weeks, after which PUVA is added.

Methotrexate and PUVA. This combination appears to be effective but requires substantial skill to administer. A 3-week course of MTX followed by a combination of PUVA and MTX was shown to rapidly clear lesions in patients with plaque, guttate, and erythrodermic psoriasis, including those in whom PUVA and/or UVB therapy had failed.

Treatment of Nails

Treatment of psoriatic nails is difficult. Systemic agents such as MTX are useful but seldom justified for nail disease alone. Topical application and intralesional injection of corticosteroids and PUVA have been reported to be effective but are not usually practical or highly effective.

REITER'S SYNDROME

(CM&S Chapter 28)

Definition

Reiter's syndrome has been classically defined as the triad of urethritis and cervicitis, arthritis, and conjunctivitis. This syndrome, which was named after Hans Reiter, who first described it, has been associated with both diarrheal illness and histocompatibility antigen HLA-B27.

Clinical Description

Reiter's syndrome, a disease of unknown etiology, occurs most commonly in men but has also been described in women and children. An association with human immunodeficiency virus infection has been described.

A patient with Reiter's syndrome typically presents with an oligoarthritis, primarily involving the lower extremity, after an episode of nonspecific urethritis or diarrhea. The eye involvement may include a sterile conjunctivitis, as well as acute anterior uveitis and iritis. Complications can also involve the cardiac, renal, and central nervous systems.

The lesions begin as erythematous papules that thicken into hyperkeratotic nodules. They occur most frequently on the soles and palms but also on the extremities, scalp, and trunk. Adjacent nail involvement frequently occurs, manifested by subungual heaped-up keratinization and possible loss of the nail. The lesions are usually asymptomatic and resolve spontaneously without scarring. Clinically, keratoderma blennorrhagicum may be difficult to differentiate from pustular psoriasis.

Balanitis circinata consists of painless, initially discrete, small vesicles on the glans penis that eventually break down and coalesce to form serpiginous borders where infection may occur. In circumcised men, these lesions become crusted and resemble keratoderma blennorrhagicum.

The stomatitis of Reiter's syndrome consists of painless superficial ulcerations or elevated erythematous gray plaques. They occur on the buccal mucosa of the cheeks, palate, and tongue and may coalesce to form a ''relief map'' appearance. They are self-limited and usually do not require treatment.

The prognosis of Reiter's disease had been suggested in the past to be favorable, but recent studies have shown that recurrences are common.

Pathology

Most of the histopathologic features of Reiter's syndrome in biopsy specimens of skin and mucous membranes are generally indistinguishable from those of psoriasis.

Diagnosis and Differential Diagnosis

The differential diagnosis of Reiter's syndrome depends on the number of presenting symptoms. The cutaneous lesions can be difficult to differentiate from psoriasis. The arthritis may present similarly to other spondyloarthropathies, such as arthritis of inflammatory bowel disease and ankylosing spondylosis if sacroiliitis is present. Differentiating Reiter's syndrome from gonococcal arthritis can be made by appropriate cultures. Also included in the differential diagnosis are acute rheumatic fever and other rheumatologic disorders.

Treatment

The treatment of Reiter's syndrome includes nonsteroidal anti-inflammatory drugs, intra-articular steroids, and physical therapy. In cases of recurring and debilitating arthritis, methotrexate and azathioprine have been used. The mucocutaneous manifestations often require no treatment. Because of the reported risk of using immunosuppressive drugs in patients with human immunodeficiency virus infection, it is prudent to avoid their use in the treatment of Reiter's syndrome in these patients.

SUBCORNEAL PUSTULAR DERMATOSIS

(CM&S Chapter 29)

Definition and Clinical Description

Subcorneal pustular dermatosis is a disorder of unknown etiology occurring in all age groups but is most frequent in women aged

40 to 60. The primary lesion is a 2- to 10-mm pustule. Large lesions can show a fluid level of pus (hypopyon). Pustules are flaccid and arise on either clinically normal or erythematous skin. They can be grouped in annular or circi-nate patterns. When the pustules are ruptured, scales or thin crusts can be seen. Healing occurs without scarring or atrophy; transient hyperpigmentation may occur.

The distribution of subcorneal pustular dermatosis favors the inguinal and axillary folds, the trunk, and the proximal parts of the limbs. The hands and feet are rarely involved, and the face and mucous membranes are always spared. Itching is absent or mild. There are no constitutional symptoms. Subcorneal pustular dermatosis is a chronic disease that usually runs a benign course for years. Acute flares, if untreated, may last for weeks or months; the patient's general health is unaffected.

Clinical and histologic variants of subcorneal pustular dermatosis may occur alone. It has also been associated with other neutrophilic dermatoses, such as pyoderma gangrenosum and Sweet's syndrome. Patients with systemic disease (e.g., myeloma, leukemia, inflammatory bowel disease, rheumatoid arthritis IgA gammopathy) may also develop subcorneal pustular dermatosis.

Pathology

The typical pathologic findings in this condition are subcorneal neutrophilic pustules.

Differential Diagnosis

The differential diagnosis of subcorneal pustular dermatosis includes impetigo, dermatitis herpetiformis, linear IgA bullous dermatosis, pemphigus foliaceus, pustular psoriasis, and pustular drug reactions.

Treatment

Dapsone, an inhibitor of the inflammatory properties of some of the neutrophils, is the mainstay of subcorneal pustular dermatosis treatment at a daily dose of 100 to 150 mg. In unresponsive patients, etretinate and psoralens and ultraviolet A light (PUVA) have been used.

PITYRIASIS RUBRA PILARIS

(CM&S Chapter 30)

Definition

Pityriasis rubra pilaris is a papulosquamous disorder of uncertain etiology that resembles psoriasis but is considerably more difficult to treat. The disease has an abrupt onset and often resolves within 3 years.

Clinical Description

Cephalad to caudad spread of lesions, ectropion, follicular papules on the dorsal aspects of phalanges and extensor aspects of wrists and thighs (''nutmeg grater'' papules), hyperkeratotic palms and soles with an orange hue, and progressive erythroderma containing patches of normal-appearing skin (''islands of sparing'') are the characteristic cutaneous features of classic adult pityriasis rubra pilaris. In addition, nail changes that may be observed in patients with type I pityriasis rubra pilaris include distal yellow-brown discoloration, onychauxis (nail plate thickening), splinter hemorrhages, and subungual hyperkeratosis. Nail plate pits (which may be seen in patients with psoriasis) are not typical for pityriasis rubra pilaris.

Pityriasis rubra pilaris has rarely been seen as the initial manifestation of internal malignancy and in association with human immunodeficiency virus infection.

Pathology

Histologic features that are characteristic of pityriasis rubra pilaris include alternating orthokeratosis and parakeratosis, broad rete ridges, hypergranulosis, narrow dermal papillae, sparse superficial perivascular lymphocytic infiltration, and thick suprabasilar plates.

Differential Diagnosis

The differential diagnosis includes psoriasis, dermatitis, cutaneous T-cell lymphoma, and erythrokeratoderma variabilis.

Treatment

The treatment of choice for pityriasis rubra pilaris is systemic isotretinoin (usually at 1.0 mg/kg per day) or etretinate (between 0.5 to 1.0 mg/kg per day); efficacy with acitretin has also been observed.

ERYTHRODERMA

(CM&S Chapter 31)

Definition

Erythroderma, which means ''red skin,'' is not a common skin condition, but, because it is a severe dermatologic disorder, it requires immediate medical attention. Erythroderma is accompanied or followed by exfoliation. Thus, *erythroderma* and *exfoliative dermatitis* are overlapping terms.

A diagnosis of erythroderma indicates that all of the skin surface is involved. However, there may be regional differences of clinical activity. Erythroderma is present continuously for days or longer, and should not be confused with temporary, physiologic, exercise-induced erythroderma.

In *primary* erythroderma, the patient is suffering from erythroderma of an unknown cause, whereas *secondary* erythroderma, which accounts for 80% of all cases of erythroderma, is part of another diagnosable dermatologic disorder.

Clinical Description

Skin Color and Texture

Erythroderma is easily recognized in whites, but it can be difficult to appreciate in black skin. Erythroderma in whites presents as slight to pronounced redness as well as a bluish hue in areas where gravitational forces lead to increased venous pressure. When the normal epidermal skin barrier is disturbed without an ensuing hyperproliferation of epidermis the skin becomes ''shiny.'' However, when exfoliation occurs, the skin looks dry and assumes a gray hue. Both conditions are accompanied by increased transepidermal water loss. Erythroderma of long-standing duration is often followed by hyperpigmentation, poikiloderma, and lichenification, and the skin becomes stiff due to edema.

Hair and Nail Growth

Diffuse hair loss is common, sometimes leading to almost total alopecia. The nails become more brittle, showing irregular growth.

Keratoderma

Up to 80% of patients with primary erythroderma develop hyperkeratosis of palms and soles, usually as an early sign of the disease.

Lymphadenopathy

Axillary and inguinal lymph glands are often enlarged. The term *dermatopathic lymphadenopathy* is used when the histologic picture shows enlargement of the paracortical areas, indicating proliferation of T lymphocytes.

Subjective Symptoms

Erythroderma is almost always accompanied by itching, which may be severe and interfere with sleep. Erythroderma occurs because of blood vessel dilatation, which leads to increased heat loss and a sensation of chilliness, resulting in shivering. Cardiac output is increased.

Course of Disease

Erythroderma of unknown origin and lasting for more than 1 month is often classified as the primary type. Approximately one third of patients who develop primary erythroderma have suffered for an average of 6 years from nonspecific eczema of the lower legs resembling stasis dermatitis. One third have a history of a positive patch test to metals, cosmetics, thiuram mix, or topical medication. Photosensitivity and contact allergies to plants are also common; however, the presence of contact allergy or photosensitivity does not necessarily indicate that erythroderma is due to these. Primary erythroderma is associated with later development of cutaneous T-cell lymphoma in approximately 10% of the patients. In these cases, erythroderma occurs years before a histologic diagnosis of cutaneous T-cell lymphoma can be confirmed.

Patients with secondary erythroderma may respond to therapy of the underlying dermatologic disorder.

Biochemical and Immunologic Findings

Patients with erythroderma often have normal blood parameters. Eosinophilia may be detected in atopics and leukocytosis in patients with generalized pustular psoriasis. Increased serum levels of IgE are frequent.

Pathology

Erythroderma is a clinical diagnosis, and there is no single histopathologic picture. In primary erythroderma the microscopic findings which are, by definition, nonspecific, range from slight vascular ectasia with sparse lymphocytic infiltrates to dense, band-like infiltrates of lymphocytes, with or without epidermal hyperplasia or spongiosis. In secondary erythroderma the histology may be, but frequently is not, diagnostic for the underlying cause, such as psoriasis, ichthyosis, seborrheic dermatitis, atopic dermatitis, pemphigus foliaceus, or pityriasis rubra pilaris.

Pathogenesis and Etiology

Secondary erythroderma accounts for approximately 80% of all cases of erythroderma.

Treatment

Secondary erythroderma needs therapy for the underlying cause. Therapy also includes careful evaluation of the water–electrolyte balance and that the cardiac status of the patient is assessed and followed. Patients with erythroderma are often diagnosed and treated as outpatients. Patients with medical complications of erythroderma, such as acute cardiovascular decompensation or sepsis, require hospitalization.

Common to any secondary diagnosis is topical therapy, which may include soaks with or without additives as well as application of potent topical corticosteroid ointment vehicles. In primary erythroderma, a standard therapeutic approach has not yet been developed. Patients are usually treated with topical regimens, including soaks, topical steroids, as well as emollients. The systemic approach is often empiric.

TRANSIENT ACANTHOLYTIC DERMATOSIS

(CM&S Chapter 32)

Definition and Clinical Description

Transient acantholytic dermatosis (Grover's disease) is an intensely pruritic, self-limited eruption of unknown etiology that occurs in individuals older than 50 years of age. Men are affected more often than women. Pruritic papules and papulovesicles occurring on the trunk and anterior thighs characterize the clinical appearance of transient acantholytic dermatosis. Although not closely clustered, the lesions are often grouped in the supraclavicular, presternal, and deltoid regions as well as the back. Lesions appear as small erythematous papules and papulovesicles on erythematous bases. Frequently, lesions appear crusted secondary to excoriation. The eruption may last from 2 weeks to 3 months and is exacerbated by heat and sweating.

Pathology

Focal acantholytic dyskeratosis, suprabasilar and intragranular acantholytic clefts, and combinations of acantholysis and spongiosis can be seen in separate foci of this condition.

Diagnosis and Differential Diagnosis

The clinical differential diagnosis of transient acantholytic dermatosis includes acne vulgaris, arthropod bites, papular urticaria, subacute prurigo (prurigo papularis), scabies, miliaria rubra, folliculitis, dermatitis herpetiformis, and seborrheic dermatitis.

Treatment

The treatment of transient acantholytic dermatosis includes an antipruritic agent, potent topical steroid creams, and maintenance of a cool, dry environment. Patients with extensive disease have been treated with isotretinoin, 40 mg per day, for 14 days, or up to 12 weeks if necessary. Other therapies include oral vitamin A, 50,000 U three times a day for 2 weeks followed by reduction to 50,000 U per day for 12 weeks. Methotrexate (25–50 mg per week) has been tried, and psoralens and ultraviolet A light (PUVA) may be effective in refractory cases.

JESSNER'S LYMPHOCYTIC INFILTRATE

(CM&S Chapter 33)

Definition and Clinical Description

Although many believe Jessner's lymphocytic infiltrate to be a distinct entity, others consider it an initial or variant stage of discoid lupus erythematosus, polymorphic light eruption, or even malignant lymphoma. Lesions are either single or multiple, papular or small and plaque-like without scaling or follicular hyperkeratosis occurring most frequently on the face and upper trunk. Not uncommonly lesions expand peripherally to become annular with clearing in the center or circinate. An individual lesion persists for days, weeks, or even months and disappears without sequelae. It may return in the same area or at other locations. About half of the patients experience itching or, occasionally, an exceptionally tender sensation. Exposure to sunlight may exacerbate the disease.

The age at onset of the disease is between 20 and 50 years, with no obvious sex predominance. It runs a cyclic and prolonged course with remissions and exacerbations occurring over a period of many years before spontaneous resolution takes place.

Pathology

The most striking feature is the presence of superficial and deep perivascular lymphocytic infiltrates and, rarely, plasma cells around dermal blood vessels and cutaneous appendages. CD8 T cells predominate and CD68-positive plasmacytoid monocytes frequently are seen.

Diagnosis and Differential Diagnosis

A diagnosis of Jessner's lymphocytic infiltrate is made after all other possible diagnoses are excluded. These include drug reaction, B-cell lymphoma, discoid lupus erythematosus, polymorphic light eruption, and erythema annulare centrifugum.

Treatment

Antimalarial agents and topical and intralesional steroids may have a beneficial but temporary effect. Thalidomide has been used with excellent results, but this drug is difficult to obtain.

FIGURATE ERYTHEMAS

(CM&S Chapter 34)

The figurate erythemas comprise a group of skin eruptions characterized by annular, polycyclic, or serpiginous migrating borders. The most important of these are erythema annulare centrifugum, erythema gyratum repens, erythema marginatum rheumaticum, erythema chronicum migrans, and necrolytic migratory erythema. The last two types are covered in Chapters 6 and 13 of this *Pocket Guide* and in Chapters 109 and 180 of CM&S, respectively.

Erythema Annulare Centrifugum

Definition

Erythema annulare centrifugum, a disease of unknown etiology, which occurs most frequently in young adults, consists of chronic recurrent annular and circinate lesions that slowly expand and usually heal within a few days to a few weeks without scarring.

Clinical Description

Asymptomatic polycyclic, annular, or serpiginous firm lesions with delicate scales on the inner margins of the rims correspond to the superficial type. The deep type consists of firm, cord-like lesions without scales.

Pathology

The two characteristic patterns are a superficial and deep tightly clustered perivascular lymphocytic infiltrate that spares the epidermis, and a spongiotic dermatitis that variably involves the deep vascular plexus.

Diagnosis and Differential Diagnosis

The differential diagnosis includes tinea corporis, lupus erythematosus, granuloma annulare, pityriasis rosacea, guttate parapsoriasis, and lymphoma.

Treatment

Therapy is seldom indicated for this asymptomatic process. If an underlying cause is found, its elimination results in resolution of the eruption. Topical corticosteroids are of some benefit.

Erythema Gyratum Repens

Definition and Clinical Description

Erythema gyratum repens is a distinctive scaling eruption most often associated with an internal malignancy in which patients present with a bizarre, recalcitrant, progressive dermatosis characterized by irregular, wavy to circinate bands with marginal desquamation that form a peculiar serpiginous or gyrate outline resembling wood grain. The eruption precedes or accompanies a malignant process in the majority of the cases and in many patients responds to the treatment of the malignant process.

Erythema Marginatum Rheumaticum

Definition and Clinical Description

Erythema marginatum rheumaticum is a rapidly spreading erythematous annular to polycyclic eruption of the trunk and proximal extremities. It is considered one of the five major criteria for the diagnosis of rheumatic fever, along with carditis, polyarthritis, chorea, and subcutaneous nodules. Erythema marginatum rheumaticum occurs in up to 18% of patients with acute rheumatic fever.

Treatment

The treatment of rheumatic fever results in resolution of the cutaneous disease.

DERMATOSES OF PREGNANCY

(CM&S Chapter 37)

Cutaneous changes during pregnancy are very common. Some of these alterations (e.g., melasma, striae distensae, spider angiomas) have a very high incidence during pregnancy and are, in a sense, physiologic. There are a number of other dermatoses that are believed to be uniquely associated with gestation. These eruptions are of concern because of their appearance, symptoms, chance for recurrence in subsequent pregnancies, and potential significance as markers of risk for fetal morbidity or mortality. The purpose of this chapter is to present an overview of the diagnosis and treatment of the most common and best defined dermatoses of pregnancy. For information regarding herpes gestationis, see Chapter 3 of this *Pocket Guide* and Chapter 77 of CM&S.

Pruritic Urticarial Papules and Plaques of Pregnancy (PUPPP)

Definition

Pruritic urticarial papules and plaques of pregnancy (PUPPP) is a relatively common, intensely pruritic dermatosis of pregnancy that typically occurs late in the third trimester in primigravidas.

Clinical Description

PUPPP typically first develops on the abdomen, especially within periumbilical striae distensae, while the umbilicus itself is usually spared in contrast to patients with herpes gestationis. PUPPP is characterized by the onset of many 1 to 2 mm erythematous, edematous occasionally vesicular papules that are extremely pruritic. Lesions often coalesce to form urticarial plaques that may involve large portions of the abdomen. Over several days, lesions often extend to involve the lower trunk, buttocks, thighs, and, at times, the legs, feet, arms, and hands. Lesions rarely develop above the breasts or on the face.

PUPPP usually begins during the latter part of the third trimester of pregnancy. Seventy percent of cases develop in primigravidas.

PUPPP usually responds to treatment within days and resolves completely after delivery; some cases clear before delivery. In contrast to herpes gestationis, PUPPP does not demonstrate a tendency to flare post partum, develop in subsequent pregnancies, or recur after exposure to oral contraceptives. PUPPP is not associated with an increased risk of fetal morbidity or mortality.

Diagnosis and Differential Diagnosis

It is important to distinguish PUPPP from the urticarial form of herpes gestationis. Early forms of herpes gestationis may be solely urticarial and mimic PUPPP to a great degree. Other disorders unrelated to pregnancy that are in the differential diagnosis of PUPPP include erythema multiforme, drug eruptions, contact dermatitis, insect bites, scabies, and common urticaria.

Treatment

The goal of therapy in patients with PUPPP is to relieve pruritus, halt progression of the eruption, and hasten its resolution. Most patients respond to frequent applications of potent topical glucocorticosteroids. As patients respond to treatment, therapy should be gradually tapered rather than abruptly stopped. Patients with extensive eruptions or those refractory to treatment with topical glucocorticosteroids usually respond to a tapering course of systemic glucocorticosteroids (e.g., prednisone, 40 mg every morning for 3 to 5 days, then tapered over the subsequent 7 to 14 days by 5 mg at 2- to 3-day intervals).

Impetigo Herpetiformis

Definition

Impetigo herpetiformis is a form of pustular psoriasis that occurs during pregnancy.

Clinical Description

Impetigo herpetiformis typically has an acute, febrile onset characterized by the development of grouped erythematous plaques that are rimmed with small sterile pustules. Lesional plaques predominate in flexural areas and expand peripherally, with new pustules forming at their leading edge. Impetigo herpetiformis may progress to involve a substantial portion of body surface area. Less frequently, involvement of mucous membranes and nails may occur.

Impetigo herpetiformis is typically associated with significant constitutional symptoms, and hypocalcemia and secondary delirium, seizures, and tetany occur without aggressive management.

Impetigo herpetiformis tends to begin in the third trimester of pregnancy and usually remits promptly after delivery but may recur in subsequent pregnancies. A number of reports have associated impetigo herpetiformis with an increased risk of maternal and fetal mortality.

Diagnosis and Differential Diagnosis

Infectious causes of pustular eruptions in pregnant patients should be distinguished from the sterile pustules of impetigo herpetiformis.

Treatment

Patients with impetigo herpetiformis require specialized care and careful monitoring for evidence of hypoalbuminemia, fluid loss, or infection. Systemic glucocorticosteroids are the mainstay of treatment; prednisone in doses as high as 60 mg per day is sometimes required to control the eruption. The dose of prednisone should be tapered slowly to avoid flares of disease in patients responding to treatment.

Prurigo Gravidarum

Definition and Clinical Description

Prurigo gravidarum is a hepatic condition that usually occurs late in pregnancy, and is believed to be hormonally induced in susceptible individuals. The initial cutaneous manifestation is pruritus, which usually precedes the onset of jaundice by 2 to 4 weeks. In severe cases, excoriations, jaundice, nausea, vomiting, and right upper quadrant abdominal discomfort may be observed. Prurigo gravidarum tends to remit soon after delivery but typically recurs in subsequent gestations. It may also recur in susceptible individuals after their exposure to oral contraceptives.

Some reports have suggested that there is an increased incidence of prematurity, stillbirth, and postpartum hemorrhage in patients with prurigo gravidarum.

Diagnosis and Differential Diagnosis

It is important to exclude other causes of pruritus during pregnancy, including scabies, drug reactions, underlying lymphomas, hepatitis, or other liver diseases.

Treatment

Therapy in patients with prurigo gravidarum is entirely symptomatic.

NEUTROPHILIC DERMATOSES

(CM&S Chapter 38)

Sweet's syndrome and bowel-associated dermatitis-arthritis syndrome are two neutrophilic dermatoses with similar, yet distinguishable, clinical features that are characterized microscopically by neutrophilic infiltrates.

Sweet's Syndrome

Clinical Description

In 1964, R. D. Sweet described a syndrome that he called an "acute febrile neutrophilic dermatosis" and that was characterized by four primary features: (1) a cutaneous eruption consisting of tender erythematous papules and plaques; (2) histopathologic features of dermal, nonvasculitic, neutrophilic inflammation; (3) fever; and (4) peripheral neutrophilia. Subsequently, other extracutaneous manifestations, including associated malignancy, have been described. The cause of Sweet's syndrome remains unknown.

Cutaneous Manifestations

The cutaneous eruption may be polymorphous. Early lesions usually consist of tender, erythematous papules that rapidly increase in size to form plaques that may be studded with pustules. The papules and plaques frequently have an irregular, "pseudovesicular" surface. This surface change has also been described as mamillated. Occasionally, vesicular and bullous lesions on an erythematous and violaceous base predominate. These latter lesions progress to frank ulceration with copious purulent discharge closely resembling pyoderma gangrenosum. Both types of lesions are typically exquisitely tender.

The lesions are most commonly located on the upper extremities, head, and neck but may occur on any cutaneous surface. If untreated, the eruption will typically resolve in 5 to 12 weeks; however, recurrent episodes are seen in one third of patients.

Extracutaneous Manifestations

Patients with Sweet's syndrome often develop fever, an upper respiratory tract or flu-like illness, myalgias, arthralgias, arthritis, and peripheral blood neutrophilia. The arthritis is nonerosive and is responsive to systemic corticosteroid therapy. Concurrent conjunctivitis and iridocyclitis occur in patients with Sweet's syndrome. Ocular involvement does not often result in permanent injury and is generally responsive to oral corticosteroids.

Malignancy-Associated Sweet's Syndrome

Malignancy occurs in approximately 20% of patients with Sweet's syndrome. The vast majority of the malignancies are hematopoietic; and of these, acute myelogenous leukemia is the most common. Unlike idiopathic Sweet's syndrome, neutrophilia and preceding symptoms of upper respiratory tract illness are less common in malignancy-associated Sweet's syndrome.

Cutaneous lesions precede or are the presenting sign of new or recurrent malignancy in approximately two thirds of patients with malignancy-associated Sweet's syndrome. Patients with malignancy-associated Sweet's syndrome frequently have more severe vesicular, bullous, and ulcerative lesions, and recurrences are more common. Both idiopathic and malignancy-associated Sweet's syndrome respond equally well to systemic corticosteroids.

Laboratory Findings

Laboratory findings are nonspecific, but leukocytosis and an elevated sedimentation rate are often seen. Other nonspecific laboratory findings include slight elevation of alkaline phosphatase and minimal transient increases in hepatic aspartate transaminase and γ-glutamyltransferase. Autoantibodies against neutrophil cytoplasmic antigens (ANCA) may also be present.

Pathology

Diffuse, dermal nodular and perivascular neutrophilic infiltrates without overt vasculitis are characteristic of well-developed papular or plaque-like lesions of Sweet's syndrome. Edema of the papillary dermis is commonly present and can result in subepidermal vesiculation.

Diagnosis and Differential Diagnosis

The clinical differential diagnosis of early papular Sweet's syndrome includes erythema multiforme, urticaria, urticarial vasculitis, erythema elevatum diutinum, cutaneous lymphoma, and leukemia. The differential diagnosis of more advanced lesions of pseudovesicular and ulcerated Sweet's syndrome includes pyoderma gangrenosum and halogenoderma, cutaneous pyoderma, deep fungal infections, atypical mycobacterial infections, and parasitic infections such as leishmaniasis.

Some patients present with cutaneous lesions that have some features of both pyoderma gangrenosum and Sweet's syndrome and have been termed *atypical bullous pyoderma gangrenosum* or *atypical Sweet's syndrome*. Close examination for extracutaneous involvement and associations, especially myelodysplastic disorders, is suggested in these patients.

Treatment

Prednisone (0.5–1.0 mg/kg/day) administered as a single daily dose is very effective, and cutaneous lesions resolve rapidly over 3 to 5 days. Extracutaneous symptoms also respond well to prednisone therapy. Systemic corticosteroids can then be tapered over 4 to 6 weeks.

Alternative therapies or corticosteroid-sparing agents include dapsone (100–200 mg/day), potassium iodide (900 mg/day), colchicine (1.5 mg/day), indomethacin, and clofazime.

Bowel-Associated Dermatosis-Arthritis Syndrome

Clinical Description

The bowel-bypass syndrome is an episodic cutaneous eruption with influenza-like symptoms that occurs in some patients after jejunoileal bypass surgery for morbid obesity, in patients with inflammatory bowel disease, and in others who have undergone Bilroth II procedures for duodenal or peptic ulcers.

The cutaneous eruption begins as small erythematous macules and progresses to urticarial papules and purpuric vesiculopustules over 24 to 48 hours. This eruption is typically distributed over the upper extremities and upper trunk. Erythema nodosum involving the lower extremities may also occur concomitantly.

Serum sickness–like symptoms of arthralgia, myalgia, malaise, chills, and fever are present and frequently precede the cutaneous eruption. Nonerosive polyarthritis and tendonitis also occur. The eruption and systemic symptoms typically last from 2 to 8 days and recur at varying intervals.

Diagnosis and Differential Diagnosis

The differential diagnosis of pustulopapular lesions of bowel-associated dermatosis-arthritis syndrome includes disseminated gonococcemia, pustular arthropod bite reactions, folliculitis, and furunculosis. Macular and papular lesions of bowel-associated dermatosis-arthritis syndrome may resemble urticaria, erythema multiforme, and Sweet's syndrome.

Treatment

Reanastomosis in patients who have had intestinal bypass surgery is curative. Prednisone (10–60 mg/day) suppresses both cutaneous and arthritic involvement. Dapsone and a variety of antibodies, including minocycline, trimethoprim, sulfamethoxazole, erythromycin, and metronidazole, are also sometimes effective. Skin lesions and constitutional symptoms frequently recur on discontinuation of therapy.

PYODERMA GANGRENOSUM

(CM&S Chapter 39)

Definition

Pyoderma gangrenosum is a chronic and recurrent ulcerative condition of the skin. Although the morphology of individual lesions is distinctive, histopathologic and laboratory findings are nonspecific and variable. Pyoderma gangrenosum is characteristically associated with certain systemic diseases; however, no underlying illness can be detected in a substantial number of cases.

Clinical Description

Pyoderma gangrenosum is most common in persons 20 to 49 years old. Lesions may occur anywhere on the body. They are more often multiple than single and are most common on the lower extremities. Lesions tend to occur at sites of trauma, although spontaneous development of pyoderma gangrenosum is common.

The fully developed lesion of pyoderma gangrenosum is an ulcer with a purulent base and a ragged, undermined, violaceous border. The disorder begins as a small papule, often in a follicular location, that rapidly develops into a pustule. Vesicles and bullae have also been described. The surrounding skin is indurated and erythematous. The central portion of the primary lesion undergoes necrosis, and the border spreads peripherally. The resulting ulcer may be shallow or deep enough to expose underlying tendons and muscles. The cyanotic, overhanging edge and its surrounding zone of erythema extend centrifugally, sometimes at a rate of 1 to 2 cm per 24 hours. The well-developed border of the ulcer may assume a round, ovoid, or serpiginous configuration. Individual lesions range from 1 to 2 cm to 20 to 30 cm and may coalesce to form even larger ulcers.

Lesions of pyoderma gangrenosum may exhibit a chronic indolent or rapidly progressive course. Pain is often significant, although other systemic symptoms are generally absent. With treatment, the ulcers reepithelialize from the margins inward, resulting in atrophic, cribriform scars with pigmentary alteration.

Associated Conditions

An underlying systemic disease is present in approximately 50% of patients. The most commonly reported associations include inflammatory bowel disease, arthritis, and lymphoproliferative disorders.

Variants of Pyoderma Gangrenosum

Bullous Pyoderma Gangrenosum. In this condition, the lesions resemble early acute lesions of pyoderma gangrenosum. Pustules and ulcers with a blue-gray bullous border have been described. The lesions tend to be distributed primarily on the face and upper extremities, and heal with a more superficial scar than typical pyoderma gangrenosum. An association with lymphoproliferative diseases has been reported. Many cases of bullous pyoderma gangrenosum are difficult to distinguish from Sweet's syndrome.

Pathology

The histopathology of pyoderma gangrenosum varies depending on the evolutionary stage of the lesion. Early lesions (papulopustules) show changes of a deep suppurative folliculitis involving the pilosebaceous unit. Changes of leukocytoclastic vasculitis, when seen, are likely secondary to the intense neutrophilic infiltrate. Ulcer beds show a suppurative dermatitis and panniculitis. The peripheral boggy, undermined margins of the ulcers show epidermal acanthosis and spongiosis with neutrophil microabscesses and massive papillary dermal edema. In the surrounding zone of erythema, a dense lymphocytic infiltrate, angioplasia, endothelial swelling, and perivascular fibrin deposition may be prominent.

Diagnosis and Differential Diagnosis

Early pustular and nodular lesions can be confused with folliculitis or furunculosis and thus should be evaluated for a possible infectious etiology. Insect bites, halogenodermas, and various forms of panniculitis can also mimic early lesions of pyoderma gangrenosum.

Ulcerative lesions of pyoderma gangrenosum should also be evaluated for a possible infectious cause. Deep mycoses, bacterial and mycobacterial infections, tertiary syphilis, chronic ulcerative herpes simplex, and infections by other unusual organisms must be considered, especially in immunosuppressed patients. Vasculitis (especially Wegener's granulomatosis), vascular insufficiency (either venous or arterial), insect bites (including those of the brown recluse spider), halogenodermas, necrobiosis lipoidica, and warfarin (Coumadin) or heparin necrosis should be excluded. The possibility of factitial ulcers must also be considered. Biopsy and appropriate cultures are essential in diagnosing pyoderma gangrenosum. Although the histopathology of pyoderma gangrenosum is characteristic rather than pathognomonic, the findings in many of the other conditions are specific.

Additional evaluation is necessary to investigate the presence of an underlying disorder. Studies of the gastrointestinal tract, serologic studies and radiographic examination, complete blood cell count, bone marrow aspirate and biopsy, and serum and urine protein electrophoresis and immunoelectrophoresis are useful in the evaluation.

Treatment

If there is an underlying systemic disorder, its treatment may improve the cutaneous disease. Adequate analgesia is required for the often excessively painful ulcers.

The treatment of pyoderma gangrenosum includes a combination of local and systemic modalities. The importance of local care cannot be overemphasized. Whirlpool baths, compresses (including saline, aluminum subacetate, and 0.25% acetic acid), topical antibacterial agents (including topical antibiotics, 20% benzoyl peroxide, and silver sulfadiazine), appropriate dressings (including the newer bio-occlusive dressings), leg elevation, and rest may be sufficient to heal small ulcers or may provide a favorable local environment for the therapeutic effect of more aggressive systemic therapies.

Immunosuppressive agents are most frequently used in the treatment of pyoderma gangrenosum. Corticosteroids may be used topically, intralesionally, or systemically. Rarely, application of superpotent topical steroids may halt the progression of early papular or pustular lesions; more often, however, intralesional steroid therapy works best in the preulcerative stage. Triamcinolone, 5 to 10 mg/mL, is delivered by multiple injections of small quantities of the solution at the periphery and base of the lesions.

For patients unresponsive to local measures or for those with rapidly progressive, widespread disease, systemic therapy is justified. Systemic administration of corticosteroids is most often used. Therapy is initiated at a dose of 60 to 120 mg prednisone daily, given as a single dose with breakfast. Patients with normal glucose-6-phosphate dehydrogenase levels may also receive dapsone, initially at a dose of 25 to 50 mg daily, increasing to 100 to 200 mg daily over 2 to 3 weeks, with appropriate hematologic monitoring. When the ulcers have stopped expanding and appear to be granulating, and the peripheral erythema has disappeared, the prednisone dose should gradually be tapered over 6 to 12 weeks.

Intermittent pulse corticosteroid therapy may be chosen as an alternative to daily administration of prednisone, since the former regimen may be associated with fewer long-term steroid-related side effects.

Cytotoxic agents may be used in patients with severe pyoderma gangrenosum. Azathioprine or cyclophosphamide may be combined with systemic corticosteroid therapy for its steroid-sparing activity, especially in patients with steroid-related side effects. Recently, cyclosporine has been reported to be successful in treating severe pyoderma gangrenosum. Required doses range from 5 to 6 mg/kg per day; as with other therapies, recurrences may be noted as the dose of the drug is tapered. Tacrolimus (FK 506), another immunosuppressive drug with pharmacologic properties and side effects similar to those of cyclosporine, also appears to have potential in the treatment of recalcitrant pyoderma gangrenosum.

Antimicrobial agents reported to be effective include clofazimine, sulfasalazine, minocycline, and rifampin.

BEHÇET'S DISEASE

(CM&S Chapter 40)

Definition

Behçet's disease is a persistent, relapsing, multisystemic disorder with prominent mucocutaneous findings. Behçet's disease is rare and has a broad range of clinical findings, the classic triad being oral aphthae, genital ulceration, and ocular disease. Its cause is not known, and only a few possible triggering or predisposing factors have been identified. It is clear that a circulating immune complex–dependent, neutrophil-mediated vasculitis is at least one of the fundamental pathogenic processes in Behçet's disease.

Clinical Description

The disorder is protean, and all organs should be considered as candidates for dysfunction when a diagnosis of Behçet's disease is contemplated. Men are afflicted more frequently than women. Symptoms arise in the third decade in a striking majority of patients. Behçet's disease occurs worldwide, but persons of Mediterranean or Japanese descent are more commonly affected than their Western European counterparts.

Orogenital Manifestations

Oral or orogenital aphthae develop in virtually every patient. The aphthae of Behçet's disease differ from common oral aphthae (''canker sores'') in that they can be large, multiple, and more frequently recurrent. Oral aphthae are often the initial manifestation of Behçet's disease. The typical primary lesion begins as a red papule that quickly develops into a shallow, circumscribed ulcer less than 1 cm in diameter. The aphthae occur in crops, persist for 1 to 3 weeks, and then resolve, only to recur days to weeks later. In some patients, aphthae are almost continuously present or may coalesce to form large ulcerations. Aphthae are most frequently found on the tongue, buccal or gingival mucosa, and lips.

Genital aphthae resemble their oral counterparts but are generally fewer in number, deeper, more painful, and have a higher tendency to scar. The scrotum is the predominant site in men, and women characteristically develop vulvar ulcers. Penile, vaginal, or perianal aphthae can also occur, but less commonly.

Cutaneous Manifestations

Many cutaneous findings have been described in association with or attributed to Behçet's disease. Primary lesions that appear to be truly attributable to Behçet's disease include sterile vesiculopustular papules and plaques, pustular vasculitic lesions, and erythema nodosum–like nodules and plaques.

Papules and plaques of Behçet's disease are most commonly acral. Papules may be pustular and purpuric with a vasculitic appearance and can be induced by minor trauma, the so-called pathergic reaction. Either an aseptic needle prick or a local injection of a minute amount of normal saline or a dilute (1 mg/mL) histamine solution can be used as the inducing stimulus. Pustular papules develop in crops, abate without treatment after 1 to 2 weeks, and become recrudescent days to weeks later.

The plaques are erythematous and edematous, and the erythema nodosum–like lesions are typically slightly infiltrated, slightly erythematous plaques that develop on the legs and buttocks, lasting 1 to 3 weeks. Erythema nodosum–like lesions also need to be distinguished clinically from subcutaneous thrombophlebitis, which develops in roughly 30% of patients with Behçet's disease.

Ocular Manifestations

Ocular disease can be the presenting feature of Behçet's disease in a minority of patients, but ocular manifestations typically lag months to years behind mucocutaneous changes. Ocular disease is common and develops in 75% to 100% of patients. Once one eye is affected, both eyes will inevitably become involved. Patients experience a blurring of vision, and the acuity loss progresses to blindness if not treated. The uveitis (iritis) that develops in the anterior chamber can progress to hypopyon without treatment. The uveitis and vasculitis that affect the posterior segment yield edema and thickening early, with vascular occlusion and retinal necrosis (resulting in blindness) later.

Joint Manifestations

Roughly 50% of all patients with Behçet's disease eventually develop articular disease. The arthritis is oligoarticular (affecting one to four joints) and nondestructive, and episodes last less than 2 months in over 80% of cases. Peripheral involvement is the rule, with knees, ankles, and wrists most commonly affected.

Other Systemic Manifestations

Behçet's disease can strike any organ. Central nervous system involvement is unusual with either an abrupt or insidious onset. Symptoms and signs are headache and meningismus, and cortical dysfunction, cerebellar signs, and cranial nerve palsies develop in patients with severe disease.

Vascular involvement presents as arterial aneurysms or venous thromboses. The latter frequently present as recurrent superficial thrombophlebitis. Gastrointestinal complaints are relatively common, occurring in roughly 50% of patients. The primary lesions are small ulcerations that resemble orogenital aphthae. Abdominal pain and gastrointestinal hemorrhage are the chief manifestations of Behçet's colitis.

Pathology

The earliest changes of induced lesions are those of leukocytoclastic vasculitis. In many patients, biopsy specimens reveal diffuse neutrophilic infiltrates with leukocytoclastic debris but with subtle or imperceptible changes of vasculitis.

Pathogenesis and Etiology

The fact that certain HLA types are overrepresented in affected patients suggests that genetic factors are important in the development of the disorder, perhaps at the level of an immunologic control mechanism. The strongest association is with HLA-B51, particularly in patients of Japanese or Mediterranean ethnicity.

Diagnosis and Differential Diagnosis

No single symptom, physical finding, or laboratory test permits a specific diagnosis of Behçet's disease. The diagnosis remains a clinical one, based on a summation of clinical criteria. New criteria developed by an international study group (Table 2–17) focus on major manifestations, exclude consideration of rare or subjective manifestations, and state acceptable clinical features to fulfill each criterion.

Since Behçet's disease is diagnosed on the basis of clinical criteria, the diagnosis of early disease is often challenging because not all manifestations have developed. It is important to exclude infection from the differential diagnosis in the evaluation of early disease. The main considerations in the differential diagnosis include neutrophilic dermatoses, infections, vesiculobullous eruptions, and erosive interface dermatitides.

TABLE 2–17. Criteria for the Diagnosis of Behçet's Disease

CRITERION	REQUIRED FEATURES
Recurrent oral ulceration	Aphthous (idiopathic) ulceration, observed by physician or patient, with at least three episodes in any 12-month period
Plus any two of the following:	
Recurrent genital ulceration	Aphthous ulceration or scarring observed by physician or patient
Eye lesions	Anterior or posterior uveitis; cells in vitreous in slit lamp examination; or retinal vasculitis documented by ophthalmologist
Skin lesions	Erythema nodosum–like lesions observed by physician or patient; papulopustular skin lesions or pseudofolliculitis; or characteristic acneiform nodules observed by physician
Pathergy test	Interpreted at 24 to 48 hours by physician

From International Study Group for Behçet's Disease. Criteria for diagnosis of Behçet's disease. Lancet 1990;335:1078–1080.

Treatment

Because Behçet's disease follows an episodic course and there are few patients with Behçet's disease even at large medical centers, most accepted therapies have been defined on the basis of anecdotal experience and open clinical trials. For patients with mucosal disease or limited mucocutaneous disease, the goal of therapy is generally palliation of symptoms. Either local or systemic therapies can be used. For patients at risk for significant morbidity, including those with ocular and neurologic involvement, systemic therapies should be aggressively employed (Table 2–18).

URTICARIA

(CM&S Chapter 41)

Definition and Clinical Description

Urticaria (hives) consists of pale to red, well-demarcated, transient, pruritic swellings involving the dermis, which vary from a few millimeters to many centimeters in size. They are often round or oval, but may coalesce into plaques with irregular borders or evolve into annular, arcuate, or serpiginous lesions. Urticarial lesions may be surrounded by an area of pallor or erythema. Individual lesions of urticaria typically last less than 24 hours, which differentiates them from other cutaneous disorders that present with a hive-like morphology. Urticaria occurring up to 6 weeks has been empirically classified as acute disease, whereas recurrent attacks of hives lasting more than 6 weeks are arbitrarily defined as chronic urticaria. While acute urticaria is more common in children and young adults, chronic urticaria is more prevalent in adults.

Urticaria may be idiopathic or a reaction to a known agent. Hives and itching usually have an abrupt presentation in acute urticaria. Respiratory or gastrointestinal complaints are generally absent or minor. The majority of patients with chronic urticaria have idiopathic disease, although they also may have one or more associated physical urticarial reactions that may be caused by heat, cold, vibration, pressure, light, and water. Fifty per cent of patients experiencing chronic urticaria will be free of their hives after 1 year, while 20% continue to experience their eruption for more than 20 years.

Types of Urticaria

Cholinergic Urticaria. Cholinergic urticaria refers to a common disease triggered by an increase in body temperature, which may occur after a hot shower or exercise. The lesions are usually smaller (2 to 4 mm) than other urticarial wheals and are either flesh colored or erythematous. Exposure to external heat has caused urticaria associated with pulsatile headaches, flushing, nausea, and dizziness. In several patients, local heat challenge has resulted in the formation of large wheals, rather than the small lesions of cholinergic urticaria, suggesting that cholinergic and heat urticaria are different syndromes. Diaphoresis and respiratory symptoms, including bronchoconstriction, may accompany cholinergic urticaria. Similar urticarial lesions may develop following periods of stress and have been termed *adrenergic urticaria*.

TABLE 2-18. Treatment of Behçet's Disease

TYPE OF THERAPY	DRUG	DOSE	INDICATION	SIDE EFFECTS/MONITORING
Local	Clobetasol proplonate ointment		Aphthae	None
	Tetracycline	250 mg/5 mL	Aphthae	None
	Viscous lidocaine		Aphthae	None
	Intralesional triamcinolone	10–40 mg/mL	Aphthae	Risk of local atrophy, Cushing's syndrome with repetitive dosage
Systemic Therapy for Limited Disease	Dapsone	100–200 mg per day	Aphthae, pustular skin lesions	Glucose-6-phosphate dehydrogenase screening before initiation of therapy; follow complete blood cell count (CBC)
	Colchicine	0.6 mg bid	Aphthae, pustular skin lesions	Gastrointestinal intolerance; follow CBC
	Methotrexate	2.5–20 mg per week	Aphthae, pustular skin lesions, arthritis	Hematopoietic, renal and hepatic toxicities; CBC, liver function tests, and serum creatinine test before initiation of and during therapy; periodic liver biopsy

Systemic Therapy for Progressive or Highly Morbid Disease			
Nonsteroidal anti-inflammatory drugs		Arthritis, aphthae, or cutaneous lesions	Gastrointestinal intolerance
Prednisone	1–2 mg/kg per day	Severe mucocutaneous or systemic disease	Cushing's syndrome with prolonged therapy
Azathioprine	1–2.5 mg/kg per day	Severe mucocutaneous or systemic disease, including ocular disease	Follow CBC
Cyclosporine	10 mg/kg per day initial dose; then 3–5 mg/kg per day	Refractory and severe mucocutaneous or systemic disease	Dose-related renal toxicity requiring complex laboratory follow-up, including blood drug levels; increased risk of infection or lipoid proliferation due to immunosuppression
Interferon gamma	100 μg per day in subcutis initial dose	Severe mucocutaneous or systemic disease	Fever and myalgias; neurotoxicity and cardiotoxicity not observed at low dosages

Cold-Induced Urticaria. Immersion in cold water and/or exposure to cold air may provoke urticaria in some patients. Lesions of cold urticaria typically appear as the skin begins to rewarm. Acquired, idiopathic cold urticaria is the most common form of this disorder and usually appears within minutes of cold exposure. Patients often develop an urticarial lesion at the site where an ice cube has been applied for 5 minutes. Acquired cold urticaria also may develop in association with a cryoprotein (cryoglobulin, cryofibrinogen, or cold agglutinin), which in some cases is due to a viral illness, paroxysmal hemoglobinuria, or syphilis. Familial cold urticaria is a rare disorder with autosomal dominant transmission in which morbilliform lesions typically appear 30 minutes after cold exposure and have a burning sensation. Systemic complaints may include fever, chills, arthralgias, and leukocytosis. The ice cube test is often negative. Headache, dyspnea, vertigo, and tachycardia may accompany severe attacks of cold-induced urticaria; however, gastrointestinal complaints and edema of the pharynx or tongue after exposure to cold foods are rare. A condition termed *cold erythema* appears to be a variant of cold urticaria and is characterized by erythema and pain at the site of cold exposure.

Pressure-Induced Urticaria. Dermatographism is defined as erythema and wheal formation occurring within minutes after firmly stroking or scratching the skin. Up to 9% of the general population may have dermatographism. Dermatographism is best thought of as a clinical entity distinct from pressure urticaria, and occurs in persons without urticaria, as well as in patients with acute or chronic urticaria and angioedema. Dermatographism can be present for years or may be a transient phenomenon associated with drug administration or scabies. Delayed dermatographism, in which lesions appear 30 minutes to several hours after skin trauma, has been reported.

Urticaria due to pressure can be delayed. Lesions of delayed pressure urticaria are often tender wheals that develop at sites of trauma such as the hand after carrying a briefcase or tightly gripping a tool, the shoulder from carrying a piece of heavy luggage by its strap, and the feet after walking or running. Lesions of delayed pressure urticaria appear 30 minutes to 9 hours after the stimulus, last an average of 36 hours, and may be associated with malaise, fever, chills, or headaches. Most patients with delayed pressure urticaria have concomitant chronic idiopathic urticaria/angioedema. Delayed pressure urticaria responds predictably only to systemic corticosteroids.

Solar Urticaria. Light-induced urticaria is a rare disorder caused by electromagnetic radiation that stimulates lesion formation within minutes to hours after exposure. Patients with this disorder rarely experience anaphylaxis, but they can be exquisitely sensitive to light.

Aquagenic Urticaria. Water may induce small urticarial wheals that appear within minutes of exposure. Coating the skin with petrolatum often prevents lesions of aquagenic urticaria, as does pretreatment with topical scopolamine, which suggests a neural component to the disease.

Contact Urticaria. Urticaria induced by contactants most often is characterized by whealing and erythema, but can manifest simply as stinging, burning, or itching after contact with a specific agent. Asthma, rhinitis, and eczematous lesions may occur in association with lesions of contact urticaria. Contact urticaria may be immune mediated or nonimmunologically based. Latex rubber is a common cause of immunologically mediated contact urticaria and has caused symptoms ranging from localized erythema and pruritus from latex gloves to anaphylaxis and death from exposure to barium enema catheter cuffs. Other low-molecular-weight chemicals that also cause IgE-mediated contact urticaria include drugs, acid anhydrides, mercaptobenzothiazole, nickel, dyes, isocyanates, and epoxy resin compounds. Cinnamates and ammonium persulfate induce contact urticaria on a nonimmunologic basis. Contact urticaria lesions may last from only a few minutes to several days.

Angioedema

Angioedema is the term used to describe deeper swellings of the skin and subcutis, which most often involve the eyelids, lips, tongue, genitalia, hands, and feet, with the larynx, gastrointestinal tract, and urinary bladder being less commonly affected. Angioedema may be acute or chronic and can occur without urticaria. Most cases are idiopathic; however, angioedema has been associated with physical and contact urticarias, as well as recurrent attacks consisting of eosinophilia, fever, and acute weight gain. Hereditary angioedema (HAE) is an autosomal-dominant disorder caused by a deficiency in C1-esterase inhibitor and is characterized by recurrent attacks of painful angioedema of the skin and mucosa of the upper respiratory and gastrointestinal tracts. Death from laryngeal edema can occur in as many as 26% of affected, untreated persons. Attacks, which may last from 2 to 4 days, are commonly initiated by minor trauma, emotional upset, infections, and exposure to sudden temperature changes. Without C1-esterase inhibitor, the complement cascade is activated, resulting in the generation of the anaphylatoxins C3a and C5a as well as other pharmacologically active chemical mediators.

Pathology

The histologic picture of urticaria includes vasodilatation, dermal edema, and a sparse to rarely dense perivascular infiltrate of T lymphocytes, eosinophils, and monocytes and a variably increased number of mast cells and neutrophils.

Pathogenesis and Etiology

A large number of studies indicate that mast cells and their mediators are central to the pathogenesis of most, but possibly not all, urticaria syndromes. Mast cells are normal residents of the skin and are known to produce and store numerous mediators. Activation of these cells by both immune and nonimmune mechanisms leads to a wheal and flare reaction like that seen in urticaria.

Mast Cells

Cutaneous mast cells are located around capillaries, lymphatics, appendages, and nerves. Their location and mediators allow them to directly affect and respond to resident dermal cells as well as inflammatory cells that traffic through the skin. They are 5 to 15 μm, ovoid to tadpole-like or even spindle-shaped cells that histologically have the appearance of a fried egg. Mast cells, which are also found in the gastrointestinal tract and lung, have characteristic 0.2 to 0.5 μm diameter secretory granules, which contain preformed mediators that are released upon activation. Mast cells express high-affinity IgE receptors FcϵRI on their surface, to which the Fc portion of IgE antibodies binds. Preformed mast cell mediators include histamine, heparin, proteoglycans, and chemotactic factors. Other mediators are formed at the time of mast cell stimulation. Mast cells also express opioid, adenosine, and beta-adrenergic receptors, but, unlike basophils, do not have H_1 histamine receptors. The normal physiologic function of mast cells is still unknown but likely involves homeostatic regulation both of nerves and blood vessels as well as host defense.

Mast Cell Mediators

Mast cells have their major effect in tissues by releasing a wide array of biologically potent mediators. Histamine, which is made predominately by mast cells, acts on many tissues through three receptors designated H_1, H_2, and H_3. Histamine mediates the "triple response" of Lewis in skin, which consists of a local vasodilation (flare); wheal formation as a result of endothelial cell contraction and increased capillary permeability; and expanding erythema, which is mediated by histamine-induced neuropeptide release. Other mast cell inflammatory mediators include heparin, proteases, TNFα, and the eicosanoids PGD_2 and LTC_4.

Mast Cell Stimulation

Mast cells can be stimulated to release their mediators through both immune and nonimmune mechanisms. Immunologic stimuli result in fusion of mast cell secretory granule membranes with the plasma membrane and subsequent release of the granule contents. Following immunologic stimulation, human mast cells become refractory to subsequent immunologic activation, thereby permitting time to generate new granule-associated mediators. While it is clear that mast cell activation can occur from exogenous agents, such as antigens and opiates, endogenous molecules, cytokines, histamine-releasing factors, neuropeptides, and autoantibodies also are important mast cell stimulators.

Pathogenesis

Antigen binding to IgE antibodies on the mast cell surface is probably the most common etiology for acute urticaria, and the antigens in these cases frequently are foods, drugs, and infectious agents. In addition to immune-mediated causes, there are possible nonimmune factors that cause urticaria and angioedema. For example, urticaria induced by contrast media appears to be nonimmunologic and is likely related to the ionic strength of the medium. Aspirin and nonsteroidal anti-inflammatory agents also cause and exacerbate chronic urticaria that appears to be mediated by nonimmune mechanisms. Anecdotal reports have linked sudden emotional stress to the onset of urticaria and angioedema, although this association is not understood. Despite the myriad reported causes of chronic urticaria, up to 90% of cases remain idiopathic.

The pathogenesis of urticaria and angioedema is not well understood, but may result from a series of pathologic events that includes mast cell activation and mediator release, stimulation of local sensory nerves, and infiltration of varying types and numbers of inflammatory cells that also release proinflammatory cytokines. The severity and duration of this inflammatory reaction are dependent upon the type and amount of mediators released, as well as the number and type of inflammatory cells that accumulate in the skin.

Diagnosis and Differential Diagnosis

Diagnosis

The diagnosis of urticaria and angioedema is usually made on the physical examination; however, a thorough history is important for not only establishing the diagnosis but also for elucidating possible causes. Screening laboratory tests and skin testing are not helpful and are not cost-effective for these disorders; however, specific tests should be obtained based on information gained from the history and physical examination. Testing for physical urticaria depends on the type of urticaria being considered. For cholinergic urticaria, patients may be challenged by exercising or by immersing an extremity in warm (42° C) water for 15 minutes. For dermatographism, stroke the skin using a retracted pen or blunt instrument. Pressure urticaria may be induced by hanging a *strap* with 15 pounds of weight on the shoulders or thigh for 20 minutes. Solar urticaria can be induced with a variety of tests to UVB, UVA, and visible light; the ice cube test is used for cold urticaria; aquagenic urticaria is tested by applying a water soaked gauze on the skin for several minutes.

Differential Diagnosis

The differential diagnosis of urticaria includes mastocytosis, systemic lupus erythematosus, serum sickness, juvenile rheumatoid arthritis, pruritic urticarial papules and plaques of pregnancy (PUPPP), dermatitis herpetiformis, bullous pemphigoid, herpes gestationis, and urticarial vasculitis. Lesions of erythema multiforme and figurate erythemas such as erythema annulare centrifugum, erythema chronicum migrans, and erythema marginatum may simulate urticarial lesions.

On rare occasions, panniculitis, cellulitis, lymphangitis, and cheilitis granulomatosa may initially mimic lesions of angioedema; however, unlike angioedema, these disorders persist for longer than 24 hours.

Treatment

The most effective treatment of urticaria and angioedema is the identification and elimination of the cause. There are a number of pharmacologic agents that are effective for the treatment of urticaria and angioedema.

Antihistamines

Antihistamines are the only currently available, specific inhibitors of a mast cell mediator and are the first line of therapy. They are most effective in acute urticaria, cholinergic urticaria, and dermatographism; somewhat effective in solar, cold, aquagenic, and chronic idiopathic urticaria; and rarely useful in delayed pressure urticaria. There are six classes of first-generation antihistamines, with the ethanolamines (diphenhydramine), ethylenediamines (tripelennamine), and phenothiazines (promethazine) causing the most sedation. Piperidines (cyproheptadine) are especially effective for cholinergic and cold-induced urticaria. Alkylamines (chlorpheniramine, dexchlorpheniramine, brompheniramine) and hydroxyzine appear to be the most useful agents in initial therapy because of efficacy, tolerance, and cost. Dosing should be continuous and is generally increased in strength every 5 to 7 days to tolerance. Most of the antihistamines may lead to weight gain, and the anticholinergic effects of traditional antihistamines can rarely lead to movement disorders after chronic use. All antihistamines, except cetirizine, undergo significant metabolism in the liver.

The second-generation, nonsedating antihistamines that have been developed have limited access to the central nervous system and tend to be more specific for H_1 receptors and less active at serotonin and muscarinic receptors. This antihistamine group is best used if the patient cannot tolerate, or is not helped by, first-generation antihistamines. The combination of two different H_1 antihistamines may prove effective in patients who are unresponsive to a single agent, and in this case, a sedating antihistamine can be taken at night, while a second-generation antihistamine can be used during the day. Both terfenadine and astemizole have been reported to cause cardiac tachyarrhythmias and prolongation of the Q-T interval as a result of accumulation of unmetabolized parent drug in patients with liver disease or those taking ketoconazole, erythromycin, and related antibiotics and antimycotics. The tricyclic antidepressant doxepin has potent anti-H_1 and H_2 receptor activity and can be effective for the treatment of urticaria. Because of its extended half-life, doxepin can be used in doses of 10 to 20 mg twice a day; however, its sedating effects may limit its use to 25 to 30 mg each night. This drug should be used with caution in patients with a history of cardiac arrhythmias, and its anticholinergic side effects may limit its use in the elderly.

Other Treatments

Adrenergic Agents. Subcutaneous epinephrine (1:1000 aqueous epinephrine) at a dose of 0.2 to 0.4 ml in adults or at 0.01 mg/kg for children is useful for treating acute episodes of urticaria and angioedema. Other agents that have been used to treat urticaria and angioedema include systemic corticosteroids, NSAIDs, colchicine, dapsone, sulfasalazine, cyclosporine, synthetic androgens, ultraviolet light, and plasmapheresis.

PERFORATING DISORDERS

(CM&S Chapter 42)

Definition and Clinical Description

The perforating disorders are a group of papulonodular skin diseases characterized by hyperkeratotic plugs or crusts in which dermal connective tissue (collagen or elastic fibers) perforates or is eliminated through the epidermis. The two prototypical diseases are *reactive perforating collagenosis* and *elastosis perforans serpiginosa*. The third perforating disease is *acquired perforating dermatosis* (Kyrle's disease), which is usually acquired in adulthood in association with diabetes mellitus or the pruritus of renal failure. In perforating folliculitis, considered by some to be the fourth perforating disorder, perforation or rupture of the follicles is found. This finding is, however, not specific, occurring in a variety of follicular diseases, including acne, bacterial and fungal folliculitis, and folliculitis from trauma and chemicals.

Reactive Perforating Collagenosis

Reactive perforating collagenosis is a rare familial disorder that begins in childhood. After superficial trauma, patients develop hyperkeratotic papules that reach a size of 5 to 8 mm over the next 3 or 4 weeks. These lesions, which often *Koebnerize*, are most commonly located on the arms and hands. The papules tend to spontaneously resolve over 6 to 8 weeks.

Acquired reactive perforating collagenosis may begin in adulthood, especially in association with diabetes or renal insufficiency, but these cases are best classified as acquired perforating dermatosis, even though the histopathology can be identical to the form arising in childhood.

Elastosis Perforans Serpiginosa

Elastosis perforans serpiginosa is a rare, pruritic, self-limited disorder beginning in childhood or early adulthood. It seems to be genetically determined, since about 40% of cases occur in association with other genetic disorders, including Down syndrome, Ehlers-Danlos syndrome, osteogenesis imperfecta, Marfan's disease, and pseudoxanthoma elasticum. Elastosis perforans serpiginosa can also occur as a complication of treatment with the drug penicillamine. Cases of elastosis perforans serpiginosa associated with renal failure or diabetes are best classified as acquired perforating dermatosis.

The lesions are hyperkeratotic 2- to 5-mm papules that tend to be arranged in a serpiginous or annular pattern, most commonly on the neck, face, or upper extremities. Most patients experience no symptoms or only mild pruritus. Like reactive perforating collagenosis, the lesions may spontaneously resolve, but they tend to persist longer, often for up to several years.

Acquired Perforating Dermatosis (Kyrle's Disease)

Acquired perforating dermatosis has been proposed as a catch-all term for those examples of perforating disease arising in adulthood, usually in association with diabetes or the pruritus of renal failure and less commonly with pruritus secondary to internal malignancy or liver disease. Acquired perforating dermatosis is far more common than the genetically inherited perforating disorders, which ordinarily begin earlier in life and without systemic disease. Kyrle described an acquired perforating disease called hyperkeratosis follicularis et parafollicularis in cutem penetrans, which also has been commonly associated with diabetes and renal failure. It seems reasonable to accept Kyrle's disease as a synonym for acquired perforating dermatosis, but the literature is confusing. Acquired perforating dermatosis is difficult to distinguish from perforating folliculitis, and some consider Kyrle's disease to represent merely end-stage hyperplastic lesions in which it is difficult to determine whether the lesions were initially centered on follicles.

Acquired perforating dermatosis, which may Koebnerize, most commonly occurs on the legs. Generalized or widely scattered hyperkeratotic papules or nodules are common.

Pathology

In all of the perforating diseases, histopathology reveals a hyperkeratotic plug, with variable parakeratosis or crusting. In reactive perforating collagenosis, collagen fibers are seen within the plug or within the epidermis. In elastosis perforans serpiginosa, elastic fibers are seen instead in the same location. In reactive perforating collagenosis, the dermal connective tissue adjacent to the plug appears unremarkable, while in elastosis perforans serpiginosa there is often increased elastic tissue in the superficial dermis.

TABLE 2-19. Differential Diagnosis of Perforating Disorders

REACTIVE PERFORATING COLLAGENOSIS AND KYRLE'S DISEASE

Folliculitis
Prurigo nodularis
Arthropod bites
Keratosis pilaris
Multiple keratoacanthomas
Pityriasis lichenoides
Guttate psoriasis

ELASTOSIS PERFORANS SERPIGINOSA (RESEMBLES OTHER ANNULAR DISEASES)

Granuloma annulare
Actinic granuloma
Porokeratosis
Discoid lupus erythematosus
Tinea

Differential Diagnosis

The differential diagnosis is listed in Table 2–19.

Treatment

Treatment is unnecessary for the genetically inherited forms of reactive perforating collagenosis and elastosis perforans serpiginosa, which generally remain mild and localized and are not problematic. For symptomatic or intensive disease, topical tretinoin, topical corticosteroids, and emollients may be successful, in addition to systemic antihistamines.

Trauma should be avoided in reactive perforating collagenosis. Elastosis perforans serpiginosa may be treated with local cryotherapy, tangential excision, electrosurgical destruction, or cellophane tape stripping.

Treatment for the more generalized acquired perforating dermatitis or extensive perforating folliculitis includes intralesional corticosteroids, oral or topical retinoids, or phototherapy. Phototherapy is a particularly good choice for patients with renal disease, since it often relieves their coexisting pruritus.

CUTANEOUS REACTIONS TO DRUGS AND BIOLOGIC RESPONSE MODIFIERS

(CM&S Chapter 43)

Definition

Adverse cutaneous reactions to systemic drugs are frequent. For commonly used agents, including nonsteroidal anti-inflammatory drugs (NSAIDs), many antibiotics, and antihypertensive agents, more than 1% and not infrequently more than 5% of the patients using these drugs for the first time will develop a reaction rash that is likely to be due to the medicine. Although only a small proportion of these reactions are likely to be life threatening or serious, it is sometimes difficult to distinguish potentially serious reactions from ones that are unsightly or uncomfortable. Cutaneous reactions to drugs are among the most frequent reasons for discontinuing treatment before the completion of a therapeutic course. Adverse reactions to topically applied medicines, erythema multiforme, Stevens-Johnson syndrome, and toxic epidermal necrolysis, which are among the most frequent and important severe adverse cutaneous reactions (see Chapter 3 in Pocket Guide and Chapters 22 and 81 in CM&S), and adverse reactions to chemotherapeutic agents (see Chapter 44 in CM&S) are discussed elsewhere.

Epidemiology

The most comprehensive analysis of overall reaction rates comes from the Boston Collaborative Drug Surveillance Program's evaluation of medical inpatients from 1975 to 1982. In this study, 2.2% of patients were affected by a drug-induced cutaneous reaction during hospitalization. Antibiotics were responsible for 75% of detected reactions. Morbilliform eruptions comprised 94% of drug rashes. Urticaria constituted an additional 5%, and the remaining 1% were drug-related pruritus. Some of the drugs with reaction rates in excess of 10 per 1,000 courses of drug therapy include ampicillin, semisynthetic penicillins, blood, penicillin G, gentamicin, cephalosporins, quinidine, erythromycin, hydralazine, and cimetidine. Because only inpatients were studied, the pattern of use is likely to be different from what would be observed among outpatients. Unfortunately, data for outpatients are largely lacking.

Diagnosing and Attribution

The clinician is frequently confronted with a patient who develops an acute skin problem while using a systemic medication. The logical and comprehensive clinical steps to be taken in assessing a reaction are outlined in Table 2–20.

Exanthematous Drug Eruptions

Exanthematous eruptions (exanthems, morbilliform eruptions, and macular and papular eruptions) are the most common of adverse cutaneous reactions to drugs. These eruptions are symmetrical and often become generalized. They consist of erythematous macules and papules, which are often most marked on dependent areas and the trunk and spread to involve the extremities and face. Mucous membrane involvement including erythema may occur. Pruritus is the most frequent associated symptom. Low-grade fever is not uncommon. With the exception of blood eosinophilia, a nonspecific

---

TABLE 2–20.   A Stepwise Approach to Assessing a Suspected Reaction to a Drug

1. Clinical diagnosis of the reaction (rash or syndrome)
   a. Exanthem (exanthem or hypersensitivity syndrome)
   b. Urticarial (urticaria or serum sickness–like reaction)
   c. Blistering eruption (e.g., erythema multiforme majus)
   d. Pustular eruption (e.g., acute generalized exanthematous pustulosis)
   e. Fixed drug eruption
2. Analysis of drug exposure
   a. Prescription drugs
   b. Nonprescription medications
   c. Herbal or traditional (holistic) therapies
3. Determination of etiologic possibilities and probabilities (e.g., drug versus infection)
4. Literature search
5. Confirmation
   a. Rechallenge—in vivo (oral or cutaneous), in vitro
   b. Dechallange
6. Advice to the patient (which drug, likelihood of reaction, future risks)
7. Reporting to state or federal regulators and drug manufacturer of severe or unusual reactions

finding that is often absent, laboratory tests are not generally helpful in diagnosis except to help exclude more serious reactions.

The eruption usually develops in the first few days and almost always within 1 or 2 weeks after beginning a first course of a drug and within a few days of re-exposure to a drug to which an individual has been previously sensitized. Reactions to chemically closely related drugs to which an individual has been previously sensitized often develop, which is a further reason to conclude that most morbilliform eruptions are probably truly allergic.

The clinician evaluating the patient must exclude the possibility that this eruption represents the initial presentation of a more serious reaction such as a hypersensitivity syndrome or the prodromal phase of toxic epidermal necrolysis. Initially, both of these serious reactions can be impossible to distinguish from a common morbilliform eruption.

The timing of the reaction in relation to presentation of antigens, the antigenic nature of the drugs that most commonly cause the morbilliform eruption, and the increased risk of these eruptions among individuals with altered immune systems (the rate of aminopenicillin eruptions is far higher in individuals with infectious mononucleosis than in uninfected persons, and the rate of cutaneous reactions to many drugs in human immunodeficiency virus [HIV]-infected individuals is about tenfold higher than in uninfected persons) suggest that morbilliform eruptions are most consistent with a type IV delayed cell-mediated hypersensitivity reaction.

Since morbilliform eruptions are responsible for about three fourths of all adverse cutaneous reactions, it is not surprising that the drugs responsible for these reactions are thought to be the same as those most commonly responsible for drug reactions. The diagnosis of morbilliform eruptions depends on the clinical presentation and an accurate history of the temporal relation of the ingestion of drugs in the few weeks to month before the onset of the eruption. Drugs initiated a few days to 1 to 3 weeks before the eruption should be most strongly suspect. Drugs that might cross-react with medications to which a patient is known to be sensitive should be carefully considered. Rechallenge with a drug or a cross-reacting drug that has previously caused a reaction usually will produce a second reaction far more rapidly than was the case for the first reaction. The differential diagnosis of morbilliform eruptions includes viral exanthems, scarlet fever, staphylococcal scarlatiniform eruption, toxic shock syndrome, acute graft-versus-host disease, and the eruptions of lymphocyte recovery and juvenile rheumatoid arthritis.

Suspect causative drugs are discontinued when this does not represent a greater risk to the patient than the eruption. The treatment of morbilliform eruptions is largely supportive. Antihistamines, topical antipruritic agents, and soothing baths all help relieve pruritus and make the patient more comfortable. Topical corticosteroids may give some relief, especially if sufficient rubbing and scratching to induce secondary eczematous changes have occurred. Systemic steroids are seldom indicated. If the causative drug is continued, patients may develop exfoliative dermatitis, or in the case of hypersensitivity syndrome more severe internal organ involvement (e.g., hepatitis, nephritis) may occur. Whether continued exposure or re-exposure to a causative drug can cause toxic epidermal necrolysis or whether the morbilliform eruption only represented the first stage of this disorder is not known.

Urticaria and Angioedema

Urticaria presents as pruritic, circumscribed, erythematous dermal papules and plaques. When inflammation is diffuse and includes deeper structures, and especially when it involves the central face, the process is termed *angioedema*. The most severe manifestation of immediate hypersensitivity is anaphylaxis. Individual lesions of urticaria generally last for less than 24 hours, but an individual can continue to develop new lesions for as long as the stimulus is present. Drug-induced urticaria and angioedema are usually symmetrical. In acute reactions, itching and compromise of respiratory or cardiovascular systems or diarrhea may occur but other symptoms such as fever are rare. Eosinophilia is relatively infrequent.

Urticaria, angioedema, and anaphylaxis are most often due to type I IgE antibody-mediated hypersensitivity. In addition to hives and pruritus affecting the skin, these immediate hypersensitivity reactions can affect the pulmonary, circulatory, gastrointestinal, and neurologic systems. Although reactions limited to the skin cause hives and itching, severe reactions involving other systems can lead to respiratory collapse, erythema, shock, and death. Reactions in previously sensitive individuals can occur within minutes (immediate reactions) or hours of re-exposure (accelerated reactions). Sometimes there may be a delay of some days between exposure and the development of urticaria and angioedema (delayed reactions).

Antibiotics, especially the penicillins and sulfonamides, and foreign proteins, including blood products and γ-globulin, are classic causes of IgE-mediated immediate hypersensitivity reaction. Other mechanisms by which drugs may produce urticaria, angioedema, and anaphylaxis include activation of complement or direct action on mast cells and basophils, with the resultant release of inflammatory mediators. Perhaps the two most frequent causes of drug-induced non–IgE-mediated urticaria and angioedema are NSAIDs and angiotensin-converting enzyme (ACE) inhibitors. Although the mechanism for nonsteroidal-induced urticaria and angioedema is not known, ACE inhibitor–induced urticaria and angioedema are a likely result of effects of kinin metabolism changes in vascular responses to bradykinin in the skin and mucous membranes in users of ACE inhibitors.

Penicillins are almost certainly the most frequent cause of drug-induced IgE-mediated urticaria and anaphylaxis. ACE inhibitors are most often responsible for cases of angioedema sufficiently severe to require hospitalization. Angioedema occurs in at least 2 per 10,000 new users of ACE inhibitors. As is the case for IgE-mediated urticaria and angioedema, the risk of these reactions is highest in the first weeks of therapy, but these reactions may occur immediately after the introduction of an ACE inhibitor or after months of use. Longer-acting ACE inhibitors are probably more likely to cause these reactions.

Allergic reactions to latex from gloves or medical devices can induce local or generalized urticaria as well as angioedema and anaphylaxis. The incidence of these reactions appears highest among persons with greatest direct exposure to latex, especially when mucosal surfaces are involved (e.g., rectal catheters).

The clinical diagnosis of urticaria is usually evident based on the classic appearance of welts or hives as well as on deeper tissue swelling with angioedema. The lesions of urticarial vasculitis are more often chronic, with individual hives lasting more than 24 hours, and this condition is frequently associated with arthritis, a low-grade fever, and an elevated sedimentation rate. The principal challenge for the clinician is to determine whether urticaria is drug induced or due to other reasons such as non-drug antigens, or is idiopathic (see Chapter 41 in CM&S). The most important step in the treatment of urticaria is withdrawal of the causative agent. If angioedema or anaphylaxis occurs, immediate therapy with epinephrine and systemic steroids may be necessary. Usually, symptomatic relief can be achieved with histamine H_1 receptor blockers (antihistamines). In contrast to the lack of efficacy of nonsedating antihistamines for most pruritic eruptions, nonsedating antihistamines are often useful in urticaria.

For IgE-mediated urticaria induced by penicillins and related compounds, radioallergosorbent test, enzyme-linked immunosorbent assay (ELISA), and scratch tests can be used to confirm the diagnosis. Positive skin test reactions in the setting of a penicillin-allergic history mean that this individual is likely to develop an IgE-mediated reaction with rechallenge.

NSAIDs, especially aspirin, zomepirac, and tolmetin, are causes of urticaria, angioedema, and anaphylaxis. Individuals with a history of nasal polyps or allergic rhinitis are at an especially high risk.

Hypersensitivity Syndrome

The hypersensitivity syndrome is a systemic reaction characterized by the onset of fever, rash, lymphadenopathy, and involvement of various internal organs. It usually begins 1 to 4 weeks after starting therapy. Most often, exanthematous eruptions including exfoliative dermatitis occur, although other eruptions including erythema multiforme, Stevens-Johnson syndrome, and toxic epidermal necrolysis may occur. Many drugs can cause this syndrome, but the most common are sulfonamide antibiotics and the aromatic anticonvulsants (phenytoin, phenobarbital, carbamazepine). Phenobarbital can cross-react in patients who have had hypersensitivity syndrome reactions to either phenytoin or carbamazepine. Hypersensitivity syndrome occurs in about 1 in 5000 exposures for these drugs.

Cross-reactions have been noted in 70% to 80% of patients taking phenytoin, phenobarbital, or carbamazepine. Valproic acid, which is different structurally from the aromatic anticonvulsants, is usually considered a safe alternative; however, patients who have had hypersensitivity syndromes to the other anticonvulsants (phenobarbital, phenytoin, carbamazepine) have been reported who have been unable to tolerate valproic acid.

Patients exposed to drugs who present with a fever and rash should be investigated for internal organ involvement. Atypical lymphocytes are often seen in the peripheral blood during the first week. This is often followed by a striking eosinophilia. Liver function tests, complete blood cell counts, urinary sediment and serum immunoglobulin studies, and chest roentgenograms are relevant and helpful. Transient-induced hypothyroidism may occur.

Diagnostic or confirmatory testing is not readily available, although in vitro testing using a mouse hepatic microsomal system appears sensitive to confirming metabolic abnormalities that often characterize most patients who develop hypersensitivity syndrome with aromatic antiepileptics and sulfonamides. Oral rechallenges are not advisable owing to the severity of these reactions.

Patients should be advised that they have had a reaction to one aromatic 5 anticonvulsant, since there is a high likelihood that a reaction may result from any of the other aromatic anticonvulsants (phenytoin, phenobarbital, carbamazepine). Patients who react to sulfonamide antibiotics are at increased risk of reacting to other sulfonamide antibiotics but do not appear to be at increased risk of reacting to some sulfonamide derivatives, such as oral hypoglycemics or diuretics. They are, however, at increased risk with other aromatic amines, including dapsone, salazopyrine, and other types of procainamide.

The risk of a severe reaction to an anticonvulsant in first-degree relatives of patients who have had reactions is increased. The abnormality appears to be a pharmacogenetic problem in drug detoxification. All physicians should be aware that a patient who gives a history of a hypersensitivity reaction or has had a first-degree relative with such a problem is at high risk of a reaction.

Serum Sickness

Serum sickness, first described in children treated with horse serum containing diphtheria antitoxin, is a type III hypersensitivity reaction mediated by the deposition of immune complexes in blood vessels and other tissues (e.g., joints, kidneys). There is subsequent activation of complement and recruitment of granulocytes and subsequent lymphocytes in the inflammatory reaction. Classically, serum sickness includes a cutaneous eruption that is most often morbilliform, with or without urticaria, and is accompanied by fever, malaise, arthralgias, and arthritis. A characteristic erythematous eruption occurs along the sides of the feet and hands. This rash may become purpuric. Renal, hepatic, pulmonary, gastrointestinal, and central nervous system involvement may also occur. In true serum sickness, serum C3 and C4 levels are decreased. Serum sickness, most often associated with exposure to foreign protein, typically begins 1 to 2 weeks after first exposure to such proteins. Foreign proteins more recently associated with the induction of this illness include horse antithymocyte globulin, immune globulin, and human diploid cell rabies vaccine.

The presence of circulating immune complexes and decreased serum C3 and C4 levels, confirm the diagnosis. On skin biopsy, perivascular inflammation without vasculitis is seen. Direct immunofluorescence reveals immune deposits, most importantly IgG, in superficial vessels. The principal differential diagnoses in these patients are acute viral and drug-induced serum sickness–like illnesses and hypersensitivity syndrome. Treatment with systemic corticosteroids is often advocated.

Serum Sickness–like Reactions

A condition clinically similar but almost certainly a result of different mechanisms is also observed after the ingestion of drugs, most notably some antibiotics, including the cephalosporins (especially cefaclor), penicillins, and sulfonamides. In contrast to true serum sickness, immune complexes, hypocomplementemia, vasculitis, and renal lesions are uncommon. These reactions typically include rash, fever, and arthralgias or myalgias and are denoted as serum sickness–like reactions.

Serum sickness–like reactions generally occur from 1 to 2 weeks after initiation of therapy and resolve on drug discontinuation. Most cases have occurred after repeated exposures to the suspect drug. Some patients who react to cefaclor have subsequently received other cephalosporins without adverse effect, although this practice does have some risk.

Treatment is usually symptomatic with antihistamines and topical antipruritics and perhaps topical corticosteroids for the rash. More severe symptoms, such as arthralgias, may benefit from a short course of oral corticosteroids. A similar clinical picture to that seen with antibiotics has been associated with administration of other types of drugs. In the absence of circulating immune complexes and activation of the complement system, these illnesses should not be considered true serum sickness.

Vasculitis

Vasculitis is defined as inflammation of and damage to blood vessel walls. Drug-induced vasculitis that typically involves small vessels may be triggered by immune deposits composed of antibodies directed against drug-related haptens.

Palpable purpuric papules, especially on the lower extremities, are the classic clinical presentation for cutaneous small vessel vasculitis, including that which is drug induced. Vasculitis may, however, be manifested with a broad range of cutaneous lesions, including urticaria-like lesions, hemorrhagic blisters, ulcers, and inflammatory nodules. Digital necrosis and vascular insufficiency are sometimes seen.

Drugs likely account for a minority of cases of cutaneous leukocytoclastic vasculitis, except in the case of intravenous streptokinase. As many as 3% of such exposed individuals develop this otherwise rare adverse reaction. The list of drugs implicated in cutaneous vasculitis is long and includes NSAIDs, quinolones, sulfonamides, zidovudine, ACE inhibitors, systemic retinoids, cimetidine, and vancomycin.

The key to diagnosing drug-induced cutaneous vasculitis is eliminating alternative etiologies for cutaneous vasculitis, especially infection and autoimmune diseases. Treatment consists of drug withdrawal. Many believe that systemic steroids are also helpful.

Anticoagulant-Induced Skin Necrosis

Anticoagulant drugs can induce hypercoagulable states with resultant vascular infarction and skin necrosis. These reactions can be life threatening. The mechanisms by which coumarin and heparin induce skin necrosis is different.

Coumarin-induced skin necrosis typically begins 3 to 5 days after initiating treatment. Initially, red painful plaques, most frequently involving areas rich in fatty tissues such as the breasts, buttocks, and hips, develop. These plaques evolve into hemorrhagic blisters, ulcers, or necrotic areas. About 1 in 10,000 individuals who receive coumarin will develop skin necrosis. Most of these individuals have deficiency of protein C or S, but only a small percentage of protein C–deficient individuals will develop this reaction when exposed to coumarin.

Coumarin-induced skin necrosis is the result of a transient hypercoagulable state caused by depressing protein C levels. Thrombi form in small cutaneous vessels, causing infarction of the skin. Treatment of coumarin-induced necrosis is discontinuation of the drug, anticoagulation with heparin, and administration of vitamin K. Protein C is also helpful.

Heparin-induced cutaneous necrosis is also the result of intravascular thrombosis and subsequent necrosis in the skin and other organisms. Localized reactions of this type at injection sites are frequent with heparin, but widespread reactions are rare. Typically, heparin-induced skin necrosis occurs 5 to 10 days after starting therapy. It also presents as red tender plaques, usually around injection sites.

Heparin-induced necrosis may be the result of induction of platelet aggregation. In both of these conditions, one initially sees fibrin plugs in blood vessels. Later, these lesions proceed to necrosis. Administration of antiplatelet aggregating drugs and anticoagulation with coumarin are helpful.

Photosensitivity

The combination of light and a drug can induce acute inflammation in the skin. This may be either as a result of direct photochemistry involving the skin, as with phototoxic drug eruptions, or because ultraviolet radiation alters the immunogenicity of a drug, resulting in formation of a new hapten and a subsequent immunologic reaction, photoallergy.

Phototoxic eruptions, which are most common, are often acute and typically resemble sunburn. Phototoxic reactions occur in anyone exposed to sufficient quantities of the appropriate wavebands of ultraviolet radiation who has sufficient levels of the drug in the skin. Ultraviolet A radiation (320–400 nm) is most often the responsible waveband, but both ultraviolet B (280–320 nm) and visible light can elicit these reactions with some drugs. Many drugs induce phototoxic reactions, including the NSAIDs, the quinolones and tetracyclines, amiodarone, and the phenothiazines.

Photoallergic eruptions are often more chronic and are usually similar in appearance to eczematous dermatitis, except for their occurrence principally in sun-exposed areas. Photoallergic reactions are most often seen with topically applied medicines. Unlike phototoxic reactions, which will not recur once the drug has been cleared from the skin even with re-exposure to light, photoallergic reactions may recur with subsequent sun exposure without reuse of the medication. A multitude of drugs, including sulfonamides, thiazide diuretics, and phenothiazines have been implicated in photoallergic reactions, as have some NSAIDs, but these reactions appear to be quite rare.

Exfoliative Dermatitis

Erythroderma or exfoliative dermatitis manifest as whole or nearly whole body skin surface erythema and scaling. It is seen in association with a variety of preexisting dermatoses as well as with lymphoreticular malignancies. Drugs have been estimated to be responsible for between one sixth and one third of cases of erythroderma. Erythroderma and exfoliative dermatitis are among the more frequent cutaneous presentations of the hypersensitivity syndrome.

A wide variety of drugs, including sulfonamides, isoniazid, ampicillin, and streptomycin, may cause erythroderma, as well as all drugs associated with the hypersensitivity syndrome.

To diagnose drug-induced exfoliative dermatitis, other causes of this condition must be eliminated (see Chapter 31 in CS&M). These include preexisting dermatoses, especially eczema, contact dermatitis, psoriasis, stasis dermatitis, pityriasis rubra pilaris, and underlying lymphoreticular malignancies. In a substantial proportion of cases, the cause of erythroderma is never determined. In addition to drug withdrawal, treatment includes the use of topical or systemic corticosteroids, antipruritics, emollients, and soothing baths.

Red Man Syndrome

Vancomycin, a frequently used antibiotic, can induce a constellation of symptoms popularly known as ''red man syndrome.'' In spite of its name, women and children can also develop this reaction. This syndrome is characterized by the sudden onset of erythema, pruritus, and, in severe cases, angioedema and intravascular collapse. It is often most marked on the neck or upper torso. The dose of vancomycin and the rate of administration appear to be the primary determinants of the occurrence of this syndrome.

Slower administration of vancomycin and use of smaller separated doses as well as pretreatment with antihistamines help lower the frequency and severity of this condition.

Fixed Drug Eruptions

Fixed drug eruptions are relatively common and distinctive. Clinically, lesions are round erythematous and edematous plaques that may include central blisters. After the acute inflammatory phase fades, gray or brown hyperpigmentation develops at the site. Sites of predilection include the face, acral areas, and genitalia. The defining features of this eruption are the postinflammatory hyperpigmentation and the recurrence of lesions at exactly the same sites with rechallenge to the causative drug. Rechallenge often results in the development of lesions at new sites as well as recurrence at prior sites. Rarely, a generalized fixed drug eruption may occur.

Among the drugs classically associated with fixed drug eruptions and still in widespread use in the United States in the 1990s are the barbiturates, sulfonamides, phenolphthalein, tetracyclines, salicylates, and NSAIDs. Since these agents can be found in combination drugs and in over-the-counter agents as well as in prescription medications, an extremely careful history is necessary to determine the likely cause. With first exposure to a sensitizing drug, the eruption usually occurs within 1 to 2 weeks. With subsequent exposures to the offending agent, the reactivation typically occurs within a few days, suggesting that this is a specialized local form of delayed hypersensitivity. Local symptoms include burning and pruritus. The hyperpigmentation may be persistent and disfiguring.

The pathologic features of fixed drug eruption are distinctive. Lymphocytes are present around the superficial vascular plexus and obscure the dermoepidermal junction and infiltrate the epidermis, where they are present in apposition to necrotic keratinocytes, while the deep plexus infiltrates also include eosinophils and neutrophils. Over time, melanophages accumulate in the dermis.

Pigmentary Disturbances

Generalized pigmentary disturbances can occur in association with the administration of a variety of drugs. Many of these pigmentary disturbances tend to be more pronounced in sun-exposed areas, suggesting that photochemical changes may account for these diseases. Chronic therapy and inflammation are also risk factors for some drug-induced pigmentations. Ingestion of heavy metals including mercury, silver, bismuth, arsenic, gold, and lead can cause pigmentary changes.

Antimalarial medications, especially quinacrine, can induce an intense yellow coloration of the skin. Sun-exposed areas are most strongly affected. Phenothiazine, amiodarone, chloroquine, and hydroxychloroquine induce a gray-purple discoloration. The former two drugs induce pigmentation in sun-exposed sites, the latter two in the mouth.

Minocycline complexed with iron induces grayish pigmentation that is most marked in sun-exposed areas or in areas of chronic inflammation in adults. Mucous membranes and acral areas may also be involved.

Usually, drug-induced pigmentary changes can be readily identified both by clinical history and appearance. If necessary, special examination to determine the nature of the material deposited in the skin can be performed (e.g., mass spectrography). The principal differential diagnosis is postinflammatory hyperpigmentation or increased melanocyte activity, which occurs in endocrinopathies or in association with pregnancy or oral contraceptive use. Cessation of drug therapy and passage of time will often lead to gradual lightening.

Acute Generalized Exanthematous Pustulosis and Pustular Drug Eruptions

Patients develop high fever and a widespread erythematous eruption and rapidly become covered by hundreds of small nonfollicular superficial pustules. Leukocytosis is almost always present. The eruption lasts 1 to 2 weeks and is followed by desquamation. Most cases appear to be drug related, especially to β-lactam antibiotics, but in a few cases, no clear precipitant is found.

Drug-Induced Pemphigus

Pemphigus can be drug induced, and the drugs most often incriminated are penicillamine and other thiol (-SH) compounds. These include captopril or drugs such as piroxicam that are metabolized to thiols. Penicillin and its derivatives have also been associated, but not cephalosporins.

Pemphigus caused by penicillamine and other thiol compounds is prone to spontaneous remission, usually presents as pemphigus foliaceus, and has an onset period of almost 1 year after drug therapy is initiated. Non-thiol drug-induced disease does not usually remit spontaneously and presents as pemphigus vulgaris with mucosal involvement.

Drug-Induced Lupus Erythematosus–like Syndrome

Some drugs are known to cause a flare of preexisting lupus erythematosus. Others induce serologic changes, such as antinuclear antibodies, induce cutaneous or subacute lupus erythematosus, or induce a lupus-like syndrome in individuals with no prior autoimmune disease. Drug-induced lupus usually differs from idiopathic lupus in that there is no sex predilection, skin involvement is less common, renal and central nervous system disease is rare, complement is normal, and antibodies to native DNA are not found. Patients may present with cutaneous findings in approximately 25% of cases. These include the malar or ''butterfly'' rash, acute or persisting photoeruptions, discoid lupus, urticarial or erythema multiforme–like lesions, and Raynaud's phenomenon.

Drugs that are strongly associated with drug-induced lupus are procainamide and hydralazine. Drugs that most frequently induce antinuclear antibodies include procainamide, hydralazine, isoniazid, α-methyldopa, chlorpromazine, propylthiouracil, acebutolol, D-penicillamine, and psoralens and ultraviolet A light (PUVA).

Lichenoid Drug Eruptions

A cutaneous drug eruption that is clinically and histologically similar to lichen planus has been associated with the ingestion of a variety of drugs (see Chapter 20 in CM&S). Many lichenoid drug eruptions occur in a photodistribution. Most frequently implicated drugs include sulfhydryl-containing drugs, especially captopril, β-blockers, gold, penicillamine, and antimalarial agents. Differentiation from lichen planus can be difficult if the lesions are not photodistributed, but the presence of eosinophils and parakeratosis histologically is helpful. Drug withdrawal and treatment with topical steroids are usually sufficient.

Cutaneous Reactions in Human Immunodeficiency Virus Infection

Patients infected with HIV develop cutaneous adverse reactions to drugs more frequently than uninfected individuals. The increased risk appears to apply to a wide range of cutaneous reactions, including the most severe ones such as toxic epidermal necrolysis and Stevens-Johnson syndrome, as well as to far more frequent eruptions, including morbilliform drug eruptions and urticaria. Reactions to sulfonamides are most frequent. Other drugs with high reaction rates include anticonvulsants, aminopenicillins, and dapsone.

CUTANEOUS REACTIONS TO CHEMOTHERAPEUTIC AGENTS

(CM&S Chapter 44)

Almost every cancer chemotherapy patient has at least one rash during his or her therapy. Most are nonspecific toxic erythemas. Chemotherapy reactions are more likely to be toxic than allergic. Oral mucosal damage and hair loss are expected responses.

Specific Reactions

Alopecia

Alopecia is probably the aspect of chemotherapy that patients fear the most. Telogen effluvium is the most common problem, usually occurring weeks to months after the induction of therapy. With higher drug doses there may be direct toxic damage to the growing hairs, resulting in anagen effluvium with thin or bayonet hairs that are easily broken off. Other more peculiar problems can occur. Hair may regrow with a different color or even texture (switching from straight to curly or vice versa).

Nail Dystrophies

Transverse ridges reflecting cyclic chemotherapeutic damage to the nail matrix and hyperpigmentation of the nails are common.

Pigmentary Changes

Pigmentary changes are often seen with chemotherapy. The oral mucosa and nails are the favored sites of hyperpigmentation. Some very unusual patterns of pigmentation may occur. Busulfan may produce diffuse bronze hyperpigmentation, mimicking Addison's disease. Fluorouracil causes several unique reactions: (1) serpentine supravenous pigmentation occurs when pigmented streaks develop over the veins used to administer the fluorouracil without extravasation or clinical phlebitis; and (2) tanning reactions may occur in which the patient tans rapidly without burning or erythema. Bleomycin causes many forms of hyperpigmentation: (1) flagellate hyperpigmentation in which the trunk shows bizarre streaks and bands of hyperpigmentation, looking as if the patient had been whipped or attacked by a marine flagellate such as a Portuguese man-of-war; (2) pressure hyperpigmentation with darkening of the knees and elbows; and (3) nail fold hyperpigmentation.

Radiation Reactions

Cutaneous "memory" may be displayed in two types of radiation reactions: radiation enhancement and radiation recall.

In radiation enhancement, agents that block repair of radiation damage such as dactinomycin and doxorubicin produce unwanted and often severe erythema in radiation portals.

In radiation recall, a unique recrudescence of radiation dermatitis occurs in radiotherapy portals weeks to years after radiation when chemotherapeutic agents, especially dactinomycin and doxorubicin, are administered.

Ultraviolet radiation may produce a series of similar reactions. Many drugs increase photosensitivity, including fluorouracil, dacarbazine, and many other drugs. Methotrexate may reactivate a prior sunburn, although with simultaneous administration of drug and sun exposure little happens.

Allergic Reactions

Urticaria, angioedema, and even anaphylaxis may occur. Often these reactions develop during the first round of chemotherapy, suggesting a toxic effect on mast cells rather than an IgE-mediated mechanism. Cyclophosphamide and asparaginase elicit specific IgE antibodies and produce an immediate type reaction.

Local Reactions

Complications of chemotherapy commonly result from extravasation. The two most severe reactions occur with doxorubicin and daunorubicin. Large cutaneous ulcers can develop if an intravenous needle or canula is misplaced or displaced. Intense pain and erythema are followed by tissue necrosis and ulceration.

In chemical phlebitis, the vein may be damaged by high local levels of a toxic agent. With both phlebitis and extravasation, the recall phenomenon may occur. When the causative agent is readministered at a distant site, the healed ulcer or vein may become inflamed again.

Acral Erythema

Fluorouracil, cytarabine, and doxorubicin may produce acral pain, burning, and erythema, often in a patterned fashion. Acral erythema is dose dependent. As both the individual and cumulative doses increase, the complication is more likely. Typically, the reaction resolves over days to weeks with desquamation and hyperpigmentation.

Inflammation of Actinic Keratosis

Inflammation of actinic keratosis lesions may occur as a complication of systemic fluorouracil therapy. Inflammation of actinic keratosis may be a sophisticated variant of radiation recall, but the mechanism of this clinical reaction is not known.

Immunologic Reactions

Some leukemic patients develop nonspecific, transient macular and papular exanthems as the peripheral lymphocyte count begins to rebound. This "eruption of lymphocyte recovery" is accompanied by a transient fever and usually occurs more than 7 days after therapy.

A number of biologic modifiers which are now employed in chemotherapy regimens such as interleukin-2, interferons, and colony-stimulating factors produce toxic erythema.

Raynaud's Phenomenon

Vinblastine and bleomycin cause true Raynaud's syndrome ulcerations.

Sclerotic Reactions

Bleomycin may cause cutaneous sclerosis as well as the better known complication of pulmonary fibrosis.

Dactinomycin Folliculitis

Dactinomycin, especially in high doses, causes an acneiform pustular facial eruption.

Contact Dermatitis

About 10% of patients treated with mitomycin-C instilled in the bladder for the treatment of superficial bladder cancer develop allergic contact dermatitis, usually of the genitalia or hands. Nurses are at risk as well. Patients frequently become allergic to mechlorethamine (nitrogen mustard) and carmustine (BCNU), used topically to treat mycosis fungoides.

C. Granulomatous Inflammation

SARCOIDOSIS

(CM&S Chapter 45)

Definition

Sarcoidosis is a multisystemic disease characterized by the presence of noncaseating granulomas in tissues. The most common organs involved are the lungs, lymph nodes, eyes, and skin, but virtually every organ may be affected. The cause of sarcoidosis is unknown, but the disease is best thought of as a granulomatous reaction to an undefined antigen.

The immunologic response of patients with sarcoidosis is classically characterized by a depression of delayed-type hypersensitivity, hyperreactive humoral immunity, and a positive Kveim-Siltzbach skin test. Other common laboratory abnormalities include an elevated angiotensin converting enzyme level, hypercalcemia, and/or hypercalciuria.

Clinical Description

Cutaneous Manifestations

Twenty-five percent of patients have skin involvement. Although the cutaneous manifestations of sarcoidosis are protean, the majority of specific lesions are usually papules or plaques. Small papules are the most common specific skin lesion present in sarcoidosis. They are typically seen on the head and neck, especially around the eyes, on the neck, and in the nasolabial folds. They may be flesh colored, red, yellow, purple, or brown and in darker races may be hypopigmented. Occasionally papular lesions may be umbilicated or may coalesce to form annular lesions. Lichenoid lesions have also been reported.

Plaques in sarcoidosis are usually few, are thick, and have a tendency to develop slowly and be recalcitrant to therapy. Similar to the papular lesions they are often found on the face and may be of various colors. Some lesions have a prominent vascular or telangiectatic component and are thus termed *angiolupoid*. Lesions on the ears, nose, cheeks, and fingers have since been termed *lupus pernio* and are often associated with upper respiratory tract disease and phalangeal bone cysts.

Other cutaneous lesions are encountered less often and consist of subcutaneous nodules, psoriasiform plaques, and erythrodermic, ulcerative, verrucous, ichthyotic, and, rarely, pustular lesions. Cutaneous changes have been noted to occur in scars and in sites of trauma.

The most common cutaneous manifestation of sarcoidosis is erythema nodosum. Erythema nodosum is a classic example of a non-specific lesion associated with sarcoidosis since its histology of a septal panniculitis, usually without vasculitis, is the same whether it is idiopathic, associated with other diseases, or seen in conjunction with sarcoid. The lesions are typically tender, red subcutaneous nodules that are most often found on the anterior tibia. The association of erythema nodosum with bilateral hilar adenopathy, fever, arthritis, and uveitis (Löfgren's syndrome) is so characteristic that biopsy confirmation is not necessary to establish the diagnosis. This presentation has a good prognosis, with resolution after several months in most cases.

Extracutaneous Manifestations

Although sarcoidosis can affect any organ, it has a striking predilection for the lung and intrathoracic lymph nodes. Other common manifestations of sarcoidosis include peripheral lymphadenopathy, anterior and posterior uveitis, conjunctival granulomas, facial palsies, meningitis, encephalopathy and seizures caused by space-occupying lesions. Central nervous system involvement is frequent in Heerfordt's syndrome or uveoparotid fever. This syndrome consists of uveitis, facial nerve palsy, fever, and parotid gland involvement.

Although involvement of the liver and spleen occurs less often, blind liver biopsy may show sarcoidal granulomas in 60% of patients. Endocrine, cardiac, hematologic, renal, and musculoskeletal involvement develop rarely.

Pathology

The characteristic histology of sarcoidosis is the presence of circumscribed collections of epithelioid macrophages with only a few accompanying lymphocytes in the superficial and deep dermis and occasionally within the subcutis. There are few giant cells, although the number of giant cells may be greater in older lesions. The Schaumann body, asteroid body, and residual body are three types of nonspecific inclusion bodies which may be found within giant cells.

Diagnosis and Differential Diagnosis

The diagnosis of sarcoidosis is established by the confirmation of noncaseating granulomas from biopsy specimens taken from two or more different organs or from one biopsy specimen plus a positive Kveim-Siltzbach test. Notable exceptions to this rule are the findings described in Löfgren's syndrome. The Kveim-Siltzbach test entails the intradermal injection of heat-sterilized sarcoid tissue followed by a biopsy of the same area 6 weeks later. A positive test shows typical sarcoidal granulomas in the biopsy specimen and is found in more than 80% of patients with active disease.

The protean cutaneous manifestations of sarcoidosis lead to an exhaustive list of differential diagnoses (Table 2–21).

TABLE 2-21. Differential Diagnosis of Cutaneous Sarcoidosis

PAPULES

Xanthelasma
Necrobiosis lipoidica
Lichen planus
Trichoepitheliomas
Adenoma sebaceum
Lupus erythematosus
Secondary lues
Acne rosacea
Granuloma annulare

NODULES

Lymphoma/leukemia cutis
Cutaneous lymphoid hyperplasia

PLAQUES

Lupus vulgaris (tuberculosis)
Necrobiosis lipoidica
Morphea
Leprosy
Leishmaniasis
Gyrate erythema

Treatment

Although there is no cure for sarcoidosis, the mainstay of treatment is systemic corticosteroids, which are reserved primarily for systemic disease or disfiguring cutaneous manifestations. Intralesional steroids for specific cutaneous lesions as well as indomethacin for erythema nodosum have also been used. Antimalarial agents, especially chloroquine, are effective in recalcitrant cutaneous disease. Immunosuppressant drugs such as azathioprine, chlorambucil, methotrexate, cyclosporine, and thymopoietin have also been used.

GRANULOMA ANNULARE

(CM&S Chapter 46)

Definition, Clinical Description, and Pathology

Granuloma annulare is an inflammatory condition of unknown etiology that is characterized clinically by dermal papules and plaques and histologically by interstitial areas of degenerative collagen with granulomatous inflammation in the dermis. There are several clinical types.

Localized Granuloma Annulare

This asymptomatic dermatosis, commonly presents as annular grouped 1- to 2-mm flesh-colored to red papules over the distal extremities. The lesions are usually multiple, but solitary lesions are also seen. Typically, children and young adults are affected. Spontaneous resolution occurs within 2 years in 50% of affected persons, although the duration may be weeks to decades, and recurrent eruptions occur in 40%.

Generalized Granuloma Annulare

Fifteen percent of persons with granuloma annulare exhibit a generalized eruption. These patients have more than 10 lesions and involvement of symmetrical multiple body regions. Both generalized and localized granuloma annulare have been associated with diabetes mellitus and thyroid disease.

Subcutaneous Granuloma Annulare (Pseudorheumatoid Nodules)

This uncommon lesion occurs predominantly in children. Sites that tend to be affected are the extremities. Histologic study shows the identical changes of granuloma annulare in the subcutaneous tissue, with large foci of degenerated collagen. Although the histology is very similar to that of a rheumatoid nodule, these lesions usually occur in otherwise healthy children, with only very few cases of subsequent rheumatoid arthritis developing.

Perforating Granuloma Annulare

This variant occurs most frequently in childhood and appears as umbilicated papules that involve the extremities.

Diagnosis and Differential Diagnosis

Localized granuloma annulare must be distinguished from necrobiosis lipoidica diabeticorum, annular lichen planus, tinea corporis, Hansen's disease, alopecia mucinosa, erythema elevatum diutinum, actinic granuloma, erythema annulare centrifugum, and erythema multiforme. The differential diagnosis of generalized granuloma annulare includes lichen planus, sarcoid, or lichen myxedematosus. Subcutaneous granuloma annulare must be distinguished from rheumatoid nodules. Perforating granuloma annulare may be mistaken for molluscum contagiosum, perforating collagenosis, elastosis perforans serpiginosa, perforating folliculitis, and sarcoidosis.

Treatment

Spontaneous resolution of localized lesions is often induced after skin biopsy. Potent topical corticosteroids, used alone or under occlusion, and intralesional corticosteroid (triamcinolone acetonide, 10 mg/mL) are frequently successful treatments. Cryotherapy is often used but may frequently result in hyperpigmentation or hypopigmentation.

The treatment of generalized granuloma annulare includes dapsone, psoralens and ultraviolet A light (PUVA), hydroxychloroquine, and isotretinoin.

RHEUMATOID NODULE, NECROBIOSIS LIPOIDICA, AND NECROBIOTIC XANTHOGRANULOMA

(CM&S Chapter 47)

Rheumatoid Nodule

Definition and Clinical Description

Rheumatoid nodules are discrete, firm subcutaneous masses with a predilection for bony prominences that typically occur in patients who have severe rheumatoid arthritis and high titers of rheumatoid factor. The pathogenesis for the development of rheumatoid nodules is unknown.

Rheumatoid nodules typically arise on areas of pressure or trauma such as extensor surfaces, the forearm, elbow, fingers, knees, feet, and scalp. They have also arisen in a variety of unusual locations, such as the epibulbar region, deep soft tissue (mimicking sarcoma), intra-articular region, temporal bone, and internal organs such as the lung and renal cortex. The nodules are usually asymptomatic, but because of their location are subject to injury and secondary infection.

Rheumatoid nodules usually accompany active and destructive rheumatoid arthritis, and patients tend to have high titers of rheumatoid factor or evidence for vasculitis. They tend to persist indefinitely, although spontaneous remission is possible. *Rheumatoid nodulosis* is a term applied to the subcutaneous nodules that occur in children who do not have arthritis and most likely have subcutaneous granuloma annnulare. Other authors have defined a syndrome consisting of multiple subcutaneous rheumatoid nodules, recurrent joint symptoms ("palindromic rheumatism"), a benign clinical course, and absent or mild systemic manifestations of rheumatoid arthritis. Additional but not essential findings are positive rheumatoid factor and subchondral cysts of small bones.

Pathology

Rheumatoid nodules and their variants are characterized by the presence of a palisading granuloma. A zone of bright red, fibrinous degenerated collagen is sometimes associated with granular basophilic material. Bordering this is a palisade of histiocytes that is sometimes admixed with giant cells.

Differential Diagnosis

The differential diagnosis of rheumatoid nodules includes Heberden's nodes, Osler's nodes, gouty tophi, and subcutaneous nodules of systemic lupus erythematosus, rheumatic fever, and seronegative ankylosing spondylitis. The histological differential diagnosis of necrobiotic palisading granulomas includes necrobiosis lipoidica, Miescher's granuloma, and granuloma annulare.

Treatment

The occurrence of spontaneous resolution of rheumatoid nodules makes assessment of response to any treatment difficult. Large or otherwise troubling lesions can be surgically removed. Apparent regression of nodules has also been achieved by injection with pred-nisolone and lignocaine. Although not well described, intralesional triamcinoline has also been successfully employed. Typically, the nodules themselves respond only sluggishly, if at all, to the "slow-acting" antirheumatic drugs such as gold, penicillamine, or hy-droxychloroquine, but their presence does not necessarily predict a poor response of other signs and symptoms of the disease to such agents. Methotrexate therapy has been reported to accelerate the development of rheumatoid nodules.

Necrobiosis Lipoidica

Definition and Clinical Description

Necrobiosis lipoidica consists of chronic yellow-brown atrophic patches that occur typically on the pretibial areas of the lower ex-tremities. Lesions begin as erythematous papules that typically ap-pear over the pretibial areas, although lesions can also occur on the forearms, trunk, or face. Over time, lesions evolve to form circum-scribed yellow-brown atrophic patches, through which one can eas-ily visualize underlying dermal vessels. Ulceration can occur readily following trauma. The Koebner phenomenon has been observed. There is reduced sensation to pinprick and light touch. Necrobiotic lesions follow a chronic course, and persistence with scarring is the rule. Squamous cell carcinoma has arisen in long-standing necro-biosis lipoidica.

Although only about 0.3% of diabetics have necrobiosis lipoi-dica, a high percentage of individuals with necrobiosis lipoidica either have diabetes mellitus (usually insulin-dependent), show an abnormal glucose tolerance test, or provide a strong family history of diabetes mellitus. There may be an association with other diabetic complications, including limited joint mobility, neuropathy, and retinopathy. The etiology of necrobiosis lipoidica is unknown. The two leading theories regarding the cause of necrobiosis lipoidica include immune complex vasculitis and blood flow abnormalities resulting from alterations of platelets and/or the microvasculature.

Pathology

There are broad zones of sclerosis with patchy granulomas or aggregates of lymphocytes and plasma cells and multinucleated giant cells. Horizontal layers of macrophages can alternate with zones of sclerosis.

Differential Diagnosis

The clinical and histological differential diagnosis includes gran-uloma annulare.

Treatment

Despite occasional successes, no treatment has thus far been reg-ularly effective in causing resolution of lesions or reversing the atrophic changes. Optimizing glycemic control appears to speed the healing of skin lesions. Intralesional, systemic, or topical fluorinated corticosteroids have been reported to promote improvement or resolution of lesions. Other therapies include the use of agents that inhibit platelet aggregation such as aspirin, dipyridamole, pentoxifylline, and fibrinolytic agents.

Necrobiotic Xanthogranuloma

Definition and Clinical Description

Necrobiotic xanthogranuloma consists of plaques and nodules, sometimes ulcerated, that occur in a variety of locations, but particularly in the periorbital region and on the trunk. Lesions are of varying coloration but usually with a xanthomatous appearance. As plaques evolve, they show marked induration but with central atrophy and sometimes ulceration. Hepatosplenomegaly, arthritis, and arthralgia may also occur.

The most significant associated finding is paraproteinemia, which has been found in most but not all patients. Most patients have IgG paraproteinemia on protein electrophoresis, but IgA paraprotein has also been detected. Lesions tend to persist without treatment, as does the paraproteinemia. Cases have evolved to multiple myeloma, and there have been reports of association with chronic lymphocytic leukemia and Hodgkin's disease. The etiology of these necrobiotic lesions is unknown.

Pathology

Findings include extensive palisaded, necrobiotic granulomas extending from the mid dermis into the subcutis. Other histologic findings include Touton giant cells, foamy macrophages, and cholesterol clefts.

Differential Diagnosis

The major differential diagnosis is necrobiosis lipoidica.

Treatment

Treatment with chlorambucil has resulted in significant improvement of lesions, while other agents such as melphalan and methotrexate are of questionable benefit. Intralesional corticosteroids may not be helpful. Radiation therapy and plasmapheresis combined with hydroxychloroquine have been used successfully in selected cases.

TATTOOS, FOREIGN BODY GRANULOMAS, AND THEIR TREATMENT

(CM&S Chapter 48)

Definition

Tattoos are the visible result of exogenous materials placed in the dermis by a tattoo artist, by a traumatic event, or by a physician for medical purposes as in the marking of radiation ports. In contrast to other foreign materials implanted into the skin, a significant granulomatous response is not usually present with tattoos. Foreign body granulomas result from the body's attempt to remove or wall off impregnated foreign material.

Clinical Description

The clinical appearance of foreign body granulomas in the skin is dependent on the reaction the particular foreign matter elicits. Potential foreign bodies are as varied as the environment around us. Glass (silica), thorns, wood splinters, suture material, and arthropods are frequent offenders. A firm, nontender, flesh-toned papule may be all that is noted. If an inflammatory reaction is incited, however, an erythematous, tender nodule may be present, whether or not an allergic response is incited.

Pathology

Histologic examination of a tattoo shows small dense clumps of ink throughout the dermis, with little alteration of other structural elements. The ink is present extracellularly, as well as within cells, and usually located in perivascular regions with either no or minimal surrounding fibrosis.

In foreign body reactions, macrophages and giant cells surround the material and are frequently accompanied by lymphocytes and plasma cells. Polarized light is often helpful for localizing foreign substances.

Treatment

For non-tattoo foreign body granulomas, the diagnostic procedure—biopsy or extraction—is often the treatment of choice, as surgical removal is usually the only curative treatment option. Intralesional steroid injections may calm the inflammatory response, but do not remove the inciting irritator. Topical application of mild acids or gentian violet, alone or in combination with dermabrasion or salabrasion; cryosurgery; surgical excision; carbon dioxide laser; and the infrared coagulator are all effective at removing tattoo ink. However, the resultant scar is often as undesirable as the tattoo itself. Excision, which may require several stages, is particularly useful for small, conveniently located tattoos, as well as for those tattoos being removed because of an allergic response to a contained ink.

Selective photothermolysis is the concept of producing preferential injury to pigment-containing structures using brief laser pulses. By using a wavelength that provides acceptably selective absorption, and a pulse duration shorter than or equal to the thermal relaxation time of the desired microscopic structure, damage is effectively contained within the targeted tissue. Using these principles, one can target endogenous chromophores (hemoglobin, melanin), as well as exogenous chromophores (tattoo ink, graphite), and leave the adjacent collagen intact, minimizing the potential for scarring.

Ultrashort pulse durations are critical for the treatment of tattoos. The high energy delivered leads to extremely high temperatures, and the resultant rapid thermal expansion exceeds the shear forces of the ink particles and they shatter.

Principles of Q-Switched Laser Treatment

Most patients are able to tolerate laser treatment of tattoos with either the Q-switched (QS) ruby, QS neodymium-yttrium-aluminum-garnet (Nd:YAG), or QS alexandrite lasers without anesthesia. The sensation is that of a snap of a rubber band. A few laser pulses may be given to assess the patient's tolerance to treatment. If anesthesia is desired, either local injections of 1% to 2% lidocaine, or topically, with EMLA (eutectic mixture of lidocaine and prilocaine) or 40% lidocaine in an acid mantle base can be used.

Given the multitude of colored inks available and the varying response to treatment, it is difficult to predict how many laser treatments are needed to clear a tattoo. Use of a wavelength well absorbed by the tattoo ink enhances the ability to treat that particular color. Other general rules for tattoos include the following: (1) amateur tattoos are easier to clear than professional tattoos; (2) older tattoos fare better than recently placed tattoos; (3) red, brown, flesh-toned, and white inks have infrequently been noted to turn a slate-gray to black color with QS laser treatment.

Wound care is similar for all QS laser systems and consists of antibiotic ointment and a clean nonstick dressing. Gentle cleansing once or twice daily with soap and water with reapplication of the ointment is sufficient and should be maintained until the crusts have healed. Strict instructions to not pick off the crusts should be given, as most cases of textural changes or scarring seem to be related to improper wound care.

Amateur tattoos respond best. Multiple wavelengths are necessary to treat multicolored tattoos. The 694-nm, 25-nsec QS ruby laser (QSRL) is best suited for green and black tattoo inks but is also absorbed well by melanin. This makes it a useful laser for treating certain benign pigmented lesions, but accounts for the hypopigmentation as a side effect of tattoo treatment. The 10-nsec QS Nd:YAG laser is available with two wavelengths: 1064 nm, which treats black ink well without pigmentary side effects; and 532 nm, which treats red tattoo ink (and epidermal pigmented lesions) but will also induce hypopigmentation. The 755-nm and 100-ns pulse duration QS alexandrite laser produces results that are not dissimilar to the ruby laser, both being short-pulsed, red-light lasers. The 510-nm, 300-nsec pulsed dye laser is effective in treating red tattoos.

D. Follicular Inflammation

ACNE

(CM&S Chapter 49)

Definition and Clinical Description

Acne vulgaris is the most common disease involving the pilosebaceous unit. The areas of skin that are most often affected are those that contain large numbers of sebaceous glands such as the face, back, and chest. Rarely, severe acne presents on the trunk either without or with only a few facial lesions. Even at the same area of skin there can be a tremendous variation of the exact localization of acne. Although presentation most often occurs in adolescence, other types of acne, including iatrogenic acne, infantile acne, occupational acne, and pomade and cosmetic acne, affect all age groups.

Acne Lesions

There are four essential features for the development of acne lesions: an increased sebum excretion rate, which is under androgen control; ductal hypercornification; colonization of the duct with *Propionibacterium acnes*; and the production of inflammation. Clinically, many patients with acne have seborrhea. In addition, it is quite likely that there is a spectrum of androgen dysfunction in patients with acne.

Comedones. Comedones, which are the clinical expression of hyperkeratosis of follicular infundibula, may be either open or closed. Open comedones (blackheads) usually take several weeks or months to develop. Although open comedones are relatively common, their absence does not negate the diagnosis of acne. Closed comedones (whiteheads), which present as small white papules, represent a distended follicular infundibulum, the orifice of which is hardly visible. Closed comedones, especially those that are microscopic (microcomedones), often precede the inflammatory phase.

Papules. Papules are palpable inflamed lesions that vary in size and redness and usually arise from normal-appearing skin.

Pustules. Pustules may be superficial or deep, varying in size from 0.1 to 3 or 4 mm. Deep pustules which are frequently tender, are more common in severe acne.

Nodules. Nodules are deep-seated lesions that take many weeks to evolve and disappear and frequently produce scarring. Nodules may ulcerate, leaving hemorrhagic crusts.

Macules. Macules are a late stage of all inflammatory lesions and certainly contribute markedly to the overall disability.

Postinflammatory Hyperpigmentation. This is a nonspecific feature of pigmented skin and is frequently seen in persons with acne. This type of hyperpigmentation contributes considerably to the cosmetic disfigurement. Hyperpigmentation is often a residuum of acne excoriée.

Scars. Scars predominantly occur in most subjects with severe deep-seated nodular acne. However, it is known that 15% of subjects with common papular pustular acne develop significant scarring.

Severe Acne Variants

Acne Conglobata

This very uncommon variant is characterized by grouped comedones, which result in deep inflammation and large abscesses that burrow from one set of grouped comedones to another. Irregular scarring occurs from the severe inflammation and tissue necrosis. Acne conglobata frequently affects males, and it is often associated with acne inversa (hidradenitis suppurativa).

Acne Fulminans

The classic features of acne fulminans are sudden onset of severe acne in an individual who has previously had only mild acne. The inflammation may be sufficient to produce ulceration. Associated toxic effects are essential for the diagnosis and often include fever, polyarthralgia, and, uncommonly, such events as erythema nodosum. Males are more frequently affected, and inflammatory acne is usually more truncal than facial. Scarring is virtually inevitable.

Gram-Negative Folliculitis

This pustular eruption occurs in subjects who have received long-term oral antibiotics for their acne. Both the acne lesions and nose should be cultured for causative organisms such as *Enterobacteriaceae*, including *Klebsiella*, *Escherichia coli*, *Serratia*, and *Proteus*.

Other Variants of Acne

There are a considerable number of other types of acne, and these must be considered despite their low incidence.

Drug-Induced Acne. Drug-induced acne is particularly seen with androgenic hormones; oral, topical, and inhaled corticosteroids; anabolic steroids; barbiturates; anticonvulsants; and other agents.

Acne Excoriée. Acne excoriée predominantly occurs in young females. Often the acne consists of papular lesions on the chin. The lesions are attacked by the patient, resulting in large areas of inflammation. This disorder merges into dermatitis artefacta.

Infantile and Juvenile Acne. Infantile and juvenile acne occurs predominantly in boys and particularly affects the face. The lesions may exhibit all the features of typical adolescent acne. Most infants have no systemic hormonal abnormalities.

Chloracne. Exogenous chemicals, especially halogenated aromatic compounds with a specific molecular shape, may cause acne. One of the most well known of these agents is dioxin. Such patients have very large comedones. Other clinical features include postinflammatory hyperpigmentation, hypertrichosis, erythema, and blepharitis. Systemic disease may also occur in the form of hepatic dysfunction with porphyria and a predisposition to systemic malignancy.

Pomade and Cosmetic Acne. Characteristic closed comedones are seen in pomade and cosmetic acne, which is due to certain chemicals that when applied to the skin promote comedone formation. Cosmetics, particularly those containing lanolin and certain vegetable oils, as well as pure chemicals, such as butylstearate, lauryl alcohol, and oleic acid, are incriminated. Animal testing (particularly of the rabbit ear) with suspected comedogenic agents can predict the comedogenicity of such chemicals.

Acne Mechanica. Mechanical friction can often localize acne to areas such as on the forehead under a football helmet, or on the chin from a chin strap.

Pathology

Acne vulgaris is caused by the retention of cornified cells in follicular infundibula, which become cystically dilated. In closed comedones the lips of follicular ostia are closely apposed, while in open comedones they are patulous.

Spongiosis with lymphocytes can be present early in inflamed acne lesions. Later lesions show rupture of follicular infundibular epithelium. Neutrophils, and later lymphocytes, macrophages, and foreign-body giant cells, accumulate at the site of rupture, where cornified material, sebum, and commensal organisms are extruded into the dermis. This suppurative and granulomatous dermatitis causes the nodular lesions of acne vulgaris.

Differential Diagnosis

Although rarely misdiagnosed, the differential diagnosis of acne includes adenoma sebaceum, boils, dental sinus, milia, perioral dermatitis, folliculitis, verruca plana, rosacea, seborrheic dermatitis, and pseudofolliculitis barbae.

Treatment of Acne

General Principles

Acne is a chronic disease, and topical therapy will be required for the duration of the condition (i.e., 8 to 12 years). This is likely to be interspersed with several months' courses of oral antibiotics or other therapies such as hormones or retinoids. It is important to emphasize the need to apply topical therapies not just to the lesions but also to the area where lesions are prone because microcomedones occur in apparently clinically normal skin. Stress aggravates acne, but it is not a major primary factor. There is no link between acne and diet.

Topical Treatment Options

Topical therapy is the mainstay of acne therapy and includes the use of topical antibiotics, benzoyl peroxide, and retinoic acid. Table

TABLE 2-22. Treatment of Acne: Typical Therapy		
COMEDONAL	**INFLAMMATORY**	**MIXED**
Tretinoin	Benzoyl peroxide	Use both types of
Isotretinoin	Clindamycin	therapies
Azelaic acid	Erythromycin ± zinc	
Erythromycin + zinc	Tetracycline	
	Azelaic acid	

2–22 outlines topical therapy appropriate for each type of acne lesion. Patients using topical therapy may develop a low-grade irritant dermatitis. True allergic contact dermatitis is rare.

Oral Treatment Options

Oral agents effective for acne include antibiotics, hormonal regimens, and retinoids. Doses of oral antibiotics are shown in Table 2–23.

There is no justification in prescribing smaller doses because there is a slower rate of improvement and a more rapid relapse on stopping oral therapy. It is not wise to mix and match antibiotics, which is likely to increase resistance to *P. acnes.*

It is important to inform patients that there is usually little response to treatment in the first month. At 2 months there should be 20% to 25% improvement; at 4 months, 60%; and at 6 months 80% to 90% improvement. The rate of response of acne to antimicrobial therapy has lessened in the past 5 years because of an increase in *P. acnes* resistance.

Side Effects. Side effects of oral antibiotic therapy include gastrointestinal upset, vaginal candidiasis, and dose-dependent light-sensitive eruption. Benign intracranial hypertension, which may present as headache, dizziness, vertigo, or nausea, is an uncommon feature of minocycline therapy. These side effects cease on stopping the therapy or on dose reduction.

Indications for Isotretinoin

Isotretinoin is used in patients with moderate to severe acne who are not responding or are only partially responding to conventional therapy. Many physicians prescribe isotretinoin 1 mg/kg, particu-

TABLE 2-23. Minimum Doses of Oral Antibiotics for Acne	
Tetracycline	500 mg bid
Oxytetracycline	500 mg bid
Erythromycin	500 mg bid
Minocycline	100 mg daily
Doxycycline	100 mg daily
Trimethoprim	200 mg bid

larly if the patient is a male adolescent with truncal acne and severe disease. Most patients require 4 months of therapy, but 15% require longer; a very small number of these patients require up to 10 to 12 months of therapy. Most patients at the end of 4 months, or at least at the end of their therapy, are virtually free from acne, and 69% remain totally free of lesions, requiring no oral therapy for their acne ever again. Male patients with more severe acne and patients with truncal acne tend to fare less well and require repeat courses. Re-treatment with isotretinoin is safe, and the response is predictable.

Side Effects. Isotretinoin is an extremely effective drug, but it has many significant side effects. It is highly teratogenic, and both a negative pregnancy test and adequate counseling on contraception are essential before initiating therapy. Pregnancy is contraindicated during and for 1 month after therapy.

Every patient on isotretinoin therapy will develop some mucocutaneous side effects. These are easily controlled by the use of simple emollients, oilated bath preparations, and, if necessary, weak or intermediate-strength steroid ointments. Secondary infection of the skin with *S. aureus* often complicates many of the mucocutaneous side effects of isotretinoin. Thus a course of an oral antibiotic such as dicloxacillin may be required.

Systemic side effects of isotretinoin include benign intracranial hypertension, myalgia, arthralgia, and, very rarely, diffuse interstitial skeletal hyperostosis. Abnormalities in liver function and fasting lipid levels have been reported but are not normally clinically significant.

Surgical Treatment of Scars

Evaluation

Scarring from acne takes many different forms. The face, the back, the chest, and even the arms can be involved. Scars can be hypertrophic or atrophic. Some scars, referred to as ice pick scars, are quite small but extend well through the dermis.

Treatment Options

Dermabrasion is the treatment of choice for sloped acne scars, but is not effective for ice pick scars. This procedure involves sanding away multiple layers of skin, leaving behind a partial dermal injury that resembles an abrasion. The wound heals by direct reepithelialization from remaining appendageal structures. Because dermabrasion relies on reepithelialization, it cannot be carried deeper than the reticular dermis and therefore is incapable of eliminating scars that extend deeper than this layer. Dermabrasion need not be denied anyone because of race or ethnicity. Darkly pigmented patients should be warned that normal repigmentation does not begin until the skin has completely healed and may not be complete for several weeks, during which time the face is pink.

Punch elevation can be successfully employed as an adjunct to dermabrasion when a scar extends too deep to effectively dermabrade but still retains normal epidermis at the bottom of the scar. This process involves drilling out the depressed scar at its margin and elevating the depressed skin to surface level. Punch elevation is usually performed before dermabrasion, which is then used to further blend the edges of the elevated skin. This technique is not indicated if the scar has a cicatricial base.

Punch grafting is employed chiefly for ice pick scars when they extend into the subcutaneous tissue or have a cicatricial base. This technique involves removing the entire ice pick scar, including the beveled component, and repairing this hole with a small skin graft, usually harvested from the retroauricular area. Dermabrasion is usually used to blend the edges of the graft.

Predermabrasion excision involves excising scars judged not to be amenable to dermabrasion and repairing them with direct suture closure. Subsequently the site is dermabraded to blend the resulting scar. *Simultaneous excision and dermabrasion* may also be used for deeper scars.

Filling substances such as Zyderm Collagen, Fibrel, and autologous collagen are useful as an adjunct to dermabrasion. These substances may be used to further elevate a depressed scar after dermabrasion. However, all of these are reabsorbed in time and must be repeated at least annually. As an adjunct to dermabrasion, fillers can be employed 3 to 6 months after the procedure to further improve scars that remain after the abrasion.

Chemical peel is particularly useful in cases in which dermabrasion is performed only over a small portion of a face or facial areas adjacent to the hairline. Chemical peel can then be used to blend the nonscarred skin or hair-bearing areas. This decreases the transition from normal to dermabraded skin. Chemical peel can also be used subsequent to dermabrasion to blend areas of permanent hyperpigmentation or hypopigmentation. Medium-depth chemical peels use trichloroacetic acid at a concentration of 35% or greater and may be combined with an epidermolytic agent such as CO_2 ice, Jessner's solution, or 70% glycolic acid to increase the depth of the peel. Phenol can be used to achieve a deep dermal chemical peel but carries the potential risk of permanent hypopigmentation, as well as renal and cardiac toxicity.

Laser resurfacing involves the use of a CO_2 laser to smooth over scars. This new technique appears as effective as dermabrasion but with a lower risk/benefit ratio.

Complications. Complications associated with dermabrasion for acne scars include hypo- and hyperpigmentation, infection, and scarring.

HIDRADENITIS SUPPURATIVA

(CM&S Chapter 50)

Definition

Hidradenitis suppurativa is a chronic, suppurative, granulomatous and fibrosing condition that affects areas of the skin rich in apocrine glands, such as the axillae, groin, and perineum. Most consider it to be primarily a disease of follicular occlusion in which apocrine glands are secondarily infected by bacteria.

Clinical Description

Hidradenitis suppurativa (apocrine hidradenitis) usually first appears at puberty, the age at onset of other acneiform conditions. Patients present with multiple cysts, scars, and suppuration of the axillary, anogenital, and sometimes inframammary areas, often accompanied by facial and truncal acne. Early cases may present as cysts or furuncles. Repeated flares with increasing numbers of lesions make the diagnosis clear. Eventually low-grade infection and chronic abscess formation with progressive scarring may become constant.

Differential Diagnosis

Lymphogranuloma venereum, granuloma inguinale, and ulcerative colitis must be considered in the differential diagnosis.

Treatment

Hygiene

Good hygiene is critical. Actively draining lesions may respond to soaks or wet dressings. Topical antibiotics in cream or powder form are useful for treatment and prophylaxis of the disease and may be substituted for deodorants, which often aggravate the condition. Tight-fitting garments should be avoided.

Dietary counseling is important for these frequently obese individuals to help prevent maceration in intertriginous zones with resulting bacterial infection that makes the disease more aggressive.

Antibiotics

Initial therapy for hidradenitis suppurativa is usually topical and systemic antibiotic therapy. Full doses of tetracycline, erythromycin, cephalosporins, and minocycline may be helpful. Long-term therapy with these agents may be required, especially if there is concomitant acne. It is often necessary to rotate antibiotics to prevent resistance. The most successful approach is to tailor antibacterial coverage to the sensitivities of regularly performed bacterial culture.

Corticosteroids

Prednisone, 0.5 to 1.0 mg/kg given daily for 10 days to 2 weeks, may be useful for severe flares. Intralesional corticosteroids (triamcinolone acetonide, 5–10 mg/mL) are especially useful for new lesions to decrease inflammation.

Isotretinoin

Isotretinoin (1–2 mg/kg) has been used in an attempt to minimize scarring and inflammation. Most patients respond to some degree; however, repeat treatment is usually required.

Surgery

When medical treatment fails, surgical intervention is often required for hidradenitis. Although incision and drainage may appear to be useful for new lesions, over the course of the chronic disease it can be harmful because new sinus tracts and fibrosis are created. Exteriorization of cysts and sinuses, which involves complete unroofing of the affected focus with careful curettage of granulation tissue, has been recommended. Individual cysts or sinuses can also be excised. Often large areas of scarred cystic tissue must be removed to control repeated infection. More serious cases may require removal of most of the axillary, anogenital, or inguinal skin, requiring split-thickness skin grafts or large flaps.

Liposuction of the axillae and inguinal areas may be performed to remove as many apocrine glands and hair follicles as possible before they become cystic. This must be done early in the course of the disease before scarring and inflammation make this procedure impossible.

ROSACEA

(CM&S Chapter 51)

Definition and Clinical Description

Rosacea, also called *acne rosacea*, is a chronic inflammatory skin condition that has a predisposition to affect the central ''flush'' areas of the face, namely, the central cheeks, nose, brow, and chin. This condition most frequently takes the form of flushing erythema with an intermittent acneiform eruption. It is characterized by erythema, telangiectases, acneiform papules and pustules, furuncles, and cysts. Some or all of these lesions may be seen in a given individual.

Rhinophyma results from chronic hyperplasia of sebaceous glands and connective tissue of the nose. It is seen almost exclusively in men over 40. The nasal tip and alae are usually distorted by large, lobulated, often pendulous masses of hypertrophic sebaceous tissue. Adjacent areas of the cheek may also be involved.

Granulomatous rosacea is a variant of papular rosacea in which there are histopathologic findings of granuloma formation with a clinical picture consistent with rosacea. Clinically, yellow-brown nodules are seen on the lateral surfaces of the face and on the neck below the mandible in addition to the medial face.

Concomitant ocular involvement may occur in up to 58% of patients with rosacea. This may take the form of blepharitis, conjunctivitis, episcleritis, iritis, and keratitis.

Constitutional findings are uncommon. These include gastritis and migraine headaches.

Vascular lesions examined microscopically reveal a nonspecific lymphohistiocytic perivascular infiltrate and telangiectases. With papulopustular lesions, ruptured follicular infundibula, perifollicular neutrophilic abscesses, and surrounding granulomatous inflammation occur. *Demodex folliculorum* is frequently found in the follicles. In granulomatous rosacea, noncaseating epithelioid granulomas surround follicular infundibula. Rhinophyma is characterized by sebaceous hyperplasia with fibrosis of the dermis and telangiectases.

Pathogenesis and Etiology

Although the precise etiology of rosacea is unknown, various factors appear to contribute to this condition. The flushing mechanism appears to be triggered by the consumption of very hot foods and beverages, highly spiced foods, or alcohol.

Environmental factors that may cause flushing are heat, cold, and wind. Sun exposure may precipitate acute episodes of flushing, but solar damage does not appear to be a necessary prerequisite for the development of rosacea.

Diagnosis and Differential Diagnosis

The differential diagnosis of rosacea is listed in Table 2–24.

Treatment

Medical Treatment

Rosacea is generally treated by avoidance of exacerbating factors (emotional stress, sunlight, wind, hot beverages, spicy foods, alcoholic beverages, and extremes of heat and cold) combined with a variety of drugs. Sunscreens should always be prescribed.

Oral tetracycline hydrochloride (250 to 1000 mg per day) or its derivatives minocycline (50 to 200 mg per day) and doxycycline (100 to 200 mg per day), are the first-line pharmacologic agents used to treat the acneiform component of rosacea. This therapy must be maintained indefinitely, since relapses are common following

---

TABLE 2-24.   Differential Diagnosis of Rosacea

ERYTHROTELANGIECTATIC ROSACEA

Lupus erythematosus
Corticosteroid-induced rosacea-like syndrome
Photodermatoses

ACNEIFORM ROSACEA

Acne vulgaris
Bromoderma or iododerma
Pustular folliculitis
Perioral dermatitis
Seborrheic dermatitis

GRANULOMATOUS ROSACEA

Acne conglobata
Amyloidosis
Sarcoidosis (lupus pernio)
Lupus vulgaris

discontinuation of therapy. Other antibiotics, such as ampicillin or erythromycin, have been used effectively when, for one reason or another, tetracycline is contraindicated, but the response rate remains highest with oral tetracycline.

Oral 13-*cis*-retinoic acid therapy has been used with excellent clinical results for treating severe, recalcitrant rosacea, but a high rate of recurrence has been noted by some authors following cessation of therapy.

In the menopausal age, estrogens or clonidine has been found to be effective in some women with severe rosacea.

Topical antibiotics such as clindamycin phosphate and erythromycin have shown some usefulness in controlling the acneiform component of rosacea. Topical metronidazole gel is more consistently effective. The gel is used alone as initial therapy for mild cases of rosacea or in combination with oral antibiotics for the initial treatment of more severe forms of rosacea. In severe cases, topical metronidazole may be used as maintenance therapy after oral antibiotics have been discontinued.

Other topical treatments that have been used alone or in combination with oral antibiotics include low-potency, nonfluorinated topical steroids, benzoyl peroxide, sulfur-containing products (Sulfacet-R, Sulfoxyl), and Vioform.

Surgical Treatment

Telangiectatic vessels may be destroyed with electrosurgery or laser surgery. The 585-nm flashlamp pumped pulsed-dye laser is useful in treating telangiectases in patients with rosacea.

Patients with rhinophyma may benefit from surgical procedures to correct the hypertrophic changes. Modalities that have been used include surgical ablation, electrosurgery (cutting current), laser surgery, and dermabrasion.

Electrosurgery

Modern electrosurgery equipment uses high-frequency alternating current to generate a variety of therapeutic waveforms. For very thin lesions, such as those involving the surface epithelium, superficial electrosurgical destruction by *electrodesiccation* or *electrofulguration* can be achieved with little, if any, scarring. *Electrocoagulation*, which penetrates more completely, is used to coagulate hair follicles, blood vessels, or more extensive skin tumors. For incision or excision of tissue, *electrosection* is the current of choice.

PERIORAL DERMATITIS

(CM&S Chapter 52)

Definition

Perioral dermatitis is a discrete eruption consisting of grouped erythematous papules, vesicles, or pustules located around the mouth with marked sparing of the skin immediately surrounding the vermilion border. It often occurs on the nasolabial folds, on the chin, around the eyelids, and in the glabellar region.

Clinical Description

The most common presentation occurs in young women between the ages of 19 and 40, but this disorder also occurs in men and children. Clinically, perioral dermatitis appears to be a combination of seborrheic dermatitis, acne, and eczema. The distribution is in the same areas of facial seborrhea, the skin often appears chapped or irritated as in eczema, and there are papules and pustules as in acne. The cause is unknown, but a nonallergic response to topical corticosteroids or to moisturizers has been suggested.

Diagnosis and Differential Diagnosis

The typical patient is a young woman with papules and vesicles sparing the vermilion border and extending to the perinasal and periorbital area. It can be difficult to make the diagnosis in patients presenting with solely periorbital or perinasal lesions. The main diseases that need to be differentiated are seborrheic dermatitis, acne rosacea, and contact dermatitis.

Treatment

All topical corticosteroids should be stopped. If the patient has been using fluorinated steroids for a long time, the dosage may need to be tapered during withdrawal by substituting a 1% hydrocortisone acetate cream for a short time period.

The treatment of choice for perioral dermatitis is oral tetracycline starting at 250 mg twice a day for approximately 6 weeks, then tapered to 250 mg per day for a few weeks and then stopped. Relapse is uncommon. In patients who have been using topical fluorinated steroids for a long period of time, 1.0 to 1.5 g of tetracycline is frequently required to control this eruption.

If the patient is unable to take tetracycline, erythromycin in the same dosage may be used but is not as effective. If oral medications are not possible or desirable, topical metronidazole, erythromycin, or clindamycin have been used successfully.

Patients with perioral dermatitis are often very intolerant of any topical medication. Because of this, it may be best to avoid topical therapy completely.

PSEUDOFOLLICULITIS BARBAE

(CM&S Chapter 53)

Definition

Pseudofolliculitis barbae is a common inflammatory disorder of the hair follicles occurring most often in the beard area of men who shave. Black men are especially affected.

Clinical Description

The primary lesions are firm, skin-colored follicular papules. Pustules or papulopustules may also be present, but they are secondary lesions. The anterior neck, submandibular area, chin, and lower jaw areas are most commonly affected, whereas the mustache and sideburn areas are usually spared. Secondary complications of secondary bacterial infection or abscess formation can lead to alopecia, scarring, and occasionally keloid formation. The severity of the disorder ranges from mild (fewer than a dozen papules and/or pustules) to severe (more than 100 papules or pustules). The hairs overlying and beneath the mandible often have a disorganized direction of growth, which makes shaving difficult. Body areas other than the beard area that are closely or repeatedly shaven, including the scalp, axillae, pubis, and legs, can also be affected.

Pathogenesis and Etiology

Shaving is the precipitating factor of pseudofolliculitis barbae, especially close shaving in individuals with tightly curled coarse hair, the type more frequently found in blacks than in whites. In black men who shave frequently, the reported incidence ranges from 45% to 83%. The curled hair is usually cut at an oblique angle during shaving, creating a sharp tip at the end of the hair that enables it to penetrate the skin. More ingrown hairs are produced when the skin is pulled taut while shaving and when shaving against the direction of hair growth.

Differential Diagnosis

See Table 2–25.

Treatment

Complete cure of pseudofolliculitis barbae is possible if shaving is discontinued. The embedded hair tips will dislodge themselves spontaneously in 2 to 6 weeks, and symptoms will resolve rapidly.

Except for mild cases, pseudofolliculitis barbae requires medical intervention during the acute pustular phase that is painful and/or pruritic. The following therapeutic approach is recommended:

1. Shaving should be discontinued for a minimum of 1 month for

---

TABLE 2-25. Differential Diagnosis of Pseudofolliculitis Barbae

Acne keloidalis nuchae
Folliculitis
Pityrosporum folliculitis
Impetigo
Tinea barbae
Acne vulgaris
Sarcoidal papules

---

mild cases, 2 to 3 months for moderate cases, and 3 to 6 months for severe cases. During this time the beard may be trimmed with scissors or electric clippers to a minimum length of 1.0 cm. The patient should be informed that when shaving is discontinued, pseudofolliculitis worsens after 1 week because all previously shaved hairs reenter the skin, creating more clinical lesions.

2. Warm tap water, saline, or Burow's solution compresses are used 10 to 15 minutes three times daily to soothe the lesions, remove any crust, stop drainage secondary to inflammation, and soften the epidermis to allow easier release of "ingrown hairs."

3. The patient should use a magnifying mirror each day to search for "ingrown hairs." Once the hair is found, its release is facilitated by carefully lifting the hair loop with a toothpick. "Ingrown hairs" should not be plucked because the broken-off hair may cause irritation or may eventually penetrate the follicular wall.

4. After the "ingrown hairs" are compressed and released, a topical hydrocortisone lotion should be applied.

5. When secondary bacterial infection is present, the appropriate systemic antibiotic should be prescribed.

6. In cases that do not improve with this regimen, 5 to 10 days of prednisone, 40 to 60 mg per day, may be indicated, provided there are no contraindications to this corticosteroid.

7. Shaving should not be resumed until all the inflammatory lesions have cleared and all "ingrown hairs" have been released.

For those who must shave, the following regimen is recommended

1. Electric clippers should be used to remove any preexisting beard hair as closely as possible without producing irritation.

2. The beard area should be washed with a nonabrasive acne soap and rough washcloth. Areas with "ingrown hairs" should be massaged with a soft toothbrush or polyester web sponge.

3. The beard area should be rinsed to remove any remaining soap, and warm water compresses should be applied to any other area to be shaved for approximately 5 minutes.

4. The patient should then use the shaving cream of his or her choice, massaging a moderate amount of lather into the area to be shaved. The lather should not be allowed to dry. If for any reason it does so, it should be reapplied before shaving. Gels seem to give a better and less irritating shave than creams or foams.

5. A sharp razor blade is chosen that cuts best with minimal irritation, and shaving is done with the grain of the hair, using short strokes while avoiding pulling the skin taut. Twice over one area is usually sufficient. In those areas where hair growth is haphazard, daily brushing of the beard with a soft brush often gives direction to the grain of the hair.

6. When shaving is completed the face should be rinsed with warm tap water and then compressed with cool to cold water for 5 to 10 minutes.

7. The patient should then use a magnifying mirror to search for any "ingrown hairs." When they are found, a toothpick should be gently inserted under the loop of the hair and the embedded hair tip lifted out.

8. The most soothing and least irritating after-shave preparation should then be applied. If burning or pruritus ensues, a topical hydrocortisone lotion should be used as the after-shave preparation.

There is a special Bumpfighter razor (American Safety Razor Co., Staunton, VA) on the market that has a single-edge blade that allows closer shaves with less irritation.

For those who find shaving too irritating or uncomfortable, chemical depilatories may be used.

Tretinoin (Retin-A) cream, gel, or solution may be used as an adjunct to shaving in patients with mild to moderate pseudofolliculitis, especially if treatment is initiated soon after the onset of the disease. There is a limited clinical response in patients with chronic and severe pseudofolliculitis. Tretinoin is postulated to work by alleviating hyperkeratosis and ''toughening'' the skin. Those who shave in the morning should apply the tretinoin at night. The use of tretinoin does not alter the previously described shaving regimen.

DISORDERS OF FOLLICULAR KERATINIZATION

(CM&S Chapter 54)

Keratosis Pilaris

Definition

Keratosis pilaris is a common skin condition in which groups of follicles demonstrate tiny keratinized plugs and varying degrees of erythema.

Clinical Description

Keratosis pilaris is so common that there is some disagreement whether it should be classified as a disease or a normal variant. In characteristic locations (extensor arms, thighs, and buttocks), groups of follicles form tiny papules surmounted by keratinized plugs, giving the skin a characteristic rough feeling. The degree of inflammation is variable; in some cases there is no erythema, and in others there is sufficient erythema to result in postinflammatory hyperpigmentation.

Treatment

Twelve percent ammonium lactate lotion with or without medium-potency topical steroids, mild keratolytics containing salicylic acid such as Epilyt, and topical retinoic acid may each be successful, but the roughness usually recurs upon discontinuing treatment.

Keratosis Pilaris Atrophicans of the Face

Definition and Clinical Description

Keratosis pilaris atrophicans of the face, also known as ulerythema ophryogenes, is classically localized to the lateral eyebrows and manifests from an early age as erythema, follicular plugging, and scarring. A similar pattern may occur on the cheeks.

Treatment

Topical steroids attenuate the erythema and the process may be slowed by combined treatment with topical retinoic acid and topical steroids.

E. Chondritis

CHONDRODERMATITIS NODULARIS

(CM&S Chapter 55)

Definition

Chondrodermatitis nodularis is a common, benign, painful lesion of the ear in which there is fibrosis of the dermis, degeneration of cartilage, or both.

Clinical Description

The patient complains of a small lump on the ear that is painful when lying on the affected side. The lesions are discrete and oval with a raised rolled edge and central ulcer or depression that usually contains a crust or scale; most are unilateral, although bilateral and multiple lesions are recognized. Any cartilaginous site on the lateral surface of the ear may be affected, although the helix in men and the anthelix in women are the most common sites. Men are more often affected, and two thirds of patients are over 60 years of age.

Pathogenesis and Etiology

The cause of chondrodermatitis nodularis is unknown, although cold injury, actinic damage, and pressure necrosis have been proposed.

Treatment

Chondrodermatitis nodularis is a benign condition, and in patients without pain-induced sleep disturbance no treatment is required. If treatment is necessary, medical therapy should be tried first and surgical excision reserved for unresponsive cases. Topical 2% lignocaine gel is applied 30 minutes before going to bed. Betamethasone valerate cream applied to the sore skin twice a day or intralesional steroids, given as triamcinolone, 0.2 to 0.5 mL, in a dose of 10 mg/mL, are occasionally effective. Blindly destructive therapies such as electrosurgery and curettage result in relapse in approximately one third of patients. Using the curette to remove necrotic cartilage after elliptical skin excision or carbon dioxide laser destruction may be more effective. There are no published results of the effect of cryotherapy. Elliptical excision results in a recurrence rate of up to 40%, usually at cut cartilage edges. Wedge excision is a deforming and unnecessary operation. Cure can be achieved by cartilage shave excision alone after incising through the skin on either side of the nodule.

RELAPSING POLYCHONDRITIS

(CM&S Chapter 56)

Definition

Relapsing polychondritis is an uncommon disease that inflames and ultimately can destroy cartilage at virtually any site within the body.

Clinical Description

In polychondritis, episodic bouts of inflammation and degeneration of cartilage and connective tissue create pain and eventuate in deformity of the pinna of the ears and nasal septum, hoarseness, nondeforming but exquisitely painful arthritis of one or a few joints, hearing loss, fever, and malaise. Less commonly, the tracheobronchial tree, heart valves, eyes, and aorta become involved. A cutaneous or systemic vasculitis can occur. Within individual patients, the degree to which the disease assumes an intermittent (i.e., relapsing) or protracted process is unpredictable.

Life expectancy is shortened in patients with polychondritis. Most deaths related to the disease are attributable to bacterial pneumonia after airway collapse or aortic insufficiency not amenable to surgical management. In patients younger than the age of 50, the presence of anemia, saddle-nose deformity, or systemic vasculitis has been statistically associated with shortened survival.

Pathology

The primary histopathologic features of relapsing polychondritis are those of a lymphocytic infiltrate that initially destroys the perichondrium and eventually the cartilage. Because the soft inferior lobe of the external ear is devoid of cartilage, only the superior cartilaginous portions display inflammation in the disease. The septum of the nose is composed of a bony and more distal cartilaginous segment, accounting for the preservation of the proximal region of the nose when the cartilage supported area collapses into the hallmark saddle-nose deformity.

Pathogenesis and Etiology

Detection of antibodies to type II collagen in the serum of some patients during highly active periods suggests that autoimmunity to this host constituent is involved.

Differential Diagnosis

Polychondritis is often initially misdiagnosed as an infectious perichondritis of the ear caused by *Pseudomonas aeruginosa*. External ear inflammation caused by trauma, exposure to cold or sunlight, Wegener's granulomatosis, and other preexisting autoimmune diseases such as rheumatoid arthritis, systemic lupus erythematosus, Hashimoto's thyroiditis, and ankylosing spondylitis should be considered in the differential diagnosis.

Treatment

Treatment of polychondritis is frequently suboptimal and leads to significant degrees of comorbidity. Prolonged administration of anti-inflammatory drugs is often necessary to improve a patient's symptoms. For initial limited and less severe attacks, a nonsteroidal anti-inflammatory drug may suffice but most patients require prednisone therapy at initial doses of 20 to 60 mg per day. The episodic or fluctuating nature of polychondritis often permits rapid tapering or discontinuation of steroid therapy. Oral methotrexate (7.5 to 15 or 20 mg a week) allows de-escalation of prednisone doses. In life-threatening situations, a cyclosporine or cyclophosphamide should be considered.

F. Vasculitis and Disorders of Vascular Reactivity

TEMPORAL ARTERITIS

(CM&S Chapter 57)

Definition and Clinical Description

Temporal arteritis (also known as giant cell arteritis) is a large vessel vasculitis of unknown etiology observed in patients older than the age of 50. Clinical criteria for the classification of temporal arteritis were recently derived and include age at least 50, new-onset localized headache, temporal artery pain on palpation or diminished pulsation, erythrocyte sedimentation rate at least 50 mm/h, and temporal artery biopsy specimen demonstrating mononuclear cell or granulomatous arteritis. The diagnosis is assigned when at least three of these criteria are met.

Early recognition and treatment may prevent sudden and irreversible visual loss, which is the most important morbidity of this illness. The usual clinical manifestations of temporal arteritis reflect its systemic nature and predilection for the extracranial vessels, which possess an internal elastic lamina. Intracranial vessels, which have little or no internal elastic lamina, are generally spared in this illness. The most common "arteritic" symptoms include headache, visual loss, scalp tenderness, and jaw claudication. Joint involvement includes polymyalgia rheumatica, which is an arthritis of the shoulders and hips that may precede, follow, or coincide with the onset of temporal arteritis. Nonspecific systemic symptoms such as fever, malaise, and weight loss are common. In fact, temporal arteritis may mimic an occult malignancy or cause a fever of unknown origin. Less common, but serious manifestations of this disease include great vessel arteritis (aortitis, or vasculitis of the aorta's immediate branches), organ system ischemia, or infarction (e.g., stroke, bowel infarction, or cholecystitis).

Palpation of the temporal artery may reveal local tenderness, beading, or lack of pulsation. In patients with concomitant polymyalgia rheumatica, joint examination will demonstrate painful shoulder and/or hip motion with or without limitation.

Dermatologic problems in temporal arteritis, which are uncommon, rarely occur without other suggestive symptoms and include scalp ulceration and necrosis, urticaria, pigmentary changes, superficial ulcerations and even gangrene of the extremities, purpura, bullae, and tongue swelling or necrosis. Lower extremity ulceration, gangrene, or neuropathy may be preceded by claudication and mistakenly attributed to atherosclerotic peripheral vascular disease.

Pathology

Temporal artery biopsy reveals segmental inflammatory infiltrates, initially including neutrophils and eosinophils, but later consisting of lymphocytes, plasma cells, macrophages, and giant cells within all layers of the vessel. The internal elastic lamina is especially affected in most cases with resultant intimal fibrosis and thickening and consequent narrowing of the lumen.

Diagnosis and Differential Diagnosis

The diagnosis should be suspected in older patients with suggestive local or systemic symptoms (new localized headache, scalp tenderness, shoulder and hip arthralgia, fever, weight loss), especially if associated with an elevated erythrocyte sedimentation rate. The dermatologic manifestations may easily be confused with trauma, bullous disease, cellulitis, atherosclerotic or other thromboembolic disease, urticarial or other vasculitis, or erythema nodosum.

Treatment

Nearly all patients with temporal arteritis will respond rapidly and dramatically to high-dose systemic corticosteroid therapy (e.g., prednisone, 1 mg/kg per day in a single oral dose), which should be tapered slowly over 6 to 8 months. Systemic, local, and the rare dermatologic manifestations of disease improve markedly within days or weeks. However, once visual loss or other end-organ infarction has occurred, it is generally irreversible.

POLYARTERITIS NODOSA

(CM&S Chapter 58)

Clinical Description

Classic Polyarteritis Nodosa

Classic polyarteritis nodosa is a systemic vasculitic process that involves the medium-sized muscular arteries in virtually all organ systems. It occurs in persons of all age groups, with a mean age at onset of approximately 45 years. The kidneys are the most frequently involved organ system, with the liver, heart, and gastrointestinal tract also involved in greater than 50% of cases. The musculoskeletal and central nervous systems are also frequently involved, but pulmonary arterial system and splenic arteries are almost always spared.

There is cutaneous involvement in up to 25% of cases of classic polyarteritis nodosa. The most frequent appearance of these lesions is as nodules, ulcerations, or the livedo reticularis pattern of erythema on the lower extremities. The deep-seated nodules are most often tender or painful. Lesions may also be seen on the trunk and upper extremities.

Pathology

There is a predominantly neutrophilic infiltrate surrounding and invading the muscular walls of medium-sized arteries. There is fibrinoid necrosis of the endothelial surface, disruption of the internal elastic lamina, and frequently thrombosis and extravasation of erythrocytes. Leukocytoclastic vasculitis is also seen in cutaneous venules.

Pathogenesis and Etiology

The classic form of polyarteritis nodosa has been associated with a wide range of antigenemias, including β-hemolytic streptococcal infection and hepatitis B surface antigens.

Diagnosis and Differential Diagnosis

The livedoid lesions and ulcerations would raise the possibility of other vasculitides, including Wegener's granulomatosis, small vessel hypersensitivity vasculitis, and superficial migratory thrombophlebitis. The tender, erythematous deep-seated nodules clinically resemble erythema nodosum, nodular vasculitis, and erythema induratum.

Treatment

In the precorticosteroid era, mortality was quite high. Five-year survival rates are now approximately 96% on combined treatment regimens including steroids (1 mg/kg/day) and cyclophosphamide (50–100 mg/day). Patients with extensive systemic involvement require high-dose steroid therapy, often for years, whereas in disease predominantly involving the skin, remission can often be attained in 3 to 6 months of lower dose steroid therapy.

Clinical and Histologic Variants

Benign Cutaneous Polyarteritis Nodosa

In benign cutaneous polyarteritis nodosa the disease is limited largely to the skin. Patients present with painful, bilateral solitary or multiple lower leg nodules in most cases. A livedo reticularis pattern, characteristic of classic polyarteritis nodosa, is also frequently seen, and ulceration is a common complication. Constitutional symptoms such as arthralgias and fever are unusual and mild when present. History of a recent infection can often be elicited.

Histologic diagnosis of benign cutaneous polyarteritis nodosa is confirmed based on a neutrophilic vasculitis involving medium-sized, muscular arteries found in the deep reticular dermis and panniculus, while the smaller vessels in the upper dermis show only a nonspecific perivascular lymphocytic infiltrate.

Because systemic vasculitis and positive hepatitis serology have been found in patients with the benign cutaneous variant, it is most likely that the variant represents a spectrum of classic polyarteritis nodosa in which the cutaneous manifestations are predominant, internal organ involvement is less pronounced, and the clinical course is more protracted.

MICROSCOPIC POLYARTERITIS, WEGENER'S GRANULOMATOSIS, AND CHURG-STRAUSS SYNDROME

(CM&S Chapter 59)

Definition

Vasculitis is inflammation of vessel walls; perivascular infiltrates of leukocytes alone without mural involvement are not definitive evidence for vasculitis.

Microscopic polyarteritis, Wegener's granulomatosis, and Churg-Strauss syndrome are closely related vasculitides. They all share necrotizing small vessel vasculitis, absence of immune deposits, and presence of antineutrophil cytoplasmic autoantibodies (ANCA). Each syndrome, however, has distinctive defining features, such as the necrotizing granulomatous inflammation of Wegener's granulomatosis and the eosinophilia and asthma of Churg-Strauss syndrome.

Microscopic polyarteritis is defined as necrotizing vasculitis with few or no immune deposits affecting small vessels (capillaries, venules and arterioles), although small or medium-sized arteries may also be affected. The absence of vascular immune deposits differentiates this disease from various forms of immune complex–mediated small vessel vasculitis, such as Henoch-Schönlein purpura, cryoglobulinemic vasculitis, hypocomplementemic urticarial vasculitis, and lupus vasculitis.

Microscopic polyarteritis differs from polyarteritis nodosa with respect to the presence of vasculitis in vessels smaller than arteries in the former but not the latter. Both diseases can cause skin nodules, but only microscopic polyarteritis causes purpura at sites of leukocytoclastic angiitis.

Wegener's granulomatosis is defined as granulomatous inflammation involving the respiratory tract, and necrotizing vasculitis affecting small to medium-sized vessels (capillaries, venules, arterioles, and arteries). Churg-Strauss syndrome is defined as eosinophil-rich and granulomatous inflammation involving the respiratory tract and necrotizing vasculitis affecting small to medium-sized vessels, and associated with asthma and blood eosinophilia.

Clinical Description

All three diseases are most common in the sixth decade of life; however, all age groups may be affected. The clinical presentations of each of these diseases are quite varied among patients because different organ system distributions of lesions occur among different patients. The initial clinical presentations often include systemic features such as fever, malaise, myalgias, and arthralgias. Major target organs for vasculitis include skin, lungs, kidneys, gut, skeletal muscle, heart, and peripheral nerves. In the latter four organs, symptoms related to inflammation give rise to abdominal pain, myalgias, myocardial infarction, and mononeuritis multiplex.

Especially in patients with Wegener's granulomatosis and Churg-Strauss syndrome, respiratory signs and symptoms are frequent. Findings include granulomatous inflammation in Wegener's granulomatosis and Churg-Strauss syndrome, eosinophilic infiltrates in Churg-Strauss syndrome, and hemorrhagic capillaritis in microscopic polyarteritis. Upper respiratory tract disease, especially destructive sinusitis, is most prominent in Wegener's granulomatosis but also occurs with microscopic polyarteritis and Churg-Strauss syndrome. Renal disease is common in all but microscopic polyarteritis.

The cutaneous manifestations are similar to those caused by other vasculitides that can involve arteries, arterioles, capillaries, and venules in the skin and subcutaneous tissue. Necrotizing leukocytoclastic angiitis affecting postcapillary venules, along with capillaries and arterioles, typically causes recurrent transient showers of palpable purpura, most pronounced on the lower extremities and buttocks. Necrotizing arteritis in the deep dermis and subcutaneous tissue most often produces tender, red nodules most frequently on the lower extremities that may be accompanied by livedo reticularis. Thrombosis of inflamed arteries may cause ischemic effects in the tissues supplied by that artery resulting in focal skin ulceration or digital infarction.

Cutaneous and subcutaneous inflammatory nodules caused by necrotizing granulomatous inflammation are most common in patients with Churg-Strauss syndrome but also occur in occasional patients with Wegener's granulomatosis.

Patients with microscopic polyarteritis have only signs and symptoms of small and medium-sized vessel vasculitis, whereas patients with Wegener's granulomatosis and Churg-Strauss syndrome have these as well as additional signs and symptoms attributable to the specific components of their syndromes. For example, patients with Churg-Strauss syndrome have a history of asthma and have blood eosinophilia.

The most specific and sensitive laboratory markers for all three diseases are ANCA (autoantibodies with specificity for enzymes in the granules of neutrophils and the lysosomes of monocytes).

Around 90% of patients with active, untreated, systemic Wegener's granulomatosis have C-ANCA (specific to proteinase). Although C-ANCA are very sensitive for Wegener's granulomatosis, they are not completely specific, because some patients with microscopic polyarteritis or necrotizing glomerulonephritis without systemic vasculitis have C-ANCA.

Approximately 80% of patients with microscopic polyarteritis have either C-ANCA or P-ANCA (specific for myeloperoxidase). Most patients with Churg-Strauss syndrome appear to have P-ANCA.

Diagnosis

Table 2–26 lists the diagnostics features of some forms of vasculitis.

TABLE 2-26. Diagnostic Features of Some Forms of Vasculitis Affecting the Skin

	PALPABLE PURPURA	CUTANEOUS OR SUBCUTANEOUS NODULES	FEATURES THAT SHOULD BE PRESENT	FEATURES THAT SHOULD BE ABSENT
Microscopic polyarteritis	++	+	Systemic necrotizing small vessel vasculitis, ANCA	Granulomatous inflammation, asthma, immune deposits
Wegener's granulomatosis	++	+	Granulomatous inflammation, ANCA	Asthma, vascular immune deposits
Churg-Strauss syndrome	++	++	Asthma, eosinophilia	Vascular immune deposits
Systemic immune complex vasculitis	+++	+	Vascular immune complex deposits	ANCA
Cutaneous leukocytoclastic angiitis	+++	0	Dermal leukocytoclastic	Systemic vasculitis, ANCA
Polyarteritis nodosa	0	+	Necrotizing arteritis	Vasculitis in vessels smaller than arteries, ANCA
Cutaneous polyarteritis nodosa	0	+++	Necrotizing arteritis in the skin	Systemic vasculitis, ANCA

0 = absent, + = occasionally present, ++ = often present, +++ = usually present.

Treatment

The cutaneous component of the disease is rarely the impetus for treatment. The most clear-cut indication for aggressive treatment is destructive pulmonary disease or rapidly progressive renal failure. With full-blown disease, combined corticosteroid—usually pulsed (7 mg/kg methylprednisolone, not exceeding 3 g for 3 days) followed by 1 mg/kg/day tapered over 3 to 6 months—and cytotoxic therapy—as either oral cyclophosphamide at 1–3 mg/kg/day for 6 to 12 months or as 6 monthly injections of 0.5–1.0 g/m²—is warranted. High-dose corticosteroid treatment alone often ameliorates the acute inflammatory injury, but the addition of cytotoxic therapy greatly improves the likelihood of long-term remission. Less severe and localized disease, however, may be controllable by corticosteroids alone.

Once microscopic polyarteritis, Wegener's granulomatosis, or Churg-Strauss syndrome is brought under control, a substantial number of patients have subsequent exacerbations that will require additional immunosuppressive treatment.

GRANULOMA FACIALE

(CM&S Chapter 60)

Clinical Description

Granuloma faciale is characterized by one to several erythematous to livid papules, plaques, or nodules of a few millimeters in size and rarely expanding to 8 cm in diameter. Most often these lesions are multiple and involve the face, eventually developing a brownish coloration with accentuation of the follicular orifices. Duration of the lesions is usually several months to years. The nose is the most commonly affected area, followed by the malar prominences and the forehead. Lesions may be asymptomatic or associated with mild pruritus or a stinging sensation.

Pathology

Characteristic findings are a mixed inflammatory infiltrate most often involving the papillary dermis, sparing the adventitial dermis, with neutrophils emanating from the blood vessel walls into the surrounding dermis admixed with eosinophils as well as lymphocytes and histiocytes. In early lesions there is evidence of small vessel vasculitis such as fibrin deposition and neutrophilic nuclear dust in and around the walls of venules.

Differential Diagnosis

The differential diagnosis of granuloma faciale includes facial infiltrates such as Jessner's lymphocytic infiltrate, pseudolymphoma, lupus erythematosus, polymorphic light eruption, and sarcoidosis.

Treatment

No therapy is uniformly effective in bringing about resolution of lesions. Treatments to consider include potent topical or intralesional corticosteroids, cryotherapy, pulsed dye or Q-switched ruby laser therapy, or dapsone.

ERYTHROMELALGIA AND FLUSHING

(CM&S Chapter 61)

Erythromelalgia and Erythermalgia

Definition

Erythromelalgia and erythermalgia are characterized by attacks of erythema due to vascular congestion and vasodilation affecting acral skin. The temperature of affected skin is elevated, and there is burning pain. Warmth intensifies the discomfort, and cold provides relief. There is often a "critical temperature," typically between 32°C (89.6°F) and 36°C (96.8°F), above which there is pain and below which there is relief.

Erythermalgia has a bilateral and symmetrical distribution, does not progress to acrocyanosis or peripheral gangrene and is refractory to treatment with low doses of aspirin.

Erythromelalgia is asymmetrical (typically in one or more toes or fingers or in the sole of the forefoot), responds to a single low dose of aspirin with complete relief for several days, can progress to acrocyanosis or peripheral gangrene, and is causally related to thrombocythemia. Prickling paresthesias usually precede, or interchange with, the attacks of burning pain and erythema.

Clinical Description

Erythromelalgia is associated with thrombocythemia, which is often a chronic myeloproliferative disorder. Secondary erythermalgia is associated with multiple disorders and vasoactive drug therapy. Because of these associations, erythromelalgia and secondary erythermalgia most affect those persons older than 40 years of age, including the very elderly. In contrast, primary erythermalgia can occur at any age, including childhood and puberty.

Pathology

Skin biopsy samples from areas of classic erythromelalgia consistently show thrombi in arterioles, without significant inflammation or involvement of venules, capillaries, or nerves. Erythromelalgia is caused by platelet-mediated arteriolar inflammation and thrombosis that occur in thrombocythemia. Histologic changes in the peripheral vasculature are usually absent in erythermalgia, suggesting a local disturbance of vasomotor regulation, either a functional abnormality in the vasculature or an autonomic neuropathy.

Treatment

Low doses of aspirin are effective in the symptomatic management of erythromelalgia. The treatment goal for secondary erythermalgia is to treat the associated disorder or discontinue the associated drug therapy.

Flushing

Definition

Flushing is a transient reddening of the face and frequently other areas, including the neck, ears, and upper chest. *Blushing* is a subset of flushing reactions associated with emotions, such as embarrassment or anxiety. *Hot flashes* refer to climacteric (menopausal) flushing.

Clinical Description

Flushing and blushing are common phenomena in healthy persons with insufficient pigmentation to totally obscure facial erythema. Because most individuals know that flushing is commonly caused by emotions or heat, few patients present with a chief complaint of flushing or blushing. More frequently, patients present with rosacea, a process exacerbated, if not caused, by frequent flushing and blushing.

Diagnosis and Differential Diagnosis

The first step in diagnosing a flushing reaction is to determine the mechanism: autonomic neural-mediated flushing, which includes eccrine sweating (''wet flush''), versus flushing from circulating agents that act directly on vascular smooth muscle (''dry flush''). The second step is to determine whether pain, paresthesias, or a burning sensation is associated with the dry flush. If so, then an antidromic sensorineural flushing reaction must be considered. If the patient has dry flushes without burning, then the third step is to determine whether the vasoactive agent is endogenous or exogenous. Exogenous, direct-acting vasodilators are discovered by asking the patient about foods, drugs, diagnostic tests, and other factors. If dry flushing cannot be associated with a drug or dietary agent, if a wide variety of agents seem to nonspecifically provoke the flushing reaction, or if it occurs spontaneously, and especially if there is a significant associated finding, such as diarrhea, headache, or pruritus, then an underlying systemic disease of which flushing may be a manifestation must be considered.

Treatment

Treatment should be targeted to the specific cause of the flushing reaction. Examples include nadolol, 40 mg, every morning to alleviate anxiety-induced tachycardia and blushing; clonidine, 0.1 mg, one-half tablet twice daily for climacteric flushing; and aspirin, 975 mg, 1 hour before taking the potent flushing-provoking agent niacin for the treatment of hyperlipidemia.

RAYNAUD'S PHENOMENON

(CM&S Chapter 62)

Definition

Raynaud's phenomenon is defined as episodic digital ischemia in response to cold or emotional stimuli and is characterized by sequential color changes (white, blue, and red) in the affected parts. Pallor is essential for the diagnosis, but attacks in patients in whom pallor does not occur can be called atypical Raynaud's phenomenon. Raynaud's phenomenon may be primary or secondary to other causes.

Clinical Description

Raynaud described intermittent attacks of pallor, cyanosis, and then rubor affecting one or more digits brought on by even a subtle lowering of temperature and occasionally by emotional upset. The prevalence of Raynaud's phenomenon is variously quoted as 5% to 30%. Most studies suggest that it is more common in women. Associated connective tissue disease may be as frequent as 13% in a hospital-based population, but in a healthy population it approximates 3%. All patients with Raynaud's phenomenon should be regarded as being at high risk of developing a connective tissue disease.

Pathology

Pathologic changes can be found in the digits of nearly all patients with Raynaud's phenomenon secondary to other causes. The presence of abnormal capillaries on nail fold microscopy or structural defects on angiography is incompatible with primary Raynaud's phenomenon and should lead to a search for an underlying cause.

Diagnosis and Differential Diagnosis

For the clinician, the principal challenge in Raynaud's phenomenon is to exclude an underlying cause. The most important causes are structural or traumatic factors, such as a cervical rib and vibration white finger, organic vascular disease, and associated connective tissue disease (Table 2–27).

Primary Raynaud's phenomenon is diagnosed according to the modified criteria of Allen and Brown:

1. Intermittent attacks of discoloration of extremities
2. Absence of evidence of organic peripheral arterial occlusion
3. Symmetrical or bilateral distribution
4. Trophic changes
5. Exclusion of any disease that could give rise to vasospastic symptoms

The prognosis of Raynaud's phenomenon depends on the presence or absence of an associated disease at time of initial assessment

TABLE 2-27. Causes of Raynaud's Phenomenon
Primary (or idiopathic) Raynaud's phenomenon
Trauma or vibration
Connective tissue disease and vasculitis
Obstructive arterial disease
Neurologic disease
Entrapment neuropathy
Reflex sympathetic dystrophy
Hematologic disease
Drugs and toxins
Ergot
β-Blockers
Methysergide
Vinblastine
Bleomycin
Oral contraceptives
Vinyl chloride
Nitroglycerin

and later progression to a systemic disease in initially apparently uncomplicated patients.

Treatment

Raynaud's phenomenon represents a therapeutic challenge. A significant number of patients remain grossly symptomatic, especially in the winter, in spite of aggressive treatment; some patients suffer pain and disability from digital ulceration and infection with the risk of gangrene and amputation despite the effectiveness of the oral calcium channel blocking agent nifedipine and the intravenous vasodilator prostacyclin. Calcium channel blocking drugs, including nifedipine, diltiazem, and nicardipine, are effective at blocking vasoconstriction in Raynaud's phenomenon. Nifedipine is the drug of first choice. Treatment can be initiated at initial doses of 10 mg three times daily or 20 mg twice daily of the sustained-release preparation. The dose can be increased steadily to control symptoms but to avoid side effects such as dizziness, headache, and leg swelling. Doses of 100 mg daily are sometimes achieved and tolerated. The dosage can be varied during the year or the drug discontinued in the summer.

Prostaglandin E, prostaglandin I_2 (prostacyclin), and iloprost (a prostaglandin I_2 analogue) as intermittent infusions are effective vasodilators in Raynaud's phenomenon. Guidelines from clinical studies as to regimens for dose, frequency, and duration of iloprost infusions are largely empiric. Five- to 10-day infusions for 4 to 8 hours a day can be used to good effect but the infusion rate is often limited by side effects such as flushing, headache, nausea, and bradycardia.

Intravenous infusions of calcitonin gene-related peptide (CGRP) have been shown to increase the acral cutaneous blood flow and promote healing of digital ulceration. CGRP is not yet commercially available.

NONINFLAMMATORY SMALL VESSEL OCCLUSIVE DISEASES

(CM&S Chapter 63)

Occlusion of the peripheral microvasculature, which can be thrombotic or embolic, is the fundamental process underlying a heterogeneous group of cutaneous and systemic disorders that are linked by a common final pathophysiologic pathway of tissue hypoxia due to vascular insufficiency. They share clinical features such as purpura, livedo reticularis, ulceration, and scarring. Despite the clinical similarities, there are distinct clinical, histopathologic, and etiopathologic differences.

Livedo Vasculopathy

Definition

Livedo vasculopathy is an idiopathic, occlusive cutaneous vasculopathy in which painful, persistent, and recurrent ulcerations develop on the lower extremities. With healing, stellate, depressed scars develop, and this characteristic clinical morphology has been termed *atrophie blanche* (white atrophy). Atrophie blanche is a nonspecific finding that is also seen as a secondary phenomenon, due to hypertensive vasculopathy, diabetes mellitus, dysproteinemic states, lupus erythematosus, and venous stasis. The terms *livedo vasculopathy, livedo (livedoid) vasculitis, segmental hyalinizing vasculitis,* and *livedo reticularis with ulceration* are synonymous.

Clinical Description

The onset of disease, which is twice as common in women, can be as early as the second or third decades of life. In patients with repetitive ulceration, increasing pain or the development of livedo can serve as a harbinger of an impending exacerbation. The earliest cutaneous lesions are erythematous to violaceous papules that ulcerate, and small ulcerations often coalesce to form larger areas of breakdown. Even as the ulcerative process continues, partial healing ensues and yields smooth, depressed, angulate, whitish areas of scarring (atrophie blanche). The natural history of the disorder consists of chronic, repetitive ulceration, with occasional spontaneous remissions. By definition, patients with livedo vasculopathy have disease limited to the skin, without systemic manifestations.

Pathology

The disorder is a vaso-occlusive process in which the lumina of many of the small vessels are occluded by fibrin thrombi, and fibrin deposits within vessel walls are also apparent.

Diagnosis and Differential Diagnosis

The diagnosis of livedo vasculopathy is made after exclusion of other conditions such as connective tissue diseases, venous stasis, the antiphospholipid syndrome, and vasculitis. The differential diagnosis can be approached by considering the causes of livedo reticularis, ulceration, or whitish scarring (Table 2–28).

Treatment

Treatments of small vessel occlusive disorders are listed in Table 2–29.

Cutaneous Atheroembolism

Definition

Atheroembolism is a more precise term for disease due to the embolism of fragments from ulcerated atheromatous plaques to peripheral vessels of the skin and viscera, otherwise cholesterol embolism.

Clinical Description

Atheroembolism, which develops only in patients with severe atherosclerosis, typically of the aortofemoral system, may be spontaneous or iatrogenic, occurring after vascular instrumentation or surgery.

The clinical findings can be subtle or florid, reflecting the size and number of the atheromatous fragments as well as their site of origin. The lesions can develop immediately after instrumentation or can occur weeks to months after the predisposing event. Purpuric or purplish discoloration of the toes and livedo reticularis are the most common findings, but upper extremity livedo reticularis can be encountered in embolism from the ascending aorta. Palpable purpuric papules or nodules suggesting vasculitis may also be seen. With larger atheroemboli, ischemic necrosis and ulceration occur and ulcers due to atheroembolism can become chronic and intractable. Any other organ system can be affected.

Pathology

The characteristic microscopic feature is an occluded blood vessel with shard-like clefts within its lumen.

Diagnosis and Differential Diagnosis

Although the clinical history and findings can lead to a suspicion of some type of vascular syndrome, microscopic diagnosis of a skin biopsy specimen is required to document cutaneous atheroembolism. Multiple biopsy specimens are usually required to demonstrate the occlusive changes in some patients because the embolus is much smaller than the cutaneous lesion.

The differential diagnosis of atheroembolism can be approached by considering the different causes of purpura, livedo reticularis, and ulceration (see Table 2–28).

Treatment

Therapy is generally directed against symptoms or is supportive (see Table 2–29).

Antiphospholipid Syndrome

Definition

The antiphospholipid syndrome has been defined as the presence of elevated titers of antiphospholipid antibodies in conjunction with venous or arterial thrombosis, recurrent fetal loss, or thrombocytopenia. The role of antiphospholipid antibodies in causing the antiphospholipid syndrome is unknown.

Clinical Description

The antiphospholipid syndrome may occur as a primary disorder or secondary to an underlying ''autoimmune'' disease such as systemic lupus erythematosus or a syndrome that closely resembles lupus erythematosus but does not completely fulfill criteria of systemic lupus erythematosus. Patients with primary antiphospholipid syndrome have significant titers of antiphospholipid antibodies but do not show clinical and hematologic evidence of systemic lupus erythematosus.

Antiphospholipid antibodies comprise a heterogeneous group of immunoglobulins encompassing lupus anticoagulants and anticardiolipin antibodies. Antiphospholipid antibodies are common in the setting of systemic lupus, with a prevalence of nearly 50%. Anticardiolipin antibodies are more prevalent than lupus anticoagulants. Antiphospholipid antibodies have also been found in patients with malignancy and infection, but an association with thrombosis in these settings has not been demonstrated.

The varied clinical manifestations of the antiphospholipid syndrome are mainly related to venous and arterial thrombosis. Vessels of any size can be affected. Nearly half of the patients present with a skin lesion as the first sign of disease. Subsequent multisystem thrombotic events develop in roughly 40% of patients with a cutaneous presentation. The extent of livedo reticularis, the hallmark finding, correlates with antiphospholipid antibody titers in patients with connective tissue disease.

Other cutaneous manifestations of the antiphospholipid syndrome include superficial thrombophlebitis, splinter hemorrhages, vasculitis-like maculopapules and nodules, and cutaneous infarcts.

Any organ system can be affected by the antiphospholipid syndrome, including thrombotic events in the deep venous system, pulmonary emboli, cerebral events (migraines, ocular syndromes, and cerebral ischemia), and cardiac ischemia. Placental vessel thrombosis and ischemia can eventuate in miscarriage precipitated by placental insufficiency. Both first- and second-trimester losses have been observed, but late intrauterine death is rare.

Cerebral thrombosis occurring in the context of livedo reticularis has been referred to as Sneddon's syndrome. The relationship between a patient's antiphospholipid antibody status and a diagnosis of Sneddon's syndrome remains controversial.

Pathology

The characteristic pathologic finding in the antiphospholipid syndrome is a noninflammatory thrombus within dermal capillaries and venules.

Text continued on page 206

TABLE 2-28. Differential Diagnosis of Cutaneous Morphologies Seen In Small Vessel Occlusive Disorders

MORPHOLOGY	DIAGNOSTIC POSSIBILITY	DISTINCTIVE CUTANEOUS FINDINGS	OTHER DISTINCT FEATURES
Livedo Reticularis			
	Atheroembolism		Histologic features
	Antiphospholipid syndrome		Positive APA or LA tests
	Polyarteritis nodosa	Associated nodular lesions	Histologic features; positive ANCA test
	Livedo vasculopathy	Stellate, whitish scars common	Histologic features
	Leukocytoclastic vasculitis		Histologic features
Erythematous or Purpuric Papules, Nodules, and Plaques			
	Antiphospholipid syndrome	Hemorrhagic bullae common	Positive APA or LA tests
	Coumarin-induced skin necrosis	Papular or nodular lesions	Recent coumarin administration
	Polyarteritis nodosa		Histologic features; positive ANCA test
	Nodular vasculitis	Nodular/ulcerative lesions common	Histologic features

202

Ulcers		
Atheroembolism		Histologic features
Köhlmeier-Degos syndrome	Papular lesions very transient	Histologic features
Atheroembolism		Positive APA or LA tests
Antiphospholipid syndrome	Digital infarcts, gangrene	Recent warfarin administration
Coumarin-induced skin necrosis		Histologic features
Nodular vasculitis		Histologic features; positive ANCA test
Polyarteritis nodosa	Livedo reticularis can be associated	Histologic features
Livedo vasculopathy	Associated livedo reticularis and stellate scarring	Histologic features
Venous stasis	Lower extremity edema, often pitting; hyperpigmentation	Histologic features
Whitish Scars		
Livedo vasculopathy	Associated livedo reticularis	Histologic features
Lupus erythematosus		DIF; ANA and other serologic studies; histologic features
Köhlmeier-Degos syndrome, fully evolved lesions		Histologic features

APA, antiphospholipid antibody; LA, lupus anticoagulant; ANCA, antineurophil cytoplasmic antibody; DIF, direct immunofluorescence; ANA, antinuclear antibody.

TABLE 2-29. Treatment of Small Vessel Occlusive Disorders

DIAGNOSIS	MODALITY	INDICATION	DOSAGE	COMMENTS
Livedo vasculopathy	Aspirin	Ulceration	162 mg–1 g qd	
	Dipyridamole	Ulceration	50–225 mg qd	With aspirin
	Ticlopidine	Ulceration	200 mg qd	
	Pentoxifylline	Ulceration	400 mg tid	
	Heparin	Ulceration	5000 U	Subcutaneous
	Tissue plasminogen activator	Refractory disease	10 mg qd × 14 days	Intravenous
Atheroembolism	Pentoxifylline	Symptoms	400 mg tid	
	Excision	Solitary ulcer		
Primary antiphospholipid syndrome	Aspirin	Thrombotic episode	80 mg qd	
	Warfarin	Thrombotic episode	Up to 20 mg qd	
Antiphospholipid syndrome with systemic lupus erythematosus	Aspirin	Prophylaxis	80 mg qd	
		Thrombotic episode		

		Prior fetal loss		
	Aspirin	Prior fetal loss	80 mg qd	Increased fetal morbidity with addition of prednisone
	Prednisone	Severe thrombocytopenia	1–2 mg k per day	Follow bleeding time
	Warfarin	Severe thrombocytopenia	Up to 20 mg qd	Improvement in platelet count may be transient
		Thrombotic episode		Maintain international normalized ratio of 3–4
Coumarin-induced skin necrosis	Vitamin K	Thrombosis	15,000–30,000 U per day	Discontinue warfarin
	Heparin	Thrombosis	1500 IU per day	
	Protein C concentrate	Thrombosis		
Köhlmeier-Degos disease	Aspirin	Active disease	325 mg–1 g qd	
	Dipyridamole	Active disease	50 mg tid	

Diagnosis and Differential Diagnosis

In the classification scheme for the secondary antiphospholipid syndrome, a definite diagnosis of the antiphospholipid syndrome requires two or more significant clinical manifestations (recurrent fetal loss, venous or arterial thrombosis, livedo reticularis, leg ulcer, transverse myelitis, hemolytic anemia, thrombocytopenia, pulmonary hypertension) and a substantially elevated serum titer of antiphospholipid antibodies. A probable diagnosis of the antiphospholipid syndrome is possible if one clinical manifestation is present along with a high serum titer of antiphospholipid antibody, or if two clinical manifestations and a low antiphospholipid antibody titer are detected. The present diagnostic criteria for the primary antiphospholipid syndrome require an appropriate clinical finding (venous or arterial thrombosis, recurrent fetal loss, or thrombocytopenia) together with moderate to high levels of an antiphospholipid antibody or a positive lupus anticoagulant test. The criteria further stipulate that the antiphospholipid antibody test must be positive on at least two occasions separated by 3 months and that a minimum of 2 years follow-up be obtained to exclude the evolution of systemic lupus erythematosus.

Antiphospholipid antibodies are a heterogeneous group of immunoglobulins with binding specificity for anionic phospholipids. Of the three tests available for detection, the lupus anticoagulant test and solid-phase antiphospholipid antibody immunoassays are used because of the low sensitivity of the Venereal Disease Research Laboratories (VDRL) test. The lupus anticoagulant test assesses a functional characteristic of antiphospholipid antibodies, while solid-phase immunoassays are dependent on antibody binding of specific, purified phospholipid antigens, including cardiolipin. Abnormal coagulation, measured with an activated partial thromboplastin time, dilute Russell's viper venom time, kaolin clotting time, or platelet neutralization procedure, is usually performed as a screening test prior to a confirmatory study that demonstrates the presence of an inhibitor that delays the coagulation of normal plasma. For the differential diagnosis, see Table 2–28.

Treatment

The present treatment recommendations are largely based on anecdotal information (see Table 2–29).

Coumarin-Induced Skin Necrosis

Definition

Coumarin-induced skin necrosis refers to a syndrome in which skin and soft tissue necrosis develops, due to capillary thrombosis and hemorrhage, during the initial days of therapy with a coumarin (warfarin) derivative. The syndrome is associated with protein C deficiency (inherited or acquired) in some instances and less commonly occurs in the context of protein S deficiency. Protein C, an anticoagulant, inhibits the conversion of prothrombin to thrombin. During the initial phase of anticoagulation, protein C levels fall more quickly than levels of the other vitamin K–dependent factors due to the protein's short half-life, and a transient hypercoagulable state ensues. *Purpura fulminans* is a broader clinical term, which has been used in reference to a clinically and pathologically similar syndrome in infants with a near absence of protein C and also in reference to severe purpura in patients with septicemia or disseminated intravascular coagulation.

Clinical Description

Women are afflicted more frequently than men, and many patients with coumarin-induced skin necrosis are obese. The initial symptoms of this syndrome, which is most common in obese women, are pain and edema which typically arise 3 to 5 days after administration of a loading dose of a coumarin derivative, and petechiae and ecchymoses rapidly develop. Hemorrhagic bullae can follow, as can widespread necrosis, which may become gangrenous. The extent of hemorrhage and necrosis is variable. Some patients present with self-limited disease, while others suffer deep soft tissue necrosis necessitating debridement or amputation.

Pathology

Noninflammatory capillary and venular thrombosis is the cardinal finding in biopsy specimens of very early skin lesions.

Treatment

Therapy should be instituted immediately to prevent the progression of necrosis (see Table 2–29).

Köhlmeier-Degos Syndrome (Degos' Disease)

Definition and Clinical Description

Köhlmeier-Degos syndrome is a rare, idiopathic vaso-occlusive disorder. The disease typically begins in the third decade of life. The earliest lesions are small (2–5 mm), slightly erythematous, asymptomatic papules, which begin to umbilicate over the next several days. The lesions occur in crops of a few to several dozen, and papules at varying stages of development are characteristic. Over 4 weeks, the centers of the lesions become progressively depressed and gain a pale, glistening, porcelain-like cast, a detachable flake of overlying, and a rim of erythema or telangiectasia. As lesions wane, a varicelliform scar remains.

Infarctive lesions of the gastrointestinal tract or of the central nervous system are most characteristic. The clinical features associated with both gastrointestinal disease and the central nervous system are highly variable. In more severe cases, infarcts can produce gastrointestinal hemorrhage, obstruction, or perforation. Postperforation peritonitis is the most frequent cause of death in fatal cases of Köhlmeier-Degos syndrome.

Pathology

Only fully developed lesions show distinctive histologic changes: a wedge-shaped area of dermal necrosis, separated from the normal dermis by an interface of lymphocytes, with an overlying, attenuated epidermis that shows vacuolar degeneration and necrotic keratinocytes.

Diagnosis and Differential Diagnosis

The diagnosis is based solely on the cutaneous morphology and supportive histologic features. For the differential diagnosis, see Table 2-28.

Treatment

See Table 2-29.

LYMPHEDEMA

(CM&S Chapter 64)

Definition

Chronic lymphedema refers to any progressive swelling resulting from the accumulation of normally removed interstitial fluid. The disorder often results from aberrant drainage of the lymphatic system. This can be due to the obstruction of lymphatic pathways or insufficient numbers of lymphatic channels to allow for the appropriate redistribution of lymph.

Classification

Lymphedema can be classified based on primary or secondary causes.

Primary Lymphedema

Primary lymphedema, most often seen in females between the ages of 10 and 25, usually result from lymphatic agenesis, hypoplasia, or obstruction. If the disorder manifests at birth, it is referred to as *congenital lymphedema* (10% of cases); after birth and before the age of 35, is referred to as *lymphedema praecox* (80% of cases); and cases that develop after age 35 are known as *lymphedema tardum* (10% of cases). Familial forms such as the hereditary version of congenital lymphedema (Milroy's disease) have been well documented.

Secondary Lymphedema

Secondary lymphedema occurs as a result of the disruption or obstruction of a previously normal lymphatic system. Damage to this system can occur in a multitude of ways including surgical removal of lymph nodes, malignant tumors such as angiosarcoma, or breast carcinoma. The latter two can extend directly or metastasize into lymphatic channels, which causes lymphatic and lymph node fibrosis, by the direct destruction of lymphatics, as seen with erysipelas or filariasis, the most common cause of secondary chronic lymphedema worldwide. Post-mastectomy angiosarcoma (Stewart-Treves syndrome) can result from chronic lymphedema.

Clinical Description

Lymphedema is generally painless, but often produces a heavy sensation. The onset is usually gradual. The most common sites of swelling are the legs, arms, face, and genitalia. Initially, the edema tends to be soft and easily depresses. As it progresses, the skin may take on more of an indurated appearance and develop thickened folds with associated hyperkeratosis. Cellulitis may occur frequently. With subsequent episodes, it becomes difficult to recognize.

Diagnosis and Differential Diagnosis

The diagnosis of chronic lymphedema is usually not difficult. A detailed history regarding radiation treatments, travel abroad, or history of previous malignancies from prostate, breast, or ovarian sources is essential in order to identify a potential cause. Renal, cardiac, pharmacologic, and psychologic causes also should be excluded.

Treatment

The treatment of chronic lymphedema consists largely of supportive measures. An important goal is to minimize inflammation and infection and enhance the emptying of distended lymphatics. Exercise, leg elevation, and compression are the mainstay of therapy. Elastic compression should be graded such that there is increased pressure (at least 30 mm Hg) distally to proximally. Low-sodium diets, gentle massage, and topical emollients can also serve as important therapeutic measures. It is essential to stress infection prevention as well as prompt diagnosis. Recurrent lymphangitis and cellulitis can be a common occurrence, and prophylactic antibiotic therapy may be necessary in some instances. Diuretics are occasionally beneficial in the short term, but their chronic use is usually discouraged. External pneumatic compression devices have been found useful in difficult to manage limbs. These devices employ variable pressure in a sequential ''milking'' action of an edematous limb from distal to proximal, in effect transferring edema fluid from dysfunctional or nonexistent lymphatics to tissues in which lymphatics are functional. Surgery should be avoided.

LEG ULCERS AND WOUND HEALING

(CM&S Chapter 65)

Definition

An ulcer is a lesion in which the epidermis and at least the upper (papillary) dermis are destroyed. Some define a chronic leg ulcer as an open wound below the knee that does not heal within a 6-week period. Leg ulceration is mainly associated with disease of the veins and arteries.

Clinical Description

Venous Ulcers

Clinical features of venous insufficiency are as follows: Chronic venous disease is an important cause of mild ankle *edema*. Patients often complain of ''aching'' or ''fullness'' in the legs, especially in the evening. *Eczematous changes of the skin (stasis dermatitis)* with erythema, scaling, weeping, and pruritus are often persistent when they occur, resulting in lichenification. *Contact dermatitis* is a common problem in patients with venous disease and/or venous ulcers. Lanolin, neomycin, bacitracin, formaldehyde, and parabens are the most frequent sensitizers. *Hemosiderin* causes a brown or brown-red *pigmentation* and petechiae in the surrounding skin. *Lipodermatosclerosis* or sclerosing panniculitis refers to dermal and subcutaneous fibrosis, resulting in a sclerotic, woody texture. It may precede venous ulceration and occurs in two stages. In the acute, inflammatory stage (when clinically apparent), erythema and scaling with some tender and warm induration are present over the medial leg. The chronic stage follows after months or years with extensive sharply demarcated fibrosis and sclerosis on the lower medial leg. Eventually, the lower third of the limb may be encircled, forming the shape of an ''inverted champagne bottle.'' *Atrophie blanche*, (livedo vasculitis or vasculopathy) consists of smooth, ivory-white plaques of sclerosis stippled with telangiectases and surrounded by hyperpigmentation. *Varicose veins* may also be present.

Venous ulcers have a characteristic appearance (Table 2–30). After repeated episodes of infection and cellulitis, chronic lymphedema may be seen. Patients with venous ulcers will often complain of aching in the limbs. The pain and swelling are relieved by elevation and exacerbated by dependency.

Pathology

Venous insufficiency is characterized by changes of venous insufficiency, which include clusters of thick-walled capillaries within a thickened, fibrotic papillary dermis, siderophages, and extravasated erythrocytes. Perivascular fibrin cuffs are often present. In leg ulcers caused by venous insufficiency, the changes described above are evident in the skin adjacent to the ulcer. Secondary vasculitis beneath ulcer beds may be seen. Ulcers due to primary vasculitis differs in that pathologic changes are distant from the ulcer. Stasis dermatitis shows, in addition to venous stasis, spongiotic dermatitis.

In leg ulcers caused by atrophie blanche, or livedo vasculitis, distinctive findings in adjacent skin include fibrin thrombi within vascular lumina, fibrin within the walls of small vessels, sparse infiltrates of neutrophils in early lesions and lymphocytes in later ones, and a sclerotic dermis.

Lipodermatosclerosis demonstrates fibrosis and thickening of the

TABLE 2-30. Important Aspects of the Ulcer and the Surrounding Skin

	VENOUS	ARTERIAL	NEUROPATHIC
Location	Medial malleolus	Distal Terminal portions of toes Bony prominences	Weight-bearing sites Toes Heel Plantar metatarsal area
Appearance			
Edge	"Shaggy" border	"Punched out"	"Punched out"
Base	Extensive granulation tissue Fibrinous debris Weeping	Minimal or no granulation tissue Gray, yellow, or black nose Dry	Deep, penetrating Suppurative drainage if osteomyelitis
Surrounding skin	Edema Pigmentation Induration Dermatitis Cellulitis	Absence of hair growth Atrophy of skin	Rim of thick callus surrounding the ulcer

subcutaneous septa and membranocystic changes in fatty lobules—large cystic spaces lined by a corrugated amphophilic membrane.

Pathogenesis

Dysfunction of a calf muscle pump system (consisting of deep and superficial venous compartments, valves, and calf muscles) can result from venous insufficiency in the deep, connecting, or superficial system; arteriovenous fistulas; or muscle dysfunction. Calf muscle pump dysfunction results in "venous hypertension." Deep venous insufficiency often occurs as a result of a previous thrombosis causing valvular damage and is a common cause of venous ulcers; however, multisystem incompetence of the valves is the most common finding.

Arterial Ulcers

Clinical Features

An arterially compromised limb can be pale or cyanotic. The skin is often dry and scaly or shiny and atrophic with brittle nails or alopecia. Arterial ulcers have a characteristic presentation (see Table 2–30).

Ischemic ulcers are usually extremely painful, especially at night and with leg elevation. The pain is often difficult to control, and improves with dependency.

Pathology

More than 90% of all arterial disease in the Western world is due to atherosclerosis, which is characterized by patchy accumulations of lipids and tissue debris within the intima of the vessel wall. These mature into lipid-rich plaques surrounded by smooth muscle cells and collagen deposition. They may eventually ulcerate, forming a thrombotic surface.

Differential Diagnosis and Diagnosis

There are many causes of leg ulcers. General categories that enter the differential include vascular diseases (e.g., venous, arterial, vasculitis, and lymphedema), neuropathic, metabolic (e.g., diabetes), hematologic (e.g., sickle cell disease, leukemia, cryoglobulinemia), trauma (e.g., factitial), neoplastic (e.g., carcinomas, metastasis), infections, panniculitis, and pyoderma gangrenosum. It is important to ascertain the etiology of an ulcer to properly manage it. The general medical history and physical examination may reveal a previous condition that may provide clues as to the etiology of the ulcer. Systemic and topical drugs, smoking, or high alcohol intake can impair wound healing. Arterial ulcers tend to develop slowly, whereas venous ulcers progress more rapidly.

Clinical Examination

Examination of the *ulcer* should take into consideration location, borders, base, discharge, and surrounding skin (see Table 2–30).

The *limb* should be assessed clinically for presence of peripheral arterial disease. The "capillary refilling time" is prolonged over the normal 3 to 4 seconds. The "venous filling time" is another simple method of testing the arterial system of the leg. It is prolonged over the normal 10 to 15 seconds, and the color of the limb will turn pink or bright red (reactive hyperemia). Neuropathic disease can be detected by testing light touch, pinprick sensations, and deep tendon reflexes.

Investigations

Laboratory investigations should include a routine blood cell count, glucose level, erythrocyte sedimentation rate, and if indicated, albumin, vitamins, trace elements (zinc), and rheumatoid factor or antinuclear antibody. Although wounds are contaminated, a baseline bacterial culture with sensitivity results is useful. Curettage or biopsy of the ulcer will give more accurate culture results.

Helpful vascular studies include *Doppler flowmeter* (to evaluate peripheral pulses), *ankle brachial index (ABI)* (to evaluate systolic ankle pressure), and *arteriography* (if vascular surgery is considered or in diabetic patients, in whom falsely high ABIs can occur).

Tests to assess venous insufficiency include *doppler ultrasound*, *photoplethysmography*, (a screening for venous disease and to differentiate between superficial and deep vein incompetence), *air plethysmography*, (to assess the calf muscle pump and to estimate the superficial venous reflux), venography, and *duplex ultrasound imaging*. An incisional biopsy of the ulcer edge should be performed in patients with recalcitrant ulcers (after 3 months of unsuccessful treatment). Other diagnostic adjuncts include patch tests, especially if a contact dermatitis is suspected, and radiologic examination of the ulcer site when osteomyelitis is suspected.

Treatment

The treatment of leg ulcers of any etiology is essentially a problem of wound healing. Wound healing is classically divided into three major overlapping stages: inflammation, granulation tissue formation and re-epithelialization, and matrix formation and remodeling. Local factors influencing wound healing include infection (10^5 bacteria per gram of tissue need to be present), foreign body, desiccation, (moist, covered wounds re-epithelialize faster), hematoma, iatrogenic factors (during surgery with crushing of the wound edges, tight sutures, and excessive tension), topical medication (e.g., povidone-iodine, hexachlorophene, chlorhexidine, benzoyl peroxide, and sensitizing antibiotics such as neomycin or gentamycin), impaired oxygenation, and aging (the elderly heal more slowly). Systemic factors influencing wound healing include deficiency states (protein, and vitamin [A and C], and trace element deficiencies), disease states (e.g., vascular diseases, renal failure, diabetes, immunodeficiency, Ehlers-Danlos syndrome, chronic pulmonary disease, chronic liver disease), and drugs, such as corticosteroids (more than 10 mg/day) anticoagulants, nonsteroidal anti-inflammatory drugs, cyclosporine, colchicine, antiprostaglandins, phenytoin, penicillamine, calcitonin, and retinoids.

Management of Leg Ulcers

The treatment of leg ulcers first includes physical methods that alleviate the consequences of the venous or arterial abnormalities. In addition, a variety of strategies may then be utilized in the attempt to encourage wound healing. Such physical modalities include elevation of the leg above the level of the heart, bed rest, external compression, (40 mm at the ankle to 30 mm at the calf is recommended), Unna's boots (semiflexible bandages impregnated with zinc oxide paste) and treating systemic causes of edema such as hypoalbuminemia, cardiac heart failure, or pulmonary hypertension.

In the management of arterial ulcers, steps to improve blood supply include elevation of the patient's head and moderate exercise to encourage the development of a collateral circulation. Sheepskins or foot cradles should be used to relieve pressure from the extremities. Foot care should aim at preventing or avoiding any traumatic event.

Analgesics to relieve the ischemic pain, angioplasty, surgical endarterectomy, and/or a bypass can be considered.

Topical Treatment

Prolonged use of topical antibiotics should be avoided, as they may encourage the growth of resistant organisms and cause dermatitis. A low to moderate potency corticosteroid ointment can be used for a few days for acute dermatitis.

Semiocclusive dressings (e.g., hydrocolloids, hydrogels, granules, polyurethane films, alginates, foam dressings, an laminates) allow ulcers to heal in a moist environment. They are not recommended in wounds that appear clinically infected.

Besides occlusive dressings, several methods can be used to debride the ulcer including *wet to dry saline dressings, gentle debridement* with a curette or scissors and forceps under local anesthesia, extensive *surgical debridement* under general anesthesia, and topical *enzymatic preparations*.

Systemic Treatment

The use of systemic antimicrobial drugs in uncomplicated venous ulcers does not significantly influence the bacteriology of the ulcers or the rate of healing. Only cellulitis or systemic infection requires systemic antibiotics. Stanozolol, an anabolic steroid with fibrinolytic properties, may be helpful in lipodermatosclerosis. Pentoxifylline, which also increases fibrinolytic activity and reduces risk of thrombus formation, may be helpful in venous ulceration and arterial disease.

Grafts

If wound epithelialization is slow, grafting should be considered. Grafting options include pinch grafting, split-thickness skin grafts, and keratinocytic/cultured autografts or allografts.

Recurrence and Prevention

Recurrence rate of ulceration is high, particularly in patients with venous insufficiency. Therefore, once resolution of an ulcer is obtained, preventive management should be emphasized. Compression stockings should be worn at all times, and there should be continuous vigilance against minor trauma. Vigorous treatment of early skin breakdown and adequate skin care are important.

PHLEBOLOGY AND SCLEROTHERAPY

(CM&S Chapter 66)

Definition

Chronic venous insufficiency, including superficial venous malfunction, is an abnormality of the peripheral venous system that reduces or prevents venous return to the heart. Chronic venous insufficiency includes superficial varicose veins with venous malfunction and accompanying venous hypertension, edema, and leg ulceration. Varicose veins are usually an integral part of venous insufficiency, arising because of venous wall weakness or defective venous valves. These defects result in reverse flow with calf muscle pump and gravitational (or hydrostatic) pressure to cause distention and pain.

Phlebology is the treatment of venous insufficiency and other venous disorders. Sclerotherapy, which is the technique for treatment of varicose veins, blue reticular veins (minor varicose veins), and telangiectatic veins, involves direct injection of a small quantity of a sclerosing solution into an abnormally enlarged or stretched vein with immediate application of compression to maintain contact of the solution with the endothelium. Within seconds to minutes, the solution disrupts the endothelium and penetrates further into the vessel wall, causing vessel wall destruction and edema. In an area of low blood flow, such as peripheral branches of the superficial venous system, sufficient contact of sclerosing solution can be made with the vessel wall to cause destructive changes. Any red blood cells remaining in the vessel lumen will form an intravascular coagulum. Within weeks to months, depending on the degree of vessel wall destruction at the time of sclerotherapy, the treated vein will either recannulate (although possibly with a smaller diameter) or undergo full-thickness sclerosis with subsequent total disappearance. Combining compression bandaging with injection markedly improves the results of sclerotherapy.

Clinical Description

Varicose veins are extremely frequent, with reports of from 30% to 60% of American women having telangiectatic leg veins. The incidence increases with age.

The most common symptom is aching of the legs. Widespread telangiectases may cause a sensation of muscle fatigue in the affected legs with localized pain over groups of telangiectases and/or small varicosities. Swelling of the ankles is a symptom of mild venous physiologic disturbance. As disease advances, swelling of the ankles is replaced with pitting edema. Symptoms and signs are made worse by prolonged standing and can be partially relieved by the wearing of support hose while standing or with rest and elevation of the legs. Often preventable complications of varicose veins include pigmentation, stasis dermatitis, subacute cellulitis, ulceration, bleeding, and thrombophlebitis.

CUTANEOUS VENULITIS (NECROTIZING VASCULITIS, LEUKOCYTOCLASTIC VASCULITIS)

(CM&S Chapter 67)

Definition

The term vasculitis describes clinical disorders in which there is segmental inflammation and, exceptionally, necrosis of the blood vessels. Syndromes are based on the gross appearance and histologic changes of the lesions, the caliber of the affected blood vessels, the involvement of specific organs, and laboratory abnormalities. The form of vasculitis that most frequently affects the skin involves venules and has been called cutaneous venulitis and leukocytoclastic vasculitis. The cutaneous vascular lesions may be a feature of an underlying chronic disorder, may develop after defined precipitating events, or may occur as a variety of idiopathic syndromes.

Clinical Description

The characteristic lesion of cutaneous venulitis is an erythematous papule that does not blanch when the skin is pressed and is known as palpable purpura. Other lesions include urticaria, angioedema, pustules, vesicles, ulcers, necrosis, and livedo reticularis. The eruption most frequently develops on the lower extremities or over dependent areas. Involvement of the face, palms, soles, and mucous membranes is uncommon. Palpable purpura persists from 1 to 4 weeks; the lesions appear in episodes that may recur over weeks to years. Lesional symptoms include pruritus or burning and, less commonly, pain.

An episode of cutaneous vascular lesions may be associated with fever, malaise, arthralgias, or myalgias. Systemic involvement most commonly occurs in synovia, muscles, peripheral nerves, gastrointestinal tract, and kidneys.

Associated Chronic Disorders

Cutaneous venulitis is associated with certain connective tissue disorders, especially rheumatoid arthritis, Sjögren's syndrome, and systemic lupus erythematosus. *Paraneoplastic vasculitis* describes patients with cutaneous vasculitis associated with malignant disorders, which include nonsolid malignancies such as Hodgkin's disease and acute and chronic myelogenous forms of leukemia, and solid tumors (less frequently) such as squamous cell bronchogenic carcinoma, prostatic carcinoma, and colon carcinoma.

Precipitating Events

Infections as well as diagnostic and therapeutic agents are known to precipitate episodes of cutaneous venulitis. The most commonly recognized infectious agents are group A hemolytic streptococci, *Staphylococcus aureus, Mycobacterium leprae*, and hepatitis B virus. Cutaneous venulitis is an uncommon presentation of a drug reaction. The most commonly incriminated therapeutic agents are penicillin, sulfonamides, thiazides, and serum.

Idiopathic Disorders

The most widely recognized idiopathic subgroup is the Henoch-Schönlein syndrome, which occurs predominantly in children and affects the skin, synovia, gastrointestinal tract, and kidneys. Urticarial vasculitis, an edematous form of venulitis, occurs most frequently in patients with serum sickness, connective tissue disorders, physical urticaria, and infections. The skin lesions appear as wheals, which may last from 3 to 5 days. Other skin manifestations include macular erythema, foci of purpura in the wheals, angioedema, livedo reticularis, nodules, and bullae. The lesions are pruritic, possess a burning or painful quality, and usually resolve without residua, although transient contusions or hyperpigmentation may develop. The episodes of urticaria are recurrent, last from months to years, and vary in frequency.

Extracutaneous manifestations include fever, malaise, myalgia, and enlargement of the lymph nodes, liver, and spleen. Episodic arthralgias are a major clinical manifestation. Other systemic involvement includes renal involvement without progression to severe impairment of renal function; gastrointestinal tract manifestations include nausea, vomiting, diarrhea, and pain; upper airway inflammation with the danger of death from laryngeal edema; eye involvement with conjunctivitis, episcleritis, iridocyclitis, and uveitis; central nervous system involvement occuring as headaches and pseudotumor cerebri. The prevalence and natural history of idiopathic urticarial vasculitis remain unknown.

Laboratory Findings

An elevated erythrocyte sedimentation rate is the most consistent laboratory abnormality. The platelet count is usually normal. Other abnormalities reflect either a coexistent underlying disorder or the involvement of an additional organ system. Acquired hypocomplementemia occurs in patients with urticarial vasculitis and in patients with palpable purpura and concomitant connective tissue diseases, cryoglobulinemia, and idiopathic forms.

Pathology

Cutaneous venulitis is a dynamic process in which fully developed lesions show infiltrates of neutrophils and nuclear dust in and around venules, in conjunction with deposits of fibrin in vessel walls and sometimes in lumina as well. The latter is a key finding in that it is evidence of damage to the walls of vessels.

Pathogenesis and Etiology

The most frequently postulated mechanism operative in the production of cutaneous venulitis is the local deposition of circulating immune complexes or the formation of immune complexes in the skin, which may activate the complement system, degranulate mast cells, and attract neutrophils that release lysosomal enzymes.

Diagnosis and Differential Diagnosis

The episodic lesions characteristic of cutaneous venulitis may be a manifestation of systemic hypersensitivity angiitis, may be associated with necrotizing angiitis of larger blood vessels, or may be restricted to the skin. Thrombocytopenia may result in purpura; however, these lesions are flat. When thrombocytopenia occurs in association with cutaneous papules due to other causes, palpable purpura may result. Palpable purpura should be considered to be vasculitis until proved otherwise by skin biopsy. The differential diagnosis also includes scurvy, disseminated intravascular coagulation, septic emboli, Rocky Mountain spotted fever, and certain forms of the progressive pigmentary dermatoses.

Treatment

The approach to the treatment of cutaneous vasculitis is based on clinical experience, open trials in small numbers of patients, and anecdotal case reports. When cutaneous venulitis is associated with a precipitating event, withdrawal of the medication or treatment of the infection results in resolution of the cutaneous lesions. If a coexistent chronic disorder is present, treatment of the underlying disease may improve the skin. Initially an H_1 antihistamine, such as dexchlorpheniramine, 2 mg four times daily, in combination with a nonsteroidal anti-inflammatory agent, such as indomethacin, 25 to 50 mg three times daily, should be administered. Depending on the therapeutic response, colchicine or hydroxychloroquine sulfate, 200 to 400 mg daily, can be added to or substituted for these agents, followed by dapsone if there is still no benefit. At this point if there is no beneficial response, a major therapeutic decision occurs since the use of more aggressive medications, such as systemic corticosteroids, azathioprine, cyclophosphamide, and methotrexate, is associated with significant side effects.

G. Panniculitis

ERYTHEMA NODOSUM AND NODULAR VASCULITIS

(CM&S Chapter 68)

Erythema Nodosum

Definition and Clinical Description

Erythema nodosum is characterized by the eruption of symmetrical, tender, erythematous nodules and plaques located predominantly over the extensor aspects of the lower extremities. This disorder usually exhibits an acute course, with spontaneous regression, without ulceration, scarring, or atrophy. Erythema nodosum has many causes and can be regarded as an inflammatory reaction pattern, like erythema multiforme, leukocytoclastic vasculitis, or erythema annulare centrifugum. All of these conditions can be precipitated by a variety of causes, which result in clinically and histopathologically indisinguishable changes.

Erythema nodosum, which is the most common type of panniculitis, can occur at any age, but most cases appear between the second and fourth decades of life, with a peak incidence between 20 and 30 years of age. In children, erythema nodosum occurs commonly in association with tuberculosis and streptococcal infections.

The typical eruption of erythema nodosum is quite characteristic. The lesions consist of symmetrical, tender, erythematous, hot, and raised nodules and plaques usually located on the shins, ankles, and knees. Usually, the lesions are bilaterally distributed. More extensive cases may involve thighs, extensor aspects of the arms, neck, and, in rare instances, the face. The size of the lesions range from 1 to 15 cm and the number from 1 to 10, but sometimes 50 or more nodules are present at the same time. Initially, lesions of erythema nodosum are bright red nodules, which over several days, become more flat, with a purplish or livid color and finally exhibit yellow and greenish appearance, often taking on the look of a deep bruise ("erythema contusiformis"). Ulceration is never seen and the nodules heal without atrophy or scarring. These two clinical features distinguish erythema nodosum from nodular vasculitis. The eruption, which generally lasts 3 to 6 weeks, may also become chronic and persistent.

Cutaneous eruption of the nodules is sometimes associated with fever of 38 to 39° C, malaise, fatigue, arthralgia, headache, abdominal pain, vomiting, cough, or diarrhea. Episcleral lesions and conjunctivitis may also appear with the cutaneous eruption.

Erythema nodosum migrans, also named subacute nodular migratory panniculitis, is a variant of erythema nodosum characterized by a single or few lesions, often grouped as large erythematoedematous plaques. The lesions are painless or less tender than those of classic erythema nodosum. The initial nodules spread peripherally, while the central area becomes paler and indurated, assuming an arciform pattern. Eventually, lesions coalesce forming large irregular areas of migratory erythema with a raised border. The disease has a prolonged clinical course.

Pathology

Erythema nodosum is classified as a septal panniculitis. The septa are always thickened and variously infiltrated by inflammatory cells that also involve the periseptal area of the fat lobules. Usually, a sparse superficial and deep, perivascular, inflammatory infiltrate is also present in the dermis, mostly composed of lymphocytes. Well-defined nodular aggregates of histiocytes surrounding a central cleft are a histopathologic hallmark of erythema nodosum. Leukocytoclastic vasculitis is not a feature of erythema nodosum.

Etiology and Pathogenesis

Erythema nodosum is considered to be a hypersensitivity response to a number of inciting factors. The variability of possible antigenic stimuli that can induce erythema nodosum indicates that this disorder is a cutaneous reactive process and that the skin has limited response capacity against very different provoking agents.

The etiologic factors that can lead to erythema nodosum are long and varied and include infections, drugs, malignant diseases, inflammatory disorders, and a wide group of miscellaneous conditions. Erythema nodosum and bilateral hilar adenopathy may be the presenting sign of sarcoidosis (Löfgren's syndrome), but also hilar adenopathy may be associated with erythema nodosum in the absence of sarcoidosis. In a variable proportion of cases of erythema nodosum, no underlying disease or triggering factor is found.

Treatment

Treatment of erythema nodosum includes elimination of the inciting factor and bed rest. Aspirin or nonsteroidal antiinflammatory drugs such as indomethacin, 25 to 50 mg three times per day, or naproxen may be added to enhance analgesia and resolution. If the lesions persist longer, potassium iodide in a dosage of 400 to 900 mg daily or a saturated solution of potassium iodide, 2 to 10 drops in water or orange juice three times per day, has been reported to be useful. Potassium iodide is contraindicated during pregnancy, because it can produce a goiter in the fetus.

Systemic corticosteroids (prednisone to 40 mg per day) are usually not indicated, especially if an underlying infectious etiology has been not completely ruled out, but intralesional corticosteroid injection (triamcinolone acetonide, 5 mg/ml) into the center of nodules may cause them to resolve. Some patients may respond to a course of colchicine, 0.6 to 1.2 mg twice a day.

Nodular Vasculitis

Definition and Clinical Description

Nodular vasculitis, or erythema induratum, is characterized by erythematous subcutaneous nodules and plaques on the posterior aspect of the legs of middle-aged patients, mainly women. Lesions usually ulcerate and heal with scarring. The course is chronic and recurrent. Individual lesions tend to involute, but new crops appear at irregular intervals, mainly coinciding with the onset of cold weather. Erythrocyanosis, heavy column-shaped calves, follicular perniosis, and cutis marmorata are frequently associated changes and may be predisposing factors. Patients are otherwise usually in good health. Like erythema nodosum, nodular vasculitis is probably a multietiologic disorder, although nontuberculous cases remain idiopathic. The pathogenesis of nodular vasculitis is unknown. Venous stasis and cold weather may be predisposing or precipitating factors.

Pathology

Nodular vasculitis is a predominantly lobular panniculitis. The infiltrate predominantly is composed of neutrophils and foamy histiocytes. Lymphocytes, epithelioid cells, and foreign body giant cells contribute to the granulomatous appearance of the infiltrate. Lobular necrosis is probably secondary to large vessel involvement, and, if the upper dermis is affected, the lesion can ulcerate. Mixed inflammatory cell infiltrates in vein walls and obliteration of lumina are the usual findings. While special stains do not reveal mycobacteria, cases associated with tuberculosis can harbor a mycobacterial genome that is detectable using the polymerase chain reaction.

Differential Diagnosis of Common Panniculitides

The differential diagnosis of both erythema nodosum and erythema induratum includes cutaneous polyarteritis nodosum and superficial migratory thrombophlebitis.

Treatment

In cases in which an association with tuberculosis is suspected (and there is at least a strongly positive Mantoux test or a positive polymerase chain reaction test for mycobacterial genome), a full course of 9 months of antituberculosis triple-agent therapy is recommended. In idiopathic cases (which constitute more than half), nonsteroidal antiinflammatory drugs and corticosteroids are classically recommended with doubtful results.

Potassium iodide is effective in approximately 50% of cases. Supporting bandages, bed rest, and attention to predisposing and precipitating factors may help.

SCLEREMA NEONATORUM AND SUBCUTANEOUS FAT NECROSIS OF THE NEWBORN

(CM&S Chapter 69)

Sclerema Neonatorum

Definition and Clinical Description

Sclerema neonatorum is an extremely rare, usually fatal disorder involving the panniculus of premature or debilitated infants in the first week of life.

It presents with the sudden onset of board-like stiffness of the skin. Nonpitting induration usually appears over the lower extremities and rapidly extends cephalad, sparing only the palms, soles, and genitalia. The outcome is usually fatal, often as a result of overwhelming septicemia, shock, and electrolyte imbalance.

Pathology

There are diffusely distributed adipose cells containing needle-shaped clefts in a radial array with little inflammatory response and fat necrosis. The crystals are doubly refractile on frozen section.

Pathogenesis and Etiology

Susceptibility to sclerema neonatorum (and also to subcutaneous fat necrosis of the newborn) may depend on an alteration in the lipid composition of subcutaneous fat, perhaps as a result of immaturity.

Differential Diagnosis

The differential diagnosis includes diffuse scleroderma, scleredema neonatorum, subcutaneous fat necrosis of the newborn, and restrictive dermopathy.

Treatment

Essential aspects of treatment consist of correcting any underlying disease, shock, dehydration, or electrolyte imbalance. The use of antibiotics is frequently necessary for intercurrent infection. Parenteral corticosteroids and exchange transfusions are controversial but may be helpful.

Subcutaneous Fat Necrosis of the Newborn

Definition and Clinical Description

Subcutaneous fat necrosis of the newborn is a condition of unknown etiology manifested by the appearance in the first few weeks of life of varying degrees of localized fat necrosis of the subcutaneous tissue and, rarely, the internal organs. It presents with bilateral red to violaceous, firm, freely movable subcutaneous nodules, which occur primarily on the cheeks, shoulders, back, thighs, and rarely as a solitary nodule. The infants appear healthy, are afebrile, and have full range of motion. Occasionally, a larger nodule may become fluctuant and drain, the necrotic material containing radial crystals on microscopic examination. Calcification can occur and be apparent radiographically.

Pathology

The normal epidermis and dermis overlie patchy areas of subcutaneous necrosis that contain needle-shaped clefts surrounded by an inflammatory infiltrate consisting of lymphocytes, histiocytes, fibroblasts, and foreign body giant cells. Patchy calcification is commonly observed within the inflammatory infiltrate.

Diagnosis and Differential Diagnosis

In general, the diagnosis of subcutaneous fat necrosis of the newborn can be differentiated by the age of onset, by other associated illness, and by biopsy. The differential diagnosis includes sclerema neonatorum and poststeroid panniculitis.

Treatment

Treatment is often unnecessary, but warm or hot application to the lesions should be avoided. In severe cases or if hypercalcemia develops, systemic corticosteroid therapy may be indicated along with dietary restriction of calcium and vitamin D. Thrombocytopenia has been rarely reported. Symptomatic care is all that is usually needed. Persistent fat atrophy may require surgery to improve appearance after resolution of the disease.

SCLEROSING PANNICULITIS

(CM&S Chapter 70)

Definition

Sclerosing panniculitis is a term that more accurately describes a form of atrophic panniculitis that had previously been labeled *hypodermitis sclerodermaformis* or *lipodermatosclerosis.*

Clinical Description

It is a relatively common finding in middle-aged or older women with venous insufficiency. In the acute stage, a poorly defined unilateral cellulitis-like area of warm, painful, edematous erythema is present usually or the medial calf near the ankle with or without findings of venous insufficiency. With progression to the chronic stage of sclerosing panniculitis, the affected area becomes progressively indurated, depressed, hyperpigmented, and less erythematous. Residual erythema at the edges of induration suggest progression of the panniculitis. The induration and associated pain are relentlessly progressive, resulting in ulceration without successful treatment. Ulcers, which are often small and multiple at first, may become confluent and large. The ulcers are difficult to heal, and when healing does occur, scarring is prominent.

Pathology

As the disease progresses, septal and periseptal subcutaneous lymphocytic infiltrates with ischemic necrosis of fat lobules progress to thickening of the septa with characteristic pale, paucicellular, ''hyalinized'' collagen progressively extending from the septum into the adipocyte lobule. The ''sclerosis'' eventually replaces most of the adipocytes.

Differential Diagnosis

The differential diagnosis of sclerosing panniculitis includes recurrent streptococcal cellulitis, sclerosis secondary to *Borrelia* infection, morphea or scleroderma, lupus profundus, and scarring as a result of trauma or thermal or chemical burns.

Treatment

Treatment options are limited and are frequently unsuccessful. Amelioration of venous insufficiency by compression stockings, elevation of the affected part, or surgery is essential.

OTHER FORMS OF PANNICULITIS

(CM&S Chapter 71)

Poststeroid Panniculitis

Definition and Clinical Description

Poststeroid panniculitis is a relatively rare complication of rapid corticosteroid withdrawal. Erythematous, subcutaneous nodules ranging from 0.5 to 4 cm in diameter develop on the cheeks, trunk, arms, or thighs, most frequently in children who are being treated for rheumatic fever within a month after the initiation of rapid oral or parenteral corticosteroid withdrawal. The nodules are firm and may be tender or pruritic. The condition resolves spontaneously, and resolution is actually hastened if corticosteroids are readministered.

Pathology

A patchy, lobular panniculitis is seen with infiltration of fat by lymphocytes, macrophages, and foreign body giant cells. The key feature is the presence of needle-shaped clefts within lipocytes.

Cold Panniculitis

Definition

In cold panniculitis, which is particularly common in children, various forms of cold injury cause the formation of tender, erythematous plaques and subcutaneous nodules.

Clinical Description

Cold injury resulting in panniculitis can occur at birth, after hypothermic cardiac surgery, on the thighs of equestrians or on the cheeks of children who suck on popsicles. The disease is self-limiting and requires no treatment.

Pathology

Cold injury produces a mixed septal-lobular panniculitis that is most pronounced near the dermal-subcutaneous junction.

α_1-Antitrypsin (Proteinase Inhibitor) Deficiency Panniculitis

Definition

The syndrome, defined by the development of painful subcutaneous nodules that ulcerate and drain, has distinctive histopathologic changes that distinguish it from Weber-Christian disease as a specific category of panniculitis. Weber-Christian disease may have been caused by this proteinase inhibitor deficiency.

Clinical Description

α_1-antitrypsin deficient individuals have an increased risk for developing emphysema, liver cirrhosis, and panniculitis. Patients with this form of panniculitis develop subcutaneous nodules or cellulitis-like lesions that are typically but not invariably painful. A history of preceding trauma can sometimes be elicited. Spontaneous ulceration and drainage are common. Diagnosis is aided by serum protein electrophoresis.

Pathology

Neutrophilic predominance, collagenolysis and elastolysis, and lobular separation are characteristic of α_1-antitrypsin deficiency.

Diagnosis and Differential Diagnosis

The tendency for lesions to ulcerate and drain helps distinguish α_1-antitrypsin deficiency from other forms of panniculitis. The two major differential considerations are Weber-Christian disease and factitial panniculitis.

Treatment

Dapsone (100 to 150 mg per day), infusions of α_1-antitrypsin inhibitor concentrate, and doxycycline are therapeutic options.

Pancreatic Panniculitis

Definition and Clinical Description

In pancreatic or enzymic panniculitis (fat necrosis), subcutaneous nodules develop, usually on the legs, in association with a variety of pancreatic diseases, including acute pancreatitis, carcinoma, or even "silent" pancreatitis.

Pathology

A neutrophilic lobular panniculitis shows fat necrosis with liquefaction and microcyst formation. As a characteristic feature, fat cells lose their nuclei and develop thick, shadowy walls, forming the so-called ghost cells.

Diagnosis and Differential Diagnosis

The association of pancreatic disease with panniculitis is key to the diagnosis. Serum amylase, lipase, trypsin, or other enzyme levels may help in reaching a diagnosis. Magnetic resonance imaging has been used to identify early changes in intraosseous fat that precede necrosis.

Treatment

Treatment is directed toward the underlying pancreatic disease and includes chemotherapy or surgical removal of tumors, drainage of pseudocysts, or repair of fistulae.

Cytophagic Histiocytic Panniculitis

Definition and Clinical Description

Cytophagic histiocytic panniculitis consists of an eruption of subcutaneous nodules and plaques that arise on the trunk and extremities. These may be associated with purpura, show spontaneous drainage, or demonstrate considerable crusting. This condition can arise in the setting of a systemic disease that consists of fever, hepatosplenomegaly, thrombocytopenia, and neutropenia. Although a benign clinical course is possible, the majority of their disease, particularly from hemorrhagic episodes or from the effects of underlying lymphoma.

Pathology

The most striking finding is a septal and lobular panniculitis associated with fat necrosis, edema, and hemorrhage. Characteristically, numerous benign-appearing histiocytes with rounded nuclei and large amounts of cytoplasm are engaged in phagocytosis of cellular elements, giving them a ''beanbag'' appearance.

Diagnosis and Differential Diagnosis

The association of panniculitis with fever, hematologic abnormalities, or organomegaly should at least suggest the diagnosis, and a generous biopsy of skin and subcutaneous tissue should be performed to look for large cytophagic histiocytes. If a particular case has these features, a search for underlying lymphoma is indicated.

Treatment

Although relentless clinical progression leading to death is common, a few cases have had a benign course and others respond to aggressive chemotherapy.

chapter 3

What Causes Blistering of the Skin?

EPIDERMOLYSIS BULLOSA

(CM&S Chapter 73)

Definition

Inherited epidermolysis bullosa (EB) is a mechanobullous disorder that includes a number of distinctive diseases that are characterized by the presence of inherently fragile skin and the tendency to develop blisters and erosions. At least 23 phenotypically different disorders are now included within this group of diseases. Some forms of EB have exclusively skin manifestations, whereas others may also involve several multiple other organs or tissues, especially those that are epithelial surfaced or lined.

Approach to Classification

The current classification separates types of EB on the basis of the ultrastructural level at which blisters form spontaneously or following mechanical trauma. Three major groups (simplex, junctional, and dystrophic EB) are defined by whether blisters form within the epidermis (epidermolytic), within the lamina lucida of the dermoepidermal junction (lamina lucidolytic), or beneath the lamina densa (dermolytic), respectively.

Subclassification is based upon other factors, such as the extent of cutaneous involvement (i.e., localized versus generalized), distribution of cutaneous lesions (acral, centripetal, inverse, other), mode of transmission (autosomal dominant, autosomal recessive, X-linked recessive), onset of disease activity (i.e., as in the delayed onset of EB progressiva), unusual course of the disease (as in the apparent self-limited nature of transient bullous dermolysis of the newborn), and presence or absence of specific cutaneous features (i.e., exuberant granulation tissue in the Herlitz variant of junctional EB).

Clinical Description

Epidermolysis Bullosa Simplex

There are at least seven recognized EB simplex (EBS) phenotypes. Most commonly, skin involvement in EBS is characterized by variably sized, tense blisters, crusts, and erosions, in the absence of obvious atrophy, scarring, milia, or nail dystrophy.

The most common form of EBS, the localized subtype referred to as the *Weber-Cockayne* variety, is characterized by blisters largely confined to the palms and soles, which occur after trauma. This disease is almost always transmitted in an autosomal dominant manner, although rare cases with apparent autosomal recessive transmission have been reported. The time of onset of apparent disease activity in Weber-Cockayne EBS is highly variable. By as early as young adulthood, some Weber-Cockayne patients develop focal extensive callosities on the palms and soles, overlying recurrent, painful, intraepidermal blisters. Blisters are usually associated with increased motor activity or ambulation, are made worse by heat or friction, are exacerbated during summer and are somewhat ameliorated as the growing child or young adult becomes more aware that friction causes blistering. With few exceptions, children with Weber-Cockayne EBS, like other individuals with inherited EB, are unable to participate in most sports, stand or walk for prolonged periods, or perform even minor mechanical labor without developing several exquisitely painful blisters. As is the case in all other forms of EBS that have been studied, approximately one-third of patients with Weber-Cockayne EBS develop localized erosions within the mouth, usually due to bottle-feeding, which are often asymptomatic and resolve with time. Clinically significant extracutaneous disease activity is characteristically absent in Weber-Cockayne EBS.

A second important EBS subtype is the generalized *Koebner* variant. This common subtype has its onset of disease activity at or shortly after birth. Nail dystrophy, milia, and scarring are more commonly observed in the Koebner than in the Weber-Cockayne variant, whereas the palms and soles are relatively spared. Extracutaneous involvement is absent in the Koebner variant.

A third major subtype of EB is EB (simplex) herpetiformis (*Dowling-Meara* variant), a subset that usually has its clinical onset at birth. This variant is usually transmitted as an autosomal dominant trait and rarely in an autosomal recessive manner. This is but one of two EB simplex subsets associated with an increased risk of death during infancy or early childhood. The two characteristic features of this important EBS variant are the presence of herpetiform (grouped) blisters and, with age, the development of confluent palmoplantar callosities, reminiscent of acquired keratoderma. As in the Koebner variant, nail dystrophy, milia, and/or scarring are frequently observed in the Dowling-Meara variant. However, extracutaneous disease activity is infrequently observed in this generalized EBS subtype.

Junctional Epidermolysis Bullosa

As in the case of all forms of inherited EB, junctional EB (JEB) is best separated into localized and generalized forms. Both are transmitted in an autosomal recessive manner. Patients with JEB exhibit blisters, crusts, erosions, atrophic scarring, and eventual dystrophy or absence of nails, although milder cases may lack one or more of these features. Milia are usually absent in JEB, regardless of the overall severity of disease activity. During infancy the cutaneous findings in JEB may be indistinguishable from that observed in any other type of EB. All patients with JEB, regardless of subtype, have some evidence of enamel hypoplasia manifested by variant-sized pits on the surface of the teeth.

Several localized forms of JEB have been described. In the most striking one, referred to as the *inversa* variant, blisters, erosions, and atrophic scars develop primarily at intertriginous sites. Symmetry of cutaneous disease activity is usually prominent. Extracutaneous involvement is primarily confined to the oral cavity and esophagus, and may be severe.

Two major forms of generalized JEB exist in which atrophic scarring is characteristically present. The most severe form of JEB is referred to as the *Herlitz* variant; other names include *EB atrophicans generalisata gravis* and *EB letalis*. A pathognomonic clinical finding is the presence of thickened areas of exuberant granulation tissue. Although any skin surface may be so involved, this granulation tissue most often is symmetrically distributed around the mouth and nostrils as well as on the posterior neck and upper and midback, and in the axillae and periungual folds of the fingers. Although findings are not usually present at birth, most patients with the Herlitz subtype have some evidence of this disfiguring complication by the first year of life. Granulation tissue serves as a chronic site for the loss of blood and protein. After many decades this granulation tissue may spontaneously involute, leaving atrophic scarring in its wake.

The skin particularly fragile in the Herlitz JEB subtype. Partial or complete scarring alopecia is commonly seen on the scalp of Herlitz patients. Nails become dystrophic early in life; later they usually are shed, leaving residual scars within the nail beds. Axillary contractures also may infrequently occur, with or without accompanying granulation tissue. Extracutaneous involvement is usually widespread and severe in the Herlitz subtype; virtually any epithelial-lined organ may be affected. Common sites include the oral cavity (resulting in marked microstomia and ankyloglossia), esophagus (leading to strictures and stenoses), and small intestine (leading to profound growth retardation or failure to thrive). Herlitz disease is also accompanied by severe anemia due to malabsorption of iron and chronic blood loss from widespread erosions on the skin and within the gastrointestinal tract. Patients with Herlitz (and non-Herlitz) disease may also develop severe tracheolaryngeal occlusion as a result of recurrent blister formation and progressive scarring. This complication, which initially presents as a hoarse cry within the first 2 years of life, is a frequent cause of death in infancy. Sepsis and arrhythmias due to electrolyte imbalance may also cause premature death in these patients.

The second major subtype of generalized JEB is known as *non-Herlitz* JEB. It has been also referred to as *EB atrophicans generalisata mitis* and *generalized atrophic benign EB (GABEB)*. Exuberant granulation tissue is not a feature of non-Herlitz JEB. Other cutaneous findings are very similar in all JEB subtypes and, with the exception of milia, may often closely resemble those observed in dystrophic EB. Except for tracheolaryngeal and/or esophageal involvement, and enamel hypoplasia, other significant extracutaneous manifestations are usually lacking in the non-Herlitz variant.

Dystrophic Epidermolysis Bullosa

Dystrophic EB (DEB) may be localized or generalized, and is transmitted as either an autosomal dominant or autosomal recessive trait. Common findings in DEB include blisters, erosions, crusts, atrophic scarring, milia formation, and dystrophy or absence of nails, although some of these features may be lacking in individual patients.

By definition, dominant dystrophic EB (DDEB) is transmitted in autosomal dominant manner and most commonly presents as a generalized cutaneous disease. Two major subtypes of generalized DDEB have been described. These have been named *Pasini* and *Cockayne-Touraine* variants, and differ only by the presence or absence, respectively, of albopapuloid lesions, which are small, white or flesh-colored papules that clinically resembles small scars, connective tissue nevi, or lichen planus. Albopapuloid lesions appear on the central trunk, and may not appear until late childhood or adolescence. Extracutaneous disease activity is usually lacking in DDEB other than esophageal or mild intraoral involvement in some cases. Patients with both forms of generalized DDEB appear to have normal life spans.

Two major subtypes of generalized recessive dystrophic EB (RDEB) exist. The *Hallopeau-Siemens* variety (RDEB-HS), which is the more severe RDEB subtype, is characterized by marked fragility of skin, and is associated with usually widespread blisters, atrophic scarring, milia, and marked dystrophy or absence of nails. It and the Herlitz variant of generalized JEB represent the two most severe forms of inherited EB. Like other generalized types of EB, widespread disease is readily evident at birth. Infants with RDEB-HS are at an increased risk of early death, as the result of sepsis or failure to thrive. Those that survive have a shortened life span. About a quarter of those surviving infancy or early childhood will develop aggressive squamous cell carcinomas of the skin by early adulthood. Other tumors, including malignant melanoma, frequently occur in patients with RDEB-HS.

Essentially any epithelial-surfaced or lined organ may blister in patients with RDEB-HS. Oral findings include severe microstomia, ankyloglossia, blistering and scarring, and rampant caries. Teeth are prematurely lost as a result of secondary destruction, further compromising the integrity of adjacent soft and hard tissues. Frequent extracutaneous findings include esophageal strictures, profound growth retardation, and severe multifactorial anemia. Infrequently, blisters, erosions, and scarring may occur on the cornea, conjunctiva, and throughout the genitourinary and lower gastrointestinal tracts. Partial pseudosyndactyly (also called mitten or claw deformities) of several of the digits of the hands and/or feet occur early in life in RDEB-HS. Most patients will have evidence of this manifestation by age 25. If untreated, some of these patients will eventually develop complete encasement of the digits by scar tissue, in association with muscular atrophy and partial bony resorption of the fingers and toes. Other acral contractures (i.e., knees and elbows) may also infrequently develop.

A second major type of generalized RDEB, the *mitis* variant, clinically resembles the Cockayne-Touraine variant of DDEB. Extracutaneous involvement, other than usually mild intraoral blistering, is uncommonly seen, life span is normal, and there appears to be no significant increased risk of skin cancers.

Immunohistochemistry and Ultrastructural Features

The inherited forms of EB produce cell-poor subepidermal blisters. In EBS, the plane of cleavage is within the epidermis. In JEB, electron microscopy shows that the plane of blistering is within the lamina lucida. All forms of DEB are typified by the presence of clefts beneath the lamina densa.

Pathogenesis and Etiology

It is now clear that most if not all forms of EBS are the result of mutations within one of a few specific keratin genes. In particular, specific point mutations in the genes for keratins 5 or 14 have been identified as the underlying molecular basis of the Weber-Cockayne, Koebner, and Dowling-Meara variants of EBS. The more severe forms of EBS have their mutations within regions of the keratin molecules most susceptible to mechanical instability, resulting in structurally fragile keratin filaments that are prone to disruption following mechanical trauma or with exposure to heat (as in warm weather). Presumably keratinocyte cytolysis and intraepidermal blistering are the end products of specific keratin abnormalities and the application of shearing forces and/or heat to the skin surface. The type VII collagen gene is indeed the site of genetic mutation in both dominant and recessive forms of dystrophic EB. Emerging data suggest that the molecular basis of JEB will be mutations within the genes for one of two anchoring filament-associated proteins, kalinin and uncein.

Differential Diagnosis

Usually there is no differential diagnosis for inherited EB in the setting of a positive family history for other identically affected individuals. During the neonatal period and early childhood, especially in the setting of an absent family history for EB, the differential diagnosis may include other blistering diseases, including herpes simplex, congenital porphyria, and incontinentia pigmenti. In addition, EB acquisita and some other autoimmune bullous diseases rarely may present in very early childhood and may clinically mimic inherited EB.

Treatment

All therapy for inherited EB remains supportive and preventive. Patients and their parents are taught to cushion the skin against pressure, injury, and infection through the chronic application of sterile gauze, nonadhesive synthetic dressings, and broad-spectrum topical antibiotics. Although as yet unproven, topical therapy with one or more recombinant growth factors might also someday prove to be beneficial in enhancing wound healing. Neither phenytoin nor retinoids appear to have a role in the treatment of EB.

Nutritional support is a keystone in the therapy of children with severe forms of EB. When oral intake is inadequate, the placement of a soft flexible intragastric feeding tube may enhance nutritional intake. If this fails, gastrostomy placement can be safely pursued, although even large intragastric feedings cannot overcome severe malabsorption due to widespread denudation of the small intestine.

Esophageal strictures occur mainly in the generalized and inverse forms of junctional and dystrophic EB. They usually can be safely improved with gentle esophageal dilatation although most patients require intermittent dilatations to maintain lumenal patency. Urethral strictures also respond to chronic manual dilatation.

Over time, web formation and mitten deformities occur in all but a few RDEB-HS patients, as well as in rare patients with JEB. Surgical degloving of these deformities is appropriate for functional impairment. In contrast, surgical correction of webbing of the feet is usually unnecessary. Other soft tissue contractures (i.e., elbows, knees) should be surgically corrected.

Split-thickness skin grafts may be used to cover chronic nonhealing erosions or ulcers in all forms of EB. Autologous or allogeneic cultured keratinocyte grafts may be similarly employed.

Patients with RDEB-HS are at high risk for the development of one or more squamous cell carcinomas and rarely malignant melanoma. Any proven cutaneous malignancies should be expeditiously excised. Local metastases similarly require immediate surgical intervention. Diffuse metastases, although usually unresponsive, may be possibly treated with radiotherapy and/or chemotherapy.

Tracheolaryngeal involvement in JEB may result in acute, fatal upper airway obstruction. Early tracheostomy placement may be life saving in patients with laryngoscopic evidence of involvement.

Dental reconstructive procedures, such as crown placement, should be instituted early in children with JEB, to offset enamel hypoplasia, which predisposes to rampant caries. Aggressive dental interventions are also appropriate in patients with RDEB-HS, who are prone to excessive caries as the result of altered intraoral soft tissue architecture and delayed clearance times for foods.

PEMPHIGUS VULGARIS AND THE PEMPHIGUS DISEASE SPECTRUM

(CM&S Chapter 74)

The term *pemphigus* refers to three autoimmune diseases that have the following characteristics in common. There is loss of epidermal cell–cell adhesion that manifests clinically as blistering and erosions of epithelial surfaces. IgG autoantibodies are bound in vivo around the plasma membranes of affected epithelia and are detected in the serum. Each form of pemphigus is characterized by specific autoantibodies that are directed against normal epithelial structural proteins. The circulating autoantibodies have been proven to be pathogenic and reproduce the essential clinical features of the disease in vivo.

There are three major forms of pemphigus that share these common elements but have distinctive clinical, histologic, and immunologic features. They are pemphigus vulgaris, pemphigus foliaceus, and paraneoplastic pemphigus.

Pemphigus Vulgaris

Definition and Clinical Description

Phemphigus vulgaris is a chronic blistering disorder of skin and mucous membranes that histologically shows detachment between cells of the basal cell layer of the epidermis and those of the suprabasilar epidermis, with IgG autoantibodies bound to the cell surface of affected epithelium and circulating in the serum. The IgG autoantibodies in pemphigus vulgaris recognize a 130-kd cell adhesion molecule of the epidermis, desmoglein 3, that is a member of the cadherin family of adhesion molecules.

Lesions of pemphigus vulgaris typically first develop in the mouth; subsequently affect the skin of the upper trunk, head, and neck; and later are seen in intertriginous areas, such as the axillae and groin. Lesions are restricted to stratified squamous epithelia, and internal organs other than the proximal esophagus are not affected. Small, flaccid bullae break easily and give rise to large painful denuded areas.

Oral lesions are painful, poorly marginated erosions that develop over a period of weeks or months. They arise in the posterior buccal mucosa, in the buccal sulci bilaterally, on the gingiva, and on the labial and lingual mucosa. In women, lesions of the cervix may occur early in the course of the disease and result in abnormal Papanicolaou smears, misdiagnosed as cervical dysplasia. Involvement of the proximal portion of the esophagus may cause substernal chest pain and dyspepsia. Pemphigus vegetans is probably a variant of pemphigus vulgaris in which chronic and persistent lesions develop into hypertrophic vegetative areas that resemble granulation tissue.

Alternatively, the onset of the disease may be explosive. Individuals will present with simultaneous development of oral lesions and extensive blistering and erosive lesions on the head, neck, and extremities. The condition may be confused with erythema multiforme or the Stevens-Johnson syndrome or other blistering skin diseases such as bullous pemphigoid.

With severe oral involvement, the pain of deglutition becomes unbearable and the intake rapidly declines. Coalescence of cutaneous lesions produces large exudative areas on the upper chest and back that have an intense burning sensation. The patient is unable to sit or lie comfortably in any position, and debilitation and exhaustion quickly ensue. The Nikolsky sign was originally described as a sign of the loss of epithelial integrity in this disease. In pemphigus vulgaris, if one presses on the top of an intact blister, the blister will enlarge laterally, or if one rubs the epithelium adjacent to a blister or erosion, the epithelium will peel off. Both of these signs have been accepted as being indicative of the Nikolsky phenomenon and are most clearly seen in patients with pemphigus vulgaris but not in those with bullous pemphigoid.

Pathology

Vesicular and bullous lesions of pemphigus vulgaris are marked by separation in a plane above the basal layer of the epidermis. The floor of the blisters is composed of a row of basal keratinocytes, which remain attached to the basement membrane, resulting in a picture likened to a "row of tombstones." If blistering occurs in hair-bearing skin, suprabasilar clefting often delves deeply into follicular epithelium.

Diagnosis and Differential Diagnosis

The diagnosis can be established by fulfilling the following criteria:

1. Clinically, there are erosions of blisters on both skin and mucous membranes.
2. Histologically, there is an acantholytic suprabasilar intraepidermal blister.
3. Direct immunofluorescence shows IgG bound to the cell surface of affected oral epithelium or skin.
4. Circulating antibodies that bind to the cell surface of squamous epithelium are detectable.

The differential diagnosis is given in Table 3–1. Low levels of "phemphigus-like" autoantibodies can be seen in penicillin allergies, after thermal burns, with dermatophyte infections, and in bullous and cicatricial pemphigoid.

Treatment

Mortality since the introduction of corticosteroids has decreased from 100% by 5 years to 5%. It is almost invariably due to complications of immunosuppressive therapy.

Therapy for pemphigus vulgaris must be directed at reducing autoantibody synthesis, because as long as significant levels of antiepithelial antibodies are present, the disease will persist. Topical treatments are of secondary importance, and long-term improvement will occur only by treatment of the hematopoietic system.

Oral corticosteroids remain the first line of treatment. About one half of patients will respond well to oral corticosteroids alone (prednisone, 1.0 mg/kg per day, with the dose tapered slowly over 6 to 9 months). Almost all individuals treated with prednisone alone will require a maintenance dosage every other day indefinitely to control their disease. Those who have resistant disease or are intolerant of

---

TABLE 3–1. Differential Diagnosis of Pemphigus Vulgaris

When only oral lesions are present:
  Aphthous stomatitis
  Erythema multiforme
  Herpes simplex
  Erosive lichen planus
  Cicatricial pemphigoid
When oral and cutaneous lesions are present:
  Stevens-Johnson syndrome/toxic epidermal necrolysis
  Bullous pemphigoid
  Linear IgA dermatitis
  Epidermolysis bullosa acquisita

corticosteroids should receive a second steroid-sparing agent, in decreasing order of efficacy: cyclophosphamide, azathioprine, chlorambucil, methotrexate, and gold.

Cyclophosphamide is an extremely effective agent, but it is also very toxic. It is more effective in reducing autoantibody synthesis and has a preferential cytotoxic affect on proliferative plasma cells. It is generally reserved for patients whose disease is most resistant to therapy and is administered in a dose of 1 to 2 mg/kg per day or by intermittent intravenous pulse. Major side effects include a predictable leukopenia, hemorrhagic cystitis caused by the toxic effects of urinary metabolites, and an increased lifetime risk of a malignancy and sterility.

Azathioprine is less toxic than cyclophosphamide but is also slightly less effective. Doses of 2 to 3 mg/kg per day are usually required to produce remission.

Treatment should always be adjusted according to the disease activity that is clinically apparent, without being unduly influenced by autoantibody titers. The antibody titers will generally be high when the disease is active and will be low or undetectable when the disease is in remission.

Pemphigus Foliaceus

Definition and Clinical Description

Pemphigus foliaceus can be subdivided into four subsets, all of which have identical immunopathologic features but arise in unique circumstances. They are idiopathic pemphigus foliaceus, drug-induced pemphigus foliaceus, pemphigus erythematosus, and a form that is endemic to regions of Brazil and Colombia, called fogo selvagem, endemic pemphigus foliaceus, or, alternately, Brazilian pemphigus foliaceus.

The cutaneous lesions of pemphigus foliaceus are similar in all subsets. Lesions are almost always restricted to the cutaneous surface. Oral mucosal lesions are rare. Lesions often first arise in the central face, the head and neck, or the upper trunk and consist of very superficial crusts and erosions. The lesions may have a seborrheic appearance, but as they spread, more of a serous exudate forms. Lesions below the elbows or knees or intact pustulovesicles are signs of very active disease. Erythrodermic cases occur more commonly in Brazil. Chronic lesions may become quite hypertrophic and resemble lesions of prurigo nodularis.

In pemphigus erythematosus, there often is both clinical and laboratory evidence of coexistent lupus erythematosus.

Pathology

Pemphigus foliaceus variants are all marked by vacuolization followed by acantholytic clefting within or just beneath the granular layer of the epidermis. These three conditions can all be considered as "superficial pemphigus," in contrast with pemphigus vulgaris, in which blistering occurs above basilar keratinocytes and can be considered "deep pemphigus."

Pathogenesis and Etiology

Autoantibodies in pemphigus foliaceus are directed against a 165-kd antigen, desmoglein I, another member of the cadherin family of cell adhesion molecules. These autoantibodies produce acantholysis throughout the epidermal granular layer.

The most commonly implicated agents of drug-induced pemphigus foliaceus include D-penicillamine, captopril, rifampin, and others.

Endemic pemphigus foliaceus occurs only in rural Brazil. Although an insect vector is suspected, it has not been proved, and the precise environmental trigger has also not been identified.

Differential Diagnosis

The differential diagnosis of pemphigus foliaceus includes pemphigus vulgaris, impetigo, staphylococcal scalded skin syndrome, pustular psoriasis, and seborrheic dermatitis.

Treatment

The mortality rate from pemphigus foliaceus is very small, possibly due to the superficial nature of the cutaneous lesions and the absence of mucosal involvement. The treatment is very similar to that of pemphigus vulgaris although one is not compelled to be as aggressive in the treatment of pemphigus foliaceus.

IgA Pemphigus Foliaceus

A rare vesicular pustular disorder has been identified and has been alternately called IgA pemphigus foliaceus or intercellular IgA vesicular pustular dermatosis. The disease clinically most closely resembles pemphigus foliaceus or subcorneal pustular dermatosis. Histopathologic features show one of two patterns: (1) a subcorneal pustule filled with neutrophils and with sparse acantholytic cells or (2) an intraepidermal pustule filled with neutrophils and occasional eosinophils and rare or absent acantholysis. Common to both forms is the presence of IgA deposited in a linear fashion on the epidermal cell surfaces. Circulating IgA autoantibodies directed against epithelium are not often detectable or are present in low titers. Both dapsone and prednisone have been used to control the disease, but neither has been proved to be uniformly effective.

Paraneoplastic Pemphigus

Definition

Paraneoplastic pemphigus is a newly described syndrome of unknown etiology associated with underlying neoplasms. The criteria that define the syndrome are as follows:

1. Mucosal erosions and a polymorphous skin eruption develop, with papular lesions progressing to blistering and erosive lesions affecting the trunk, extremities, and palms and soles in the context of an occult or known neoplasm.

2. Cutaneous histopathologic changes consist of vacuolar interface dermatitis, keratinocyte necrosis, and intraepidermal acantholysis.

3. Direct immunofluorescence demonstrates deposition of IgG and complement in the epidermal intercellular spaces and often granular/linear complement deposition along the epidermal basement membrane zone.

4. Serum autoantibodies bind the cell surface of skin and mucosae in a pattern typical for pemphigus but also bind to simple, columnar, and transitional epithelia.

5. These serum autoantibodies immunoprecipitate a complex of four high-molecular-weight proteins from keratinocytes. The antigens represent desmoplakins I and II and the bullous pemphigoid antigen.

Clinical Description

The most constant clinical feature is the presence of intractable stomatitis, which is usually the earliest presenting sign, and it is the one feature that is persistent and resistant to therapy. The cutaneous lesions of paraneoplastic pemphigus are quite variable and change according to the stage of the disease. Blisters on the extremities are sometimes tense, resembling those seen in bullous pemphigoid or erythema multiforme. Lesions on the trunk are often arcuate, resembling those seen in linear IgA dermatitis. Lichenoid lesions may be the primary cutaneous signs of the disease or may develop in chronic lesions that had previously been blistered. These lesions consist of infiltrated erythematous papules and plaques. In chronic disease, this lichenoid eruption may predominate over blistering on the cutaneous surface. Both blisters and lichenoid lesions affecting the palms and the soles are common. Some individuals who have chronic lichenoid skin lesions also have painful ulcerative paronychial lesions. The malignancies most commonly associated with paraneoplastic pemphigus are non-Hodgkin's lymphoma, chronic lymphocytic leukemia, Castleman's disease, thymoma, spindle cell neoplasms, and Waldenström's macroglooulinemia.

Pathology

The histopathology of lesions of paraneoplastic pemphigus is as varied as the clinical features. Findings include nonspecific inflammation, suprabasilar acantholysis, vacuolar interface dermatitis with necrosis of basilar keratinocytes, and areas of dense band-like lymphocytic infiltrate in the papillary dermis depending on the type of lesion biopsied. Intact cutaneous blisters reveal suprabasilar acantholysis.

Differential Diagnosis

The differential diagnosis of paraneoplastic pemphigus includes pemphigus vulgaris, erythema multiforme, chemotherapy induced stomatitis, herpes simplex virus infection, pemphigus erythematosus, cicatricial or bullous pemphigoid lichen planus, epidermolysis bullosa acquisita, and linear IGA dermatosis.

Treatment

Individuals with benign tumors such as thymoma or Castleman's disease should have them surgically excised. In the majority of patients who are freed of tumor burden the disease will improve substantially or clear completely.

In patients with malignant neoplasms there is no clear effective therapy. Oral prednisone, 1 mg/kg per day, will produce partial improvement but not complete resolution of lesions. Many other agents have been tried, but none have been reliably effective.

BULLOUS PEMPHIGOID

(CM&S Chapter 75)

Definition

Bullous pemphigoid is an acquired autoimmune subepidermal blistering disease of the skin, in which IgG and C3 bind to the epidermal basement membrane, and circulating IgG antibodies are directed against the epidermal basement membrane zone (BMZ).

Clinical Description

Bullous pemphigoid usually begins after age 60. The characteristic cutaneous lesions in bullous pemphigoid include tense blisters that may occur on normal-appearing skin or on an erythematous base. The blisters may range from vesicles to large bullae many centimeters in diameter. The distribution of skin blisters may include the entire skin surface, although the most common sites are the flexor surfaces of the arms and legs, the groin, the axilla, and the lower abdomen. Along with tense blisters, patients may present with erythematous macules, papules, or urticarial plaques. The degree of pruritus in bullous pemphigoid may vary from nonexistent to severe, and generalized pruritus may be the presenting symptom.

Oral mucous membrane involvement may occur but is rarely the presenting feature. The mucosal lesions in bullous pemphigoid are often transient, of minimal consequence, almost always limited to the oropharynx, and nonscarring. Patients with bullous pemphigoid generally do not have a history of any obvious precipitating factor related to their disease. There are, however, convincing reports of furosemide- and phenacetin-induced bullous pemphigoid. Discontinuation of the offending medication allowed disease resolution, and rechallenge led to new blister formation.

There have been numerous reports of bullous pemphigoid occurring in association with malignancy. Several large series of patients with bullous pemphigoid have been evaluated, and the results reveal that there is generally not a significantly increased incidence of malignancy in patients with bullous pemphigoid.

If left untreated, patients with bullous pemphigoid typically have disease that will persist for months to years. They may have spontaneous remissions and exacerbations, and recurrent disease is often less severe than the initial episode. As many as 75% of patients will achieve prolonged clinical remission without further therapy after an initial course of glucocorticosteroid treatment. The mortality rate is relatively low even in the absence of systemic glucocorticosteroid treatment, but the disease can be fatal during the active stage, particularly in elderly or debilitated patients.

As many as 15% to 20% of patients with bullous pemphigoid have localized disease, with a predilection for lesions on the lower extremities or on the palms and soles. Localized disease is more responsive to therapy and may be controlled with topical corticosteroids.

Pathology

The hallmark of bullous pemphigoid is a subepidermal blister with a normal epidermis and a variable dermal infiltrate composed predominantly of eosinophils.

Linear deposits of both IgG and C3 at the epidermal basement membrane are found in the large majority of patients with bullous pemphigoid. Biopsy specimens obtained from perilesional skin or from urticarial unblistered skin will generally provide the best results for direct immunofluorescence.

Most patients with bullous pemphigoid have circulating IgG anti–basement membrane zone antibodies. There is no correlation between antibody titer and disease activity in bullous pemphigoid. To accurately distinguish bullous pemphigoid from epidermolysis bullosa acquisita, special studies such as indirect immunofluorescence utilizing salt-split skin are required. This treatment induces a split at the level of the lamina lucida. Bullous pemphigoid antibodies will bind to the roof only or to the roof and base, whereas epidermolysis bullosa acquisita antibodies will bind solely to the base of the split skin.

Differential Diagnosis

Several other immunologically mediated skin diseases may mimic bullous pemphigoid and need to be considered in the differential diagnosis. These include cicatricial pemphigoid, herpes gestationis, epidermolysis bullosa acquisita, dermatitis herpetiformis, and linear IgA bullous dermatosis.

Treatment

The major form of therapy for generalized bullous pemphigoid is the administration of systemic glucocorticosteroids. The majority of patients have a reasonably rapid response to therapy.

Most therapeutic regimens are based on clinical experience. No controlled prospective studies comparing patients treated with systemic glucocorticosteroids with nontreated control patients are available. Mild disease usually responds to lower doses of prednisone, and localized disease may respond to topical steroid treatment or to intralesional corticosteroids. For generalized disease, moderate doses of prednisone are effective. Although extensive clinical experience supports the utility of immunosuppressive agents, especially azathioprine, in the treatment of patients whose disease cannot be controlled with glucocorticosteroids alone or in whom high-dose systemic glucocorticosteroid therapy cannot be tolerated or is contraindicated, a controlled study failed to demonstrate any benefits of treatment with azathioprine and corticosteroids as compared with corticosteroids alone.

Some patients, those with neutrophil predominant disease, can be successfully treated with sulfapyridine or dapsone. In certain patients, particularly in those with contraindications to systemic glucocorticosteroids, a combination of oral erythromycin or tetracycline (2 g per day) and niacinamide (1.5 to 2.5 g per day) is a worthwhile alternative.

Steroid Management of Bullous Pemphigoid

Localized disease is managed with high-potency topical steroids. When patients present with generalized disease that is relatively mild, low-dose prednisone (approximately 0.5 mg/kg per day, in a single morning dose) is successful. For those patients with generalized more severe disease, treatment with moderate-dose prednisone (0.75 to 1.25 mg/kg per day, in a single morning dose) is usually effective. Once the disease is under control, often within 3 weeks, the prednisone dose should be tapered in 10-mg increments weekly to an alternate-day regimen to minimize steroid side effects. The alternate-day dosage is tapered in 10-mg increments until the dosage is at 20 mg prednisone on alternate days and, assuming that there is no major disease flare during this taper, the taper is continued in 5-mg increments until the patient is off therapy.

CICATRICIAL PEMPHIGOID

(CM&S Chapter 76)

Definition

Cicatricial pemphigoid is a rare, chronic subepithelial blistering disease of middle-aged and elderly individuals that predominantly affects mucosal surfaces, most often the eyes and mouth, and is thought to be mediated by autoantibodies directed against an antigen in the epithelial basement membrane. The inflammatory lesions heal with scarring, and this, more than the primary lesions, is the source of morbidity and even mortality associated with cicatricial pemphigoid.

Clinical Description

Cicatricial pemphigoid affects predominantly mucous membranes with less frequent cutaneous involvement. Oral and ocular mucosa are most often involved, but other mucous membranes including nasal mucosa, pharynx, larynx, esophagus, genitalia, and anus may be affected. Some patients may have only mucous membrane involvement with one or more affected sites, while others may have cutaneous and mucous membrane disease.

Oral lesions are a frequent manifestation of cicatricial pemphigoid (noted in 85% to 100% of patients). The lesions often present as slowly healing erosions without pseudomembranes that have sharply defined margins. Occasionally, intact blisters are noted, but they often are quickly broken. Cicatricial pemphigoid may involve any portion of the oral mucosa and is a frequent cause of desquamative gingivitis.

Ocular involvement is seen in 64% to 80% of patients and is characterized by conjunctivitis with symptoms of irritation and tearing. Signs of active disease include a conjunctivitis with a violaceous erythema and subconjunctival fibrosis. The fibrosis leads to the gradual shrinkage of the conjunctival sac, with eventual symblepharon formation. Inturning of eyelashes (trichiasis) secondary to cicatricial entropion can cause corneal damage with resultant decrease in vision and eventual blindness, found in up to one third of patients with eye involvement followed for an average of 6 years.

Cutaneous lesions have been observed in approximately 25% of patients. Two types of skin lesions occur—erythematous plaques that develop recurrent blisters and heal with atrophic scars, usually on the head and neck; or vesicles and bullae that appear on the trunk and extremities and heal without scarring, similar to bullous pemphigoid.

Genital, nasal, and pharyngeal mucosa are involved in about 20% of patients. The fibrosis that occurs as the inflammatory lesions heal may lead to urethral stenosis in men and narrowing of the vaginal introitus and fusion of the labia minora in women, while pharyngeal involvement causes a sore throat and difficulty swallowing.

Esophageal involvement is uncommon, occurring in under 5% of patients, but can be the cause of dysphagia and odynophagia and result in esophageal strictures and predispose patients to regurgitation and aspiration pneumonia.

Pathology

The characteristic histopathologic features of a biopsy specimen taken from a bulla of skin or oral mucous membrane include a subepithelial blister with a mixed inflammatory infiltrate consisting of lymphocytes, neutrophils, and eosinophils in the dermis or lamina propria. In keeping with the formation of superficial scarring in cicatricial pemphigoid, the plane of separation is below the lamina densa. In contrast to the case in bullous pemphigoid or epidermolysis bullosa acquisita, anchoring fibrils are preserved and not obscured or destroyed by immunoglobulin deposition. Perilesional biopsy specimens of mucous membranes, skin, or conjunctiva are preferable to biopsy specimens of lesional skin and most often show linear deposition of IgG and complement along the basement membrane zone (BMZ). Deposition of IgA has also been found in up to half of biopsy specimens, and in some cases linear IgA may be the only immunoreactant present along the BMZ.

Diagnosis and Differential Diagnosis

A diagnosis of cicatricial pemphigoid should include three criteria: (1) a consistent clinical picture of scarring blisters and erosions, usually affecting mucous membranes to a greater extent than keratinized skin; (2) histopathologic findings showing subepithelial blister formation and/or inflammatory infiltrate either of neutrophils and eosinophils or in scarring variants, plasma cells, and lympho-cytes; and (3) direct immunofluorescence studies of perilesional biopsy specimens showing linear deposition of IgG and comple-ment and/or IgA along the BMZ.

Ocular involvement alone can resemble viral conjunctivitis and ocular rosacea. In cases in which either multiple mucous mem-branes or both mucous membranes and a cutaneous eruption are present, the differential diagnosis includes bullous pemphigoid, pemphigus vulgaris, erythema multiforme, erosive lichen planus, linear IgA dermatosis, and epidermolysis bullosa acquisita.

Treatment

Treatment is generally dictated by the organs involved and at-tendant anticipated morbidity. For example, if only oropharyngeal lesions are present, treatment may be limited to topical or intrale-sional steroids, possibly short courses of oral corticosteroids or dap-sone. However, severe or progressive eye disease, esophageal or laryngeal involvement, and potential morbidity that includes blind-ness or asphyxiation warrants a more aggressive approach, includ-ing the use of oral steroids and immunosuppressive agents.

Topical therapy is helpful in removal of necrotic tissue to mini-mize infectious problems, discomfort, and inflammation. Diluted solutions of either hydrogen peroxide or povidone-iodine can be used to gently cleanse the oral cavity several times daily, including after meals. Topical anesthetics such as viscous lidocaine or diluted diphenhydramine elixir can be used before meals for comfort. The use of corticosteroids topically in the oral cavity helps reduce in-flammation.

Intralesional corticosteroids may be helpful in healing persistent mucous membrane erosions (triamcinolone acetonide, 5 to 7.5 mg/mL injected into the periphery of lesions every 2 weeks).

Systemic medications useful in the treatment of cicatricial pemphigoid include oral corticosteroids, dapsone, cyclophos-phamide, and azathioprine. Oral corticosteroids, in the range of 1 mg/kg per day of prednisone, are often the first systemic medication used. Patients usually require moderately high daily doses of pred-nisone to maintain control and alternative-day therapy is often in-sufficient. Because corticosteroids are simply suppressive, the pa-tients may be subjected to the numerous side effects of prolonged steroid therapy.

Second-line systemic therapy includes dapsone, cyclophospha-mide and azathioprine. There are various regimens for the use of dapsone, but in general it is begun at less than the therapeutic dose, 25 to 50 mg daily, and increased to 100 to 150 mg daily as tolerated. Both cyclophosphamide and azathioprine, which are able to induce disease remission, are used in a dose of 1 to 2 mg/kg/day.

Surgical intervention may be needed to deal with the scarring outcome of the disease, but it is essential to remember that complete control of cicatricial pemphigoid needs to be achieved before any surgical procedure is undertaken.

HERPES GESTATIONIS

(CM&S Chapter 77)
Definition

Herpes gestationis, otherwise known as pemphigoid gestationis, is a rare autoimmune disease that occurs exclusively during pregnancy or the immediate postpartum period. It is characterized by intensely pruritic urticarial lesions and tense blisters and appears to be mediated by a specific anti–basement membrane zone (BMZ) IgG, which activates complement, causing the infiltration and degranulation of eosinophils. The herpes gestationis antibody is specific for a 180-kd transmembrane component of the hemidesmosome. The appearance of the herpes gestationis antibody, as demonstrated by immunofluorescence, is the sine qua non for herpes gestationis.

Clinical Description

Classically, herpes gestationis presents during the second or third trimester of pregnancy or in the immediate postpartum period as a rapidly progressive, intensely pruritic, urticarial eruption on the abdomen that usually evolves within days into a generalized pemphigoid-like eruption, sparing the face, mucous membranes, palms, and soles. Tense blisters occur within urticarial plaques or on clinically normal skin. Most cases flare at the time of delivery, then spontaneously regress over weeks to months. The disease tends to recur during subsequent gestations, and 25% of women experience flares with use of oral contraceptives.

The disease typically presents as pruritus alone or pruritic urticarial lesions that start most commonly on the abdomen. Progression to clustered, tense, vesiculobullous lesions is nearly invariant and usually occurs within days to weeks of the initial onset of pruritus. Facial involvement is distinctly uncommon, and mucosal disease is nearly nonexistent. The clinical presentation and course can be extremely variable. Patients may experience spontaneous resolution during the later part of gestation, only to flare at the time of delivery. Exacerbation at the time of delivery is characteristic, occurring in at least 75% of patients. As the disease begins to resolve, recurrence during menstruation is common. The majority of patients experience spontaneous regression over the weeks to months following delivery, with or without treatment.

The newborn may be affected with mild cutaneous involvement approximately 10% of the time, but typically the disease is self-limited, resolving spontaneously over days to weeks.

There is controversy about whether there is an increase in fetal morbidity or mortality associated with herpes gestationis. Although the perception persists from a review of reported individual case reports that there is significant fetal morbidity and mortality associated with herpes gestationis, no increase in spontaneous abortions or fetal mortality has been noted in most recent studies. There is, however, a slight tendency for small-for-gestational-age births and a tendency for prematurity.

Women with a history of herpes gestationis have an increased prevalence of autoimmune diseases, such as Graves' disease, Hashimoto's thyroiditis, and pernicious anemia, diseases that are associated with the same HLA antigens of herpes gestationis—HLA DR3 and DR4.

Pathology

The histopathologic features of herpes gestationis are similar to those of bullous pemphigoid.

The sine qua non for the diagnosis of herpes gestationis is the immunofluorescent finding of C3 during active disease, with or without IgG, in a linear band along the BMZ of perilesional skin.

Diagnosis and Differential Diagnosis

In the classic appearance of a pemphigoid-like eruption associated with pregnancy, herpes gestationis is readily apparent. The urticarial phase of herpes gestationis may be easily confused with pruritic urticarial papules and plaques of pregnancy (PUPPP). Erythema multiforme, allergic contact dermatitis, and drug eruptions are also in the differential diagnosis.

Treatment

Topical steroids and antihistamines are usually ineffective but may suffice until delivery. Systemic steroids remain the cornerstone of therapy. Most patients respond to 0.5 mg/kg of prednisone daily. Maintenance therapy, generally at a lower dose, may or may not be required throughout gestation; many patients experience spontaneous regressions during the third trimester only to flare again with parturition. There is no evidence that the use of systemic steroids adversely affects fetal outcome.

None of the alternatives to steroids (dapsone, pyridoxine, ritodrine) or adjuvants (gold, methotrexate, cyclophosphamide, plasmapheresis) are useful before term, and the experience with each has been variable at best. There is no compelling argument to be made for induced delivery, except for the management of symptoms. Although the pruritus and blisters of herpes gestationis are exasperating, there is no clear evidence that the presence of herpes gestationis poses a significant risk to mother or child.

EPIDERMOLYSIS BULLOSA ACQUISITA

(CM&S Chapter 78)

Definition

Epidermolysis bullosa acquisita is an acquired immune mediated subepidermal bullous disease characterized by skin fragility and blisters over trauma-prone sites, in which IgG deposits localize below the lamina densa of the dermoepidermal junction. Diagnostic criteria include that the patient have an acquired blistering disorder without a family history of blistering diseases.

Clinical Description

Although it was initially thought that epidermolysis bullosa acquisita always presented as a noninflammatory mechanobullous eruption reminiscent of porphyria cutanea tarda, it is now clear that the clinical presentation can be quite variable. The initial presentation, typically between ages 40 and 50, is often a disseminated inflammatory bullous eruption more reminiscent of bullous pemphigoid than porphyria cutanea tarda or hereditary forms of epidermolysis bullosa. Disseminated pruritic macules, papules, urticarial plaques, and vesicles appearing on sheets of inflammatory skin may be the initial clinical presentation of some patients. Later in the course of the disease, noninflammatory mechanobullous lesions involving trauma-prone regions of the body (e.g., elbow, knee, and extremities) predominate more reminiscent of inherited forms of dystrophic epidermolysis bullosa or porphyria cutanea tarda. The bullous lesions heal with scarring and formation of milia. Blindness, nail dystrophy, and cicatricial alopecia are also sometimes observed as sequelae of the lesions.

The course of the disease is usually chronic with periods of partial remissions and exacerbations. Spontaneous resolution rarely occurs, but in some patients the intensity of the disease appears to decrease with time.

Epidermolysis bullosa acquisita is often associated with other autoimmune disorders, such as diabetes mellitus, inflammatory bowel disease, and systemic lupus erythematosus. These patients have an increased frequency of the haplotype DR2 of class II HLA.

Pathology

Blisters of epidermolysis bullosa acquisita are subepidermal with a variable dermal infiltrate. Direct immunofluorescence shows IgG and C3 at the dermoepidermal junction of perilesional skin (approximately 1 cm from a blister) in most patients with epidermolysis bullosa acquisita, sometimes accompanied by IgM or IgA. Indirect immunofluorescence is positive in a minority of patients. Immunoelectron microscopic examination of perilesional skin demonstrates IgG deposits below the lamina densa. The cleavage plane of the blister at the dermoepidermal junction may take place at two different levels — within the lamina lucida correlated with a dense inflammatory cell infiltrate in the dermis, or below the lamina densa associated with minimal clinical or histologic inflammation. Patients with epidermolysis bullosa acquisita have decreased numbers of anchoring fibrils at the dermoepidermal junction, similar to patients with inherited forms of dystrophic epidermolysis bullosa.

Pathogenesis and Etiology

Epidermolysis bullosa acquisita is immunologically characterized by IgG autoantibodies against a component of the dermoepidermal junction. The target of the autoantibodies is type VII collagen, a major component of anchoring fibrils that are structures located below the lamina densa of the basement membrane beneath stratified squamous epithelium. These structures are thought to play a role in the adherence between the basement membrane and the papillary dermis.

Diagnosis and Differential Diagnosis

Diagnostic criteria of epidermolysis bullosa acquisita include the following: an acquired subepidermal blistering disorder; cutaneous lesions consisting of blisters, erosions, milia, and scars in trauma-prone sites; an absence of family history for bullous disorders; linear IgG and C3 deposition in the dermoepidermal junction; and exclusion of all other blistering disorders. The wide spectrum of clinical presentations dictates that a wide range of diagnostic possibilities be considered when the patient is initially seen, including blistering disorders of genetic, immunologic, metabolic, and iatrogenic origin.

Immunofluorescence testing of salt-split skin specimens can be used to distinguish epidermolysis bullosa acquisita from other blistering diseases. In epidermolysis bullosa acquisita, the autoantibodies react to the dermal side of the salt-split skin. By contrast, the autoantibodies from bullous pemphigoid serum react to the epidermal side of salt-split skin.

Treatment

Treatment of epidermolysis bullosa acquisita is difficult owing to the poor response observed with prednisone and standard immunosuppressive agents that are usually helpful in the treatment of bullous pemphigoid. However, a logical strategy based on the clinical presentation of the patient may help in formulating a treatment plan. If the patient presents with a disseminated inflammatory blistering eruption, prednisone at 1 to 2 mg/kg or higher may be helpful initially. If the patient has predominantly a noninflammatory mechanobullous syndrome, the response to systemic steroids is often unsatisfactory but such treatment should still be attempted. In these cases, the addition of dapsone or high-dose cyclosporine (above 6 mg/kg/day) may be helpful.

DERMATITIS HERPETIFORMIS

(CM&S Chapter 79)

Definition

Dermatitis herpetiformis is a chronic, intensely pruritic, papulovesicular eruption characterized by the presence of granular deposits of IgA at the dermoepidermal junction of the skin, an associated gluten-sensitive enteropathy, and an increased frequency of HLA-A1, HLA-B8, HLA-DR3, and HLA-DQw2.

Clinical Description

Dermatitis herpetiformis manifests as erythematous papules or vesicles (rarely with urticarial plaques or bullae), often with multiple erosions with and without crusts. These lesions typically appear symmetrically on extensor surfaces, particularly on the shoulders, elbows, buttocks, sacrum, knees, and posterior hairline. A hallmark of the disorder is an intense pruritus, a result of which is only crusted and eroded lesions are present and the primary papulovesicular lesions may not be seen.

Dermatitis herpetiformis most often presents in the second or third decade. The clinical course is typically one of remissions and exacerbations, although the remissions rarely persist. If patients adhere to a gluten-free diet, however, the skin lesions as well as the gastrointestinal abnormalities can be controlled.

Sixty percent to 70% of patients with dermatitis herpetiformis have, on biopsy of the small bowel, histologic features qualitatively identical to those seen in patients with gluten-sensitive enteropathy without any skin disease. Avoidance of dietary gluten, a protein found in various grains such as wheat, rye, and oats, results in a return of the small bowel morphology to normal. Small bowel biopsy specimens of patients with dermatitis herpetiformis reveal a histologic picture that is identical to that seen in patients with isolated gluten-sensitive enteropathy, although usually less severe. The clinical manifestations of the enteropathy in patients with dermatitis herpetiformis are often minimal; 5% to 10% have clinical symptoms such as diarrhea, bloating, and abdominal pain.

Dermatitis herpetiformis may be associated with an increased risk for lymphoma and other malignancies. The cumulative incidence of malignancy in patients with the disorder is 6.4%, resulting in an increased relative risk of 2.3.

Dermatitis herpetiformis is also associated with the frequent occurrence of other autoimmune diseases, including thyroid disease, gastric atrophy and hypochlorhydria, dermatomyositis, myasthenia gravis, rheumatoid arthritis, systemic lupus erythematosus, and Sjögren's syndrome.

Pathology

Neutrophils localized to the dermal papillae are present in the earliest lesions of dermatitis herpetiformis, later followed by the appearance of clefts at the dermoepidermal junction. Even in the early lesions, the routine pathologic features are not unique for dermatitis herpetiformis, having been reported in biopsy specimens from patients with bullous pemphigoid, linear IgA dermatosis, or bullous systemic lupus erythematosus. The diagnosis should be confirmed by direct immunofluorescence on normal-appearing, perilesional skin.

Immunopathology

Seventy percent to 90% of patients with the clinical characteristics of dermatitis herpetiformis have granular IgA deposits at the dermoepidermal junction, often in the dermal papillae, while 10% to 30% have linear deposits of IgA. Patients with linear deposits of IgA do not have gluten-sensitive enteropathy or the increased haplotype associations. Thus, the diagnosis of dermatitis herpetiformis is reserved for patients with the characteristic clinical presentation and granular deposits of IgA below the epidermal basement membrane.

Differential Diagnosis

The differential diagnosis includes erythema multiforme, bullous pemphigoid, transient acantholytic dermatosis, papular urticaria, scabies, insect bites, and neurotic excoriations.

Treatment

The major forms of therapy include medical therapy with either dapsone or sulfapyridine and dietary therapy with the avoidance of gluten. Because compliance with a gluten-free diet is extremely difficult, dapsone or sulfapyridine has become the treatment of choice in most cases. The starting dose of dapsone for the majority of patients is 100 mg per day; most patients will have symptomatic relief within 24 hours. Maintenance doses of 100 to 200 mg per day are sufficient to control the eruption in most patients and to avoid the side effects of dapsone but do not alleviate gastrointestinal symptoms, nor do they reverse the morphologic changes in the gut.

The main complication of dapsone therapy is hemolysis, which occurs to some degree in all patients but can be catastrophic in patients with glucose-6-phosphate dehydrogenase deficiency. Testing of baseline glucose-6-phosphate dehydrogenase values is recommended in blacks, Asians, and persons of southern Mediterranean origin. Methemoglobinemia is seldom a severe problem but may be tolerated poorly in patients with glucose-6-phosphate dehydrogenase deficiency, methemoglobin reductase deficiency, or cardiopulmonary decompensation. Recommendations for the follow-up of patients on dapsone are as follows: (1) baseline complete blood cell count and liver function tests; (2) a complete blood cell count weekly for the first month, monthly for the next 5 months, and semiannually thereafter; and (3) liver function tests every 6 months.

Sulfapyridine, also useful treatment, is poorly absorbed from the gastrointestinal tract, and it is less effective in controlling the cutaneous eruption. Most patients require 500 to 2000 mg of sulfapyridine per day to achieve adequate control. A gluten-free diet appears to be effective in treating both the cutaneous manifestations and the gastrointestinal abnormality while allowing a reduction or complete elimination of drug therapy. Compliance is difficult.

Gluten is a ubiquitous protein, present in wheat, oats, rye, and barley. Rice and corn, however, do not contain gluten. The patient needs to be carefully educated, with the assistance of a dietician, if success is to be achieved. Institution of a gluten-free diet in patients already on dapsone allows patients to reduce or eliminate their dependence on this drug.

LINEAR IgA BULLOUS DERMATOSIS

(CM&S Chapter 80)

Definition

Linear IgA bullous dermatosis is a distinct subepidermal vesiculobullous eruption occurring in adults, defined on the basis of a unique immunopathology that consists of linear deposition of IgA along the cutaneous basement membrane. Chronic bullous disease of childhood is a subepidermal vesiculobullous disease originally considered separate from linear IgA bullous dermatosis. However, circulating IgA antibody binds to the same antigen seen in patients with linear IgA bullous dermatosis and deposition of immunoreactants in the lamina lucida, suggesting that, on a molecular basis, this is the same disease occurring in a different age group.

Clinical Description

The average age at onset is after 60 years of age, but it may present throughout adult life. Clinical manifestations are variable, and patients present with findings consistent with dermatitis herpetiformis and/or bullous pemphigoid. They may have subepidermal tense bullae often indistinguishable from bullous pemphigoid, but not infrequently the lesions appear in herpetiform but asymmetrical arrangements on erythematous and/or normal-appearing skin. Oral lesions are present in more than 70% of cases, whereas in dermatitis herpetiformis they are uncommon.

Pathology

Distinguishing between dermatitis herpetiformis and linear IgA bullous dermatosis can be nearly impossible; linear IgA deposition at the dermoepidermal junction is the diagnostic feature.

Diagnosis and Differential Diagnosis

Linear IgA bullous dermatosis is difficult to diagnose clinically and is often confused with dermatitis herpetiformis and bullous pemphigoid. By definition, linear IgA bullous dermatosis is separated from dermatitis herpetiformis and bullous pemphigoid on the basis of its direct immunofluorescence; linear IgA deposition along the BMZ in perilesional skin biopsies is characteristic of linear IgA bullous dermatosis, in contrast to dermatitis herpetiformis, which shows granular deposition of IgA in dermal papillary tips, and bullous pemphigoid, which shows linear deposition of IgG along the cutaneous BMZ.

Circulating anti-BMZ antibodies of IgA class can be demonstrated in 60% to 70% of linear IgA bullous dermatosis sera, whereas patients with dermatitis herpetiformis have not been shown to have a circulating antibody that binds to skin and 60% to 70% of patients with bullous pemphigoid demonstrate circulating IgG class antibody. Other bullous diseases that should be considered in the differential diagnosis include erythema multiforme and bullous lupus erythematosus.

The incidence of gluten-sensitive enteropathy in linear IgA bullous dermatosis has been reported in the literature to range from 0% to 24%. Linear IgA bullous dermatosis has a much lower prevalence of histologic small bowel abnormalities than dermatitis herpetiformis. Drug-induced linear IgA bullous dermatosis has been reported as well, with the drugs implicated including captopril, lithium, vancomycin, and diclofenac sodium.

Treatment

The majority of cases of chronic bullous disease of childhood respond to either sulfapyridine or dapsone therapy. Sulfapyridine, which has less significant side effects than dapsone, is started at 70 mg/kg per day, in divided doses, not to exceed 100 mg/kg per day. If sulfapyridine is unsuccessful, dapsone is begun at 1 to 2 mg/kg per day, increasing at weekly intervals until the symptoms are adequately controlled. The dosage of dapsone is not to exceed 3 to 4 mg/kg per day.

The majority of patients with linear IgA bullous dermatosis respond to dapsone, although sulfapyridine and, rarely, prednisone are required. The average dose of dapsone to control the eruption is 100 mg daily, but doses as high as 300 mg daily may be needed. Initially, dosing should begin at 25 mg, and the dose is increased every 1 to 2 weeks until control is achieved.

The course of the disease is characterized by persistence for several years, but eventual spontaneous remission is likely in 10% to 60%.

TOXIC EPIDERMAL NECROLYSIS

(CM&S Chapter 81)

Definition

Toxic epidermal necrolysis is defined as extensive detachment of full-thickness epidermis most often related to an adverse drug reaction. Because of many resemblances to Stevens-Johnson syndrome, toxic epidermal necrolysis is often considered as the most severe form of the so-called erythema multiforme spectrum. However, there is no consistent agreement on the boundary between toxic epidermal necrolysis and Stevens-Johnson syndrome and between Stevens-Johnson syndrome and erythema multiforme. The current concept is to separate an erythema multiforme spectrum (erythema multiforme minor plus erythema multiforme major) from a Stevens-Johnson syndrome/toxic epidermal necrolysis spectrum. The first disorders are often recurrent and postinfectious with low morbidity and no mortality. The second disorders are usually severe drug-induced reactions with high morbidity and poor prognosis. A consensus has been reached on a graded classification within the Stevens-Johnson syndrome/toxic epidermal necrolysis spectrum. Stevens-Johnson syndrome is defined as comprising cases with mucosal erosions plus widespread purpuric macules and epidermal detachment affecting less than 10% of the skin; overlap Stevens-Johnson syndrome/toxic epidermal necrolysis as cases with widespread purpuric macules and epidermal detachment of between 10% and 30%; and toxic epidermal necrolysis as cases with widespread purpuric macules and epidermal detachment above 30% or those rare cases in which there is more than 10% detachment without any discrete lesions.

Mucocutaneous Pattern

The disease usually begins as nonspecific symptoms; fever, sore throat, and burning eyes occur 1 to 3 days before the onset of cutaneous and mucous membrane lesions. A burning or painful rash starts symmetrically on the face and in the upper part of the body and rapidly extends. Most frequently, the initial individual cutaneous lesions form poorly defined macules with darker purpuric centers, or atypical targets, progressively merging on the chin, chest, and back. Less frequently, the initial manifestation may be an extensive scarlatiniform erythema. The maximal extension of the lesions is usually observed in 3 or 4 days, sometimes in a few hours. Occasionally, extension may last for a week. Sometimes the lesions are distributed in photoexposed areas. Most characteristic of toxic epidermal necrolysis is the appearance of a sheet-like loss of the epidermis within the regions involved by the confluent erythema. The epidermis is raised by flaccid blisters, which spread on pressure. The Nikolsky sign is positive over large areas. Detachment of the full thickness of the epidermis over pressure areas such as the back of the shoulders and the buttocks or on traumatized sites will reveal a dark red, oozing dermis. In other areas, the pale necrotic epidermis remains over the dermis with a wrinkled appearance. The entire surface of the skin can be involved with all of the epidermis sloughing off. The hairy portion of the scalp is never affected. The extent of the detachment of the epidermis should be noted daily and expressed as the percentage of body surface area involved, using the same tables as for burns.

Mucous membrane involvement is present in nearly all patients (85%–95%), preceding the skin lesions by 1 to 3 days in about one third of the cases. Several sites are usually affected, in the following order of frequency: oropharynx, eyes, genitalia, anus. Widespread painful erosions, identical to those of Stevens-Johnson syndrome, cause crusted lips, increased salivation, impaired alimentation, photophobia, and painful micturition. Ocular lesions need special attention and daily examination by an ophthalmologist, since they carry a high risk of sequelae. In the acute phase, redness and soreness of the eyes are conspicuous. The eyelids are often stuck together, and attempts to separate them result in the loosening of the eyelashes and the epidermis of the eyelids. Pseudomembranous conjunctival erosions are usual with a tendency to form synechiae between eyelids and conjunctiva. Keratitis and corneal erosions are less frequent. A sicca syndrome may appear during the first few days.

Visceral Involvement

High fever is usual and may persist until there is complete skin cicatrization, even in the absence of superinfection. A sudden drop in temperature is more indicative of severe sepsis than is fever. Asthenia, skin pain, and anxiety are extreme. Agitation and confusion are not uncommon, often heralding hemodynamic complications or sepsis. Systemic involvement is usual in toxic epidermal necrolysis.

Gastrointestinal Tract. Disseminated mucosal erosions lead to dysphagia and sometimes to bleeding. The prevalence of esophageal involvement is probably grossly underestimated, since dysphagia from oropharyngeal lesions may mask dysphagia of esophageal origin. Half of patients with toxic epidermal necrolysis have liver inflammation. Overt hepatitis is present in about 10%.

Respiratory Tract. Tracheal and bronchial erosions may develop. Pulmonary edema is frequent. Adult respiratory distress syndrome sometimes precipitated by infection is one of the main complications of toxic epidermal necrolysis.

Blood. Anemia and lymphopenia are present in most patients. Neutropenia, indicating a poor prognosis, is observed in about 30% of patients.

Consequences of Extensive Epidermolysis ("Acute Skin Failure")

Many of the visceral manifestations observed in toxic epidermal necrolysis are the same as in extensive burns. They result from skin loss and are proportional to the surface of epidermal destruction. The concept of ''acute skin failure'' may help one to understand both the severity and the multiplicity of organ failure resulting from widespread skin loss.

Fluid Loss. The blister fluid of toxic epidermal necrolysis contains approximately 40 g/L of proteins and electrolytes, similar in concentration to that of plasma. The total daily cutaneous fluid loss averages 3 to 4 L in adult patients with epidermal necrolysis over 50% of their body surface area. Electrolyte, fluid, and protein losses result in a reduction of intravascular volume.

Infection. Destruction of the mechanical barrier and alteration of the normal host defense mechanisms, in combination with the fact that necrotic epidermis and exudates supports the growth of a wide spectrum of microorganisms, makes patients with widespread skin erosions very susceptible to systemic infection from both exogenous and endogenous sources. Severe systemic infections are the main cause of death in toxic epidermal necrolysis. During the first few days, skin lesions are usually colonized by *Staphylococcus aureus*. Later they are invaded by gram-negative rods from the digestive flora, especially *Pseudomonas aeruginosa*. Sepsis may be caused by access lines inserted near or through skin lesions or from digestive flora without concomitant skin colonization.

Impaired Thermoregulation. Fever and shivering occur even in the absence of overt infection. Hypothermia is infrequent and usually a harbinger of severe infection and irreversible septic shock.

Increased Energy Expenditure. Energy expenditure increases with the extension of skin lesions to reach twice the basal metabolism when 50% or more of the body surface is involved; protein loss may reach 150 to 200 g per day; and inhibition of insulin secretion and/or insulin resistance in peripheral tissues are frequent, resulting in elevated plasma glucose levels and often in overt glycosuria.

Course and Sequelae

The naked dermis bleeds easily and becomes covered with dark crusts. Regrowth of epidermis begins after a few days, sometimes while the disease is still spreading to the lower parts of the body. Most of the skin surface is reepithelialized in 2 to 3 weeks. Areas subject to pressure and periorificial skin often remain eroded and crusted for 1 to 3 more weeks. These localized lesions do not preclude hospital discharge.

Usually, erosions heal without scarring, but scarring may occur over sites of pressure or infection and dyspigmentation is inevitable. Nails are frequently shed, and regrowth may be abnormal and occasionally absent. Many patients complain of increased sweating.

Mucous membrane erosions sometimes persist for months after epidermal healing and may leave atrophic scars, phimosis in men and vaginal synechiae in women.

Ocular sequelae are the most severe, affecting 20% to 40% of survivors. A few patients have lacrimal duct obstruction resulting in watery eyes, but most have a sicca syndrome, indistinguishable from that observed in Sjögren's syndrome with inturned eyelashes, epithelial proliferation with squamous metaplasia, and neovascularization of the conjunctiva and the cornea. This leads to a "post-toxic epidermal necrolysis" ocular syndrome with punctate keratitis and formation of a corneal pannus with associated photophobia, burning eyes, visual impairment, and even blindness.

Prognosis

Toxic epidermal necrolysis is a disease of severe morbidity and high mortality. The fatality rate averages 30%. Sepsis, mainly from *S. aureus* and *P. aeruginosa* and adult respiratory distress syndrome, is the most important cause of death. Four variables are particularly important prognostic factors: (1) patient's age, (2) percentage of denuded skin, (3) blood urea nitrogen level, and (4) neutropenia.

Pathology

Early stages of toxic epidermal necrolysis are histopathologically indistinguishable from those of erythema multiforme; there is vacuolar change at the dermoepidermal junction with individual necrotic keratinocytes and a sparse infiltrate of lymphocytes, both at the junction and around vessels of the superficial plexus. The typical advanced lesions show necrosis of the whole epidermis, detached from a slightly altered dermis.

Pathogenesis and Etiology

Toxic epidermal necrolysis is most often drug induced. Several case reports have suggested that some cases are secondary to infection. The occurrence of toxic epidermal necrolysis as the most severe form of acute graft-versus-host (GVH) reaction is generally accepted.

Responsible Drugs

The vast majority of cases are related to chemicals systemically administered as drug therapy, while an offending drug is found in 70% to 90% of cases. In large homogeneous series of toxic epidermal necrolysis, a few drugs accounted for the majority of cases. These "classic culprits" are antibacterial sulfonamides (e.g., cotrimoxazole), aromatic anticonvulsants (phenobarbital, phenytoin, carbamazepine), some antibiotics (e.g., aminopenicillins), some nonsteroidal anti-inflammatory agents (e.g., phenylbutazone, oxyphenbutazone, isoxicam, piroxicam), and allopurinol.

Associated Diseases

Patients infected with human immunodeficiency virus have higher risks of cutaneous reactions to drugs. Many cases of toxic epidermal necrolysis have been reported in these patients, reflecting an extended exposure to sulfonamides and a higher risk of reaction than for other users of the same drugs. Patients with systemic lupus erythematosus also have an increased incidence of toxic epidermal necrolysis.

Diagnosis and Differential Diagnosis

Clinical morphology and histopathologic evaluation of lesions are required to separate early toxic epidermal necrolysis from exfoliative erythroderma, acute generalized exanthematous pustulosis, and generalized fixed drug eruption.

Treatment

There is no specific treatment. Because of the unproven hypothesis of an allergic reaction to drugs, some authors still believe that systemic corticosteroids are helpful in the treatment of toxic epidermal necrolysis. The data, although uncontrolled, suggest that corticosteroids are more detrimental than useful in toxic epidermal necrolysis and should be avoided.

The main principles of therapy are the same as for major burns (Table 3–2).

BLISTERING AND PUSTULAR DISORDERS OF THE NEONATE

(CM&S Chapter 82)

Many diseases can cause blisters and/or pustules in the neonate. Conceptually, these diseases are best classified into infectious causes, transient skin lesions, and uncommon and rare causes.

TABLE 3-2. Treatment of Toxic Epidermal Necrolysis

PRIMARY EMERGENCY CARE

Withdraw any suspect drug.
Avoid skin trauma.
Insert a peripheral venous line.
Begin administration of macromolecular solution.
Direct the patient to a burn unit or an intensive care unit.

SYMPTOMATIC THERAPY

Evaluation of Severity

Extent of epidermal lesions: actual detachment plus blisters and areas of positive Nikolsky's sign; use burn tables or the "rule of nines"
General status: daily weight, respiration rate, urinary output

Fluid Replacement

Use peripheral veins when possible.
Fluid requirements are two thirds to three fourths of those recommended for burns of same extent, 4-6 L per day, including 1-2 L macromolecular solutions.

Antibacterial Policy

Sterile handling of patients
Topical antiseptic solutions (silver nitrate, chlorhexidine)
Nonadherent dressings (skin grafts?)
Bacterial sampling of altered skin
Systemic antibiotics only if high suspicion of sepsis

Nutritional Support

Nasogastric tube, 3000-4000 calories per day, high-protein diet

Pulmonary Care

Aerosols, bronchial aspiration

Reduce Caloric Losses

Raise environmental temperature to 30°-32° C.
Use air-fluidized bed and warmed antiseptic solutions.

Eye Lesions

Provide for daily examination by an ophthalmologist.
Antiseptic/antibiotic eye drops every 2 hours
Disrupt synechiae with a blunt instrument.

Other Supportive Therapies

Heparin
Tranquilizers
Analgesics

Infectious Causes

Staphylococcal Pyoderma

Superficial *Staphylococcus aureus* infection, often acquired in the neonatal nursery, may begin in the first days to weeks of life, often with vesicles, pustules, crusting, or bullae in the diaper area. The diagnosis can be made with Gram stain of exudate and confirmed with bacterial cultures. Oral antibiotics, such as dicloxacillin, 12.5 to 25 mg/kg per day, or cephalexin, 25 to 50 mg/kg per day, divided in four daily doses for 7 to 10 days, are the drugs of choice.

Listeriosis

Listeria monocytogenes can cause a rash, usually present at birth, consisting of widespread erythematous or purpuric macules, often in conjunction with pustules on an erythematous base. Affected infants are typically born after a maternal fever, often in association with premature delivery induced by maternal infection. Gram stain of the infant's skin may show gram-positive rods. Cultures of the blood, gastric aspirate, placenta, and maternal vagina and lochia are usually positive. Affected infants should be immediately started on intravenous ampicillin and an aminoglycoside, pending culture results, since the mortality rate is as high as 50%.

Ecthyma Gangrenosum

Ecthyma gangrenosum, a cutaneous manifestation of *Pseudomonas aeruginosa* infection, usually associated with pseudomonas septicemia, is relatively rare in neonates, usually occurring in the setting of a severe predisposing illness, such as gastrointestinal surgery. Lesions usually present as pustules or areas of cellulitis that rapidly ulcerate. The perineum is the most common site of involvement. Diagnosis can be made with Gram stain and bacterial cultures. Cephalosporins such as ceftriaxone or ceftazidime and an aminoglycoside are used parenterally, pending results of bacterial sensitivity studies.

Congenital Candidiasis

In congenital candidiasis, a relatively rare condition, the entire cutaneous surface of the neonate is exposed to *Candida*, either by microscopic breaks in the amniotic membranes or after the membranes have ruptured.

Lesions are usually either present at birth or develop in the first week of life. The varied lesional morphologies include erythematous papules, diffuse erythema, with or without scale, and small vesicopustules. Virtually any part of the skin may be affected with sparse or extremely widespread lesions.

Potassium hydroxide preparation from affected skin demonstrates budding yeast and pseudohyphae. Examination of the placenta may also reveal yellow-white papules on the umbilical cord.

Topical therapy with an imidazole cream is usually adequate for infants weighing over 1500 g. Those weighing less than 1500 g have a much greater risk for developing systemic candidiasis and are usually treated with parenteral agents such as amphotericin B after cultures have been obtained.

Aspergillosis

Cutaneous aspergillosis may develop in very premature infants, presenting as erythematous papules that rapidly evolve into pustules and ulcerations. Potassium hydroxide preparations may demonstrate septate hyphae, but if deep or crusted ulcerations are present, then skin biopsy may be necessary for diagnosis.

Herpes Simplex Virus Infection

Subtle or inconspicuous skin lesions may herald the onset of infection, and failure to treat promptly can have disastrous consequences. The average age at diagnosis is 11 to 13 days, with a mean of 5 days of symptoms before diagnosis. Skin lesions are present at the onset of symptoms in only one third of cases but appear in more than 50% of affected infants at some point during the course of disease. Other presenting findings include irritability, lethargy, temperature instability, and poor feeding. A maternal history of genital herpes simplex infection is present in approximately one third of cases.

The most characteristic skin lesions are grouped vesicles on an erythematous base, but such grouping may be lacking in neonates. Vesicles quickly evolve into pustules, crusts, or erosions.

Intrauterine herpes simplex, a much rarer, more serious form of HSV infection, is usually due to a primary maternal herpes infection during pregnancy. Affected infants are often born prematurely and have microcephaly and chorioretinitis. The majority have skin lesions either at birth or within the first few days of life, including vesicles, widespread bullae resembling epidermolysis bullosa, and aplasia cutis–like lesions on the scalp.

Rapid diagnostic tests such as the Tzanck preparation and fluorescent or immunoperoxidase antigen detection are helpful in making a presumptive diagnosis while awaiting viral culture results.

The differential diagnosis of neonatal or intrauterine HSV infection depends on the specific clinical presentation. Vesicular lesions may resemble incontinentia pigmenti, congenital varicella, and acropustulosis of infancy. Dermatomal lesions may mimic herpes zoster. Pustular lesions may resemble congenital candidiasis, erythema toxicum neonatorum, congenital self-healing histiocytosis, and listeriosis. Widespread blistering may resemble epidermolysis bullosa, although a few vesicles or pustules are usually present.

Acyclovir, 30 mg/kg per day given intravenously, is the treatment of choice.

Varicella

Twenty-five percent of infants of mothers with primary varicella infection during the last 3 weeks of pregnancy develop neonatal varicella infection. Infection is most severe if maternal infection occurs within 7 days before to 2 days after delivery, owing to lack of protection with maternal antibodies. Onset usually occurs between 5 and 10 days of age, with widespread vesicles. The diagnosis is usually obvious because of the maternal history of chickenpox, but it can be confirmed with direct immunofluorescent stains and viral culture. Untreated neonatal varicella developing between 5 and 10 days of life has a mortality rate as high as 20% to 30%. Varicella-zoster immune globulin should be given to exposed neonates, and intravenous acyclovir should be used in affected infants.

Scabies

Scabies is rare in neonates but has been reported in infants as young as 3 to 4 weeks of age. Vesicles and pustules may be prominent findings, particularly on the insteps of the feet and hands.

Diagnosis can be confirmed with a scabies preparation. The treatment of choice in young infants is permethrin cream 5%, which should be applied to all areas of the skin including the scalp and face.

Transient Disorders

Erythema Toxicum Neonatorum

Erythema toxicum neonatorum, an entity of unknown etiology, is the most common cause of pustules in the neonate, occurring in 20% to 60% of term infants, but the condition is rare in premature infants and in those weighing less than 2500 g. Lesions usually develop between 24 and 48 hours after birth. Most affected infants are otherwise healthy.

Erythematous macules, wheals, papules, and pustules occur in various combinations. The papules and pustules are usually 1 to 2 mm in size, superimposed on an erythematous base varying in size up to several centimeters. Vesicles occasionally precede the development of pustules but are uncommon. A few to several dozen lesions may be present, typically involving the face, torso, and proximal extremities, although any area, except the palms and soles, may be involved. The rash waxes and wanes, with resolution of lesions except one or two over hours and the development of new ones in different areas.

The diagnosis is usually made clinically and can be confirmed if Wright's stain of the exudate from a pustule demonstrates eosinophils, a finding that is sensitive, but not specific, since other neonatal vesiculopustular diseases such as incontinentia pigmenti and acropustulosis of infancy may also have eosinophils. The condition is self-limited and resolves without treatment.

Transient Neonatal Pustular Melanosis

Transient neonatal pustular melanosis, a disease of unknown etiology, is a relatively common condition, occurring in 2% to 5% of term black neonates, and less than 1% of white neonates. Unlike erythema toxicum, lesions are virtually always present at birth. In the initial stage of the eruption, superficial, fragile pustules varying in size from 1 to 10 mm but usually 2 to 3 mm, are usually superimposed on uninflamed skin. Lesions may be located anywhere, including the palms and soles, but are most common on the forehead, behind the ears, under the chin, on fingers and toes, and on the torso. As lesions evolve, hyperpigmented macules with a collarette of scale are noted, eventually resolving into a melanotic macule that slowly fades over weeks to months.

The diagnosis is usually made clinically, based on the characteristic lesional morphology and the presence at birth. The Gram stain is negative. Wright's stain demonstrates keratinous debris with neutrophils and occasional eosinophils. No treatment is necessary.

Miliaria

Miliaria is a relatively common finding in neonates, especially in warm climates. Miliaria crystallina, occasionally present at birth, represents blockage of the sweat ducts, which occurs at the level of the stratum corneum, resulting in tiny flaccid vesicles. Most cases of miliaria rubra are postnatal and often occur following excessive warming (e.g., in an incubator or warmer), in areas of occlusive dressings, or with swaddling or overdressing in warm weather. The blockage is deeper, with a resultant inflammatory response and erythematous papules and pustules.

The most common locations are the forehead, upper trunk, and volar aspects of the upper arms. The diagnosis is usually made clinically. No specific treatment other than avoidance of excessive heat is necessary in most cases.

Sucking Blisters

Sucking blisters, which result from vigorous in utero sucking, occur in 1 in every 250 live births and are always present at birth. Characteristic bullae, which are occasionally bilateral, flaccid, and often hyperpigmented, are located on the radial forearm, wrist, hand, dorsal thumb, and index finger. If the bulla has ruptured, an oval or linear erosion may be present before healing. The diagnosis is usually made clinically because of the presence of the lesion(s) at birth and the characteristic location(s).

Neonatal Acne

Acne is a common condition in young infants. It is virtually never present at birth but often develops after 1 to 2 weeks. Although most neonatal acne is comedonal, pustules and papules may occur. The characteristic location and the presence of comedones make it easy to differentiate the condition from other causes of blisters and pustules. No treatment is necessary except in severe cases.

Skin Changes Due to Perinatal and Neonatal Trauma

Perinatal and neonatal trauma, either iatrogenic or spontaneous, may lead to erosive skin lesions. Rapidly healing superficial erosions in the diaper area in neonates have been ascribed to either perinatal trauma or the minor trauma of normal diaper care. The most common iatrogenically induced skin lesions in neonates are erosions secondary to fetal scalp electrodes.

Uncommon and Rare Causes

Acropustulosis of Infancy

Acropustulosis is an uncommon cause of blisters and pustules characterized by acral vesicles and pustules at birth or thereafter, most commonly in pigmented races. Crops of intensely pruritic vesicles and pustules develop on the palms and soles, dorsal hands and feet, and sides of the fingers and toes and occasionally are present on the wrists and ankles. Lesions are initially tense but begin to flatten and develop scales and postinflammatory hyperpigmentation, usually over 5 to 10 days. New crops occur every 2 to 4 weeks.

Scabies is the major alternative diagnosis; inquiry about any family members with rashes, as well as scraping of lesions, searching for mites, eggs, or feces, is imperative. Biopsy demonstrates an intraepidermal vesicle and neutrophils or eosinophils in the blister fluid.

The disease usually improves spontaneously within 1 to 2 years, but severe itching may require symptomatic treatment for active disease. Very potent topical corticosteroids and/or oral antihistamines may be helpful. Dapsone, 2 mg/kg per day, may be effective but should be used with caution, especially because of the risk of methemoglobinemia.

Transplacentally Transferred Dermatoses

Mothers with either herpes gestationis or pemphigus vulgaris may give birth to infants with a generalized blistering eruption as a result of transplacentally transferred IgG.

chapter 4

What Diseases Are Caused by Environmental Exposure or Physical Trauma?

BASIC PHOTOBIOLOGY, PHOTOTOXICITY, AND PHOTOALLERGY

(CM&S Chapter 83)

Basic Photobiology

Electromagnetic radiation emitted by the sun that reaches the surface of the earth is divided into ultraviolet (UV) light (290–400 nm), visible light (400–760 nm), and infrared radiation (>760 nm). UV radiation is responsible for the vast majority of photodermatoses; a notable exception is porphyrin-induced photodermatoses, which are associated with exposure to Soret band radiation (400–410 nm).

UV light, by convention, is further divided into UVC, UVB, and UVA. The shortest UV wavelength, UVC (200–290 nm), is absorbed in the atmosphere and is of no biologic significance. UVB (290–320 nm) is responsible for cutaneous erythema seen in sunburn reaction. UVA, which is further subdivided into UVA-II (320–340 nm) and UVA-I (340–400 nm), is the action spectrum of almost all of the photosensitivity reaction induced by exogenous agents.

The longer the wavelength, the higher is the dose required to produce a given biologic response. This is reflected in the determination of minimal erythema dose (MED), a commonly used photobiologic test to evaluate the dose of UV radiation needed to induce minimally perceptible erythema on the skin. For a fair-skinned white person, the MED of UVA (MED-A) is 20 J/cm^2, while the MED of UVB (MED-B) in the same individual would be 20 mJ/cm^2, a difference of one thousandfold!

Phototoxicity and Photoallergy

Definition

Phototoxicity and photoallergy are cutaneous photosensitivity disorders associated with concomitant exposure to a photosensitizer and the appropriate range and dose of electromagnetic radiation. The photosensitizer can be a topical or a systemic agent. The range of radiation eliciting the cutaneous response is referred to as the action spectrum, which usually, but not invariably, corresponds to the in vitro absorption spectrum of the photosensitizing agent.

Phototoxic agents and photoallergens are most often exogenous agents (Table 4–1), except for porphyrinogens. All individuals exposed to adequate doses of phototoxic agents and radiation develop cutaneous lesions (e.g., 8-methoxypsoralen and UVA [PUVA]). In contrast, photoallergy, a manifestation of a delayed hypersensitivity reaction, develops only in "allergic" individuals (e.g., musk ambrette and UVA).

Clinical Description

Patients with phototoxicity present with lesions on areas exposed to the sun, such as the forehead, tip of nose, dorsa of hands, and occasionally, the nails. There is sparing of areas covered by clothing and other sun-protected areas, such as the submental area, postauricular area, and inner aspects of arm and forearm. However, in severe cases (of both phototoxicity and photoallergy), extension to the covered areas can occur.

Lesions usually appear within hours of exposure and peak at 24 hours and are associated with burning and stinging. Phototoxic lesions range from erythematous patches to edematous plaques to vesicles and bullae. They resolve with desquamation and hyperpigmentation.

The lesions in photoallergy are usually acute to subacute erythematous papulovesicular eruptions involving the sun-exposed areas of skin, and the most common symptom is pruritus. Lichenoid

TABLE 4–1. Common Systemic Phototoxic Agents

TYPE OF AGENT	GENERIC NAME
Antibacterial	Nalidixic acid
	Quinolones
	Tetracyclines
	Sulfanilamide
Antihistaminic	Diphenhydramine
Antimalarial	Chloroquine
	Quinine
Antimitotic	Dacarbazine
	5-Fluorouracil
	Vinblastine
Antisporiatic	Psoralens
Cardiac	Amiodarone
	Nifedipine
	Quinidine
Diuretic	Furosemide
	Thiazides
Hypoglycemic	Sulfonylureas
Nonsteroidal anti-inflammatory	Piroxicam
Psychotropic	Phenothiazines
	Tricyclic antidepressants

lesions, consisting of violaceous or hyperpigmented flat-topped papules and plaques, may also be a manifestation of photosensitivity. Since this is a delayed hypersensitivity response, photoallergy occurs only in previously sensitized individuals, in whom the eruption typically begins 24 to 72 hours after exposure to a photoallergen and sunlight.

In the vast majority of patients, photosensitivity resolves on the discontinuation of the photosensitizers; however, evolution into chronic actinic dermatitis may occur.

Pathology

Phototoxicity is characterized by the presence of scattered necrotic keratinocytes, slight spongiosis, dermal edema, and infiltrates consisting of lymphocytes, macrophages, and neutrophils.

Histologic changes in photoallergy are similar to those in allergic contact dermatitis, including epidermal spongiosis, dermal edema, and dermal infiltrates consisting of lymphocytes, macrophages, and occasional eosinophils.

Diagnosis and Differential Diagnosis

Phototoxicity and photoallergy can be differentiated by history, clinical manifestations, histologic changes, and photobiologic features. Phototoxicity has no incubation period; therefore, lesions can develop even after the first exposure. These lesions appear within 24 hours after exposure to the phototoxic agent and radiation; the exception is furocoumarin-induced phototoxicity, which may appear 24 to 48 hours after exposure. The doses of the phototoxic agent and radiation needed are relatively high. In contrast, photoallergy has all the characteristics of a delayed hypersensitivity reaction. An incubation period is needed, which is usually 7 to 10 days for the first exposure and 1 to 2 days for subsequent ones. In photosensitized individuals, the doses of the photoallergen and radiation needed for development of lesions are small.

Treatment

Identification and discontinuation of a photosensitizer and avoidance of sun exposure are the most important aspects of the management of these patients. Acute flare can be treated with topical corticosteroids; compresses can be used for vesicular lesions. An oral antihistamine is helpful for the pruritus. Short courses of oral corticosteroid (60 to 80 mg of prednisone per day, tapered in 10 to 14 days) should be reserved for the most severe acute eruption.

PHOTODAMAGE AND PHOTOAGING

(CM&S Chapter 84)

Definition

Photodamage and photoaging are the deleterious effects on normal skin caused by the ultraviolet (UV) component of terrestrial sunlight. UVB radiation (290–320 nm) is responsible for most of the acute and chronic photodamage to normal skin. The depth of penetration of UV light depends on the wavelength. Most of the shorter but relatively more powerful UVB radiation is absorbed in the epidermis, and even in fair skin only 10% penetrates beyond this barrier. However, about 50% of incident UVA radiation (320–400 nm) traverses the epidermis and reaches a depth of 0.1 to 0.2 mm in the papillary dermis. Since the shorter wavelengths are more biologically active, most of the acute and chronic photodamage is to be expected in the epidermis and upper layers of the dermis.

The obvious clinical deleterious effects of terrestrial sunlight on normal skin include sunburn, tanning, altered immunity, photoaging, and photocarcinogenesis. In this chapter the discussion is limited to acute and chronic photodamage in normal skin.

The most clinically apparent symptom of acute photodamage is sunburn. It starts to appear within 2 to 6 hours, reaching its maximum intensity after 15 to 24 hours. The degree of erythema varies with wavelength. Of terrestrial sunlight, wavelengths around 290 nm (UVB) are the most erythemogenic. UVA is 1000 times less erythemogenic. The threshold dose required to produce just perceptible erythema is called the minimal erythema dose (MED) and is routinely used as a reflection of effectiveness in describing the UVB protection of sunscreens. The MED varies with skin type; and for fair-skinned whites, the MED is approximately 25 mJ/cm². Sunburn is histologically associated with typical changes, including the appearance of necrotic keratinocytes and depletion of Langerhans' cells.

In most fair-skinned individuals, erythema is followed by increased pigmentation or tanning. Tanning can be seen from 48 to 72 hours after UV light exposure and represents true melanogenesis. Tanning is a protective response to injury from UV radiation.

Photoaging changes are the deleterious alterations caused by chronic sun exposure that superimpose themselves on the normal chronologic aging process. The clinical changes are quite distinct from the normal intrinsic aged skin.

Clinical Description

Chronically sun-exposed skin has unique clinical and histologic features that are not observed in chronologically aged, sun-protected skin.

Clinical changes in old, sun-protected skin are relatively subtle and consist primarily of fine wrinkling, laxity, and a variety of benign neoplasms. In photoaged skin, the following changes are superimposed on the alterations of intrinsic aging: coarsening, deep wrinkling and furrowing, roughness or dryness, laxity and sagging, sallowness, mottled hyperpigmentation (composed of solar lentigines, flat seborrheic keratoses, and freckles) and hypopigmentation, telangiectasia (particularly obvious over the cheeks), purpura and stellate pseudoscars (both common over the forearms and the back of the hands), and ultimately a tendency to develop premalignant and malignant neoplasms (Table 4–2).

Photoaged skin may display different phenotypes of photodamage. Some individuals have relatively few wrinkles and extensive hyperpigmentation (common in Far East Asians), others have

TABLE 4-2. Intrinsic Aging and Photoaging: Clinical Differentiation

	INTRINSIC AGING	PHOTOAGING
Skin texture	Smooth	Rough, leathery
Wrinkling	Fine	Fine and coarse
Color	Pale	Yellowish
		Mottled hyperpigmentation
		Telangiectasia, purpura
Neoplasms	Benign	Premalignant and malignant

extensive fine and coarse wrinkling, and a third group displays numerous actinic keratoses. Relatively common neoplastic lesions on sun-exposed skin include basal cell carcinomas, actinic keratoses, keratoacanthomas, squamous cell carcinomas, solar lentigines, and lentigo maligna, which is a form of melanoma in situ. Elastotic degenerative changes, senile comedones, and infundibular follicular cysts may form in the periorbital region, a combination known as Favre-Racouchot disease.

Pathology

Wrinkles. Traditionally, wrinkles are considered largely the result of gravitational or conformational forces that are not preceded or even accompanied by permanent or recognizable changes under the microscope. The epidermis contributes to coarse wrinkles, by forming a groove of parallel surface and undersurface, above a corresponding groove of a locally thinned, solar elastosis, papillary dermis. The skin markings, however, can be recognized as depressions and grooves on the surface of the epidermis.

Solar Elastosis. Basophilic "degeneration" of the uppermost reticular dermis consists of the swelling, coarsening, and late homogenization of connective tissue fibers in upper dermis.

Actinic Vasculopathy. The superficial aspects of dermal arterioles facing the skin surface may appear thickened, with disorganized and fragmented internal elastic membrane, an intimal fibroplasia, and early microcalcification.

Tumors. The spectrum of neoplasia associated with photodamage is broad and includes tumors of most compartments of the skin. Epithelial tumors seen more frequently in aged skin, mainly as a result of photoaging, include solar (senile) lentigo, seborrheic keratosis and lichenoid keratosis, actinic keratosis, keratoacanthoma, basal cell carcinoma, squamous cell carcinoma, and squamous cell carcinoma in situ (Bowen's disease). Severely sun-damaged skin is often riddled by atypical intraepidermal proliferations of melanocytes, frank lentiginous malignant melanoma in situ (lentigo maligna), and malignant melanoma. Connective tissue neoplasms can be produced by actinic damage such as malignant fibrous histiocytoma or atypical fibroxanthoma.

Pigmentary Disorders. Sun damage-induced alterations of the pattern of melanin deposition include ephelides (freckles), solar (or senile) lentigines, and pigmented actinic keratoses.

Prevention

When discussing measures to protect normal skin against sunburn, caused more readily by UVB than by UVA wavelengths, one has to take into account the variation of UVB intensity in sunlight and the influence of season, time of the day, latitude, altitude, and reflectance of surfaces such as water. For instance, at noon in summer, skin can burn 100 times faster than at noon in winter. The UVB intensity is highest from 11 A.M. to 1 P.M. In Northern Europe, the UVB percentage is five times less than at the equator. Since UVB is absorbed by the atmosphere, it is easier for skin to burn at higher altitude. Although the progressive thinning of the ozone layer may in the future increase the UVB component of sunlight, it is not clear if this will be counterbalanced by pollution in the atmosphere.

Measures that can be taken to protect the skin from sunburn are making use of shade and avoiding direct sunlight, especially from 11 A.M. to 1 P.M., which constitutes nearly half of the daily UV light. Wearing appropriate clothing is often the simplest and most practical way of protecting the skin. The most important factor in determining the protective value of the clothing is the density of the weave. The more tightly woven a material, the better the protection. Adequate protection of the face can be obtained by wearing a hat with a brim of at least 7.5 cm. Another useful photoprotectant is window glass, which blocks virtually all UVB and at least half of all UVA energy. The use of sunscreens in the prevention of photodamage is discussed under Sunscreens, later in this chapter. Briefly, sunscreens containing only UVB filters or UVB sunscreens are usually sufficient to protect against sunburn. Para-aminobenzoic acid (PABA) and its esters are the most widely used UVB filters in the United States. In Europe, they are mostly replaced by camphor derivatives and cinnamates. These UVB sunscreens are assigned a sun protection factor (SPF). This SPF is defined as the ratio of the amount of sun exposure required to produce a minimal erythema reaction through a sunscreen product film to the amount of energy required to produce the same erythema without any sunscreen application. A sunscreen with an SPF of 15 will filter more than 92% of the UV radiation responsible for the erythema. In actual use, the SPF is often substantially lower, probably because the amount used is less than the recommended standard amount. Other factors are transpiration and exposure to water. Sunscreens should be applied in a sufficient amount (15 g for a thin person, 30 g for a well-built person), and may need to be reapplied after swimming or sports activities.

Not everyone has the same sensitivity to sunlight. Within a normal population six skin prototypes (type I to type VI) have been described, determined by the skin pigmentation or constitutional pigment content and facultative pigmentation or the capacity to become pigmented above the constitutional pigment content. The characteristics of the different skin types are given in Table 4–3. The higher the skin type, the better the endogenous protection offered by melanin against the harmful effects of sunlight.

In contrast to sunburn, the relationship between photoaging and chronic sun exposure is often not recognized, especially during childhood, when most of the lifetime exposure occurs. Effective protection of the face, neck, and hands during the first 18 years of

TABLE 4-3. Classification of Skin Types		
TYPE	**DESCRIPTION**	**THOSE AFFECTED**
I	Never tan, always burn	Whites (Celtic type)
II	Usually tan, always burn	Whites
III	Always tan, sometimes burn	Whites
IV	Always tan, rarely burn	Whites
V	Sunburn and tanning after extreme UV light exposure	Dark-skinned races (e.g., Latinos, Native Americans)
VI	Sunburn and tanning after extreme UV light exposure	Blacks

life may reduce photocarcinogenesis, and presumably also photoaging, by 80%.

Treatment

Treatment of Sunburn

There is no agent that will block the sunburn reaction; thus, treatment is limited to reducing the pain. Symptomatic treatment includes cooling the skin with cold compresses, shower, or bath. Topical anesthetics, calamine lotion, which cools the skin through evaporation, and high-potency corticosteroid creams may be of help.

Treatment of Photoaging

Medical Therapies

Although it is often claimed by cosmetic manufacturers that various creams and lotions (or even pills) containing natural and often exotic substances have the potential to decrease wrinkling, it has never been shown that their impact on human skin extends beyond a temporary emollient action.

The application of topical all-*trans*-retinoic acid or tretinoin (Retin-A) in concentrations ranging from 0.025% to 0.1% has been reported to partially reverse some of the structural alterations associated with photodamaged skin. A dose-dependent decrease of tactile roughness and of fine and, to a lesser degree, coarse wrinkling and dyspigmentation as well as an increase in pinkness of the skin has been documented after at least 6 to 10 months of treatment. Histologically, there is abundant evidence that topical retinoids produce certain dose-related changes in epidermal structure, such as an increase in epidermal and granular layer thickness, compaction of the stratum corneum, reduction of melanin content, elimination of epidermal dysplasia, and restoration of keratinocyte polarity. Restoration after dermal photodamage has not been easily demonstrable by light microscopy, but increased collagen type I synthesis after topical tretinoin therapy has been seen.

Topical tretinoin appears to be most effective when used at high concentrations (0.1% cream) for prolonged periods. Most patients experience a transient irritant dermatitis during the first weeks of therapy, especially with the higher concentrations or with solution- or gel-based topical agents. Intermittent night-time applications of a small amount of 0.025% tretinoin cream early on may allow a gradually increasing tolerance of the product.

Surgical Therapies

Surgical therapy for sun-damaged skin is designed to produce a controlled partial-thickness injury to the skin, removing varying amounts of epidermis and producing some effect on dermal collagen. A normal wound healing response after the injury produces (depending on the depth of injury) epidermal regeneration by migration from adnexal structures and replacement of new dermal connective tissue, resulting in a decrease of wrinkles, removal of actinic keratoses and lentigines, decrease in solar elastosis, and overall improvement of skin texture.

Three methods are currently available: Surgical planing or *dermabrasion*; *chemical peeling*, application of a caustic chemical to the skin; and *laserbrasion* or laser skin resurfacing, CO_2 laser vaporization of damaged skin. The dermabrasion technique does not differ significantly from that used in the treatment of acne scarring. Laser resurfacing uses pulsed and scanned CO_2 lasers to remove skin layer by layer in a highly controlled fashion.

Classification of Chemical Wounding Agents. Chemical peeling agents are commonly divided into superficial, medium, and deep (Table 4–4). These classifications are based on the depth of wound produced when these agents are applied to the skin. Analogous depths can be produced with dermabrasion and laser resurfacing.

Patient Selection and Indications. The key to a good result in chemical peeling for both patient and physician is successful patient selection. A systematic classification of patient photoaging types has been developed (Table 4–5). Patients are classified as photoaging types I through IV, depending on the degree of wrinkling seen in the skin, particularly the face. In general, the lighter peels and abrasions are appropriate for photoaging type I and II patients and the medium and deeper peels and abrasions for photoaging type III and IV patients.

The Fitzpatrick sun-reactive skin type (see Table 4–3) classification gives a very good indication of potential dyschromia after epidermal/papillary dermal injury, the likelihood of developing postinflammatory hyperpigmentation during the short-term postoperative period, and the potential for permanent hypopigmentation resulting from destruction of melanocytes. As a general rule, patients with Fitzpatrick skin types I through III will tolerate peeling or abrasion without significant risk of color change. Although both dermabrasion and peeling may be undertaken in Fitzpatrick skin types IV through VI, the risk of pigmentary change is certainly high enough that the patient should be warned that there is a significant risk of color change in the peeled skin.

Superficial Peels—α-Hydroxy Acids. α-Hydroxy acids are a group of nontoxic organic compounds that are derived from food products. In low, 5% to 10% concentrations, the α-hydroxy acids diminish corneocyte cohesion. In concentrations greater than 50%,

TABLE 4-4. Classification of Peeling Agents

TYPE	AGENT	DEPTH OF PEEL
Superficial	Trichloroacetic acid (10%–25%), Combes (Jessner's) solution: resorcinol, 14 g; salicylic acid, 14 g; lactic acid, 85%, 14 mL; ethanol 95%, 100 mL α-Hydroxy acids (glycolic acid) 30%–70%	0.06 mm (stratum granulosum to superficial papillary dermis)
Medium	Phenol 88% (full strength) Trichloroacetic acid (35%–50%) ($\pm$a second agent, e.g., carbon dioxide snow)	0.45 mm (papillary to upper reticular dermis)
Deep	Baker's phenol formula (open or taped): phenol 88% 3 mL; croton oil, 3 drops Septisol, 8 drops; distilled H_2O 2 mL	0.6 mm (midreticular dermis)

TABLE 4-5. Glogau Photoaging Classification

TYPE I—"NO WRINKLES"	TYPE II—"WRINKLES IN MOTION"
Early photoaging Mild pigmentary changes Minimal wrinkles Younger patient age: 20s or 30s Minimal or no makeup	Early to moderate photoaging Early senile lentigines Keratoses not visible Parallel smile lines beginning Patient age: late 30s or 40s Usually wears some makeup

TYPE III—"WRINKLES AT REST"	TYPE IV—"ONLY WRINKLES"
Advanced photoaging Obvious dyschromia, telangiectasia Visible keratoses Wrinkles at rest Patient age: 50s or older Always wears heavy makeup	Severe photoaging Yellow-gray color of skin Prior skin malignancies Wrinkled throughout Patient age: sixth or seventh decade Cannot wear makeup: "cakes and cracks"

they cause epidermolysis and have been used in the treatment of acne and actinic damage such as wrinkles and keratoses. Under the supervision of a physician, a 50% to 70% solution (usually glycolic acid) is applied and left intact for up to 7 minutes, at which time water or a 5% to 10% solution of sodium bicarbonate is applied to wash the face.

The degree of erythema and discomfort produced depends on the strength of the solution and the length of time the solution is permitted to stay in contact with the skin. Minimal erythema is followed by inconspicuous desquamation. Desquamation begins within a matter of 3 days and resembles a mild sunburn. Recovery is usually complete within 5 days. The α-hydroxy peel is often frequently repeated within days of recovery.

The effects of multiple α-hydroxy acid peels are not well established and may be restricted to mild improvement in those disorders residing chiefly in the epidermis, such as comedonal acne, superficial keratoses, and epidermal variants of melasma. The long-term clinical effects of these agents are minimal at best. Permanent changes in the mid-dermal architecture probably do not occur, and patients seeking correction of clinical problems related to such defects must turn to deeper peels for results.

Superficial Peels—Trichloroacetic Acid. One or two applications of 20% to 25% trichloroacetic acid solution to the entire face produce minimal and transient frost and mild erythema but do result in a temporary burning sensation. The skin turns brown in 24 to 48 hours, and on the third to fifth day exfoliation begins. Reepithelialization is complete within a week. Repeated applications may produce deeper wounding.

The indications for superficial peeling with trichloroacetic acid in the 20% to 25% range are similar to those of the α-hydroxy acids: superficial keratoses, mild epidermal dyschromia, and comedone formation. Repeated applications may effect some change in the upper papillary dermis, giving a smoothing effect of the very mildest wrinkles at most.

Medium-Depth Peels—Trichloroacetic Acid, Combined Agent Peels, and Phenol. Medium-depth peeling refers to application of a caustic agent or combination of agents that will routinely produce an injury that penetrates to the upper reticular dermis. These peels are usually performed as a single therapeutic procedure to treat actinic keratoses, dyschromia, and milder forms of wrinkles or scars.

Trichloroacetic acid 50% and plain phenol 88% provide the ''standard'' medium-depth peeling agents against which other techniques can be measured. A single application produces an even frost that appears within 10 to 15 seconds and fades to erythema within an hour. The pain from 50% trichloroacetic acid is intense but fades within several minutes, while that from 88% phenol fades more slowly but is not as intense as the pain produced by the deep-peeling formulas such as the Baker-Gordon formula. With medium-depth peels, edema and crusting appear within 48 to 72 hours and with frequent water rinses and antibiotic ointment concludes within 7 to 10 days. Erythema remains and fades slowly for 4 to 6 weeks, during which time protection from UV light is important to avoid irregular pigmentation.

To achieve deeper penetration using these agents, immediate reapplication produces a second or denser frost. This is useful where deeper wrinkles escape the effect of a single application frost (e.g., along the vermilion of the upper lip).

Thirty-five percent trichloroacetic acid may be combined with prior treatment of the skin with CO_2 ice or with prior application of Jessner's solution as a keratolytic before application of 35% trichloroacetic acid in an effort to achieve deeper penetration of the dermis.

Use of full-strength phenol 88% requires appropriate monitoring because of the potential systemic cardiotoxicity.

Deep Peels—Baker-Gordon Formula. The Baker and Gordon saponated phenol formula (Table 4–3) reliably produces an injury that goes to the midreticular dermis. The solution applied to the skin produces almost instant frosting, accompanied by a deep and persistent burning sensation that lasts for several hours. Anesthesia or light sedation combined with regional nerve block anesthesia of the face is commonly utilized to abate the discomfort of the procedure. Monitoring is required. The technique of application requires treating the face in segments to help to avoid acute phenol toxicity. The face is taped for 24 hours, followed by repeated showering or washing with copious amounts of water and application of a topical antibiotic ointment three to four times a day. Secondary infection is the inevitable and unhappy consequence of inadequate postoperative care.

Crusting should be held to a minimum with frequent soaks and topical antibiotic ointment. Ideally the skin should be reepithelialized within 12 days. The post-peel erythema that accompanies deep peeling takes weeks to months to fade.

Conditioning of Skin Before and After Peel. Topical application of tretinoin for a month before surgery appears to accelerate the healing of skin in both dermabrasion and chemical peeling. In patients with Fitzpatrick type II, III, and IV skin, addition of hydroquinone 2% to 6% applied daily appears to establish a more even color and is also widely used as a prepeel treatment. Both agents may be routinely restarted as soon as epithelialization is complete.

Complications of Chemical Peeling. The risks of chemical peeling correlate directly with the depth of injury produced during the peel. Superficial peels can produce transient postinflammatory pigmentation but may produce more serious sequelae if secondary factors, such as infection, are introduced. Medium-depth peels can cause pigment changes, persistent erythema, fine textural changes in the skin, and, rarely, true scarring. Deep peels have a range of potential effects including dyschromia, scarring, prolonged erythema, textural changes such as atrophy, milia, temperature sensitivity, flushing, cardiac arrhythmias (phenol), laryngeal edema, psychiatric decompensation, and secondary risks such as bacterial infection, activation of latent herpes simplex, unmet patient expectations, and litigation.

SUNSCREENS

(CM&S Chapter 85)

Sun Protective Factor (SPF)

The SPF is defined as the ratio of the time of UV radiation exposure necessary to produce the minimal erythema dose (MED) in sunscreen-protected skin to the time for unprotected skin.

Substantivity

Substantivity is the characteristic of a sunscreen that reflects how effectively the advertised degree of protection is maintained under adverse conditions including repeated water exposure or sweating. According to the FDA, a sunscreen is declared *water resistant* if it can maintain its original SPF after two 20-minute immersions. A sunscreen is *waterproof* if it retains its protective integrity after four 20-minute immersions.

Active Sunscreen Ingredients

Protectants Against UVB

Para-Aminobenzoic Acid. *Para*-aminobenzoic acid (PABA) one of the earliest sunscreens, is now used infrequently as a sunscreen for a variety of reasons. Its absorption peak at 296 nm is relatively far from UVB-induced erythema peak at 307 nm. It is poorly soluble in water and must be used as a 5% to 15% solution in alcohol. After application, PABA penetrates the stratum corneum effectively, where it is trapped and remains bonded through hydrogen bonding to epidermal proteins. This greatly enhances its substantivity but also increases the risk for contact or photocontact dermatitis. Sensitivity of this sort is seen in up to 4% of the population. PABA can cause a stinging sensation when applied and stains both cotton and synthetic fabrics. After photo-oxidation, this can leave a permanent yellow discoloration.

PABA Derivatives. PABA esters are created by addition of hydrocarbon groups to the PABA molecule. Many of these molecules are an improvement over PABA in that they are water soluble and do not penetrate the stratum corneum. The most widely used of the PABA derivatives is padimate O, or octyl dimethyl PABA. Its absorption peak is more desirable at 300 nm in nonpolar solvents, ranging to 316 nm in polar solvents. Padimate O is relatively stable chemically, making it less likely to stain clothing. Padimate A (amyldimethyl PABA) is similar to padimate O and is also used in combination with other agents. Neither ester stains clothing, although both can cause stinging when applied.

Salicylates. These agents are *ortho*-disubstituted aromatic compounds with a peak absorption around 300 nm. Two compounds of this type—octyl salicylate and homomenthyl salicylate (homosalate)—are approved in the United States. Although not very effective as sunscreens, they have the benefit of being exceptionally stable, essentially nonsensitizing, and water insoluble, leading to high substantivity. They are also useful as solubilizers of other poorly soluble sunscreen ingredients such as the benzophenones. They are used commonly in "PABA-free" products.

Cinnamates. 2-Ethylhexyl *p*-methoxycinnamate (absorption maximum 310 to 311 nm), 2-ethoxyethyl-*p*-methoxycinnamate (UV absorption maximum 310 nm), diethanolaminemethoxycinnamate, and octyl-methoxycinnamate are available in the United States. These are effective in blocking UVB but have poor substantivity and are generally found in combination with other agents. Cross-sensitization is seen with other cinnamates, found in balsam of Peru, balsam of Tolu, coca leaves, and cinnamon oil.

Protectants Against UVA

Benzophenones. Benzophenones are aromatic ketones that absorb predominantly in the UVA portion of the spectrum between 320 and 350 nm. Oxybenzone, for example, has an absorption maximum of 326 nm in polar solvents compared with 352 nm in nonpolar solvents. Benzophenone-3 (sulisobenzone) and dioxybenzone are also approved for the U.S. market. Oxybenzone is frequently implicated as the etiologic agent in photocontact allergy, although reactions have also been reported with dioxybenzone.

Dibenzoylmethanes. Dibenzoylmethanes are substituted diketones that undergo keto-enol tautomerism on absorption of UV radiation. The keto form of the dibenzoylmethanes has a UV absorption maximum of 260 nm, whereas the enol form absorbs above 345 nm. Parsol 1789 (avobenzone or 4-t-butyl-4′-methoxy-dibenzoylmethane) with an absorption maximum at 355 nm is the only agent of this class available in the United States. Although these compounds are capable of a high degree of UV absorption, they are unstable and can undergo photoisomerization to compounds that are not protective. Parsol 1789 has been shown to have a loss of protective power as high as 36% due to photodegradation. Even Parsol 1789 does not provide significant protection against UVA radiation close to 400 nm.

Physical Blockers

Physical blocking agents such as zinc oxide, titanium dioxide, iron oxide, kaolin, ichthammol (ichthyol), red veterinary petrolatum, talc ($MgSiO_2$), and calamine (FeO_2) are composed of particles of a size that scatter, reflect, or absorb solar radiation in the UV, visible, and even infrared ranges. Zinc oxide 20%, titanium dioxide 20%, and iron oxide 1% have been spectrophotometrically demonstrated to reduce transmittance in the UVA and visible ranges to a maximum of approximately 20%. However, a combination of the zinc and iron oxides together is synergistic, effectively reducing transmittance in the UVA and visible ranges as low as 1.5%.

Older physical blockers have the disadvantage that they are comedogenic, must be applied in a relatively thick layer, and melt in the sun, staining clothing. They are opaque and therefore visible, making them cosmetically undesirable for many individuals. These formulations have found a market in young persons who apply brightly pigmented products in limited areas. However, this does not provide protection for untreated areas. Because of their efficacy and broad-spectrum coverage, physical blockers are potentially important for persons with certain photosensitivity disorders.

Recently developed micronized preparations now available in the United States provide an excellent option within this class of sunscreens. Micronized physical blockers are suspensions of finely ground material such as titanium dioxide that reflect at wavelengths shorter than the visible spectrum. Since they do not reflect in the visible spectrum, they are invisible and thus more cosmetically acceptable. Micronized titanium dioxide is chemically stable and does not cause any photoallergic or contact dermatitis.

Micronized sunscreens are more effective at the shorter wavelengths. A major difficulty in formulating micronized sunscreens is in preventing agglomeration of the particles. If this occurs, the portion of the spectrum reflected will shift into the visible range and the product will have characteristics of traditional opaque physical blockers.

Vehicle

The choice of vehicle for a sunscreen is important for several reasons. First, the proper vehicle can enhance a sunscreen's substantivity or ability to remain on the skin and be effective. Second, the wrong vehicle can act as a skin irritant, can induce a phototoxic or photoallergic reaction, or may be comedogenic. Finally, a solvent may modify the sunscreening agent because of its polarity and thereby dramatically shift the absorption spectrum of the agent toward or away from the desired range.

Systemic Photoprotection

Over the years, a variety of systemic agents have been investigated as oral agents for sunscreening purposes. The appeal is three-fold. First, oral agents are convenient. Second, they provide coverage for the entire body. Finally, oral agents are likely to eliminate the concern over substantivity—so critical for topically applied products. Included in the list of these products are PABA, antihistamines, aspirin, indomethacin, retinol, ascorbic acid, α-tocopherols (e.g., vitamins A, C, and E), corticosteroids, psoralens, beta-carotene, and antimalarials. The last three are used in some individuals afflicted with certain photosensitivity dermatoses. Otherwise, these agents have been disappointing for persons with normal skin.

Sun Protective Clothing

Although UVB is partially reflected by clothing, lightweight fabrics typically worn in summertime do not even provide an SPF of 15. Once damp from sweat or water, the SPF of these fabrics decreases. The weave of a fabric does not appear to dramatically affect the flux of solar radiation through garments. In fact, it has been shown that a tightly woven cotton fabric provides less protection against UV exposure than a shirt of white knitted fabric. Sun-protective wear tested in vivo to provide an SPF of more than 30 regardless of color or moisture content is now commercially available. Such special fabrics are useful for some photosensitivity sufferers. However, practitioners should be aware that some fabrics provide protection through an applied coating that may lose efficacy over time.

Other Barriers

Window glass effectively blocks UV radiation below 320 nm, usually providing protection against UVB. Sufficiently tinted windows and the plastic interleaf found in vehicle windshields may filter most or all UVA. However, front and side window tinting to protect individuals with UVA-sensitive skin is illegal in many areas because of concerns about reduced driver visibility and limited ability for law enforcement officers to see what is happening inside a vehicle with closed windows.

Sun Protection

Sun Protection for Normal Skin

It is well established that chronic exposure to UVB leads to dele-terious effects on human skin, including photoaging and nonmela-noma skin cancers. Application of a UVB-blocking sunscreen does decrease the risk for development of nonmelanoma skin cancer. Patient sunscreen guidelines are described in Table 4–6.

Also, all individuals should be encouraged to stay indoors or seek shade during the peak hours of solar radiation flux from 10 A.M. to 2 P.M. A hat or a sun visor is useful. Patients with pale complexions should be reassured that ''fair'' skin is attractive. Those who insist on darker skin should use a self-tanning lotion containing dihydrox-yacetone (DHA). Tanning salons should be avoided since intense UVA exposure provides limited protection and induces photoaging and photoallergic reactions.

Individuals who spend a significant amount of time outdoors, particularly in areas of high solar flux, should be cautioned about the short- and long-term skin risks from UV exposure and should be advised as to how to properly protect themselves.

Finally, this information should be disseminated to children at an early age. Childhood is typically the time of life when maximal sun exposure occurs. Childhood sunburns are implicated in increasing risk for malignant melanoma and nonmelanoma skin cancer and thus should be assiduously avoided.

Sun Protection for Photosensitive Skin

A variety of skin disorders occur as a result of, or can be exacer-bated by, exposure to solar radiation. In general, persons with pho-tosensitivity disorders (including polymorphous light eruption (290–365 nm), porphyria (400–410 nm), solar urticaria (290–515 nm), chronic actinic dermatitis (290–360 nm), persistent light reac-tion (290–400 nm), lupus erythematosus (290–340 nm), xeroderma pigmentosum (290–340 nm), vitiligo, and albinism should be dis-couraged from sunlight exposure. If this is impractical or unaccept-able, it is advisable to phototest them and then provide protection against the appropriate action spectrum using a chemical blocker, physical blocker, or sun protective clothing as necessary.

In general, persons with photosensitivity dermatitis also tend to be supersensitive to chemicals. Many ultrahigh SPF sunscreens are available in the United States. These products use high concentra-tions of several agents together and, particularly for those with preexisting photosensitivity dermatitis, may cause chemical irrita-tion and sensitization.

THE IDIOPATHIC PHOTODERMATOSES

(CM&S Chapter 86)

Photosensitive disorders are primarily divided into idopathic photodermatoses, which without light exposure do not develop, and into photoaggravated dermatoses, which are provoked (occasion-ally) by light exposure but that most often develop in its absence.

TABLE 4–6. Skin Types and Recommended Sunscreen Protective Factors

TYPE	CHARACTERISTIC	EXAMPLES	SUGGESTED SPF	
			Routine Day	Outdoor Activity
I	Always burns easily, never tans	Celtic or Irish extraction; often with blue eyes, red hair, and freckles	15	25–30 (waterproof)
II	Burns easily, tans slightly	"Fair-skinned" individuals; often have blond hair	12–15	25–30 (waterproof)
III	Sometimes burns, then tans gradually and moderately	Most whites	8–10	15 (waterproof)
IV	Burns minimally, always tans well	Latinos and Asians	6–8	15 (waterproof)
V	Burns rarely, tans deeply	Middle Easterners, Indians	6–8	15 (waterproof)
VI	Almost never burns, deeply pigmented	Blacks	6–8	15 (waterproof)

When the clinician is presented with a patient who has a problem on exposed cutaneous sites yet is uncertain of the role of sunlight, careful clinical examination is invaluable. Sparing of the relatively shaded sites, hair-bearing scalp, and retroauricular, infranasal, submental, and periorbital areas, combined with involvement of those maximally exposed sites, which include the ''V'' of the neck, dorsum of the hand, and rim and lobe of the ear, all point toward photosensitivity. Specific examinàtion for clothing-protected cutoff lines at collar and cuffs is also of particular value.

Behavioral avoidance of responsible wavelengths involves advice appropriate for the degree to which an individual is affected. Baseline management includes avoiding midday exposure and wearing protective clothing, including hats, gloves, and thick cotton, long-sleeved shirts and slacks. To those less affected, controlled gradual sunlight exposure allowing the build-up of natural pigment and, possibly, adaptation of the cutaneous immune system allows near-normal exposure during summer months. In those severely affected, artificial phototherapy hardening with narrow or broadband ultraviolet light B (UVB) or psoralens and UVA (PUVA) or immune suppression with azathioprine or cyclosporine may be considered.

Polymorphic Light Eruption

Definition and Clinical Description

Polymorphic (polymorphous) light eruption is most likely a group of photosensitive diseases rather than a single disease entity that can be induced by UVB, UVB and UVA, or UVA alone. This condition is the most common photodermatosis seen, with a worldwide prevalence in the range of 10% to 20%. Females seem particularly prone to be affected by this condition, which has a familial tendency of up to 50%. The majority of cases present in the first three decades of life.

A wide range of morphology is encountered, although individual patients consistently describe the same type of presentation. Most patients report pruritic erythematous papules in sunlight-exposed sites during the sunshine season. Others may experience vesicles, plaques, and hemorrhagic and erythema multiforme – like presentations.

In the majority, the condition is confined to spring and summer. Some patients describe hardening, which is an increased tolerance following UV summer exposure. The amount of sunlight required to induce polymorphic light eruption depends on the time of day, month of year, and such factors as sun barrier use and type of clothing worn. Although there are those who react within minutes of exposure, others require a gap of up to 2 to 3 days before emergence of the condition. With avoidance of sunlight, healing without scarring is complete within 1 to 2 weeks.

A characteristic clinical feature in some patients is the relative sparing of those normally exposed sites (face and hands), which is usually explained on the basis of natural desensitization. The severity of polymorphic light eruption varies greatly from one patient to another. Some have one or two episodes per year when exposed to large amounts of sunlight, while others are profoundly sensitive, requiring only minutes of exposure during the winter months.

Pathology

The common histopathologic denominator in lesions of polymorphic light eruption is superficial (and in late lesions, deep) perivascular lymphocytic infiltrates. Edema of the papillary dermis is seen in papular lesions.

Diagnosis and Differential Diagnosis

A range of conditions must be considered in the differential diagnosis, including lupus erythematosus, actinic prurigo, solar urticaria, and hydroa vacciniforme. Serology should be performed in any patient with polymorphic light eruption to rule out lupus erythematosus.

Treatment

With a wide range in severity, the therapy of polymorphic light eruption varies accordingly. Changes in behavior and clothing and application of a broad-spectrum sunscreen are adequate for the majority of patients. Systemic treatment with corticosteroids has been used with relative success to prevent severe polymorphic light eruption. Recently, however, a more physiologic approach has been taken through desensitization programs using broad- or narrow-(Philips TL-01) spectrum UVB or PUVA to artificially induce hardening.

Actinic Prurigo

Definition and Clinical Description

Actinic prurigo is a perennial photoeruption that affects all sun-exposed sites and is particularly common in Native American tribes. Actinic prurigo frequently has a positive family history. It is most active during the sunshine months and often has no apparent relationship to sunlight in the mind of the patient. The eruption initially appears as red and indurated papules and may progress to small blisters. Over days or weeks, a chronic papulonodular state develops that heals with scarring. All exposed sites are affected, and marked sparing of some exposed sites as seen in polymorphic light eruption is unusual. Covered sites may also be involved, although to a lesser extent than light-exposed areas. Lower lip cheilitis is particularly common in North American patients with actinic prurigo.

Diagnosis and Differential Diagnosis

When the presentation is classic, the diagnosis is straightforward. However, mild forms may be difficult to distinguish from early-onset polymorphic light eruption. Phototesting reveals the majority to have abnormal responses to UVB, UVA, or visible wavelengths.

Treatment

The management of actinic prurigo is difficult. Avoidance of sunlight, supplemental clothing, and a broad-spectrum sun barrier preparation may be of assistance. When the eruption arises, sedative antihistamine use and topical steroids may help resolution. In some patients, desensitization using either UVB or, in adults, PUVA can help provide summertime protection. If there is no response to such measures, thalidomide has been used successfully, although great care is required to monitor toxic effects, including motor neuropathy. Spontaneous resolution occurs most commonly in early adult life.

Idiopathic Solar Urticaria

Definition and Clinical Description

Solar urticaria is an uncommon, although not rare, condition characterized by a whealing response that follows ultraviolet or visible skin irradiation. Often described by patients as arising with sudden onset, typically the history is of a pruritic urticaria emerging within half an hour of sunlight exposure. Sharp clothing cut-off features and relative sparing of covered sites are the rule. Solar urticaria settles within 1 to 2 hours, although a persistent erythema may be present for 1 to 2 days.

Diagnosis and Differential Diagnosis

Diagnostic phototesting is of great value. UVB, UVA, and visible waveband involvement are seen either singly or in combination.

Treatment

Treatment is proportional to disease severity. For mild cases, appropriate sun barrier use and sunlight avoidance may suffice. If not, nonsedative antihistamine use is likely to produce total or partial benefit in up to 70% of cases of solar urticaria. A combination of H_1 and H_2 blockade may provide further benefit. Artificial induction of hardening may be achieved with careful use of PUVA or UVB therapy.

Photodermatoses Related to DNA Abnormalities

Xeroderma Pigmentosum

See Chapter 168 in CM&S and Chapter 11 in this text.

Photoaggravated Disorders

Under certain circumstances, a range of diseases of diverse etiology may be aggravated by sunlight in patients who otherwise seem to react normally (Table 4–7).

TABLE 4-7. Photoaggravated Dermatoses

Atopic dermatitis
Photosensitive psoriasis
Lupus erythematosus
Lichen planus
Dermatomyositis
Herpes simplex
Cutaneous lymphocytoma and Jessner's lymphocytic infiltrate
Erythema multiforme
Acne vulgaris
Pemphigus
Chronic benign familial pemphigus (Hailey-Hailey disease)
Bullous pemphigoid
Darier's disease
Transient acantholytic dermatosis
Disseminated superficial actinic porokeratosis
Pellagra

CHRONIC ACTINIC DERMATITIS

(CM&S Chapter 87)

Definition

Chronic actinic dermatitis is synonymous with the photosensitivity dermatitis and actinic reticuloid syndrome. These unifying terms are used interchangeably and encompass the conditions previously known as photosensitive eczema, photosensitivity dermatitis, actinic reticuloid, and persistent light reactivity, now thought to be different variants of the one disease process. Chronic actinic dermatitis is characterized by persistent eczema or pseudolymphomatous changes induced by ultraviolet (UV) radiation exposure.

Clinical Description

Chronic actinic dermatitis is an uncommon disorder that occurs predominantly in middle-aged to elderly individuals, of which 80 to 90% are male. It is extremely rare in subjects younger than the age of 50 years. The eruption predominantly affects light-exposed sites, notably the face, scalp, back and sides of neck, upper chest, and dorsa of hands and forearms, classically sparing the upper eyelids, submental area, the skin protected by the earlobes, and the skin creases and finger webs. However, in more severely affected individuals, it may spread to light-protected sites. With long-standing disease, eyebrow and scalp hair may become stubbly and prematurely gray and areas of hyperpigmentation or hypopigmentation may develop. Onset of the eruption following UV radiation exposure may be insidious, delayed by hours to days. Although generally most severe between spring and early autumn, the condition may persist into winter. Thus, both the patient and the unwary physician may not recognize the relationship to UV light exposure. Contact and photocontact dermatitis occur in association with chronic actinic dermatitis in 75% of cases, and a history of endogenous eczema is obtained in up to about 15% of patients.

Pathology

The histologic changes vary with the severity of the disease. At the mild end of the spectrum the changes are of a subacute or chronic spongiotic dermatitis, whereas in the pseudolymphomatous or actinic reticuloid response the density and depth of the infiltrate are greater and atypical Sézary-like lymphocytes are also seen, sometimes clustering in the epidermis to resemble Pautrier microabscesses. T lymphocyte infiltrates are CD8-positive predominant, in contrast to mycosis fungoides, in which CD4-positive cells predominate.

Diagnosis and Differential Diagnosis

The diagnosis of chronic actinic dermatitis is made on the following criteria:

1. Clinical features of eczema with or without pseudolymphomatous change, predominantly but not necessarily exclusively on light-exposed sites. Urine, stool, and blood porphyrins are normal, and circulating antinuclear, anti-SSA (Ro), and anti-SSB (La) antibodies are absent.
2. Minimal erythema responses at 24 hours of unaffected skin to monochromatic or broadband irradiation are reduced. Lesions characteristic of the disease may also thereby be induced. The abnormal response occurs to UVB in all patients, to UVA also in 90%, and to visible wavelengths as well in 10%.
3. Histopathology, if performed, of nonspecific eczema with pseudolymphomatous change in the more severe variants.

Chronic actinic dermatitis may be clinically indistinguishable from allergic contact dermatitis, particularly to airborne allergens, from oral drug photosensitivity, with thiazides and quinine being most commonly implicated, and from photoallergic contact dermatitis to sunscreens. Light-exacerbated atopic and seborrheic dermatitis and cutaneous T-cell lymphoma must be also differentiated.

Treatment

Reports of cutaneous lymphoma arising in patients with chronic actinic dermatitis have not been substantiated. Chronic actinic dermatitis is nonetheless a disabling and persistent disease, and spontaneous remission occurs only occasionally. Good disease control may thereby be achieved in the majority of cases by avoiding exposure to causative UV wavelengths, avoiding contact and photocontact allergens and with systemic treatment with either azathioprine up to 150 mg/day, cyclosporine 3 to 5 mg/kg/day, or PUVA.

PSYCHOCUTANEOUS DISORDERS

(CM&S Chapter 89)

Psychological factors often play an important role in the diagnosis and management of patients who present with a chief complaint pertaining to their skin. The interaction between the mind and the skin may take many different forms:

1. Many chronic, recurrent, inflammatory skin diseases, such as eczema, psoriasis, and acne, are exacerbated by emotional stress.

2. In many cutaneous disorders, such as vitiligo or alopecia areata, the psychosocial impact of disfigurement is the main morbidity.

3. Dermatologists see patients who have no real cutaneous disorder but who present with self-induced lesions; patients have delusions of parasitosis, trichotillomania, neurotic excoriations, or factitial dermatitis.

4. Patients present with only cutaneous sensory complaints, such as chronic idiopathic pruritus, formication, burning, and stinging, without diagnosable underlying medical, dermatologic, or psychiatric disorders.

5. Certain psychopharmacologic agents, such as amitriptyline (Elavil) and doxepin (Sinequan) are widely used to treat purely dermatologic conditions such as post-herpetic neuralgia, urticaria, and pruritus.

6. Psychosocial factors such as improvement in quality of life may eventually become the gold standard against which the value of dermatologic therapeutics may be measured, because of the fact that, for most skin disorders, one cannot use the usual measures of outcome such as survival, physical disability, or quantitative improvement in laboratory tests to demonstrate the value of an intervention by a dermatologist.

Delusions of Parasitosis

Definition

In delusions of parasitosis, a monosymptomatic hypochondriacal psychosis in which the patient presents with an encapsulated somatic delusion, patients mistakenly believe that they are infested by insects, worms, or other organisms.

Clinical Description

Most patients complain of formication (i.e., crawling, biting, and stinging sensations). These patients characteristically bring in various specimens of alleged parasites in small containers. The self-induced skin lesions may frequently resemble moon craters because these patients gouge their skin deeply to try to extricate the ''parasites.''

Diagnosis and Differential Diagnosis

Monosymptomatic hypochondriacal psychosis can be distinguished from schizophrenia by its circumscribed psychopathology. Patients with monosymptomatic hypochondriacal psychosis are usually normal in their psychosocial functions with the exception of their somatic delusion. Recreational drugs such as amphetamine and cocaine also induce formication. Delusions of parasitosis can also be encountered as one aspect of an underlying psychiatric condition such as organic brain syndrome, depression, or schizophrenia.

Treatment

The mainstay of therapy for delusions of parasitosis due to mono-symptomatic hypochondriacal psychosis is pimozide (Orap), an antipsychotic medication with a side effect profile similar to other high-potency antipsychotic agents, such as haloperidol (Haldol). Treatment can be started with as small a daily dose as 1 mg orally and increased by 1 mg (i.e., half a tablet) every 5 to 7 days as tolerated, up to 4 to 6 mg orally per day. The main side effect of pimozide in this type of usage is pseudoparkinsonian (extrapyramidal) side effects, such as stiffness and restlessness. These can be controlled with diphenhydramine (Benadryl), 25 mg orally three times a day as needed or benztropine mesylate (Cogentin), 1 to 2 mg orally four times a day as needed. In this type of low-dose usage tardive dyskinesia is unlikely to be a problem. Once the patient shows a response to pimozide, the dosage should be maintained at a steady therapeutic level for 1 to 2 months before it is gradually tapered and eventually discontinued.

Trichotillomania

Definition

Trichotillomania refers to a condition in which the patient pulls out his or her own hair.

Clinical Description

Trichotillomania, which can be seen in any age group, is characterized by the presence of a relatively well-circumscribed patch of incomplete alopecia where a few to many remaining hairs of varying lengths are seen. This condition often involves the frontal or vertex area of the scalp but occasionally can involve the scalp diffusely. Frequently, the condition also involves the eyebrows and eyelashes and, in rare occasions, pubic hair. The hairs are either plucked out or twisted until the hair shaft breaks. Because these findings can be superimposed on those of inflammatory alopecias, such as alopecia areata, a diagnosis of trichotillomania should also be based on the absence of evidence of another cause of alopecia.

Diagnosis and Differential Diagnosis

The most common psychopathology that leads to trichotillomania is obsessive-compulsive disorder; the patient obsesses about pulling hair and has a compulsion to pull out hair. Patients with obsessive-compulsive disorder characteristically have good insight into the destructive and irrational nature of their problem. Even so, many of these patients cannot refrain from pulling out their hair.

Treatment

Anti–obsessive-compulsive medications such as clomipramine (Anafranil) or fluoxetine (Prozac) are used widely to treat trichotillomania.

Clomipramine is a tricyclic antidepressant that inhibits the reuptake of serotonin. The starting dose is 25 mg orally at bedtime. The dose is gradually increased every 5 to 7 days until the desired therapeutic response is obtained (usually at 75 to 100 mg per day), which may not become evident until after several weeks of treatment. In addition to the usual side effects such as sedation, anticholinergic effects, and weight gain, clomipramine also causes nausea, seizures, and sexual dysfunction more frequently than other tricyclic antidepressants.

Fluoxetine (Prozac) is a nontricyclic antidepressant with more specific serotonin reuptake blocking activity than clomipramine. Fluoxetine is available in 20-mg capsules, and the usual dose for treating depression is 20 to 40 mg per day; for obsessive-compulsive disorder it is 20 to 60 mg per day. Side effects common to tricyclic antidepressants are not likely to be encountered. Side effects such as diarrhea, agitation, anxiety, and rash may occur.

Behavioral therapy or psychotherapy may enhance the success rate of the overall treatment plan. Without patient motivation and vigilance, the use of psychopharmacologic medication alone is unlikely to extinguish a long-standing compulsive tendency.

Neurotic Excoriations

Definition

Neurotic excoriation is a term used to describe psychogenic excoriations of the skin. In contrast to patients with factitial dermatitis in which a more elaborate means such as the use of pointed objects, acid, or lighted cigarette butts are employed to induce skin lesions, neurotic excoriations are induced with only the use of the fingernails.

Clinical Description

Patients with neurotic excoriations usually present with multiple excoriations in easily reachable areas of the body. The lesions are often located on the face, extensor aspects of the extremities, and reachable areas of the back. Often, there is sparing of the upper, lateral back in a symmetrical configuration resembling the shape of butterfly wings corresponding to the areas of the back that are not reachable.

Diagnosis and Differential Diagnosis

The psychopathologies usually encountered in patients with neurotic excoriations are depression, anxiety, and obsessive-compulsive disorder. In contrast, patients with factitial dermatitis present with different, and in some ways more serious, psychopathologies, such as psychosis or borderline personality disorder.

Treatment

The treatment of choice for the depressed ''neurotic excoriator'' is the tricyclic antidepressant doxepin (Sinequan), a very effective antipruritic. Doxepin is started at a dose of 25 mg, and increased by 25-mg increments every 5 to 7 days until the patient reaches the antidepressant dosage range of 100 to 300 mg. To avoid sedation, the drug can be taken as a once-a-day dose at bedtime.

A possible alternative to doxepin is desipramine (Nopramin, Pertofrane) used in a dose of 100 to 150 mg per day. Even though desipramine is much less sedating and also has less anticholinergic and cardiac side effects, it also has very little antihistaminic effect and, therefore, the antipruritic effect of doxepin is lost.

If the psychopathology of a neurotic excoriator is "stress" or "emotional tension," the use of antianxiety agents should be considered. Alprazolam, a very effective, quick-acting benzodiazepine, is started at a dose of 0.125 mg three or four times per day as needed. For long-term use, there is a possibility of addiction; therefore, it is advisable to limit alprazolam use to 2 to 3 weeks. If the patient requires long-term treatment with an antianxiety agent, the nonaddicting, nonsedating anti-anxiety agent buspirone (BuSpar) may be preferred, because it has no withdrawal symptoms and does not react with alcohol or benzodiazepines.

Factitial Dermatitis

Definition

In factitial dermatitis, the patient uses elaborate means such as sharp objects, caustic chemicals, or the injection of toxic substances to induce skin lesions.

Clinical Description

Because of the bizarre clinical appearance of factitial dermatitis characterized by the presence of certain features such as sharp edges and unnatural configurations in an easily accessible area, there is usually no difficulty distinguishing these lesions from those of real skin diseases or from neurotic excoriations. The exact appearance of the lesions depends on the particular method the patient uses to produce the lesion.

Diagnosis and Differential Diagnosis

Certain types of underlying psychopathologies such as malingering, psychosis, and personality disorders characterized by self-destructive behavior (e.g., borderline personality disorder) are often encountered among patients with factitial dermatitis.

Treatment

Because of the difficulty in managing patients with these more intractable underlying psychopathologies, these patients should be managed by mental health care professionals even though patients with factitial dermatitis frequently resist such a referral.

INSECT BITES AND STINGS

(CM&S Chapter 91)

Insect Bites

Definition

An insect bite consists of the damage done by the bite of an insect and the human response to that bite. Bites are often the result of a blood meal that is necessary for a particular insect to complete its life cycle. For this reason, some bites are hemorrhagic. As part of the biting process, some tearing of flesh may be noted, especially among the more vicious biting insects. Some insects are able to inject material from their saliva and thus transmit disease while they bite. Others defecate as they feed and act as disease vectors because the feces contain the infecting organism.

Clinical Description

There are four different patterns of insect bites. Erythematous papules, sometimes with central puncta, are the hallmark of insect bites. They may be individual, linear, or grouped, and their distribution may help to elucidate the causative agent. A second pattern is the presence of vesicles, often clustered together, 2 to 3 cm apart. Giant urticaria with wheals up to 20 cm across is a third pattern. Hemorrhagic nodular or bullous lesions may be present, especially if the insect is a vicious biter. There may be symptoms of itching or pain at the time of the bite, although some insects seem able to produce an anesthetic bite.

Pathology

Insect bites are characterized histopathologically by a superficial and deep infiltrate of lymphocytes and eosinophils, both around vessels and interstitially. In vesicular reactions to bites, spongiotic microvesicles are present, often accompanied by papillary dermal edema and sometimes by small subepidermal vesicles.

Chronic or long-standing lesions can show dense infiltrates of lymphocytes, including immunoblasts and plasma cells. This picture sometimes simulates lymphoma or granulomatous dermatitis and can be produced by retained insect parts.

Differential Diagnosis

The diagnosis of insect bites is usually straightforward. There can be confusion with "itchy red bump disease," sometimes termed *prurigo papularis.*

Treatment

The treatment of insect bites includes local use of cool compresses, evaporating shake lotions such as calamine lotion, and topical steroids. Antihistamines are often helpful. Systemic steroids are reserved for severe or recalcitrant disease.

In addition to the treatment of the individual, consideration should be given to the eradication of breeding sites for the insects involved. Insect repellants such as Deet (*N,N*-diethyl-m-toluamide) are useful. Variations on the chemical structure has produced newer repellants, such as *N,N*-diethylphenylacetamide. A more effective substance may be Elimite, a synthetic chlorinated pyrethrum sold as a 5% lotion for use on scabies. It is also sold as a 0.5% solution as Permanone or Coulston's Permethrin Tick Repellent and is used on clothing as well as topically on individuals who are at risk for insect bites. Permethrin is actually a toxicant and not a repellant. It resists washing, and it remains active on the skin for several days and on clothing for 1 month or longer.

Insect Stings

Definition

A sting involves the insertion of a stinger, usually from the abdomen of the insect, into the skin. The stinger may or may not remain in the skin. If it does, it results in the death of the insect. Honeybees, wasps, and yellow jackets are the most common stinging insects.

Clinical Description

Severe reactions may occur when many stings inject large amounts of toxin. The most serious reaction is anaphylaxis in which the sting produces swelling, collapse, and death from respiratory failure.

Pathology

In the usual uncomplicated sting, there is dermal edema and an infiltrate of lymphocytes and neutrophils. Later, the lymphocytes increase as the edema subsides, and then eosinophils, plasma cells, and histiocytes appear later.

Diagnosis and Differential Diagnosis

Diagnosis is usually by history. The erythematous papule may resemble other bites, but if a honeybee is involved, a stinger may remain in place.

Treatment

In instances of small local reactions, cool compresses, elevation, or antihistamines are sufficient. Toxic reactions may require specific treatments. Generally, allergic individuals should be provided with a self-injectable supply of 1:1000 solution of epinephrine. The subcutaneous injection of epinephrine may be lifesaving. Other treatment for shock, such as support of blood pressure and antishock trousers, may be needed.

Fire Ant Stings

Definition

Fire ants were imported into the southeastern United States in the 1920s and 1930s. They have spread gradually over an enlarging area of the Southeast. They build mounds in the ground and are capable of producing multiple stings.

Clinical Description

Fire ant stings are unusual because of the pustular reaction. The ant bites an area of skin and holds on with its powerful mandible. It then bends around and stings with the stinger in its abdomen. The stinger may penetrate several times around a central bite as the ant rotates, causing a classic central erythematous bite and a series of peripheral pustules. These require several days to disappear.

Pathology

An intraepidermal pustule, consisting mostly of neutrophils lymphocytes, and eosinophils forms. The dermis contains a dense mixed cellular infiltrate.

Differential Diagnosis

The differential diagnosis of a fire ant sting includes pyoderma or pustular psoriasis.

Treatment

There is no effective treatment for these stings. Local cool compresses and antihistamines may be helpful, but avoidance would seem to be the best therapy. Secondary infection is common, so that the use of antibiotics may be helpful.

Caterpillar Dermatitis

Definition and Clinical Description

Disease is produced when the caterpillar comes in contact with the skin. This may be intentional, as when children play with caterpillars, or unintentional, as in occupational or accidental contact.

Most caterpillar contacts present as an erythematous macule that evolves into a wheal. The lesion may occur immediately or may be delayed 2 to 10 hours. Wheals may evolve into papulovesicles that persist for several days.

Pathology

The histopathology of caterpillar dermatitis is nonspecific with spongiosis, vacuolar change, edema of the papillary dermis, and a mixed lymphohistiocytic infiltrate.

Pathogenesis and Etiology

Some of the setae or hollow hairs normally found on the backs of caterpillars are modified to become poisonous hairs when in contact with poison glands. They are thought to produce most of the reactions by injecting toxins into the skin.

Differential Diagnosis

Other bites, from mites, fleas, or flying insects, are in the differential diagnosis.

Treatment

Treatment is mostly symptomatic. Topical steroids and antihistamines are useful. Systemic steroids and narcotics have been used to treat pain of caterpillar dermatitis.

Arachnid Bites

Definition

Bites by spiders, otherwise known as arachnidism, seem to hold a particular terror for humans. All spiders bite and have toxins. Few are powerful enough to penetrate human skin. In the United States, only the brown recluse spider and the black widow are significant causes of disease.

In addition to bites, spiders can produce urticaria and itching. Usually, this is due to urticating hairs, particularly the abdominal hairs on tarantulas. With the exception of these urticating hairs, tarantulas, despite their large size and menacing appearance, do not cause significant skin disease.

Brown Recluse Spider Bites (Loxoscelism)

In the United States, *Loxosceles reclusa* is the most common of these spiders. The spider has a characteristic violin-like pattern on the back of the thorax, giving rise to the name "fiddle-backed spider."

Clinical Description

The initial spider bite is followed by burning pain. Erythema appears within a short time, followed by a central zone of ischemia. Edema occurs over the whole area, and, after about 48 hours, the central area becomes dusky and then necrotic. The total area of necrosis may not be evident until the seventh day. An eschar forms and is shed painlessly after about 3 weeks.

Some patients with necrotic loxoscelism may develop systemic symptoms: headache, fever, dizziness, nausea, vomiting, diarrhea, sweating, and nervousness. A generalized morbilliform or scarlatiniform eruption may occur. Severe systemic symptoms may occur, including hypotension, shock, hemolysis, jaundice, disseminated intravascular coagulation, renal failure, convulsions, pulmonary edema, and death.

Pathology

Brown recluse spider bites are characterized histologically by severe edema, dermoepidermal separation, and diffuse and perivascular neutrophilic and eosinophilic infiltrates. Panniculitis and scarring can be seen in resolving lesions.

Differential Diagnosis

The pain and spreading erythema with central ischemia and necrosis — the "red, white, and blue sign" — is quite characteristic. Differential diagnosis includes the bites of other arthropods. The severe necrotic response may mimic pyoderma gangrenosum.

Treatment

Prednisone, 80 to 100 mg daily, may prevent the area of necrosis from spreading. Systemic symptoms similarly benefit from early steroid use. Large doses, given early and tapered rapidly, seem to be the best way to use systemic steroids.

Dapsone (20 mg daily), surgical excision, and grafting are useful treatment options. Narcotics may be needed to control pain. Cleaning out old boxes and newspapers probably reduces brown recluse populations but must be done with care to avoid bites. Insecticides may be helpful, since few spiders have a defense against them.

Black Widow Spider Bite: Latrodectism

Definition and Clinical Description

The female *Latrodectus mactans,* the black widow spider, is 8 to 15 mm in length, with a bright red hourglass or button on the abdomen. A painless bite is followed in about 10 minutes by severe, intense pain, beginning first in the regional lymph nodes and spreading centrifugally. Swelling and tenderness at the bite site follow, and then headache, backache, and colicky abdominal pain. Symptoms diminish in 24 hours and rarely last over 3 days.

Differential Diagnosis

The symptoms are characteristic if spider bite is suspected. An acute abdominal event, such as appendicitis, may be ruled by the absence of tenderness, normal pulse, and absence of distention.

Treatment

A specific antivenom is available and should be given as soon as possible in a dose of 5 mL subcutaneously or intravenously. If necessary, an additional 5 to 10 mL should be given 1 hour later. Calcium gluconate intravenously gives immediate but brief relief. Ice may retard the absorption of the toxin. Muscle relaxants may help.

Tick Bites

Definition

Ticks consist of the mouthparts and eight legs. There are hard ticks, or Ixodidae, in which the mouthparts project beyond the shell, and soft ticks, or Argasidae, in which the body of the tick completely conceals the mouthparts.

Ixodid ticks require a blood meal for developmental changes from larva to nymph and again from nymph to adult. There may be a long interval between the blood meal and the next stage. Argasid ticks may not require blood meals as frequently.

The tick attaches itself to skin first by a cutting or tearing movement of the mouthparts and then by secreting a cement that keeps it anchored in place. Saliva with cytolytic and anticoagulant properties is secreted, and the tick feeds, often increasing its size 10 times or more over several days. When the tick is sated, the hold is loosened and the tick falls to the ground.

Clinical Description

The bite is occasionally symptomatic, but in most instances, it is painless. An erythematous papule may result, which sometimes has surrounding numbness. This may subside, or may progress to a nodule, with marked inflammation, bullous lesions, or even central necrosis. Systemic symptoms have been reported, including fever, restlessness, edema, and gastrointestinal symptoms.

Tick paralysis occurs within hours of a tick bite. A rapid ascending paralysis is noted, up to and including bulbar paralysis and death, unless the tick is found. When the tick is removed, the symptoms disappear in the reverse order. Recovery may be slower. The cause of the paralysis is unknown.

Many diseases may be transmitted by ticks, several of which are listed in Table 4–8.

Pathology

There is a dense infiltrate of neutrophils, with occasional eosinophils. Pseudoepitheliomatous hyperplasia can be seen, along with coagulation necrosis of the dermis in the area of the tick's mouthparts. Lymphocytes and then, later, plasma cells and histiocytes arrive.

Differential Diagnosis

If the tick is still attached, the differential diagnosis is one of suddenly growing tumors. Patients may suspect melanoma, since the engorged tick may appear blue-black. If the tick has already released, the differential diagnosis includes other bites, nodular scabies, and lymphocytoma cutis.

Treatment

Ticks must be removed carefully to avoid leaving mouthparts in the wound. Gentle pulling may work but must be done with care to avoid rupture of the mouthparts. Application of ointment to the tick will cause the tick to release in a few hours. A punch biopsy will remove the tick with certainty. The residual inflammatory area may be treated with strong topical steroids and/or intralesional injections of triamcinolone acetonide.

Protection from ticks can be afforded by using permethrin, either as a spray or impregnating it into clothing. This seems more effective than the use of DEET.

TABLE 4–8. Vectors of Diseases of Dermatologic Importance

DISEASE	CAUSE	VECTOR (COMMON NAME)
Yellow fever	*Yellow fever virus*	Mosquito
Epidemic typhus	*Rickettsia prowazekii*	Body louse
Murine (endemic) typhus	*Rickettsia mooseri*	Rat flea
Rickettsialpox	*Rickettsia akari*	Mouse mite
Rocky Mountain spotted fever	*Rickettsia rickettsii*	Lone Star tick, dog tick
Bartonellosis	*Bartonella bacilliformis*	American sand fly
Bubonic plague	*Yersinia pestis*	Rat flea
Lyme disease	*Borrelia burgdorferi*	Deer tick
Tularemia	*Francisella tularensis*	Lone Star tick, dog tick
Relapsing fever	*Borrelia recurrentis*	Ticks (Europe, Asia, Africa)
African trypanosomiasis		Tsetse fly
American trypanosomiasis (Chagas' disease)	*Trypanosoma cruzi*	Reduvid bug, kissing bug, cone nose bug
Onchocerciasis	*Onchocerca volvulus*	Black flies
Loiasis	*Loa loa*	Deer fly
Malaria	*Plasmodium* spp.	Mosquito
Filariasis	*Wuchereria bancrofti*	Mosquito
Old World leishmaniasis	*L. donovani, L. tropica*	Sand fly
American leishmaniasis	*L. mexicana, L. brasiliensis*	American sand fly
Myiasis	*Dermatobia hominis*	Mosquito

MYIASIS AND TUNGIASIS

(CM&S Chapter 92)

Furuncular Myiasis

Definition

Myiasis is the deposition of a living larva into the skin of an animal. The larva goes through several stages in the tissue and eventually emerges, drops to the ground, and pupates. In most situations, animals are the customary hosts and humans are accidental hosts.

Clinical Description

The clinical presentation is that of one or several raised, inflamed papules, each with a central opening. The papules are 2 cm or more in size, and the patient may have a sensation of movement within the papule. In the center of the opening, a small white circle can be seen that is the breathing tube (spiracle) of the fly.

Etiology

Myiasis is caused by a variety of flies: *Dermatobia hominis* in the extreme southern United States, Mexico, and Central and South America; *Cuterebra* botflies are the most likely source of myiasis in persons who have not traveled outside the United States; and the tumbu or mango fly, which is found in tropical Africa.

Treatment

The injection of anesthesia such as lidocaine will allow the warble to be extracted with a pair of forceps. Alternatively, a formal excision can be accomplished. The native methods of extraction are based on the fact that the spiracle must be exposed to the air for the larva to breathe. Therefore, occlusion of the spiracle will cause the larva to migrate in such a way as to allow the spiracle to again reach the surface. Pork fat, mineral oil, liquid paraffin, and petrolatum are all effective occlusive agents.

Tungiasis

Definition

Tunga penetrans, the burrowing flea, one of the smallest species, is known worldwide in tropical areas. When the flea finds an appropriate host, the female burrows into the skin, with her head reaching down to the papillary dermis. She breathes through spiracles in her hindmost segments. As she takes in nourishment, her abdomen swells. The eggs mature and are extruded, after which the body collapses, the flea dies, and is usually extruded.

Clinical Description

The patient presents with thickened, crusted areas on particularly calloused skin, such as the soles of the feet and around the nails, but less often on the hands.

At first, only a black dot can be seen. Then, an erythematous papule appears as the flea enlarges. Secondary infection often occurs, producing cellulitis and regional adenopathy.

CUTANEOUS EFFECTS OF HEAT AND COLD

(CM&S Chapter 93)

Heat and Heat Injury

Heat is a form of energy that may be transmitted by direct contact (conduction), by a warm medium such as heated air or water (convection), and from a heated body in the form of infrared radiation (radiant heat). Despite different means of transmission, the final product (heat energy) is the same, manifesting as an increase in temperature.

Infrared radiation is the invisible portion of the electromagnetic spectrum adjacent to the long wavelengths, or red end, of the visible light range that extends up to the microwave range. It consists of a wavelength from 0.75 to 1000 μm (0.75 μm = 750 nm). Infrared radiation can penetrate from 0.7 to 30 mm into tissue, sufficient to transmit through the chest wall.

Clinical Syndromes Related to Infrared Radiation

Erythema ab igne

Definition. Erythema ab igne is a localized dermatosis caused by repeated exposure to increased temperatures insufficient to produce a burn.

Clinical Description. Erythema ab igne appears as a reticulated pigmentation and telangiectasia over sites chronically exposed to heat. It is commonly seen in countries without central heating, where it tends to occur on the legs of elderly women who sit close to gas or electric heaters or in the lumbar region in patients who apply hot water bottles or electric heating pads for backache. Erythema ab igne may progress to squamous cell carcinoma.

Pathogenesis and Etiology. Chronic infrared radiation produces thermal elastosis manifested by an increase in the number and thickness of elastic fibers, which form dense accretions similar to those in solar elastosis. It also may induce epidermal changes ranging from hyperkeratosis and slight keratinocyte atypia to frankly invasive squamous cell carcinoma.

Treatment. There is no effective treatment for erythema ab igne. In patients with active disease, however, further damage can be prevented by altering the causative behavior.

Heat as Therapy

Heat has been demonstrated to be effective in the treatment of psoriasis, atopic eczema, and infectious diseases such as warts, chromomycosis, sporotrichosis, leishmaniasis, and atypical mycobacteria.

Cold and Cold Injury

Humans and animals adapt to cold by several mechanisms, including cutaneous vasoconstriction to conserve heat and maintain core body temperature; shivering, increased basal metabolic rate, and exercise to generate heat; and behavioral modifications to supply insulation through the use of adequate clothing and housing. Inasmuch as a primary function of the skin is thermoregulation, temperature-induced alterations in cutaneous blood flow result in wide variations in skin temperature (20° to 40° C) without ill effects. Extreme cold for a prolonged period results in cold injury.

Diseases of Cold Exposure

Frostbite

Definition. Frostbite is localized tissue injury that results from acute freezing of tissue on exposure to extreme cold, that is, temperatures below the freezing point of intact soft tissue (28° to 14° F, $-2°$ to $-10°$ C).

Clinical Description. Frostbite affects the extremities preferentially (toes, feet, fingers, and hands) and as well as exposed areas such as the face (ears, nose, and cheeks). After the initial tingling, dull pain, or feeling of burning on exposure, the affected part becomes white, waxy, hard, and anesthetic with loss of sensation of cold and pain.

Tissue damage becomes more apparent on rewarming. Erythema and mild pain lasting for a few hours may be the only sequelae in mild cases. More severely affected individuals experience burning pain and paresthesias associated with redness, swelling, and blistering, followed by formation of hard black eschar. Destruction of the epidermis, dermis, and deeper tissues may occur with later onset of gangrene and tissue loss. Depending on the severity of the cold exposure, muscles and nerves may be damaged, leading to paralysis, and even bone may be injured. Damage to nerves and blood vessels may result in persistent paresthesias, hypersensitivity to cold, hyperhidrosis, sensory loss, and compromised tissue nutrition, lasting for months or even years.

Critical environmental conditions are the ambient temperature and the duration of exposure. Environmental factors that increase the rate of loss of heat from the skin, especially strong wind velocity (wind chill), high altitude, and contact with good conductors such as water or metal, result in greater severity of injury for the same duration of exposure. Predisposing host factors include inadequate or constrictive clothing, nicotine use, physical immobility, impaired mental state, previous cold injury, old age, presence of systemic diseases, and peripheral vascular disease, particularly arterial insufficiency.

Diagnosis and Differential Diagnosis. The diagnosis is made on the history of exposure to extreme cold, in the presence of predisposing factors, and on the clinical appearance. Other causes of cold-related erythema, blister formation, and gangrene must be excluded.

Treatment. Frostbite has traditionally been classified according to the degree of injury. However, because the initial clinical appearance of frostbitten tissues may be deceiving, the extent and severity of tissue damage are difficult to predict. Therefore, the more simple designation of superficial versus deep injury is now used. To prevent unnecessary removal of viable tissue, conservative management is recommended until the full extent of tissue damage becomes apparent.

The principles of cold injury can be applied to treatment of frostbite: slow thaw, as used in cryotherapy, increases tissue damage; therefore, rapid rewarming should be performed. When available facilities allow, and after ascertaining that the victim is not suffering from hypothermia (rectal temperature in the normal range taken with a thermometer capable of registering hypothermic temperatures), rapid rewarming by immersion in water at 40° to 42° C (104° to 108° F) for 15 to 30 minutes until the most distal tissue is flushed and soft is recommended. Exposure to higher temperatures is contraindicated. On field conditions, further mechanical trauma must be avoided, in particular by rubbing the affected part.

After thawing, treatment goals should be the preservation of viable tissue and the prevention of infection. Bed rest with elevation and open nonocclusive sterile wound care are recommended. Twice-daily soaking for 20 minutes in a warm whirlpool bath with a mild antiseptic is advocated to gently debride, prevent infection, and encourage joint mobility. Adequate analgesics and tetanus prophylaxis should be administered. Prophylactic antibiotic use and vasodilator and thrombolytic agents are controversial. The prompt and early administration of heparin and infusion of low-molecular-weight dextran appear to have proved beneficial.

Early favorable prognostic signs include rapid return of skin warmth and sensation, erythema, edema, and vesicles with clear fluid. Unfavorable prognostic signs include cold, pale, anesthetic skin, absence of edema, and sanguineous or absent vesicles.

Immersion Foot (Trench Foot)

Definition. Immersion foot is the preferred term used for non-freezing injury to the feet. It typically occurs in the setting of prolonged exposure to cold temperatures above freezing in combination with a damp, usually occlusive, environment and prolonged immobility and dependency of the limbs.

Clinical Description. The clinical signs and symptoms of immersion foot depend on the temperature at which the exposure occurs. Four distinct phases have been described associated with cold temperatures: exposure; prehyperemic with cold, blue, and numb feet; hyperemic with warm, edematous, and painful feet that may last for as long as 10 weeks; and posthyperemic with cold sensitivity and hyperhydrosis that may persist for many years. Exposure to warmer temperatures results in less tissue destruction and sensory disturbance and more rapid complete recovery. The soles of the feet become cool, white, wrinkled and painful and may demonstrate associated edema and maceration. On removal from moisture, symptoms begin to resolve within 2 days, and healing is complete within 2 weeks with minimal to no sequelae.

Susceptibility to the development of immersion foot is variable. Exacerbating factors include thick soles, immobility and prolonged dependency of the limbs, constrictive footwear, footwear that is permeable to water and grit, and footwear that causes perspiration and increased maceration. Smoking and peripheral vascular disease contribute to the severity of the tissue damage. Previously a finding associated with military campaigns, immersion foot is a serious problem of the homeless.

Diagnosis and Differential Diagnosis. Diagnosis is based on a history of exposure to cool/wet conditions associated with use of constrictive footwear in the setting of immobility with accompanying venous stagnation and on the presence of compatible clinical findings in a symmetrical, localized distribution limited by the level of submersion or occlusion. Differential diagnosis includes causes of arterial vascular occlusion as well as cutaneous infections that involve the feet such as bacterial cellulitis, dermatophyte infection, and interdigital erythrasma.

Treatment. The best treatment is prevention. Adequate foot care with sufficient time to dry the feet after immersion is essential. Once immersion foot has occurred, supportive care, including bed rest, air drying and elevation of the feet, and appropriate analgesics, should be instituted. Secondary infection should be treated with systemic antibiotics.

Diseases of Abnormal Sensitivity to the Cold

Perniosis (Chilblains)

Definition. Chilblains (perniosis) are localized erythematous inflammatory lesions that occur as an abnormal reaction to cold temperatures above freezing in combination with high humidity (cold damp environment), which exacerbates conductive heat loss.

Clinical Description. The onset of perniosis is in the autumn or early winter when the humidity is high. Individual lesions are red or purple, tender, pruritic patches, papules, or plaques that may blister or ulcerate. They occur especially on the fingers and toes, heels, lower legs, thighs, nose, and ears, usually in a bilaterally symmetrical distribution. A typical course is self-limiting over 3 weeks or so. The condition in severely affected individuals may persist throughout the winter and may be unremitting even in the summer months.

Chilblains may be familial, and the lesions are often superimposed on a background of acrocyanosis and/or erythrocyanosis. Chilblains occur particularly in children but can develop at any age. They are infrequently seen in the United States compared with Northern Europe, probably because of warmer living and working conditions and the more prolific use of well-insulated clothing.

A particular type of perniosis (erythrocyanosis with nodules and pernio, or equestrian panniculitis) has been described in young, mainly female, patients who are horse riding enthusiasts and wear tight-fitting, poorly insulating breeches, but it has also been noted to occur in both men and women who wear tight-fitting pants and ride slow-moving vehicles open to the cold, wind, and rain, such as golf-carts, delivery vans, and tractors. Infiltrated erythrocyanotic plaques are distributed symmetrically on the outer aspects of obese thighs; occasionally, there is ulceration and follicular plugging.

Pathology. Lesions typically demonstrate necrotic keratinocytes, intense edema of the papillary dermis, a superficial and deep perivascular mononuclear cell infiltrate, and a lymphocytic vasculitis in roughly one half of specimens.

Pathogenesis and Etiology. In contrast to normal individuals in whom moderate cold exposure induces cutaneous vasoconstriction, which is succeeded by vasodilation in an attempt to maintain perfusion, a persistent cold-induced constriction of the large cutaneous arterioles and a persistent dilatation of the smaller, more superficial, vessels occurs in individuals who are afflicted by perniosis.

Differential Diagnosis. The diagnosis is based on a compatible history and consistent clinical picture. The differential diagnosis includes acrocyanosis, cryoglobulinemia, chilblain lupus erythematosus, and peripheral vascular insufficiency.

Treatment. Prophylactic measures include wearing warm clothing and living in warm housing conditions. Vasodilator calcium channel blockers (especially nifedipine) are effective therapy and prophylaxis for acral idiopathic perniosis. Nicotinic acid derivatives and minoxidil topically applied are also effective in some patients.

Acrocyanosis

Definition. Acrocyanosis is a persistent erythrocyanotic discoloration of the hands and feet, often with a mottled pattern, which is accentuated by exposure to cold temperatures above freezing.

Clinical Description. The changes of acrocyanosis may be transient after cold exposure but frequently persist during the winter and even throughout the summer months. The face may also be involved. There is often a positive family history, suggesting a genetic basis for this condition. The disorder usually starts in adolescence and persists into adult life. Perniosis, erythrocyanosis, and livedo reticularis may occur simultaneously with acrocyanosis. Discoloration is related to arteriolar reactivity, the cause of which is unknown.

Diagnosis and Differential Diagnosis. The diagnosis is based on the clinical finding of persistent cyanotic discoloration in the presence of normal peripheral pulses and absence of venous occlusion. The differential diagnosis includes severe, usually secondary, Raynaud's phenomenon and perniosis.

Treatment. There is no medical cure for this condition, but treatment includes an increase in ambient temperature, physical exercise, and use of insulated gloves and shoes. Synthetic vasodilator therapy usually is not effective, but nicotinic acid derivatives and minoxidil applied topically can be beneficial.

Erythrocyanosis

Definition. Erythrocyanosis is persistent dusky erythema and cyanosis occurring usually over areas with a thick layer of subcutaneous fat, such as the thighs and lower legs, and less commonly over the buttocks and forearms.

Clinical Description. Erythrocyanosis may occur with or independent of acrocyanosis. Dusky, frequently deeply red-purple discoloration of the skin occurs most commonly in adolescent girls on the lower legs and on the thighs and buttocks of obese prepubescent boys. Nodular lesions resembling chilblains or erythema induration may occur after acute cold exposure. The disease may persist indefinitely and may be accompanied by progressive thickening, edema, and fibrosis. Spontaneous improvement may occur.

Differential Diagnosis. The differential diagnosis includes deep perniosis, superficial thrombophlebitis, erythema induratum, and varicose eczema, depending on the affected site.

Treatment. Warm clothing, exercise, weight reduction, and elastic support hose may all be helpful. Vasodilators are ineffective.

Livedo Reticularis (Reticularis Multiplex, Dermatopathic Pigmentosa Reticularis, Inflammatio Cutis Racemosa, and Livedo Racemosa)

Definition. Livedo reticularis is a cyanotic mottled discoloration of the skin with a characteristic net-like pattern.

Clinical Description. The mottled cyanotic discoloration of livedo reticularis most commonly occurs on the lower limbs, but the upper limbs and trunk may also be affected. Tingling and numbness of the skin may commonly occur on exposure to cold, which also intensifies the severity of cyanotic discoloration.

Physiologic Livedo Reticularis (Cutis Marmorata). This physiologic mottled cyanotic transient reaction to cold may be seen in up to 50% of normal children and in some adults. The mottling is diffuse and mild and usually symptomless. Chilblains, acrocyanosis, and erythrocyanosis may be associated. This condition and idiopathic livedo reticularis may represent a spectrum of disease.

Congenital Livedo Reticularis (Cutis Marmorata Telangiectatica Congenita). This is a rare developmental defect of the skin that presents at birth as asymmetrical and severe lesions with atrophy of the skin. It is not usually associated with other disorders. Although no treatment is effective, the condition may improve spontaneously with age.

Acquired Idiopathic Livedo Reticularis. This condition occurs predominantly in young adult and middle-aged women. Although mild degrees appear to be common and harmless, in the more rare severe cases it is associated with severe ulceration, usually in winter. The mottling usually has its onset in the third or fourth decade of life and is at first transient on exposure to cold; subsequently, permanent discoloration can occur. Tingling and numbness of the skin and sometimes edema may be present.

A rare group of patients with livedo reticularis have widespread and severe livedo reticularis associated with arterial disease in peripheral, cerebral, and coronary vessels, with or without renal involvement, associated with the presence of lupus anticoagulant and/or antiphospholipid anticardiolipin antibodies. The course progressively worsens over several years with intermittent cerebral and other vascular occlusive episodes and a poor prognosis. Histologically, the small arteries show an endarteritis obliterans or luminal thrombi. This constellation of abnormalities has now become known as the antiphospholipid syndrome or Sneddon's syndrome.

Pathogenesis and Etiology. Livedo reticularis may be physiologic, idiopathic, or secondary—associated with intravascular obstruction or vessel wall disease (Table 4-9). The histologic changes of endarteritis are found in the small arterioles and venules of livedo reticularis of any degree of severity.

TABLE 4-9. Classification of Livedo Reticularis

I. Physiologic
  A. Cutis marmorata
II. Idiopathic or primary livedo reticularis
  A. Congenital
    1. Cutis marmorata telangiectatica congenita
  B. Acquired idiopathic
    1. Uncomplicated
    2. With winter ulceration
    3. With summer ulceration
    4. With systemic vascular involvement
III. Secondary livedo reticularis
  A. Intravascular obstruction
    1. Stasis
    2. Paralysis
    3. Cardiac failure
    4. Amantadine therapy
    5. Occlusive disease
      a. Emboli
      b. Oxalosis
      c. Compressed air
      d. Thrombocythemia
      e. Cryoglobulins
      f. Cold agglutinins
  B. Vessel wall disease
    1. Arteriosclerosis
    2. Arteritis
      a. Polyarteritis nodosa
      b. Connective tissue disease

Diagnosis and Differential Diagnosis. Underlying causes and associated diseases must be excluded before making a diagnosis of idiopathic livedo reticularis.

Treatment. Uncomplicated idiopthic livedo reticularis does not require measures other than protection from and avoidance of cold. Severe cases, including those with ulceration, may be helped by prolonged anticoagulant and ''antithrombotic'' therapy.

Secondary Livedo Reticularis

Secondary livedo reticularis has many causes, and it tends not to be widespread or symmetrical but patchy and asymmetrical, reflecting a more limited arterial change. Full investigation is required to seek secondary causes. The treatment of secondary livedo reticularis is that of the underlying condition.

Cryoglobulinemia

Definition. Cryoglobulinemia is the presence of cold precipitable immunoglobulins in the peripheral blood. Cryoglobulins can be monoclonal or polyclonal. So-called mixed cryoglobulins are complexes of IgM and either IgG or IgA. Cutaneous lesions similar to those of cryoglobulinemia are produced by cold precipitable fibrinogen (cryofibrinogenemia).

Clinical Description. The cutaneous manifestations of cryoglobulinemia are varied. Purpura, livedo reticularis, cold urticaria,

Raynaud's phenomenon, and ulceration of the legs may occur after cold exposure.

The disease may be primary (idiopathic), occurring in the absence of any other detectable pathology, or may be associated with lymphoproliferative disorders. It can also occur in association with collagen diseases, carcinomatosis, Lyme disease, rheumatoid arthritis, leprosy, subacute bacterial endocarditis, syphilis, and vasculitis.

Pathology. In monoclonal cryoglobulinemia and in cryofibrinogenemia, the lumens of dermal venules can be distended by homogeneous eosinophilic deposits. Inflammatory cell infiltrates are present only if the deposits result in anoxic damage to either vessel walls or the adjacent dermis. In mixed cryoglobulinemia, immunoglobulin complexes lodge in vessel walls, resulting in leukocytoclastic venulitis.

Diagnosis and Differential Diagnosis. A search for all the known causes of cryoglobulinemia (myeloma, macroglobulinemia, lymphoma associated with single-complement cryoglobulins) is indicated together with the characterization of the nature of the cryoglobulin protein (which may be IgG, IgA, or IgM) before regarding the disease as primary or idiopathic.

Treatment. The cause of the cryoglobulinemia should be treated, but treatment can be unsatisfactory where the cause cannot be removed. Anticoagulants and systemic steroids may be beneficial, and in recalcitrant cases plasmapheresis may be a valuable recourse.

RADIATION DERMATITIS

(CM&S Chapter 94)

Definition

Radiation injury is subclassified into acute effects, which are manifested within minutes to a few weeks after radiation exposure, and chronic or late effects, which are manifested months to years later.

Clinical Description

Acute Radiation Injury

After either a single exposure to ionizing radiation exceeding 10 Gy (1000 rad) or multiple, closely spaced exposures exceeding the same dose level, the skin develops a reaction that is similar to a thermal burn. Its clinical manifestations include erythema, edema, and pruritus. This type of reaction begins within 2 to 7 days after exposure, peaks within 10 to 14 days, and gradually subsides, and eventually clears in most instances. With exposure to higher doses of ionizing radiation, a more severe radiation injury takes place, characterized by intense erythema, which becomes violaceous, edema, vesiculation, erosion, and superficial ulceration associated with burning, tingling, and pruritus. This moderately severe inflammatory response subsides within 4 to 8 weeks. Permanent postinflammatory pigmentary abnormalities are common. Telangiectasia and other atrophic changes may develop. Radiation doses leading to deep ulceration and necrosis are usually accidental.

Chronic radiodermatitis generally occurs years after radiation exposure and results from relatively short but intense courses of radiation therapy, such as those used in the treatment of cutaneous malignancy. Chronic radiodermatitis has also resulted from gradual but excessive occupational exposure or from overdoses of radiation received during the treatment of nonneoplastic conditions such as acne, hirsutism, or eczematous disorders. The clinical manifestations of chronic radiodermatitis include cutaneous atrophy, telangiectasia, partial or complete destruction of cutaneous appendages, pigmentary changes, and sclerosis of underlying tissue.

An absorbed dose of at least 20 cGy is necessary for the development of postirradiation malignancy. The incidence of basal cell carcinoma in irradiated sites is higher than that of squamous cell carcinoma.

Pathology

Histologically, acute radiodermatitis is characterized by individually necrotic keratinocytes, ballooning and spongiosis of the epidermis, vacuolar change at the dermoepidermal junction, effacement of the rete ridges, and many abnormally large nuclei. Dermal changes include edema, vasodilatation of blood vessels, and swelling endothelial cells.

In chronic radiodermatitis the inflammatory changes may be minimal or absent. The most striking feature of chronic radiation injury is sclerosis of the dermis-thickened bundles of reticular dermal collagen with diminished spaces between them and homogenization of the papillary dermis. Large, stellate cells termed *radiation fibroblasts* are often found in the dermis. The walls of dermal blood vessels can be so markedly thickened that the lumen may be partially or totally occluded.

chapter 5

What Disorders Change the Structure of the Dermis?

SCLERODERMA AND CHEMICALLY INDUCED SCLERODERMA

(See CM&S Chapters 98 and 99)

Definition

Scleroderma, a disease of unknown etiology, is the result of an excess deposition of collagen in the dermis. It occurs in both local and systemic forms. The local forms are linear scleroderma and morphea, which typically occurs as confined patches of scleroderma. The systemic forms of scleroderma occur in a limited and a diffuse cutaneous pattern. Limited disease was previously referred to as CREST syndrome, an acronym for *c*alcinosis, *R*aynaud's phenomenon, *e*sophageal involvement, *s*clerodactyly, and *t*elangiectasia. Because all of these features can also be found in diffuse disease, the term CREST syndrome has been largely abandoned.

Clinical Description

Scleroderma is a rare autoimmune disease of unknown etiology that affects women about three times more often than men, and is most frequent from 40 to 60 years of age. Cutaneous involvement is usually prominent and may be highly disabling. Internal organ involvement, particularly of the heart, lung, and kidney, is associated with an increased mortality. Thickening of the skin is the major diagnostic feature of systemic sclerosis. Internal organ involvement without skin disease is rare. In a case of unequivocal scleroderma the skin is thick, tight, immobile, and difficult to pinch. Early in the course of the disease, the changes may be more subtle. The fingers are usually the first structures to be affected, presenting with pain and frequently associated with Raynaud's phenomenon. This almost universally precedes or begins concomitantly with skin involvement. The disease may spread to the arms, face, and other areas, but newly involved areas are not necessarily contiguous. The skin changes evolve sequentially through edematous, sclerotic, and finally atrophic phases, although they may not be apparent on physical examination.

The degree of skin involvement correlates with prognosis. Areas of skin that are the last to become involved are often the first to improve.

Hand involvement may lead to digital flexion contractures, resulting in inability to grip or pinch, and can be disabling. Skin tightness over the joints of the fingers mechanically predisposes to ulcerations. Ulcerations of the distal pulp, believed to be due to vasospasm, may be followed by more severe ischemic changes that can lead to gangrene and digital amputation, a complication found with greater frequency in patients with limited disease. Calcifications in the soft tissue of the digits can also contribute to this problem.

The face is a common site of involvement in scleroderma; the nose often appears tight and shiny, the mouth may have a decreased aperture and its perimeter may be surrounded by perpendicular creases. Small telangiectases, common over the face and hands, may also appear in the mouth and the upper respiratory and gastrointestinal tracts.

Raynaud's phenomenon, which is defined as blanching or color change of the hands followed by tingling and/or numbness after exposure to cold temperature or emotional upset, is present in over 90% of patients with systemic sclerosis and about 5% of the general population. Raynaud's phenomenon tends to be more severe in limited cutaneous disease. The feet and the nose may be involved in severe cases.

Involvement of the internal organs determines the mortality of systemic sclerosis. Renal disease is frequently subclinical and is manifested by proteinuria and hypertension. Renal crisis is an acute rise in serum creatinine level accompanied by a microangiopathic hemolytic anemia and severe hypertension that, left untreated, results in chronic renal failure and death. A rising blood pressure and serum lactate dehydrogenase level are two important signs of possible impending renal crisis.

Pulmonary involvement in scleroderma is the most common life-threatening factor in this disease. The lungs can be involved in two ways: pulmonary fibrosis and pulmonary arterial hypertension. Pulmonary hypertension is more common in patients with limited cutaneous disease and portends a poor prognosis.

The most frequent signs of cardiac involvement in scleroderma are heart blocks and arrhythmias associated with pericardial effusion and myocardial fibrosis. The gastrointestinal tract is the most common internal system affected by scleroderma. Esophageal dysmotility with decreased contractility of the distal two thirds of the esophagus and a decrease in lower esophageal sphincter tone are characteristic. These lesions produce dyspepsia and dysphagia with patient complaints of heartburn and of solid food "getting stuck" in the mid chest. Acid suppression with H_2 blockers and tilting the head of the bed at a 45-degree angle are advisible. Stasis of the small and large bowel due to collagen infiltration produces bacterial overgrowth manifested by diarrhea and, in severe cases, malabsorption with weight loss or chronic constipation.

Pathology

The histopathologic features of fully developed lesions of scleroderma in the skin are indistinguishable from those of morphea.

Early lesions show superficial and deep, perivascular, and sometimes interstitial infiltrates of lymphocytes, along with fewer numbers of macrophages and occasional eosinophils. As the condition progresses, collagen bundles of the reticular dermis are thickened. The eccrine coils in normal skin are surrounded by adipocytes; as scleroderma progresses, these are replaced by thickened bundles of collagen, and in time, there are only sparse inflammatory infiltrates, and epithelial adnexal structures often wither away completely.

Diagnosis and Differential Diagnosis

To diagnose systemic sclerosis according to the American College of Rheumatology, patients are required to have either proximal scleroderma (proximal to the digits) as a major criterion or to have at least two minor criteria, which are sclerodactyly, digital pitting scars, or bibasal pulmonary fibrosis. In practical terms, symmetrical skin thickening involving the hands, a history of Raynaud's phenomenon, and a positive antinuclear antibody test are usually all that is needed to make the diagnosis (in the absence of features of other collagen vascular diseases). In patients with Raynaud's phenomenon with no skin thickening, serology coupled with capillary microscopy examination is helpful for predicting who will develop scleroderma; patients with scleroderma or those with Raynaud's phenomenon who will develop disease frequently have a tortuous nonhomogeneous appearance to their capillary loops, with areas of loop dropout.

The differential diagnosis of scleroderma includes early rheumatoid arthritis, gout, reflex sympathetic dystrophy, bilateral eosinophilic fasciitis, scleredema, scleromyxedema, carcinoid tumors, porphyria cutanea tarda, and sclerodermoid chronic graft-versus-host disease.

Environmental exposure to chemicals such as polyvinyl chloride, bleomycin cancer chemotherapy, liquid silicone injections for breast augmentation, implantation of silicone gel-filled envelopes, and L-tryptophan ingestion produce findings that may closely mimic scleroderma.

Chemically induced scleroderma appears to differ in several ways from the more common idiopathic variants. Both toxic oil and the L-tryptophan–associated illnesses have acute components, manifested by respiratory symptoms in the former and myalgias in the latter, that do not occur in scleroderma. In addition, Raynaud's phenomenon and positive antinuclear autoantibodies, which occur in 90% of idiopathic scleroderma patients, are seen much less commonly in chemically induced scleroderma. Finally, in general there is some clinical improvement after the withdrawal of the inducing chemical, in both patients exposed to toxic oil and patients exposed to pathogenic lots of L-tryptophan.

Treatment

There is no Food and Drug Administration–approved treatment for systemic sclerosis. Some patients may improve over a period of years without treatment; however, spontaneous remissions are rare. The 5-year survival in several subgroups is 50% or less. Average survivals decrease further with lung, cardiac, or renal involvement.

Careful attention to the vasospastic components of the disease and local organ involvement is warranted. Several medications are effective in preventing Raynaud's phenomenon, the most effective being calcium channel blockers. Nifedipine, starting at 30 mg/day, can be increased if necessary over a period of weeks up to 90 or occasionally 120 mg daily. Patients must be warned of potential symptoms of hypotension or peripheral edema. To prevent distal digital pulp ulcerations and infection, the concomitant use of pentoxifylline, dipyridamole, and a calcium channel blocker may be effective. Existing ulcerations must be kept clean and protected from trauma. Loosely wrapped bio-occlusive dressings over the joints can be helpful. Severe flexion contractures may be cautiously approached with surgical release.

Internal organ involvement needs to be monitored closely. Treatment of the global disease is difficult and controversial. D-Penicillamine, which inhibits the cross linkage of collagen, may be clinically effective. Although the evidence for efficacy of D-penicillamine is weak, it should probably be used as a first-line agent in patients with diffuse disease. D-Penicillamine can be initiated at a dose of 250 mg daily, and increased by 250 mg every 6 to 8 weeks depending on the rapidity of the disease; 750 mg for more than 6 months appears to be the minimally effective dose. Blood cell counts and urine should be monitored monthly. Up to 30% of patients are discontinued from D-penicillamine therapy owing to adverse effects, which include skin eruptions, proteinuria, and peripheral cytopenia. Mild early rashes may be cautiously treated with antihistamines while D-penicillamine therapy is continued.

Corticosteroids are indicated for patients with scleroderma who have concomitant myositis. Encouraging prospective data needing further confirmation exist for several other treatments, including interferon gamma, cyclosporine, and extracorporeal photochemotherapy.

MORPHEA

(CM&S Chapter 100)

Definition

Scleroderma has been defined as "chronic hardening and thickening of the skin, which may be a finding in several different diseases, occurring in a localized or focal form and as a systemic disease." *Morphea* is "localized scleroderma," in which the primary changes of scleroderma are in the skin. The different types of morphea have different clinical presentations and various levels of involvement in the skin. Some feel that morphea is a disease spectrum encompassing sclerosing processes ranging from superficial (lichen sclerosus et atrophicus) to deep (morphea profunda). Mild systemic involvement may occur, but transition from morphea to systemic scleroderma is rare. The exact mechanism and etiology in morphea are still unknown. Common to all forms of morphea is overproduction of collagen by lesional fibroblasts.

Clinical Description

Lichen Sclerosus et Atrophicus

The lesions of lichen sclerosus et atrophicus are characterized by shiny white plaques that are often preceded by violaceous skin discoloration. The lesions can involve the trunk and extremities but also have a predilection for the anogenital area, especially in women.

Lichen sclerosus et atrophicus may be seen in patients with generalized morphea, and histologic changes resembling lichen sclerosus et atrophicus can occur in the papillary dermis above the typical ones of morphea, suggesting that the two entities overlap.

Morphea

The lesions in morphea en plaque involve only one or two sites and often begin insidiously with slightly erythematous patches that gradually evolve into indurated, dusky, or hypopigmented plaques with a surrounding violaceous zone of inflammation. Morphea en plaque may become more widespread, beginning insidiously with localized plaques on the trunk that gradually increase in size and become confluent. Atrophoderma of Pasini and Pierini is characterized by asymptomatic, hyperpigmented atrophic patches on the trunk, with a depressed center and a well-demarcated "cliff-drop border," without marked inflammatory or sclerotic changes. Most regard this condition as an end-stage of morphea. In guttate morphea, multiple, 1-cm or less, oval lesions develop most often on the trunk.

Linear morphea is most common in children and primarily affects the extremities, especially the legs. It presents as discrete linear induration, not necessarily in a dermatomal distribution. En coup de sabre is a special variant of linear morphea that involves the head. Less often facial hemiatrophy develops, which occasionally results in atrophic facial distortion, sometimes with associated electroencephalographic abnormalities and seizures.

Subcutaneous Morphea, Morphea Profunda, and Pansclerotic Morphea of Childhood

Some patients with morphea have deep, bound-down, sclerotic plaques that are deeper than ordinary morphea, which largely affects the dermis. In subcutaneous morphea, the onset of the sclerosis is relatively rapid, often occurring over a period of several months. Plaques are generally mildly inflamed, hyperpigmented, bound-down, symmetric, and somewhat ill defined.

Patients with morphea profunda have involvement of sclerosis in the deep dermis, subcutaneous tissue, fascia, and superficial muscle, deeper than the involvement with subcutaneous morphea and eosinophilic fasciitis. These patients may also have typical dermal morphea. Patients respond to antimalarial agents, systemic corticosteroids, or other anti-inflammatory agents.

Pansclerotic morphea of childhood is an aggressive and mutilating form of morphea. Its onset usually occurs before the age of 14 years, and it typically involves the extensor aspect of the extremities, but it can also affect the trunk, with sclerotic plaques that extend deeply to involve subcutaneous tissue, fascia, muscle, and bone.

Pathology

In lichen sclerosus et atrophicus, an interface dermatitis is seen initially, followed by fully developed lesions characterized by hyperkeratosis, with follicular plugging and pronounced edema and homogenization of the collagen bundles in the papillary dermis with a lymphocytic infiltrate below the homogenized area. In the superficial morphea variants, there is thickening of the collagen of the dermis and dermal–subcutaneous junction with narrowing of the spaces between them, and an inflammatory infiltrate in perivascular and interstitial distribution.

In linear morphea, either only the dermis and dermal-subcutaneous junction are affected or the subcutaneous tissue, panniculus, and even the muscle and the periosteum are affected, similar to morphea profunda. In the deeper morphea variants, the inflammation and sclerosis may reach as deep as bone; the differences in the different subtypes are in the levels of involvement. Changes identical to those of morphea profunda are often present in patients with eosinophilic fasciitis, which primarily involves the fascia.

Differential Diagnosis

The differential diagnoses for localized plaques include stasis dermatitis with fibrosis, forms of panniculitis, pretibial myxedema, porphyria cutanea tarda, and injection-induced sclerosis. The differential diagnosis of deep morphea includes scleromyxedema, scleroderma, premature aging syndromes, graft-verus-host reaction, and eosinophilic fasciitis.

Treatment

Some patients with morphea en plaque, atrophoderma of Pasini and Pierini, guttate morphea, and localized lichen sclerosus et atrophicus have spontaneous remission. No specific treatment is needed. Emollients are recommended for dry skin. If the lesions are spreading or painful, antimalarial agents are considered.

In patients with generalized morphea, linear morphea, bullous morphea, and generalized lichen sclerosus et atrophicus, the lesions may be progressive, and use of anti-inflammatory medications is reasonable. Antimalarial agents may be useful. In cases of antimalarial intolerance, non-steroidal anti-inflammatory drugs or systemic steroids are used.

In deep morphea variants, progressive involvement is common and requires both systemic steroids and antimalarial agents.

KELOIDS AND HYPERTROPHIC SCARS

(CM&S Chapter 101)

Definition

A keloid is a firm, benign, frequently pruritic or painful protuberant scar that commonly develops after injuries in certain familial and racial groups. Keloids typically project beyond the site of the original injury and contain abnormally thickened collagen bundles. A hypertrophic scar is a raised scar that may develop in any racial group after injuries at anatomic locations where there is high tension, such as the presternum, shoulders, knees, and ankles.

Clinical Description

Both keloids and hypertrophic scars have an increase in the total amount of collagen that is normally present. Keloids have a particular predilection for developing on the upper trunk, arms, and neck, especially after burn injuries, surgical procedures, and vaccinations, and they are uncommon on the hands, feet, eyelids, genitalia, and mucous membranes. Keloids may also form "spontaneously" on the mid chest in the absence of any known prior injury. They do not spontaneously resolve; instead, they grow relentlessly until they extend beyond the wound margins onto the normal adjacent skin. Keloids may be asymptomatic, but are commonly pruritic and may even be the source of significant discomfort or pain. Blacks and individuals of Mediterranean descent are at the greatest risk for developing keloids. However, keloids may form in any individual at any time.

Although it may be difficult at times to differentiate them from keloids, hypertrophic scars tend to approximate the size of the original wound and are typically asymptomatic. Hypertrophic scars are commonly seen in patients with cystic acne. They usually spontaneously soften and flatten over a period of time.

Pathology

Hypertrophic scars are exaggerations of "normal" scarring. Keloid scars have, in addition to areas resembling ordinary scars, discrete zones that contain thick, homogeneous-appearing "keloidal" collagen bundles that are often separated by mucin.

Treatment

The most important aspect in the treatment of both keloids and hypertrophic scars lies in initially attempting to minimize the risk of formation after any surgical procedure. By reducing wound tension, intraoperative tissue injury, and providing a tensionless closure, the risk of inducing the formation of abnormal scar tissue can be greatly minimized. However, once a keloid or hypertrophic scar has developed, the treatment is frequently very similar, although keloids are more difficult to manage. Generally, the most effective approach to the management of keloids and hypertrophic scars often combines medical, surgical, and radiologic techniques.

Medical Techniques

External Pressure

Long-term (4 to 6 months) use of external compression with elasticized garments, stretchable dressings, or pressure earrings on both keloids and hypertrophic scars can help prevent additional growth of scar tissue and may also be useful postoperatively to reduce the potential for recurrence after excision of keloids.

Topical, Intralesional, or Systemic Medications

Corticosteroids. Intralesional corticosteroids, the most important medical treatment, directly suppress collagen synthesis, accelerate the rate of collagen breakdown, reduce inflammation that might otherwise stimulate more fibrosis, and antagonize the action of transforming growth factor-β, a stimulator of collagen and extracellular matrix protein production by fibroblasts. To be effective, the corticosteroids, usually as triamcinolone acetonide in a concentration of 40 mg/ml, must be injected directly into the bulk of a very firm keloid or hypertrophic scar. Pretreatment with liquid nitrogen spray cryosurgery can facilitate the injection process by causing edema and decreasing the density of the scar.

Side effects include temporary hypopigmentation at or around the injection site and atrophy of the surrounding skin if the drug is not injected precisely into the scar.

Cytotoxic and Immunosuppressive Drugs. Oral mechlorethamine (nitrogen mustard) and methotrexate, either alone or combined with surgical excision, have been reported to be effective in reducing recurrence rates.

Silicone Gel Dressings. Simple application of a cross-linked polydimethylsiloxane polymer in a sheet that has been reinforced with a polyester mesh into surgical dressings substantially reduces the size and local symptomatology of both hypertrophic scars and keloids. These dressings work best when they are placed on the surface of the skin without external pressure for a minimum of 12 hours per day for 2 to 4 months.

Interferon. Interferon gamma and interferon alfa-2b injected intralesionally at a dose of 0.01 to 0.1 mg of recombinant interferon gamma three times per week for 3 consecutive weeks have both been reported to be useful in the treatment of keloids and hypertrophic scars. Further work is required to accurately establish effective treatment intervals and dosages.

Surgical and Radiologic Approaches

Cryosurgery

Cryosurgery used alone is performed using a contact probe in a single freeze–thaw cycle for 30 seconds. This procedure is repeated every 20 to 30 days as needed.

Simple Surgical Excision

To achieve the best results, a combination of excision plus cryo-surgery, intralesional corticosteroid injections, pressure, or radiation therapy may be required. Simple excision followed by undermining and tensionless primary closure is probably the best alternative, but it is only useful for treating relatively small lesions in locations where skin tension is minimal. Because tension is extremely important in determining the ultimate outcome, when simple surgical excision is used for the treatment of keloids and hypertrophic scars, great attention should always first be given to determine the best orientation for the excision so as to minimize tension on the repaired wound to decrease the incidence of recurrence.

When combining simple surgical excision plus intralesional corticosteroids, they should be injected into the scar preoperatively at 2-week intervals for several times and postoperatively at least four times after the completion of surgery. Ten milligrams of triamcinolone acetonide can also be injected into the wound edges before final wound closure. Buried suture material such as polyglycolic acid should be used because of its low tissue reactivity. The skin surface should be repaired using either monofilament nylon or polyester suture because of the elasticity and low tissue reactivity of these materials. The sutures should be left in place for 10 to 14 days, since the use of intralesional corticosteroids will interfere with the normal rate of development of tensile strength, and early suture removal may result in wound dehiscence.

Ionizing Radiation

The use of ionizing radiation therapy alone either delivered through superficial x-ray, electron beam, or interstitial implantation or in conjunction with surgical intervention may be helpful in the management of certain keloids and occasionally hypertrophic scars to reduce the risk of regrowth.

Laser Surgery

Controlled studies have failed to show a distinct advantage to using CO_2 or argon lasers in the treatment of keloids and hypertrophic scars, but recent studies have demonstrated that the pulsed dye laser (585 nm) is effective treatment for hypertrophic scars and some keloids.

DUPUYTREN'S DISEASE

(CM&S Chapter 102)

Definition and Clinical Description

Dupuytren's disease is a hand disorder of unknown etiology that is characterized by progressive fibrosis of the palmar aponeurosis and its extensions into the digits. Dupuytren's disease has also been called palmar fasciitis or palmar fibromatosis. It is an inherited disease and is most likely to occur in patients with a Northern European ancestry (especially Celts). Dupuytren's disease has been associated with epilepsy, alcoholism, diabetes mellitus, and trauma.

Patients with Dupuytren's disease often have bilateral involvement of the upper extremities, the presence of knuckle pads, fibromatosis of the plantar fascia of the feet, and fasciitis of the dorsal penis (Peyronie's disease). If fibrosis is advanced, the overlying skin and underlying flexor tendons are involved, resulting in contracture and deformity. Contracture most frequently involves the ring finger, and the small finger is also often affected. The long and index fingers are occasionally affected, but the thumb is seldom involved.

Early clinical manifestations of Dupuytren's disease in the palm or digits may include the presence of nodules, pits, and cords without joint contracture. As fibrotic cords develop, however, metacarpophalangeal and proximal interphalangeal joint contracture often results. Knuckle pads may be found on the dorsal aspect of the hand at the level of the metacarpophalangeal joint or on the dorsal aspect of the digit at the level of the proximal interphalangeal joint; knuckle pads may be present even when joint contracture is not. Biopsies, incisions in skin altered by Dupuytren's disease, or partial excisions of involved skin or fibrotic cords often result in aggravation and acceleration of fibromatosis and should be avoided.

Pathology

In both palmar and plantar fibromatosis and knuckle pads, the deep dermis or subcutis is replaced by fascicles of spindled fibroblasts separated by bundles of collagen.

Differential Diagnosis

The differential diagnosis of Dupuytren's disease includes ainhum and pseudoainhum.

Treatment

In general, reassurance and observation are appropriate initially if there are no joint contractures and no skin, hygienic, or pain problems associated with the presence of fibrotic tissue. Fasciectomy, the mainstay of treatment, may be indicated if the patient is unable to place the entire palm and palmar surface of each finger on a flat surface simultaneously.

Premature fasciectomy may be associated with early recurrence or progression of fibrosis. Complications associated with delayed fasciectomy include skin deficiency requiring skin grafts, joint stiffness, prolonged edema, pain, wound dehiscence, the loss of palmar skin after hematoma formation resulting from extensive dissection, the recurrence of fibrosis or deformity, and irreparable contracture formation that may require amputation.

ANETODERMA

(CM&S Chapter 103)

Definition and Clinical Description

Anetoderma is a disorder characterized by multiple, well-localized areas of flaccid skin that show histologic loss of elastic fibers. The typical developed lesion consists of a well-circumscribed, small (few millimeters to few centimeters), bag-like outpouching of shiny wrinkled skin that, on palpation, has the characteristic sensation of passage into a herniation defect. Anetoderma is subdivided into primary (idiopathic) and secondary forms: in the primary variant lesions occur in otherwise normal skin; in the secondary variant lesions occur at the site of a previous dermatosis. Examples of conditions that have produced secondary anetoderma include acne, varicella, syphilis, cutaneous lymphomas, granulomatous diseases, xanthomas, and urticaria pigmentosa. Anetoderma must be differentiated from other focal conditions that exhibit either a clinical laxity (or sometimes an atrophy or a protuberance) or a histologic reduction in elastic tissue.

Differential Diagnosis

The differential diagnosis includes atrophoderma, striae, lichen sclerosus et atrophicus, focal dermal hypoplasia, neurofibromas, connective tissue nevi, corticosteroid injection–induced atrophy, and other elastolytic conditions, such as cutis laxa.

Treatment

The current therapy for primary anetoderma is restricted to surgical excision of cosmetically unacceptable lesions; appropriate treatment of secondary anetoderma is largely directed at prevention of future lesions by curtailment of the underlying disorder.

CUTIS LAXA

(CM&S Chapter 104)

Definition and Clinical Description

Cutis laxa is a cutaneous feature of several rare disorders caused by the loss of dermal elastic fibers. This group of disorders, which are both inherited and acquired, cause the skin to hang loosely from lack of recoil. The facial appearance of persons so affected is particularly striking and often referred to as a bloodhound facies. The corners of the mouth sag, giving the individual a mournful appearance. Involvement of the eyelids includes blepharochalasis and ectropion. These manifestations are common to all types of cutis laxa. What differentiates the various inherited and acquired types of cutis laxa are the associated systemic abnormalities.

Inherited Forms of Cutis Laxa

There are three inherited forms of cutis laxa. Two are autosomal recessive, and one is autosomal dominant. The autosomal recessive forms include cutis laxa with emphysema and cutis laxa with retarded development. Cutis laxa associated with emphysema carries the worst prognosis. Cutis laxa is evident at birth with generalized skin laxity, which progresses with age, and normal birth weight. Emphysema may begin in the first few months of life. This complication is associated with recurrent pulmonary infections, cor pulmonale, and death often before age 2 years. Other complications include abnormalities of the great vessels, GI tract, and bladder.

The autosomal dominant form of cutis laxa has a variable age of onset and clinical manifestations that are milder than the recessive form. Facial involvement is common, as is looseness of the "inverse" skin areas such as the neck axillae and popliteal fossae. Associated abnormalities include bronchiectasis, emphysema, pulmonary artery stenosis, inguinal hernias, uterine prolapse, and gastrointestinal diverticula. As with the recessive form the voice is often described as hoarse or deep.

Acquired Forms of Cutis Laxa

Acquired cutis laxa, which usually begins in adulthood, occurs as a generalized progressive disease typically associated with internal manifestations that result from the loss of elastic tissue support. Progressive skin laxity may vary somewhat in distribution, but facial involvement is prominent. Systemic problems include emphysema, diverticula of the gastrointestinal and genitourinary tracts, inguinal hernias, and rectal prolapse. Gastrointestinal involvement is the most common internal manifestation and is often asymptomatic. Death from aortic rupture or emphysema is reported. Inflammatory skin lesions are present in many individuals before or concurrent with the onset of cutaneous laxity.

Pathology

Histologic sections of cutis laxa stained with hematoxylin and eosin are normal. Elastic tissue stains reveal either reduced numbers of elastic fibers or their absence from the papillary and reticular dermis.

Diagnosis and Differential Diagnosis

The differential diagnosis of cutis laxa includes other conditions associated with wrinkled sagging skin such as anetoderma, perifollicular elastolysis, mid-dermal elastolysis, and granulomatous slack skin.

Treatment

There is no effective treatment for the cutaneous manifestations of any of the forms of cutis laxa other than corrective surgery to improve the cosmetic appearance and correct the blepharochalasis.

chapter 6

What Infections and Infestations Affect the Skin?

SKIN INFECTIONS CAUSED BY STAPHYLOCOCCI, STREPTOCOCCI, AND THE RESIDENT CUTANEOUS FLORA

(CM&S Chapter 105)

Cutaneous infections usually occur when trauma, inflammatory skin diseases, excessive hydration, or other processes disrupt the protective mechanisms of the skin. The organisms causing these infections may be part of the resident cutaneous or mucosal flora, or they may originate from sources external to the host. Many pyogenic infections in humans occur from *Staphylococcus aureus* and *Streptococcus pyogenes*, which normally reside on the skin or mucous membranes of some persons.

The main location for *Staphylococcus aureus* is the anterior nares, which it colonizes in about 30% of the normal population. Carriage elsewhere is uncommon. *Staphylococcus aureus* is present on normal skin in less than 5% of the population, but in diseased skin, such as in patients with atopic eczema, skin cultures are positive in nearly all patients. *Streptococcus pyogenes* often inhabits the nasopharynx of healthy persons, but cutaneous colonization is rare.

Impetigo

The most superficial cutaneous infection caused by *Staphylococcus aureus* and *Streptococcus pyogenes* is impetigo. Once regarded as primarily of streptococcal origin, most cases of nonbullous impetigo are due solely to *Staphylococcus aureus*, some to a combination of both organisms, and few to *Streptococcus pyogenes* alone. Impetigo, which is considerably more common in children than adults, usually develops on exposed areas of the skin, especially the face and distal extremities, and typically follows trauma, such as abrasions, insect bites, excoriations from scratching pruritic areas, and cuts. It is more common in hot, humid climates. Poor hygiene is also a predisposing factor, as are crowded living conditions.

Impetigo usually starts as red papules that transform into vesicles and pustules, which, because they are located in the superficial epidermis, rupture readily to create thick, adherent, honey-colored crusts surmounting an enlarging, erythematous base. The lesions, which are often numerous, may be pruritic but are not usually painful and are sometimes associated with tender regional lymph node enlargement. On the face impetigo is commonly periorificial, and in any location the lesions may coalesce to form large areas of exudation and crusting. Cultures of impetigo will usually yield the responsible pathogens but are often unnecessary in clinically obvious cases.

Sometimes, impetigo is self-limited, but treatment will relieve symptoms more rapidly, halt the formation of new lesions, and promote more prompt resolution for those already present. Systemic antimicrobial therapy is very effective. Treatment should be directed against both *Staphylococcus aureus* and *Streptococcus pyogenes*. In most locales oral erythromycin remains effective, but resistant staphylococci may be frequent, and alternatives include dicloxacillin or an oral first-generation cephalosporin such as cephalexin or cephradine. The best topical agent is mupirocin, which, when applied three times a day for 7 to 8 days, is equivalent in efficacy to oral erythromycin. Widespread lesions, involvement of several family members, and the inability to eradicate streptococci from the respiratory tract, which may sometimes be a reservoir for reinfection or spread of the organism to others, make topical treatment less advantageous. This later limitation of topical therapy is especially of concern in epidemic situations or when the streptococci are ''nephritogenic strains,'' those uncommon isolates of *Streptococcus pyogenes* capable of initiating poststreptococcal glomerulonephritis. Cutaneous infections caused by *Streptococcus pyogenes* do not lead to another nonsuppurative complication, acute rheumatic fever, which occurs only after respiratory infections with the organism.

Unlike the nonbullous form, bullous impetigo is strictly due to certain strains of *Staphylococcus aureus*, primarily phage II, group 71, which produce a toxin, exfoliatin, that causes cleavage in the granular layer of the epidermis. When produced in the localized skin infection of bullous impetigo it causes vesicles and bullae to form on an erythematous base. When generalized, this toxin is responsible for the staphylococcal scalded skin syndrome. Intact bullae may be present often only as erosions, which may coalesce to form large, clearly demarcated areas surrounded by erythema.

Appropriate therapy for bullous impetigo is an oral agent active against *Staphylococcus aureus*, such as erythromycin, a first-generation cephalosporin, or dicloxacillin. Topical mupirocin is an alternative. In areas where the risk of impetigo is high, its frequency can be reduced in children by applying topical neomycin-bacitracin prophylactically to areas of minor trauma.

Ecthyma

Ecthyma refers to an infection resembling impetigo but located deeper in the skin. It is caused by *Streptococcus pyogenes*, *Staphylococcus aureus*, or a combination of the two, and it produces ulceration that reaches the dermis and heals with scarring. It usually occurs in patients with preceding trauma, frequently in the setting of poor hygiene, and commonly affects the lower extremities, often with several lesions. It begins with pustules and vesicles that deepen, leading to ulcerations typically covered with thick, adherent crusts with surrounding erythema. Treatment should be an oral anti-microbial agent with activity against both *Staphylococcus aureus* and *Streptococcus pyogenes*, such as dicloxacillin.

Folliculitis

Folliculitis, inflammation of the epithelium of the hair follicle, is a common dermatologic problem with several different causes, including several infections. Organisms beneath an obstructed follicular ostium can proliferate, causing follicular inflammation and purulence. Sometimes, *Staphylococcus aureus* is isolated from the pus. Staphylococcal folliculitis has been most common in children, appearing usually on the scalp or extremities. Erythematous papules or pustules surrounding hairs may occur singly or in crops; this disorder responds promptly to systemic antistaphylococcal antimicrobial therapy.

Furuncles and Carbuncles

When staphylococci infect the hair follicle at a deeper level than in folliculitis, the inflammation extends to the dermis, causing furuncles or carbuncles. An inflammatory nodule develops, topped by a pustule through which a hair emerges. Individual lesions, called furuncles or boils, can appear anywhere on the hairy skin but are most common on the legs and face. Infection involving several adjacent follicles (carbuncles) typically occurs on the back of the neck. Moist heat, which may promote drainage, is often satisfactory therapy for small furuncles; incision and drainage are required for larger furuncles and for carbuncles. Unless substantial surrounding cellulitis or fever is present, systemic antistaphylococcal antibiotics are usually unnecessary.

Recurrent Staphylococcal Skin Infections

Some patients are afflicted by recurrent episodes of staphylococcal skin infections. Although diabetics, dialysis patients, intravenous drug abusers, and individuals with immunologic diseases are predisposed, most patients have no obvious underlying disorder and are probably chronic staphylococcal nasal carriers who disperse the organisms onto the skin, where trauma, often mild and inapparent, allows the staphylococci to invade the skin and cause infections. Attempts to eliminate staphylococcal carriage are generally ineffective. The most effective topical medication is mupirocin, which often eliminates *Staphylococcus aureus* for long periods even after the course of application has ended. Unfortunately, widespread or protracted use has led to the emergence of resistance to the drug. Effective oral antibiotics include rifampin and the fluoroquinolones, such as ciprofloxacin, but resistance to these agents is a major concern when they are used alone. Clindamycin, probably the best antimicrobial agent for this purpose, is given as a single 150-mg tablet daily for 3 months.

Erysipelas and Cellulitis

Erysipelas and cellulitis are acute, rapidly spreading, nonsuppurative infections of the skin and underlying soft tissues but not including the muscle. Erysipelas is more superficial than cellulitis and involves predominantly the upper part of the dermis. Cellulitis affects the deep dermis and subcutaneous fat. The diagnostic difference, sharp delineation in erysipelas but less clear differentiation in cellulitis, is frequently difficult to appreciate, and, for many, the term *erysipelas* applies only to facial involvement. Erysipelas so defined is most common in the elderly. It may occur after obvious facial injury or without any apparent cause, and typically affects the cheeks, often spreading across the nasal bridge to form a butterfly pattern. From this area and other common sites such as the forehead and ears, the process may spread to the eyelids. It is usually a painful, sometimes pruritic, bright-red, spreading edema on which vesicles, bullae, and exudation may develop. It is hot and tender to the touch. Fever and chills are common, but not invariable, accompaniments. Erysipelas is considered to be a streptococcal infection, usually due to group A (*Streptococcus pyogenes*) but sometimes to other groups, such as G and C.

Cellulitis commonly involves the extremities, particularly the calf area. Preceding trauma, an ulcer, other damaged skin from which the infection emanates, and lymphedema are predisposing factors. Classically, a small fissure in the skin, particularly in the toe webs from tinea pedis, is the source of infection. As in erysipelas, fever and chills may accompany, or even precede, the cutaneous findings, but many patients are afebrile and do not appear seriously ill. The skin is red, hot, and edematous; the margin of the inflammation is irregular; and, as in erysipelas, vesicles, bullae, and exudation of fluid from the surface of the lesion may occur.

The clinical diagnosis of cellulitis is usually simple. The differential diagnosis includes venous thrombosis, and acute gout.

A definitive bacteriologic diagnosis of erysipelas and cellulitis is difficult to obtain. Culture of a needle aspirate, skin biopsy, or blood are usually negative.

Treatment of erysipelas and cellulitis includes local measures and antimicrobial agents. The affected inflamed area should be elevated, and cool, moist dressings may help relieve discomfort.

Because erysipelas is nearly always streptococcal, the treatment of choice remains penicillin, given by mouth or parenterally, depending on the severity of the infection and the ability of the patient to take oral medications. Benzathine penicillin, as a single, 1.2 million-unit intramuscular dose, is very effective for outpatient management. In severely ill patients requiring hospitalization, intravenous aqueous penicillin G is the drug of choice; a first-generation cephalosporin (e.g., cefazolin), clindamycin, and vancomycin are alternatives.

Many clinicians are concerned about the possible role of *Staphylococcus aureus* in cellulitis and employ an agent active against both pathogens. For oral therapy, erythromycin, dicloxacillin, clindamycin, and a first-generation cephalosporin such as cephradine or cephalexin are reasonable choices. Parenteral therapy for hospitalized patients could include an antistaphylococcal penicillin such as nafcillin or oxacillin or a first-generation cephalosporin such as cefazolin.

Patients treated for erysipelas or cellulitis often appear to worsen in the first 1 or 2 days of antimicrobial therapy. These apparently worrisome features are probably due to the dying organisms suddenly releasing enzymes. No change in antimicrobial therapy is necessary, and improvement is usually evident within a day or so.

Some patients have recurrent episodes of erysipelas or cellulitis. Each attack probably causes some lymphatic damage from inflammation and scarring, which may increase the likelihood of further episodes. Lymphatic injury from other causes, such as surgery and any long-standing or permanent cutaneous injury such as from a preceding saphenous venectomy imposes a similar risk.

In patients with recurrent cellulitis in the same location, any remediable predisposing skin condition, such as tinea pedis, eczema, or dry skin should be treated. If recurrences continue, effective prophylactic programs include monthly intramuscular injections of benzathine penicillin, or oral penicillin or erythromycin given daily or for 1 week once a month.

Resident Flora As Cutaneous Pathogens

Cutaneous Abscesses

Staphylococcus aureus is isolated in only about 25% of cutaneous abscesses. The location of the abscess determines the identity of the infecting flora. *S. aureus* is present in more than 50% of finger paronychiae, breast abscesses in puerperal women, and axillary abscesses. It is isolated in 20% to 40% of breast abscesses in nonpuerperal women, toe paronychiae, and abscesses of the hands, buttocks, extremities, trunk, and inguinal areas.

When *S. aureus* is not the cause, the bacteriology is usually anaerobes alone or a mixture of aerobic and anaerobic organisms, typically members of the resident regional flora or transients from contiguous mucous membranes. Abscesses of the perineal area and buttocks regions commonly grow fecal flora, such as anaerobic gram-positive cocci, streptococci, and *Bacteroides* species. Abscesses of the head and neck typically yield *Staphylococcus epidermidis*, *Propionibacterium* species, and anaerobic gram-positive cocci.

Cutaneous abscesses are usually tender, erythematous, fluctuant masses, sometimes with a purulent top. Removal of the pus by incision and drainage is the appropriate therapy; leaving the resultant cavity open, packing it with gauze, or suturing the incision are therapeutic alternatives with different proponents. Gram stain and culture of the pus are usually unnecessary, as is antibiotic therapy, which should be reserved for those patients with extensive surrounding cellulitis, seriously impaired host defenses, cutaneous gangrene, or systemic manifestations of infection.

Erythrasma

Erythrasma is characterized by red to brown scaling patches. It is apparently caused by coryneforms, most likely *Corynebacterium minutissimum*. Usually producing no symptoms, erythrasma tends to affect intertriginous areas such as the groin, submammary regions, axillae, and toe webs, probably because the high moisture content, friction, and maceration damage the stratum corneum, allowing this organism to proliferate. Diabetes mellitus, increasing age, obesity, and residence in tropical climates are predisposing factors. The most common form of erythrasma, which may occur in 20% or more of the population, affects the toe webs, especially the fourth interspace, producing scaling, fissuring, and maceration. Elsewhere, the typical lesions are irregular, scaly, slightly brown or erythematous patches with well-demarcated borders.

Because these infecting organisms produce porphyrins, the involved areas fluoresce coral-pink to orange-red with ultraviolet light from Wood's lamp. This test confirms the diagnosis; cultures are not rewarding.

Vigorous washing with soap sometimes suffices as treatment. Another approach is topical therapy with azoles, except ketoconazole, which have activity against some gram-positive bacteria as well as fungi. Topical erythromycin, clindamycin, and Whitfield's ointment are also effective, as is oral erythromycin.

Trichomycosis Axillaris

Yellow, red, or black waxy nodules forming on axillary hair characterize trichomycosis axillaris. They may fluoresce various colors under Wood's light. Similar lesions occasionally occur on pubic or facial hair. This process is produced by large colonies of coryneform bacteria coating the cuticular layers of the hair and perhaps elaborating enzymes that partly destroy the superficial hair keratins. The disorder occurs primarily in patients who have poor personal hygiene, sweat excessively, and do not use deodorants. Shaving the hair and using axillary deodorants are usually successful in treating the disease. Topical clindamycin or erythromycin may also be effective.

Axillary Odor

Studies on axillary flora indicate that common isolates are gram-positive cocci (including *Staphylococcus* and *Micrococcus* species) and coryneforms. Persons with a coryneform-dominant flora have a more intense axillary odor. Sterile apocrine sweat has no smell, but when incubated with lipophilic or large-colony coryneforms, axillary odor is reproduced. A principal action of many axillary deodorants lies in their antibacterial properties.

Pitted Keratolysis

Pitted keratolysis is the presence of pits 1 to 7 mm in diameter on the soles or, less commonly, collarettes on the palms. Patients are usually asymptomatic, but pruritus, burning, pain, and tenderness may be present, as may a cheesy malodor. Scaling, erythema, and fissuring may occur, and sometimes the pitted areas coalesce to form larger erosions and erythematous plaques. Pitted keratolysis seems to occur in association with increased moisture from occlusive footwear, frequent contact with water, or excessive sweating. Coryneform bacteria appear responsible for this disorder and may produce enzymes that digest keratin to create the pits or erosions in the stratum corneum. Several therapies seem to be effective, including topical azoles such as miconazole and clotrimazole (which are active against many gram-positive bacteria); topical erythromycin or clindamycin; antiseptics, such as glutaraldehyde and formaldehyde; and oral erythromycin.

Interdigital Toe Space Infections

Interdigital toe space infections or ''athlete's foot'' usually begins as scaling and fissuring. Although some of the infections are erythrasma, dermatophytes are present in about 85% of cases and the normal flora is increased in density. As the infection becomes more severe and maceration develops, the normal flora, especially large-colony coryneforms including *Brevibacterium epidermidis* and *Corynebacterium minutissimum*, continues to proliferate, and other bacteria become more prevalent, including gram-negative bacilli and *Staphylococcus aureus*. Cultures for dermatophytes are positive in about 60%. As ''athlete's foot'' becomes more severe, characterized by redness, maceration, itching, and malodor, cultures yield less dermatophytes, more numerous normal flora, a marked increase in gram-negative bacilli and large-colony coryneforms and the occasional presence of *Pseudomonas*.

In mild interdigital infections dermatophytes are the main cause, and antifungal agents should suffice in most cases. In moderately severe infections, all azoles, which are active against both fungi and the bacteria, are the treatment of choice. Drying the interspaces by removal of footwear, separation of the toes, and application of astringents such as aluminum chloride may also be helpful in severe cases.

STAPHYLOCOCCAL TOXIN-MEDIATED SYNDROMES

(CM&S Chapter 106)

Toxic Shock Syndrome

Clinical Description

Staphylococcal toxic shock syndrome (TSS) is characterized by sudden onset of high fever associated with vomiting, diarrhea, headache, pharyngitis, profound myalgia, and significant hypotension. It is caused by infection with certain toxin-producing strains of *Staphylococcus aureus* in persons lacking protective antibodies at the time of infection. Toxic shock syndrome toxin-1 (TSST-1) is one of the significant mediators of pathogenicity in TSS. Multisystem organ involvement is an additional characteristic feature that results from both poor tissue perfusion and direct damage from mediators. Potentially fatal complications include refractory shock, oliguric renal failure, ventricular arrhythmia, disseminated intravascular coagulation, and adult respiratory distress syndrome. Although initially described in menstruating women, TSS can occur in patients of either sex, of any age, and within various settings of occult, trivial, or severe staphylococcal infection.

Both cutaneous and mucocutaneous findings are prominent in TSS. A diffuse, flexurally accentuated, scarlatiniform exanthem appears early in the illness. The eruption initially may appear over the trunk, but inevitably it spreads to the arms and legs. Petechiae, vesicles, and bullae are uncommon. Erythema and edema of the palms and soles occur frequently. ''Strawberry tongue'' may occur along with intense erythema of the mucous membranes and conjunctivae.

Generalized desquamation with prominent sheet-like peeling of the hands and feet usually occurs between 10 and 21 days after presentation. A late-onset, pruritic, generalized macular and papular skin eruption, appearing 9 to 13 days after initial onset of symptoms, has been described. Reversible patchy alopecia and shedding of fingernails may also occur. The diagnosis requires the identification of clinical criteria, as delineated by the case definition (Table 6–1).

Pathology

Characteristic histopathologic findings include sparse infiltrates of lymphocytes, neutrophils, and sometimes eosinophils around vessels of the superficial plexus and small foci of spongiosis, some of which have clusters of necrotic keratinocytes accompanied by neutrophils.

Differential Diagnosis

The differential diagnosis of TSS includes Kawasaki disease, erythema multiforme, Rocky Mountain spotted fever, rubeola, leptospirosis, and enteroviral infections. In recent years, cases of a severe TSS-like streptococcal disease have appeared, associated with reemergence of type A (and type B) pyrogenic exotoxin-producing streptococci.

Treatment

Prompt intervention is the key to the successful management of the shock and the resulting multiorgan involvement in TSS. Removal of infected foreign bodies, drainage of infected sites, and institution of penicillinase-resistant antistaphylococcal antibiotics are essential to eradicate the focus of toxin-producing organisms.

TABLE 6-1. Clinical Features of Toxic Shock Syndrome

Fever, with temperature greater than 38.9°C (102°F)
Diffuse macular or scarlatiniform skin eruption
Desquamation, 1 to 2 weeks after onset of illness
Hypotension
Involvement of three or more organ systems:
  Gastrointestinal (usually vomiting and diarrhea)
  Muscular
  Mucous membrane erythema
  Renal
  Hepatic
  Hematologic (platelet count less than 100,000/mm³)
  Central nervous system
Efforts should be made to rule out other treatable causes of
  illness (i.e., Rocky Mountain spotted fever, leptospirosis)

Massive volume replacement may be needed in the setting of severe intravascular volume depletion accompanied by both a decrease in vasomotor tone and capillary leakage. Cardiovascular support may be necessary, including both inotropic and antiarrhythmic measures. Pediatric patients may require ventilatory support for respiratory distress more often than adult patients. Metabolic acidosis, hypomagnesemia, hypocalcemia, and hypophosphatemia may accompany renal disease, requiring aggressive monitoring and management.

Systemic corticosteroids have been used in the management of severely affected hypotensive patients who are not responsive to removal or drainage of the focus of infection and several hours of fluid administration. Administration of immune globulin (400 mg/kg as single dose infused over 2 to 3 hours) is a rational approach to providing specific neutralizing antibody to patients with TSS who typically lack immunity to TSST-1 (or enterotoxins).

Staphylococcal Scalded Skin Syndrome

Clinical Description

Staphylococcal scalded skin syndrome (SSSS), also known as Ritter's disease, is a potentially life-threatening but treatable, toxin–mediated manifestation of localized infection with certain strains of staphylococci. SSSS results from the effects of one of the two epidermolytic toxins: ET-A and ET-B.

Bullous impetigo, the most common expression of the SSSS spectrum, is caused by a localized skin infection with epidermolytic toxin–producing staphylococci. Bullous impetigo is rarely associated with systemic illness, occurs predominantly in children, but is also seen in adults. The lesions of bullous impetigo contain staphylococci.

Infections leading to SSSS typically originate in the nasopharynx and frequently go unrecognized. Other primary foci of infection leading to SSSS have included the umbilicus, urinary tract, conjunctivae, and blood. Sudden onset of fever, irritability, cutaneous tenderness, and scarlatiniform erythema herald the syndrome. The erythema is often accentuated in flexural and periorificial areas. This generalized involvement leads to the clinical appearance of scalded skin. Flaccid blisters and erosions develop within 24 to 48 hours. The blisters and erosions yield no organisms when sampled for bacterial culture. Important clinical clues to diagnosis include prominent denudation in areas of mechanical stress, easy disruption of skin with firm rubbing (Nikolsky's sign), and skin tenderness. Occasionally, erythema and desquamation occur without bulla formation. A facies with conjunctival inflammation and circumoral erythema evolving to prominent crusting is characteristically seen a few days into the course of the skin disease. Recovery from SSSS is common, but sepsis as well as serous fluid and electrolyte disturbances can lead to morbidity and mortality.

Epidemiology

SSSS is predominantly a disease of infancy and early childhood, with most cases seen before the age of 5. Factors responsible for the age distribution include renal immaturity leading to decreased toxin clearance in neonates and lack of immunity to the toxins.

Pathology

Bullous impetigo is characterized by a blister whose roof is composed of the granular and cornified layers and whose cavity contains neutrophils. SSSS is an acantholytic intraepidermal blistering process, in which clefts appear in the granular layer or just beneath the stratum corneum. The histopathologic differential diagnosis includes the superficial forms of pemphigus, bullous impetigo, SSSS, and subcorneal pustular dermatosis

Differential Diagnosis

The differential diagnosis of SSSS is identical to that of TSS.

Treatment

Therapy for SSSS in affected patients should be directed toward eradication of staphylococci from the focus of infection, which generally requires intravenous penicillinase-resistant antistaphylococcal antibiotics. Antibiotics, supportive skin care, and appropriate attention to fluid and electrolyte management in the presence of disrupted barrier function will usually ensure rapid recovery. Control measures should be applied, including strict enforcement of chlorhexidine hand washing, oral antibiotic therapy for infected workers, and mupirocin ointment for eradication of persistent nasal carriage.

SKIN INFECTIONS CAUSED BY UNUSUAL BACTERIAL PATHOGENS

(CM&S Chapter 107)

Endogenous Skin Infections

Haemophilus influenzae Infections

Haemophilus influenzae are pleomorphic, gram-negative, coccobacillary organisms. They are primarily respiratory tract pathogens. Most severe infections with *H. influenzae*, including meningitis, pneumonia, epiglottitis, and cellulitis, are caused by encapsulated type b strains. Greatest susceptibility to *H. influenzae* type b infection occurs at 3 months to about 3 years of age.

In healthy young children, *H. influenzae* is frequently part of the upper respiratory tract flora. Cellulitis caused by *H. influenzae* type b usually accompanies an upper respiratory tract infection or otitis media. Typically in a young child with an upper respiratory tract infection an edematous and erythematous area develops on the face or upper body accompanied by high fever. The margins of the skin infection are usually indistinct. In infants, a characteristic purplish cellulitis has been described. Marked tenderness and swelling may develop. The presence of buccal cellulitis is frequently accompanied by otitis media; the mechanism of this association is unclear. The patients are often acutely ill with a high fever, leukocytosis, and lethargy. Bacteremia is present about one half of the time. During the illness, one must be on the lookout for complications of *H. influenzae* sepsis, including meningitis.

H. influenzae type b cellulitis is unusual in adults. It usually begins with pharyngitis and may progress rapidly to dysphagia, neck swelling, and erythema. Although the purplish hue of the cellulitis has also been reported in adults, most cases are indistinguishable morphologically from common streptococcal cellulitis.

Immunization against *H. influenzae* type b with conjugated ribosylribitol phosphate polymers, the capsular antigen of the organism, has decreased the incidence of infections with the organisms, including cellulitis.

Streptococcus pneumoniae *Infections*

Streptococcus pneumoniae, or the pneumococcus, is the most common cause of bacterial pneumonia and frequently a part of the respiratory flora in healthy adults. Although it is an aggressive pathogen, it infrequently infects the skin. Most of the cases occur in chronically ill or immunocompromised patients and manifest as soft tissue infections, including cellulitis. Characteristics of pneumococcal cellulitis include face or upper body involvement, brawny erythema, bullae, a purplish color, and pneumococcal bacteremia.

Pseudomonas aeruginosa *Infections*

Pseudomonas aeruginosa is a ubiquitous, gram-negative, aerobic bacillus responsible for frequent and often distinctive skin infections. It is found widely in wet areas in the environment. In healthy persons the organism colonizes moist parts of the body such as web spaces or the external auditory canal about 5% of the time and the bowel flora up to 20% of the time. Even a larger percentage of hospitalized patients are colonized. *P. aeruginosa* becomes pathogenic when local tissue conditions foster overgrowth or when altered host defenses become permissive. The infections vary from life-threatening septicemia to serious localized infections such as otitis to the more common manifestations of bacterial overgrowth in moist cutaneous areas. Skin lesions secondary to *P. aeruginosa* septicemia may be diagnostic.

Paronychiae typically occur in those persons with occupational chronic water immersion of the hands, such as bartenders or nurses. Acute paronychiae are often caused by *S. aureus* and characterized by pain, swelling, erythema, and purulence. In chronic infection, *P. aeruginosa* and *Candida albicans* are usually etiologic. Chronic paronychiae are characterized by intermittent tenderness and erythema, resulting in often extensive nail dystrophy. In the case of *Pseudomonas,* green to blue discoloration of the nail may be seen either diffusely or in bands reflecting intermittent infectious activity.

Pseudomonas overgrowth in moist, intertriginous areas such as toe web spaces is usually characterized by superficial erosions with exudation. The typical fruity smell of *P. aeruginosa* or the pigment production may be evident. In the moist external auditory canal, *Pseudomonas* organisms often overgrow, causing inflammation with swelling, discomfort, and discharge. This ''swimmer's ear'' or external otitis is common.

When external otitis becomes invasive, it may involve the cartilage of the pinna, causing intense swelling and pain. In its most severe form the infection spreads to the soft tissues at the base of the skull, often causing multiple cranial neuropathies and osteomyelitis of the base of the skull. Although this scenario is usually seen in diabetics, normal elderly patients may also be afflicted. Minor trauma or a surgical procedure can trigger conversion of a pesky external otitis to an invasive, life-threatening infection, sometimes called malignant external otitis. Early treatment can be life saving.

Pseudomonas folliculitis is a common infection occurring in persons exposed to closed-cycle recreational water sources such as hot tubs or pools. The organisms are able to resist relatively high temperatures and chlorine levels, making them very difficult to eradicate. The clinical picture is characterized by erythematous papulopustular lesions on the trunk and proximal extremities 2 to 4 days after exposure. Prolonged exposure with maceration of the skin is a risk factor. *Pseudomonas* colonization of the skin does not result in folliculitis unless there is concomitant superhydration of the skin from occlusion. External otitis or intertriginous infection may be seen along with folliculitis. Malaise and low-grade fever have been reported.

In the normal host, *Pseudomonas* folliculitis is usually self-limited. Immunocompromised patients with *Pseudomonas* folliculitis rapidly develop progressive infection and require aggressive treatment.

Gram-Negative Folliculitis

Gram-negative folliculitis is the term used to describe the infection of facial lesions of acne vulgaris with various gram-negative bacilli. It is usually seen in patients on long-term oral antibiotic treatment for acne. Lactose-fermenting Enterobacteriaceae such as *Escherichia coli* or *Klebsiella aerogenes* are responsible for superficial pustules in 80% of the patients. *Proteus* species cause deep nodular lesions in about 20% of patients. *P. aeruginosa* may also cause gram-negative folliculitis; often this is associated with *Pseudomonas* external otitis. Usually, discontinuation of the long-term antibiotic therapy and specific systemic antibiotic treatment for the offending gram-negative bacillus is curative.

Wound Infections

Clostridium perfringens and other clostridial species cause a characteristic wound infection—anaerobic cellulitis. The rapidly spreading infection occurs postoperatively, after dirty surgery or a wound resulting in devitalized tissue. The infection usually results in the accumulation of large amounts of tissue gas, causing crepitus, swelling, and often very little other cutaneous change. This type of clostridial cellulitis is readily cured with minor debridement and antibiotics. If muscle becomes involved, the clinical picture is dramatically altered and a pesky cellulitis becomes a life-threatening infection, clostridial myonecrosis, or gas gangrene. The transition is usually marked by the development of severe pain. The patient with clostridial myonecrosis is acutely ill and may require extensive debridement to remove all involved muscle.

Necrotizing fasciitis is an aggressive cellulitis centered in the superficial fascia and subcutaneous tissue. The causative organisms are Enterobacteriaceae, *Bacteroides fragilis*, *Streptococcus pyogenes*, and *Vibrio vulnificus*. The outstanding characteristic of necrotizing fasciitis is the extensive undermining of the tissue caused by the necrosis in the superficial fascia. Because nerves and blood vessels that penetrate the fascia are often damaged, clinically one sees patchy necrosis and anesthesia of the overlying skin. Necrotizing fasciitis must be considered when the cellulitis is atypical or does not respond to appropriate treatment for the usual streptococcal cellulitis.

Fournier's gangrene is a unique necrotizing fasciitis that usually involves the genitalia of middle-aged men, but any age male can be infected. The illness, which often occurs in diabetics, may be explosive in onset and progression. The infection can spread anteriorly up the abdominal wall or posteriorly through the perineum. Most of the patients have predisposing trauma, which may be perianal suppuration, local trauma, or perineal surgery. Usually, mixed bowel organisms are etiologic in Fournier's gangrene.

Exogenous Skin Infections

Vibrio vulnificus *Infections*

V. vulnificus is a noncholera vibrio that grows in saltwater. The organism is found widely in warmer coastal waters and infects up to 10% of raw shellfish on the market in the United States. *V. vulnificus* is virulent in normal as well as compromised hosts.

Two distinct clinical syndromes caused by *V. vulnificus* predominate. The first is a bacteremia following ingestion of the organism, almost always related to consumption of raw oysters. Seeding of the soft tissues regularly occurs during *V. vulnificus* bacteremia with resultant bullous cellulitis. Fasciitis, myositis, and necrotic skin ulcers are also reported during bacteremia. As with other causes of gram-negative septicemia, shock is common and, when it occurs, the end result is usually fatal. Most of the patients with primary *V. vulnificus* bacteremia have liver disease (usually cirrhosis).

Gastroenteritis without bacteremia is seen with *V. vulnificus* ingestion, as well as with other vibrios such as *V. parahaemolyticus*, *V. damsela*, and non-01 *V. cholerae*. Consequent bacteremia and its sequelae are essentially limited to impaired hosts.

The second clinical syndrome of *V. vulnificus* infection occurs when wounds are contaminated by sea water, often related to trauma during water sports or fishing. The severity of infection varies from a mild cellulitis to cellulitis with bullae and gangrenous areas to necrotizing fasciitis. Bacteremia with its severe sequelae may also occur when wound infection is primary.

Erysipelothrix rhusiopathiae *Infections*

Erysipelothrix rhusiopathiae, a pleomorphic gram-positive rod, is another organism responsible for skin infection following trauma in a marine environment, as well as occupational infections. From animals the organisms contaminate the environment. There the organisms can persist in water (including sea water) for weeks. Infection following trauma is seen in fish, meat, and poultry handlers as well as farmers.

Skin infection is the usual manifestation of infection with *E. rhusiopathiae,* although rarely systemic disease is reported. The usual manifestation is erysipeloid, a distinctive cellulitis. Lesions usually begin on the fingers or hands at sites of trauma. Purplish-red indurated plaques develop and extend peripherally, often with central clearing. Hemorrhagic vesicles may occur in the involved area. There may be stiffness of joints in the area and local pain. The infection spreads slowly and usually runs a self-limited course over about 3 weeks. The pace of the infection is slow compared with erysipelas, from which the name erysipeloid was derived. Occasionally there is associated fever, malaise, regional lymphadenopathy, and diffuse arthralgias. The rarely occurring systemic disease is associated with endocarditis about 90% of the time.

Bite-Associated Infections

Soft tissue infections frequently follow animal or insect bites. When secondary wound infections occur, the usual etiologic agents of pyodermas, namely, *Staphylococcus aureus* and *Streptococcus pyogenes,* are the cause. There are, however, a few exogenous bacteria that cause characteristic infections following bites. Lyme borreliosis and the skin lesions of erythema migrans that may result from the bite of an infected deer tick are discussed in Chapter 6 (Chapter 109 in CM&S). *Yersinia pestis* infection, or plague, is secondary to rat flea bites; usually no skin lesions are seen in plague.

The salivary flora of dogs and cats is complex, and bite wound infections are frequently polymicrobial. *Pasteurella multocida,* a gram-negative coccobaccillus, is present in the mouth of the majority of cats and is frequently present in dog saliva. It may cause serious epizootic infection in a variety of animals. Often within hours after a bite, pain, swelling, erythema, and purulent or serosanguineous drainage result from infection with the organism. The hand is frequently infected because it is the most common bite site, and local complications of osteomyelitis, tenosynovitis, or arthritis may occur. Low-grade fever, lymphadenopathy, and, rarely, bacteremia are seen.

Tularemia (rabbit fever or deer fly fever) is caused by infection with *Francisella tularensis,* a small gram-negative coccobaccillus that is widely distributed in animals and insects. It is spread by contact with infected animal fluids, usually those of rabbits. Humans become infected by the cutaneous route, probably through inapparent breaks in the skin rather than by penetration through intact skin. Less commonly, the organism enters through pulmonary or ocular mucous membranes. Vector-borne tularemia is becoming increasingly important. Bites of insect vectors, usually the tick or deer fly, and, rarely, bites from other animals, including cats, are responsible. In 75% to 85% of the patients, cutaneous inoculation yields an inflammatory papule or an area of cellulitis that ulcerates and crusts. Fever, chills, headache, and painful regional lymphadenopathy complete the usual clinical presentation. Several other clinical syndromes of tularemia are seen in the absence of cutaneous lesions, including glandular, typhoidal, oculoglandular, and oropharyngeal tularemia.

Disseminated Skin Infections

Good examples of systemic infections that involve the skin in a characteristic way are the cutaneous abscesses or the purulent petechiae that may occur secondary to high-grade bacteremia in staphylococcal endocarditis. Skin lesions are commonly seen during episodes of endocarditis of various causes. Most often, the skin lesions reflect vasculitis rather than metastatic infection. Osler's nodes, Janeway lesions, and the petechiae seen in endocarditis are all secondary to manifestations of a vasculitis.

In acute meningococcemia, three types of skin lesions are seen: (1) early, a transient urticarial or macular eruption may occur; (2) later, one may see the purpura of disseminated intravascular coagulation; and (3) the most characteristic skin lesions in meningococcemia are purulent petechiae. These are manifestations of a septic vasculitis with fibrin thrombi in the lumina of venules, organisms, and polymorphonuclear leukocytes in vessel walls and sparse perivascular infiltrates of neutrophils without leukocytoclasis. Extravasation of red blood cells yields petechiae that develop gray to yellow centers as the organism multiplies and more white blood cells accumulate.

The clinical picture in disseminated gonococcal infection is characteristic and often the only way to make the diagnosis. In women, it is manifested by the abrupt onset of fever, chills, and joint pain, usually at the time of menses. An acral eruption occurs, characterized by a small number of lesions that tend to be concentrated near joints; it consists of erythematous papules that evolve into hemorrhagic vesicles. Migratory tenosynovitis completes the usual clinical picture. Since blood cultures and cultures of the skin lesions may be negative, it is essential to recognize and think of this clinical picture. Cultures of the uterine cervix, if done during the episode of disseminated gonococcal infection, will often be positive for *Neisseria gonorrhoeae*. Biopsy of a papulopustule in a patient with gonococcemia reveals thrombi in small vessels and dense dermal infiltrates of neutrophils, which accumulate in an edematous papillary dermis. Organisms are exceedingly rare, and tissue staining with Gram stain is almost always negative. Immunofluorescent examination has shown gonococcal antigens in pustular lesions, however.

Several types of skin lesions may occur during the course of *Pseudomonas* septicemia. The organism has a predilection to settle and multiply in the walls of small vessels, especially veins, in the skin, causing a necrotizing vasculitis, usually with sparing of the intima. The overgrowth of organisms in *Pseudomonas* septicemia can be so dramatic that they are visible as basophilic encrustations that obscure the walls of blood vessels in biopsy specimens. In some immunosuppressed hosts, this picture is seen in the absence of inflammatory cells. There is extravasation of red blood cells and often extensive perivascular edema and necrosis with consequent interference with blood supply. Organisms spread through the vessels and invade the skin. This process results in the several different morphologic types of skin lesions, which include:

1. Vesicles and bullae.
2. Ecthyma gangrenosum, which is a sharply demarcated, painless, indurated, necrotic ulcer or eschar with surrounding erythema, is often present in the anogenital area or other apocrine gland areas.

3. Macules, papules, and focal gangrenous cellulitis may also occur.

In typhoid fever due to *Salmonella typhi*, rose spots are regularly seen. It is unusual to see rose spots in other enteric fevers. They occur early in the course during the acute febrile period. They are raised, pink, blanchable, nontender papules a few millimeters in size. Crops of 10 to 20 lesions occur, usually on the trunk, and they fade gradually over several days. Biopsy reveals a dilated dermal vessel infiltrated with macrophages that may contain intracellular organisms.

One does not usually think of syphilitic skin lesions as due to bacteremic spread to the skin, but indeed secondary lesions are just that. After the primary lesion or chancre, there is a spirochetemia, and organisms are deposited in the dermal vessels. The various skin manifestations of secondary syphilis reflect multiplication of the organisms in the skin and the subsequent tissue response.

Bacteremic spread of *V. vulnificus* to the skin causing often multiple areas of cellulitis has been referred to earlier.

Diagnosis

The staphylococcal and streptococcal pyodermas discussed in Chapter 6 (Chapter 105 of CM&S) constitute the majority of bacterial skin infections. One should be concerned about a different infectious process in three clinical situations: (1) when the infection does not fit the clinical picture of the typical pyoderma, or the infection does not respond promptly to standard therapy for staphylococcal or streptococcal cutaneous infections; (2) when the host is impaired in his or her ability to combat infections; and (3) when there is an epidemiologic history of potential exposure to an unusual cutaneous pathogen.

Treatment

The principles of treating cutaneous bacterial infections are the same as those that apply to all bacterial infections: (1) accumulations of pus must be drained; (2) necrotic tissue must be debrided; and (3) antibiotic treatment must be guided ultimately by sensitivity determinations but initially by an educated guess. Treatment recommendations for many of the infections discussed are presented (Table 6–2).

SYPHILIS AND THE TREPONEMATOSES

(CM&S Chapter 108)

Definition

Syphilis is an acute or chronic infectious disease caused by the spirochete *Treponema pallidum*. It is usually sexually transmitted during infectious stages of the disease, except in the case of congenital syphilis, which is spread from mother to fetus. Classically, the disease passes through four stages: primary stage, secondary stage,

TABLE 6-2. Treatment of Some Uncommon Cutaneous Bacterial Infections

INFECTION	TREATMENT
Haemophilus influenzae cellulitis	Ampicillin/clavulanic acid, second-generation cephalosporin
Pseudomonas infections	Fluoroquinolones
Gram-negative folliculitis	Stop anti-acne antibiotic; treat based on results of sensitivity studies
Clostridial cellulitis	Debridement and penicillin
Necrotizing fasciitis	Debridement and antibiotics
Vibrio vulnificus cellulitis	Debridement and antibiotics
Aeromonas hydrophila cellulitis	Debridement and antibiotics
Erysipelothrix rhusiopathiae infection	Penicillin
Pasteurella multocida infection	Penicillin
Tularemia	Aminoglycoside, doxycycline

latent stage, and tertiary stage. Syphilis may be spread sexually during the primary, secondary, and early latent phases. During pregnancy, however, syphilis in all stages is potentially infectious to the developing fetus.

Clinical Manifestations

Primary Syphilis

After an incubation period of 9 to 90 days (average of 3 weeks), the primary stage appears. It is characterized by the chancre, which emerges at the point of inoculation usually on the genitalia as single or multiple lesions. The chancre begins as a papule and soon erodes and becomes a painless, indolent, punched-out and clean, ulcer with a scanty, yellow, serous discharge. The base is finely granular and hard, and the entire lesion is indurated or rubbery. There is regional nonsuppurative adenopathy. Anorectal chancres superficially resemble an anal fissure with pain and bleeding on defecation. Bilateral inguinal adenopathy makes a chancre more likely. In women, the labia are the most common sites, but they may occur anywhere.

The lips are the most common site for chancres of the oral cavity. Painless chancres of the tongue and tonsils (often unilateral, displacing the uvula) may also occur and may present with cervical adenopathy.

Secondary Syphilis

The secondary stage follows the onset of the chancre by 3 to 6 weeks, or about 6 to 8 weeks following infection. The chancre is present in about 25% of cases of secondary syphilis but usually is healing. The signs and symptoms of secondary syphilis are protean. Early symptoms consist of an influenza or flu-like syndrome consisting of headaches, lacrimation, nasal discharge, sore throat, generalized arthralgia, generalized lymphadenopathy, and occasionally hepatosplenomegaly. Adenopathy usually precedes the cutaneous eruption. The bilateral symmetrical eruption tends to be more profuse on the upper extremities and upper trunk than on the abdomen and lower extremities and is painless and often nonpruritic. Mucous membrane lesions (mucous patches) and alopecia may be found. Skin lesions tend to follow the skin tension lines, especially on the trunk. There is a special predilection for the palms and soles. These lesions are discrete and sharply demarcated rather than confluent and have a coppery hue. The eruption is most commonly macular, papular, and/or pustular but may show any morphology except a vesicular or bullous eruption. It may last a few weeks to as long as 12 months, followed by a period of latency, which may be interrupted by relapse.

The pattern of eruption is related to the duration of infection. The earliest cutaneous expression of secondary syphilis is the macular or erythematous eruption, which tends to spare the face, palms, and soles. Individual lesions are oval 1- to 2-cm patches that may coalesce. The rash is transient and fades within 2 weeks.

The macular stage is the forerunner of the classic coppery-red maculopapular eruption. This eruption is generalized, involving the middle of the face, chest, back, abdomen, the flexors of the forearms and arms, the palms and soles and, to a lesser extent, the lower extremities. The mucous patches that appear on the moist surfaces of the genitalia are oval lesions with a slightly raised border within which is a shallow ulcer or erosion covered by a grayish-white membrane. On the tip and sides of the tongue, mucous patches show more ulceration than elsewhere in the mouth.

Papular lesions of secondary syphilis appear next. They are fewer in number and larger. They may be *follicular* and associated with a nonscarring, nonerythematous patchy alopecia of the scalp and beard and eyebrows, *lenticular* (small, generalized, flat-topped), *papulosquamous*, *corymbose* (a central larger papule surrounded by smaller papules), or *nodular*.

Papular lesions tend to be of a darker-red to reddish-brown color and more indurated with a greater tendency toward postinflammatory hyperpigmentation. Papular lesions are almost invariably found on the palms and soles. The papular lesions on the moist areas of the body are called condylomata lata. They are elevated, reddish-brown or gray, flat-topped, moist, and teeming with spirochetes.

Pustular lesions follow and are less common. They may be generalized, resembling chickenpox or generalized impetigo. The patient is sicker, with fever, headaches, and arthralgia. The lesions are frequently seen around the fingernails and toenails, as well as on the palms and soles. The lesions teem with treponemes.

Annular syphilis, seen often in dark-skinned persons, tends to be papular and may appear and disappear without treatment. The lesions of recurrent secondary syphilis tend to be larger, more discrete, and darker in color than the earlier manifestations.

Secondary syphilis may involve virtually any organ system. Characteristic visceral associations include *hepatitis* (alkaline phosphatase level is usually more elevated than the transaminases), *gastritis*, *renal disease* (usually presenting as nephrotic syndrome), and *musculoskeletal* symptoms (tenosynovitis, symmetrical polyarteritis, periostitis, or, rarely, syphilitic osteomyelitis).

Latent Syphilis

Latency is defined as acquired or congenital syphilis that is without signs or symptoms (of early or late symptomatic syphilis) and characterized by repeated reactive reagin and treponemal tests, and a nonreactive spinal fluid. Early latent syphilis is defined as syphilis under 1 year's duration, if there is a history of untreated primary or secondary syphilis, or of lesions consistent with primary or secondary syphilis within the past year or if the patient has had a nonreactive reagin test within the past year. Early latent syphilis is potentially infectious and encompasses the first 2 years of infection. About 25% of patients with untreated latent syphilis will have the reappearance of mucocutaneous lesions, usually within the first year of infection.

Late Mucocutaneous Syphilis

Late syphilis of the skin may appear from 5 to 10 years or as long as 20 years after the primary infection. The lesions may be nodular, noduloulcerative, or gummatous and are chronic, painless, asymptomatic, asymmetrical, indolent, slow growing, and progressively destructive. They are hard and indurated, with sharply demarcated borders. Nodular lesions are reddish brown, appear asymmetrically in clusters or large plaques, and form annular or arciform lesions with central scarring. They may involve any area of the skin, including the scalp, palms, and soles. Noduloulcerative lesions represent lesions that have ulcerated. Gummas tend to be solitary lesions. They usually develop at sites of trauma, deep in the dermis. Ulceration may occur. Lesions may spontaneously heal. Gummas may be seen in many other organ systems, most commonly, the bones, upper respiratory tract, and mucous membrane of the mouth. Involvement of the nasal bones/cartilage and palate may lead to a saddle-nose deformity and perforation, respectively. The long bones, especially the tibia, skull, and the sternal end of the clavicle, are also involved.

Epidemiology

In the United States, there was a dramatic drop in reported primary and secondary syphilis after World War II with the development of penicillin. In the late 1950s and 1960s, this trend reversed. Rates fell in the early 1980s due to changes in sexual behavior among gay men with the onset of the acquired immunodeficiency syndrome epidemic. In 1985, the incidence of syphilis began to increase dramatically among heterosexual men and women, especially in the black population, with an associated increase in congenital syphilis.

Transmission

Syphilis may be contracted in one of five ways: sexual exposure, kissing a person who has lesions of primary or secondary syphilis on the lips or in the oral cavity, prenatally, through transfusion or needle sharing by intravenous drug users, and by accidental direct inoculation.

Pathology

The pathologic findings of syphilis depend on the stage of the disease and the type of lesion sampled. Infiltrates containing plasma cells and spirochetes are common to all three stages. Swollen endothelial cells are classic but nonspecific.

Chancres are often flanked by epithelial hyperplasia with dense infiltrates of lymphocytes and plasma cells at the base of the ulcer and vascular thrombi just beneath the ulcer. Spirochetes tend to be numerous and can be demonstrated with an appropriate silver stain, such as the Warthin-Starry, or by immunoperoxidase staining.

Macules of secondary syphilis feature superficial and deep perivascular infiltrates of lymphocytes, macrophages, and plasma cells without epidermal change, or accompanied by slight vacuolar change at the dermoepidermal interface.

Papules and plaques of secondary syphilis most often show dense superficial bandlike and deep infiltrates of lymphocytes, macrophages, and plasma cells with psoriasiform epidermal hyperplasia and hyperkeratosis. As lesions age, macrophages become more numerous, and granulomatous foci are often present. Condylomata lata have spongiform pustules within areas of papillated epithelial hyperplasia that teem with spirochetes.

Laboratory Tests

The diagnosis of syphilis is usually confirmed by one of four methods.

The Darkfield Examination

The darkfield examination may be performed on any exudate from a suspicious genital ulceration, wet lesion, umbilical cord in congenital syphilis, or the aspirate of an enlarged lymph node. *T. pallidum* is a slender, motile, spiral organism 7 to 14 μ long and 0.25 μ thick. The spirals are evenly spaced and are about 1 μ apart.

Nontreponemal Tests (The Reagin Blood Test)

The Venereal Disease Research Laboratory (VDRL) test and the Rapid Plasma Reagin (RPR) test measure antilipid antibodies formed by the host against the lipid on the treponemal cell surface. They are less sensitive and less specific than the treponemal tests (see below) but are used as screening tests and are also essential in assessing the effectiveness of treatment and the detection of possible relapse or reinfection. These tests may not be reactive early in primary syphilis. A very high titer antibody in secondary syphilis may cause a false-negative reaction (prozone phenomenon). This can be avoided by diluting the serum. A positive result should always be confirmed by a specific treponemal test.

Treponemal Tests

These tests use *T. pallidum* or a portion of it as the antigen. The FTA-ABS is an indirect fluorescent antibody test in which the patient's serum is placed on a slide to which a suspension of *T. pallidum* has been fixed. Then, a fluorescein-labeled antihuman globulin is added that binds specifically to the patient's serum antibodies adhering to the *T. pallidum*, resulting in a visible reaction under fluorescent microscopy. The microhemagglutination assay for *T. pallidum* is gradually replacing the FTA-ABS because it is easier to perform and less expensive and has about the same sensitivity and specificity. Treponemal tests usually remain positive for life and therefore are not useful in diagnosing other than the initial episode of syphilis.

The biologic false-positive (BFP) reaction is a positive RPR or other reaginic serologic test, usually of low titer, $< 1:8$, with a negative treponemal test in a patient without a history of syphilis. The acute reaction (reactive for less than 3 to 6 months) occurs in many infectious diseases, immunizations, and pregnancy. Chronic BFP reactions (more than 3 to 6 months) occur in connective tissue diseases, chronic liver disease, multiple blood transfusions/intravenous drug usage, advancing age, and Lyme disease.

Differential Diagnosis

Primary Syphilis

The differential diagnosis is that of a patient with a genital ulcer. Multiple pathogens may be seen in genital ulcers. The differential diagnosis includes *herpes simplex, traumatic erosions and ulcerations, allergic contact dermatitis, fixed drug eruption, chancroid, granuloma inguinale*, and *lymphogranuloma venereum.*

Secondary Syphilis

The rash of secondary syphilis may be macular, maculopapular, papular, papulopustular, pustular, or relapsing with annular macular or papular rings. The differential diagnosis is principally that of the papulosquamous eruptions and includes *pityriasis rosea, lichen planus, psoriasis*, and *drug eruptions.*

Late Mucocutaneous Syphilis

The differential diagnosis of late mucocutaneous syphilis includes cutaneous tuberculosis, sarcoidosis, granuloma annulare, skin carcinoma, leprosy, deep fungal infection, and halogenoderma.

Treatment

See Table 6–3. The drug of choice for the treatment of syphilis is penicillin. All syphilis patients should be tested for human immunodeficiency virus (HIV) disease, since HIV infection may increase the risk of treatment failure or early central nervous system relapse. Therapeutic alternatives to penicillin are recommended for early syphilis, late, and late latent syphilis if the central nervous system is not involved.

Patients should be seen every 3 months for the first year, every 6 months in the second year, and yearly thereafter to ensure a serologic cure. The quantitative RPR titer should decline fourfold by the

TABLE 6-3. Treatment Recommendations for Syphilis

EARLY SYPHILIS (PRIMARY, SECONDARY, AND EARLY LATENT)

Benzathine penicillin G, 2.4 million units intramuscularly weekly for 2 weeks; a total of 4.8 million units
Penicillin allergy: doxycycline, 100 mg orally every 12 hours, or tetracycline, 500 mg every 6 hours for 14 days

LATE SYPHILIS (EXCLUDING NEUROSYPHILIS), LATE LATENT SYPHILIS, OR SYPHILIS OF UNKNOWN DURATION

Benzathine penicillin G, 2.4 million units weekly for 3 weeks; a total of 7.2 million units
Penicillin allergy: doxycycline, 100 mg orally every 12 hours, or tetracycline, 500 mg every 6 hours for 28 days

third month and eightfold by the sixth month in patients with their first episode of syphilis. Many patients with primary syphilis will be nonreactive at 12 months, and at 24 months with secondary syphilis. Titers decline more slowly if there has been previous treatment or reinfection.

Special considerations must be taken for pregnant patients.

The Jarisch-Herxheimer Reaction

The Jarisch-Herxheimer reaction is a brief, self-limited flu-like syndrome occurring 2 to 6 hours following penicillin treatment of some cases of primary, many cases of secondary, and some cases of early latent syphilis. The chancre or rash may be exacerbated. This reaction lasts for several hours, and is believed to be the breakdown of the spirochetes.

Neurosyphilis

Involvement of the central nervous system in syphilis occurs early in the disease. Patients with primary or secondary syphilis frequently have cerebrospinal fluid involvement which usually resolves. Ten per cent of males and 5% of females with untreated syphilis develop neurosyphilis.

Neurosyphilis can occur at any stage of syphilis after the primary stage. Neurosyphilitic manifestations include meningeal syphilis (within the first year—cranial palsies and ophthalmic findings are common), meningovascular syphilis (occurs 5 to 12 years after infection—focal central nervous system findings), parenchymatous neurosyphilis, which includes general paresis (occurs 15 to 20 years after initial infection with dementia/psychiatric manifestations), and tabes dorsalis (occurs 20 to 25 years after infection and causes posterior columnar abnormalities).

A positive nontreponemal test in the cerebrospinal fluid is sufficient for the diagnosis of neurosyphilis. Unfortunately, only 50% to

70% of patients with late syphilis have a positive serum nontreponemal test.

Congenital Syphilis

Congenital syphilis occurs when spirochetes from an infected, untreated mother enter the placenta and the fetal circulation. Congenital syphilis is divided into two stages—early and late. It is early congenital syphilis if the disease is found within the first 2 years of life, and late congenital after this time. Spontaneous abortion is the most common outcome of syphilis in the second and early third trimester.

Infants of women who meet any of the following criteria should be evaluated for congenital syphilis: untreated syphilis or inadequate treatment, treatment of syphilis with erythromycin, treatment less than 1 month before delivery, inadequate response to treatment, or appropriate treatment before pregnancy but insufficient serologic follow-up. Serologic testing of the mother and child at delivery are recommended. Evaluation of children of women noted above should include a complete physical examination, nontreponemal serology of the infant's sera, cerebrospinal fluid evaluation, long bone radiographs, and pathologic evaluation of the placenta using specific antitreponemal antibody staining. Determination of specific antitreponemal IgM could be considered.

Early Congenital Syphilis

The manifestations of early congenital syphilis resemble acquired secondary syphilis. Neonates may be premature, emaciated, and pot bellied; however, most infants appear healthy at birth. In two thirds, the early signs appear in the third to eighth week, and in nearly all cases by the third month. The prognosis is poor. The findings of early congenital syphilis include snuffles (bloody mucousy nasal discharge), rhagades (deep fissures radiating around the mouth), meningovascular manifestations, iritis, chorioretinitis, hoarse cry, osteochondritis, generalized lymphadenopathy, hepatosplenomegaly, anemia, thrombocytopenia, hypoalbuminemia, edema, and skin lesions (similar to acquired secondary syphilis including mucous patches and condylomata lata; palmar/plantar bullae and pustules are also seen).

Late Congenital Syphilis

This stage occurs in children age 2 years or older. The findings of late congenital syphilis include frontal bossing, saddle nose, periostitis of long bones including the tibia (saber shins) and clavicle, Hutchinson's teeth (wide-spaced, notched incisors and canines), Mulberry molars (lower first molar with multiple cusps in a circle), eighth nerve deafness, interstitial keratitis, and Clutton's joints (doughy periarticular swellings due to sinovitis).

Congenital neurosyphilis presents in a pattern similar to acquired syphilis. Meningitis appears in the first year, meningovascular syphilis in the first two years, and general paresis or tabes dorsalis between age 6 and 21, usually in adolescence.

Syphilis and Human Immunodeficiency Virus

In general, HIV-infected patients exhibit the same manifestations as non–HIV-infected ones with similar treatment responses; however, patients with HIV may be more likely to present with secondary syphilis (53% vs. 33%) and to have a chancre persisting when they had secondary syphilis (43% vs. 15%). Unusual clinical manifestations of syphilis in HIV include florid skin lesions to few atypical ones. Also, the serologic response may be greater, impaired, or delayed, and HIV-infected patients may develop neurosyphilis even after appropriate therapy.

Endemic Treponematoses (Endemic Syphilis, Pinta, and Yaws)

These three diseases are caused by spirochetes morphologically identical to *T. pallidum*. They are spread nonsexually, affecting primarily children. They are endemic to certain geographic regions, especially rural regions where malnutrition and poor hygiene are common.

Endemic Syphilis

Endemic syphilis is caused by *T. pallidum* subspecies *endemicum*. It is found primarily among nomadic tribes in Southwest Asia, especially Saudi Arabia, and sub-Saharan Africa. Children ages 2 to 15 years represent the main reservoir. It is spread from a lesion or saliva to the skin or mouth via contaminated drinking vessels or infected saliva or by contaminated fingers. Early-stage lesions are primary and secondary lesions very similar to venereal syphilis. Late-stage disease consists of late latent disease and tertiary lesions. Primary lesions are often in the oropharynx and usually undiagnosed. Presentation is usually in the secondary stage with mucous patches, shallow relatively painless oral ulcerations, angular stomatitis, condylomata lata, nonpruritic skin eruptions, and generalized adenopathy. Osteoperiostitis of the long bones may cause leg pains. Late disease is usually latent but may present as gummas of the skin, bones, or cartilage, with destruction of the nose and palate and bone pain (especially tibial). Neurologic and cardiac involvement are rare, but uveitis may occur.

Diagnosis

The diagnosis must be considered in persons from endemic regions. Serology for syphilis is positive, and biopsies or smears of active lesions demonstrate spirochetes. Distinction of early lesions from venereal syphilis is largely clinical. Late lesions must be differentiated from yaws, leishmaniasis, histoplasmosis, rhinoscleroma, rhinosporidiosis, tuberculosis, leprosy, and Wegener's/lethal midline granuloma.

Pinta

Pinta, caused by *T. carateum*, is prevalent in remote tropical regions of Central and South America. Transmission is through injured skin or mucous membranes. Pinta affects the skin only.

Early pinta is characterized by primary and secondary lesions. The primary lesion appears 1 week to 2 months after inoculation (average 10 days) as a small scaling papule on the lower legs, face, arms, or trunk. It expands over several months to a plaque of about 10 cm. It may then resolve or persist into the secondary stage. Secondary lesions (pintids), appearing 2 to 6 months or even longer after the primary stage, are identical to the primary lesion, but usually smaller. They are frequently hyperpigmented or hypopigmented, hyperkeratotic (psoriasiform), and asymmetrical. Lesions tend to fade, intermix, and relapse, forming polycyclic plaques. There is generalized lymphadenopathy.

Late (tertiary) pinta develops 2 to 5 or more years after the early lesions, and tends to be generalized and symmetrical. Tertiary lesions are less erythematous and hyperkeratotic, may be atrophic, and are more dyspigmented.

Serologic tests become positive 2 to 4 months after the appearance of the primary lesion. Early pinta must be distinguished from tinea, psoriasis, pellagra, and eczematous eruptions. Dyspigmented lesions must be distinguished from vitiligo, tinea versicolor, leprosy, lupus erythematosus, pityriasis alba, and lichen planus actinicus/erythema dyschromicum perstans.

Yaws

Yaws, caused by *T. pallidum* subspecies *pertenue*, is found in Africa, Southeast Asia, South and Central America, and areas of the Pacific. Yaws is spread by direct contact with broken skin so exposed areas, mainly the legs, are the most common sites of involvement. Children under 15 remain the principal reservoir and the most commonly affected.

The primary stage consists of the primary lesion, or "mother yaw," occurring between 9 and 90 days (average 21) after inoculation. It begins as a painless red papule that enlarges, develops a crust, and then ulcerates. The surface may resemble a raspberry (*framboesia*). These lesions heal spontaneously after a few weeks to months. Associated features include fever, joint pain, and lymphadenopathy.

The secondary lesions, or "daughter yaws," are widespread multiple papules and ulcers that often cluster around the primary lesion, periorificially and in the axillae and groin. On the soles, they are often hyperkeratotic and painful, resulting in a crab-like gait (*crab yaws*). This papillomatous stage averages 6 months for the first crop of papillomas, and subsequent outbreaks may last another 6 months or longer, up to 5 years. Secondary yaws is followed by a latent period. Tertiary yaws develops in about 10% of untreated patients, and is characterized by nodular, hyperkeratotic, and plaque-like cutaneous lesions, juxta-articular nodules, as well as gummatous lesions. Bony involvement includes gangosa (a deforming rhinopharyngitis), goundou (production of exostoses of the maxilla), and a deforming osteoperiostitis mainly of the long bones.

Both primary and early secondary lesions of yaws are said to show dense diffuse dermal infiltrates of lymphocytes, plasma cells, macrophages, and eosinophils, coupled with psoriasiform papillated epidermal hyperplasia and intraepidermal spongiotic vesiculation and spongiform pustules. Late secondary lesions resemble those of late secondary syphilis. The diagnosis can be made by demonstrating the spirochete by silver stain or biopsy or darkfield examinations with serologic confirmatory tests for early lesions.

Differential Diagnosis

Early yaws must be distinguished from topical ulceration, venereal syphilis, leishmaniasis, ecthyma, scabies, eczema, psoriasis, and keratodermas. The bony lesions may mimic venereal and endemic syphilis, tuberculosis, and osteomyelitis, whereas the nasopharyngeal lesions may resemble leprosy, leishmaniasis, deep fungal infections, and tuberculosis.

Treatment of the Endemic Treponematoses

A single intramuscular injection of benzathine penicillin is the recommended treatment for yaws, pinta, and endemic syphilis. Adults are given 1.2 to 2.4 million units and children under 10, 0.6 to 1.2 million units.

LYME BORRELIOSIS

(CM&S Chapter 109)

Definition

Lyme borreliosis is a complex, multisystemic disorder caused by infection with the spirochete *Borrelia burgdorferi*. It has protean manifestations that are acute or chronic. The most striking signs and symptoms involve the joints, central and peripheral nervous systems, heart, and skin.

Clinical Description

Epidemiology

Ixodes ticks are the primary vectors for Lyme borreliosis, and the disease occurs in areas where these ticks are endemic. *I. scapularis* (*dammini*) is the major vector in the eastern and *I. pacificus* in the western United States. *I. ricinus* is the major vector in Europe. The disease is most common in the northeast, upper midwest, California, and Oregon. It occurs on all continents except Antarctica.

The white-footed mouse is the main reservoir for *B. burgdorferi*. The nymph, the most infectious form of the vector, develops into an adult on the white-tailed deer. Humans are incidental hosts. In some parts of the eastern United States, up to 60% of *I. dammini* may be parasitized by *B. burgdorferi*, compared with only 1% to 2% of *I. pacificus* in the west.

The bite of an infected tick is painless. Spirochetes are transmitted to the host after 1 to 3 days of attachment. If the tick is removed promptly, transmission of infection may be avoided. Because of its very small size, the nymph may not be noticed and removed in time to prevent infection.

Stages of Lyme Disease

The manifestations of infection with *B. burgdorferi* vary from early to late in the course. Like syphilis, Lyme disease has primary, secondary, and late stages.

Stage 1 disease begins 3 to 30 days after a tick bite, which is recalled by fewer than one half of patients. The disease is characterized by flu-like symptoms and, initially, vague, migratory joint complaints. Erythema chronicum migrans (ECM), which is diagnostic, is present in up to 75% of patients. It classically starts as an erythematous papule at the bite site and then evolves into an annular, erythematous ring. The lesion clears spontaneously within weeks or months in most cases. Although they are usually annular with central clearing, they may remain as an enlarging, bluish-red plaque or develop central vesiculation, necrosis, or both.

Stage 2 begins after weeks or months and primarily involves the nervous and cardiovascular systems. Regional or generalized lymphadenopathy may be present. Multiple annular, erythematous lesions, simulating secondary syphilis and lymphadenosis benigna cutis, may occur.

Stage 3 disease develops weeks or months after primary infection and chiefly involves the musculoskeletal and nervous systems and eye. A late cutaneous manifestation is acrodermatitis chronica atrophicans.

An orderly progression from one stage or another is not often found and some patients may have symptoms or findings of several stages simultaneously; therefore, manifestations of Lyme disease are categorized here by their effects on each organ system.

Musculoskeletal System

In about 60% of untreated cases (especially children) the patient may develop arthritis later in the course of the disease. The arthritis tends to involve the large joints, especially the knee, and be intermittent. Many cases may resolve; however, 10% may develop chronic, erosive oligo-arthritis. The radiographic features are similar to other inflammatory arthritides and are not diagnostic for Lyme disease.

Cardiovascular System

Cardiac manifestations occur in about 8% of patients with Lyme disease, with the most common finding being fluctuating degrees of atrioventricular block. The involvement is usually transient, but high-grade block may require a temporary or, at times, a permanent pacemaker. Myopericarditis, mild left ventricular dysfunction, pancarditis, and cardiomyopathy may occur.

Nervous System

Neurologic disorders may occur in 15% of untreated patients with Lyme disease. The disease may involve the peripheral or central nervous system. Patients in early-stage disease may have aseptic meningitis, cranial nerve palsies (especially Bell's palsy), radiculitis, and encephalitis. The cerebrospinal fluid typically reveals a lymphocytic pleocytosis, and spirochetes may be cultured. The triad of meningitis, cranial neuritis, and radiculoneuritis is virtually unique to Lyme disease and is almost diagnostic in a patient from an endemic area. Patients with late or chronic Lyme disease may have encephalitis, encephalopathy, chronic neuropathy, and entrapment neuropathies such as carpal tunnel syndrome.

Ophthalmologic Manifestations

A variety of ophthalmologic manifestations can occur at any stage of the disease. The most common finding is conjunctivitis seen early in the course of the disease. Other manifestations include iritis, iridocyclitis, optic neuritis, exudative retinal detachments, panophthalmitis with blindness, papilledema with and without pseudotumor cerebri, diplopia due to cranial nerve palsies, and Argyll Robertson pupils.

Specific Cutaneous Manifestations
Acrodermatitis Chronica Atrophicans

Acrodermatitis chronica atrophicans has been reported in Europe for many years but is rare in the United States. It is characterized by two stages: early inflammatory and late atrophic. Early lesions are erythematous nodules or plaques, which may have central clearing. These lesions progress slowly over months or years. Eventually, atrophic, poikilodermatous areas develop with subcutaneous nodules, sclerosis, and fibrous bands that may result in joint immobility. Erythema chronicum migrans may precede the appearance of acrodermatitis chronica atrophicans.

Lymphadenosis Benigna Cutis

Lymphadenosis benigna cutis is the term used for lesions of cutaneous lymphoid hyperplasia in which lymphoid follicles are present. It occurs in Lyme disease, especially in Europe, and presents as reddish violaceous nodules and plaques.

Pathology

Several histologic changes may be found in erythema chronicum migrans. Most commonly, there is a superficial and deep perivascular and interstitial lymphoplasmacytic infiltrate. Specimens from the centers of lesions may resemble an arthropod bite reaction. A third pattern may have only lymphocytes. Spirochetes may be demonstrated with silver stains.

In the early inflammatory stage of acrodermatitis chronica atrophicans, dermal edema and telangiectasia with perivascular lymphocytes and plasma cells are present. Later, there is epidermal atrophy, loss of appendages, and a sclerosis resembling morphea.

In lymphadenosis benigna cutis, the changes are identical to those seen in the follicular pattern of cutaneous lymphoid hyperplasia.

The pathogenesis of the various manifestations of Lyme borreliosis is not well understood. Some changes are due to the host inflammatory response to the organism, while others may be due to the triggering of autoimmune reactions.

Diagnosis and Differential Diagnosis

Initially, the differential diagnosis includes a viral illness or a connective tissue disorder. At this stage, the diagnosis is primarily based on clinical grounds (i.e., confirming erythema chronicum migrans) since serologic tests may not become positive for a number of weeks. An acute tick bite reaction must be distinguished from erythema chronicum migrans; the former occurs within 1 day, is usually less than 2.0 cm in diameter, and regresses within several days rather than expanding. Other differential diagnoses of erythema chronicum migrans include cellulitis, contact dermatitis, fixed drug eruption, tinea, and spider bite. The definitive diagnosis is made on demonstration of the spirochete with a silver stain.

Serum antibodies to *B. burgdorferi* may be measured. IgM antibody appears first and usually declines in 4 to 6 months; persistence of IgM antibody or reappearance at a later time may predict continued infection and a greater risk of complications. IgG antibodies appear later and remain elevated in patients with long-term infection.

Unfortunately, there is no standardization of these serologic tests, and thus interpretation is difficult. There also may be cross-reacting antibodies in patients with other diseases.

Treatment

The best antibiotic treatment for the various manifestations of Lyme disease is unsettled. In general, early Lyme disease is treated with oral regimens of doxycycline or amoxicillin. Erythromycin may be used in children or patients unable to take tetracyclines or penicillin. Late manifestation of the disease and meningitis require parenteral therapy.

Prevention

Personal protection remains the most effective means of reducing infections and involves the use of permethrin-based repellents, the wearing of appropriate clothing, and a careful search for and prompt removal of ticks. As yet, there is no firm recommendation for prophylactic antibiotic treatment of all tick bites, even in endemic areas.

CHANCROID, GRANULOMA INGUINALE, AND LYMPHOGRANULOMA VENEREUM

(CM&S Chapter 110)

Chancroid

Definition

Chancroid, or soft chancre, is a painful ulcerative genital disease caused by sexual transmission of *Haemophilus ducreyi*. Genital lesions are often associated with tender inguinal lymphadenopathy, which may progress to suppuration and bubo formation.

Clinical Description

Epidemiology

Chancroid is endemic in many tropical and subtropical countries, particularly in Africa and Southeast Asia. Chancroid has historically been a relatively rare sexually transmitted disease (STD) in the United States; however, with an increased flow of immigrants, there has been an increase of chancroid in the United States. There is a higher incidence of HIV seropositivity in patients with chancroid.

Clinical Manifestations

Initial entry of *H. ducreyi* into the skin occurs through minor abrasions. The incubation period ranges from 3 to 14 days (usually 4 to 7 days). The first manifestation of infection is a small, inflammatory papule, which progresses within 2 or 3 days to a pustule that rapidly ulcerates. The classic chancroidal lesion consists of one or more well-demarcated, nonindurated, tender ulcerations with ragged, undermined edges and surrounding erythema. Autoinoculation of adjacent skin results in characteristic "kissing lesions." A gray or yellow, necrotic, often foul-smelling exudate usually overlies the friable, granulomatous base, which bleeds easily when scraped.

In males, the disease most commonly involves the distal prepuce, frenulum, and coronal sulcus. In females, ulcers are more superficial and most often located on the labia, fourchette, vestibule, and clitoris and in the perianal area. Painless cervical and vaginal lesions are also possible.

In approximately 50% of patients, chancroid is associated with painful inguinal, usually unilateral lymphadenopathy. Suppuration with bubo formation occurs in about 25% of cases.

Pathology

The base of the chancroidal ulcer reveals three distinct zones. The superficial zone contains necrotic tissue, fibrin, erythrocytes, neutrophils, and the causative bacteria. The middle zone is an area of neovascularization and thrombosed vessels. The deepest zone consists of a dense infiltrate of lymphocytes and plasma cells. Bacteria can be demonstrated by either Giemsa or silver stains.

Pathogenesis and Etiology

H. ducreyi is a short, compact gram-negative bacillus (1.5 × 0.5 μm) with rounded ends that often grows in chains. It is a facultative aerobe located both extracellularly and within neutrophils.

Diagnosis and Differential Diagnosis

STDs such as herpes simplex, syphilis, lymphogranuloma venereum, and granuloma inguinale may mimic chancroid. The differential diagnosis also includes non-STDs such as Behçet's disease, extraintestinal Crohn's disease, and fixed drug eruption.

Gram staining of an ulcer specimen may reveal gram-negative coccobacilli singly or in a "school of fish" formation, in which the bacilli are arranged in long parallel columns between cells or shreds of mucus; however, this test has poor sensitivity and specificity since this "typical" Gram stain is seen in only 5% to 36% of culture-proven cases.

Definitive diagnosis of chancroid requires cultural isolation of *H. ducreyi* using Nairobi medium. Ulcers are cleaned with sterile, nonbacteriostatic saline and gauze, and specimens are obtained from the base and undermined margins using a cotton swab. Isolation of *H. ducreyi* from inguinal bubo aspirate may be attempted, but it is generally less successful.

Treatment

Untreated chancroidal ulcers may persist for 1 to 3 months, whereas appropriate antimicrobial therapy results in resolution within 7 to 14 days. The current recommendations are ceftriaxone sodium, 250 mg intramuscularly in a single dose, or oral erythromycin, 500 mg four times daily for 1 week. Alternative regimens include ciprofloxacin, 500 mg twice daily for 1 to 3 days; oral amoxicillin/clavulanate, 500 mg/125 mg three times a day for 1 week; and trimethoprim-sulfamethoxazole, 160 mg/800 mg orally twice daily for 1 week (except Thailand). Treatment also includes prophylactic aspiration of buboes, particularly if they are fluctuant.

Granuloma Inguinale

Definition

Granuloma inguinale (donovanosis, granuloma venereum) is a rare, chronic, indolent disease characterized by anogenital and inguinal ulcerogranulomatous lesions. It is generally considered to be caused by sexual transmission of *Calymmatobacterium granulomatis*.

Clinical Description

Epidemiology

Granuloma inguinale primarily occurs in small endemic foci located in tropical and subtropical areas of the world. In the United States, most cases have been reported from southern and southeastern states.

Clinical Manifestation

Four morphologic variants of granuloma inguinale have been described: ulcerovegetative, nodular, hypertrophic, and cicatricial. In *ulcerovegetative* disease (the most common), papules or small nodules appear at the site of initial infection after an incubation period ranging from less than 2 weeks to 3 months. These nodules rapidly erode to form one or more painless ulcerations with a raised, rolled, sharp border and a clean, "beefy red" base containing exuberant, friable granulation tissue. Ulcers slowly spread by direct extension and by autoinoculation of adjacent skin that results in "kissing lesions." In the *nodular* variant, lesions are soft, erythematous papules with a granulation tissue–like surface. *Hypertrophic* granuloma inguinale consists of large, vegetating masses that may closely resemble condyloma acuminatum or latum. Finally, the rare *cicatricial* form is characterized by expanding scarring plaques.

Lesions in men occur most commonly on the prepuce, coronal sulcus, or perianally (in homosexuals); women usually present with labial lesions, although the vagina and cervix may also be involved. Infection often spreads to the inguinal lymph nodes causing swelling and ulceration, but true inguinal lymphadenopathy does not occur.

Scarring and fibrosis may be prominent, and infrequent complications include phimosis, destruction of the penis, lymphedema, and an elephantiasis-like swelling of the external genitalia in women. Fatal intrapelvic and disseminated disease may occur. Rarely extragenital mucocutaneous lesions occur.

Pathology

Characteristic features include an infiltration of histiocytes containing 1- to 2-μm intracytoplasmic bacilli known as Donovan bodies. These are best demonstrated with Warthin-Starry or Giemsa staining, in which their two polar bodies give them a safety-pin–like appearance. Plasma cells and microabscesses are common.

Pathogenesis and Etiology

C. granulomatis is a small (1 to 1.5 mm × 0.5 to 0.7 mm) gram-negative pleomorphic bacillus with a characteristic safety-pin appearance due to bipolar condensations of chromatin. *C. granulomatis* has not been successfully grown on conventional solid media; thus, culture is rarely performed.

Diagnosis and Differential Diagnosis

The differential diagnosis includes primary and secondary syphilis, penile carcinoma, chancroid, condyloma acuminatum, and anogenital amebiasis; 30% to 45% of patients with granuloma inguinale also have positive syphilis serology.

The diagnosis is based on clinical appearance in conjunction with supportive laboratory findings. Since cultural isolation is not practical, the definitive diagnosis is established by direct visualization of the causative bacteria (Donovan bodies) within histiocytes in either crush preparations or biopsy specimens stained with Giemsa, Wright, Leishman, or Warthin-Starry silver stain. Hematoxylin-eosin does not demonstrate the organisms well.

To prepare a crush preparation, the lesion is cleaned with saline, and the tissue is removed from the leading edge of the ulcer using a scalpel, forceps, scissor, or punch biopsy. The deep portion of the moist specimen should be crushed between two slides immediately to avoid desiccation, which may lower yield owing to rupture of histiocytes. The impression is then air dried and stained.

Biopsy specimens stained with Giemsa or Warthin-Starry stains are also diagnostic in more than 95% of cases.

Treatment

Treatment recommendations are based on empiric observations since in vitro antibiotic sensitivity testing of *C. granulomatis* has not been done. Granuloma inguinale responds best to lipid-soluble anti-biotics that achieve a high intracellular concentration and are effective against gram-negative bacilli. Therapy is typically continued for 2 to 3 weeks or until healing is complete. The antibiotic of choice is tetracycline, 500 mg orally four times a day; however, resistance has been reported. Alternative regimen is oral trimethoprim-sulfa-methoxazole, 160 mg/800 mg twice daily. Erythromycin, lincomy-cin, sodium methicillin, and norfloxacin may also be helpful. Gran-uloma inguinale is less responsive to therapy in patients co-infected with HIV. HIV testing should be done on all patients with granu-loma inguinale.

Lymphogranuloma Venereum

Definition

Lymphogranuloma venereum is a systemic disease caused by the sexual transmission of specific serotypes of *Chlamydia trachomatis*.

Clinical Description

Lymphogranuloma venereum is classically divided into three clinical stages. The primary stage is characterized by the appearance of a small (5 to 6 mm), painless genital lesion after an incubation period of 3 to 30 days. This lesion may be a shallow papule, erosion, ulcer, or herpetiform lesion or a nonspecific urethritis or cervicitis if internally located. The primary lesion goes unnoticed by more than 60% of patients. In men, it is most commonly located on the glans, coronal sulcus, or scrotum or in the urethra. The typical locations in females are the labia, posterior vaginal wall, and cervix. Rarely, extragenital areas are involved. Primary anorectal infection charac-terized by purulent or bloody diarrhea and tenesmus may occur in men or women who practice receptive anal intercourse. The primary lesion heals after a few days but may persist for 2 to 4 weeks.

The second stage, termed the *inguinal syndrome*, usually devel-ops within 2 to 6 weeks of the appearance of the primary lesion (range 10 days to 6 months). This stage is characterized by painful, inflammatory inguinal and femoral lymphadenopathy, and bubo formation. The pathognomonic "groove sign" occurs in 15% to 20% of patients as the result of nodal enlargement above and below the inguinal ligament. Constitutional symptoms are common. Ery-thema nodosum may also be seen.

Complications include fistulae formation, matting of nodes, fi-brosis, lymphedema, and eventual elephantiasis. Most men present with classic second stage disease; however only one third of women develop inguinal adenopathy, since their lymphatic drainage is often to deep iliac and perirectal nodes. This may result in lower abdomi-nal or back pain.

The destructive tertiary stage, known as the *genitoanorectal syn-drome*, occurs more commonly in females, probably owing to unrecognized and thus untreated second stage disease. It is charac-terized by proctocolitis, lymphorrhoids (perirectal lymphatic hyper-plasia), perirectal abscesses, ulcerations, fistulae, rectal stric-tures, and lymphatic fibrosis resulting in elephantiasis and labial hypertrophy.

Pathology

The histopathology of the initial papule is nonspecific. Biopsies of the lymph nodes may reveal stellate microabscesses, the center of which are composed primarily of neutrophils and occasional macrophages; epithelioid cells surround the center in a palisade formation. Chlamydial organisms can be shown by direct immunofluorescence with an antichlamydial antibody.

Pathogenesis and Etiology

This STD is caused by the L1, L2, and L3 serovars of *C. trachomatis*.

Diagnosis and Differential Diagnosis

Diagnosis is based on characteristic clinical features and appropriate laboratory confirmation. Today, laboratory diagnosis most commonly involves serologic testing using the complement fixation (CF) test and the microimmunofluorescence (MIF) test. Positive results usually develop within 2 weeks of the onset of infection. If clinically appropriate, a single CF titer of more than or equal to 1 : 64 is believed to be diagnostic of lymphogranuloma venereum. Lymphogranuloma venereum may also be diagnosed on the basis of a fourfold increase in titers. Antibodies to various chlamydial species and serotypes may cross-react. However, CF titers are rarely higher than 1 : 16 in association with routine chlamydial urethritis, cervicitis, or conjunctivitis. The MIF test is the most accurate serologic assay and is more sensitive than the CF test.

The "gold standard" of diagnosis is cultural isolation and typing of lymphogranuloma venereum–related *C. trachomatis* from a fluctuant lymph node, although this is difficult to achieve.

The differential diagnosis of lymphogranuloma venereum includes other causes of lymphadenopathy and genital ulceration, such as syphilis, herpes simplex, chancroid, and tumor. Other concomitant STDs are common and should be excluded, including HIV infection.

Treatment

The current drug of choice for treatment of lymphogranuloma venereum is oral doxycycline, 100 mg twice daily for 21 days. A 3-week course of tetracycline, 500 mg four times a day, is also acceptable first-line therapy. Alternatively, erythromycin or sulfisoxazole, both in a dosage of 500 mg four times daily, may be used. Constitutional symptoms resolve rapidly; however, buboes typically require several weeks to heal. Fluctuant lymph nodes should be aspirated, and incision and drainage may be needed for abscesses. Disease in patients with HIV infection may be less amenable to therapy.

TUBERCULOUS MYCOBACTERIAL INFECTIONS OF THE SKIN

(CM&S Chapter 111)

Definition

Mycobacteria are acid-fast, nonmotile, non–spore-forming anaerobic rods. They are usually stained by the Ziehl-Neelsen method, demonstrate acid-fastness, a distinguishing feature of this genus not found in any other bacteria of medical significance.

The genus *Mycobacterium* contains many members, including *M. tuberculosis* and *M. leprae.* and nontuberculous mycobacteria (atypical mycobacteria) that can be pathogenic to humans, as well as a number of harmless commensal organisms.

Mycobacterium tuberculosis *and* Mycobacterium bovis

The human type *(M. tuberculosis)* and the bovine type *(M. bovis)* are the most important tubercle bacilli in human disease. *M. tuberculosis,* spread by droplets, is responsible for most cases of human tuberculosis worldwide. In primary tuberculosis, there is a single focus of infection in the lung with hilar nodes, which usually resolves spontaneously and causes no symptoms, although in a few cases the infection can spread to bones, joints, kidneys, or meninges. In postprimary tuberculosis, reinfection by bacilli is usually from an exogenous source (although reactivation of primary lesions can occur), and involvement of the apices of the lungs and regional lymph nodes is common. *M. bovis* is usually conveyed to humans through infected cow's milk and commonly involves the cervical glands, infected through the pharynx, and the abdominal glands, infected from the intestines. Pasteurization of milk has made this infection rare.

Cutaneous Tuberculosis

Tuberculosis of the skin is caused by *M. tuberculosis, M. bovis, and occasionally the bacillus Calmette-Guérin (BCG), which is an attenuated strain of M. bovis.*

Clinical Description

The clinical manifestations of cutaneous tuberculosis are legion, and are dependent on the source of infection and the immune response of the host. The clinical types are broadly classified into four categories of infection: (1) inoculation of cutaneous mycobacteriosis from an exogenous source, (2) cutaneous mycobacteriosis from an endogenous source, (3) cutaneous mycobacteriosis from hematogenous spread, and (4) the tuberculids.

Inoculation Tuberculosis — Exogenous Source

Tuberculous Chancre

A chancre occurs after the inoculation of *M. tuberculosis* into the skin of a patient with no previous exposure to mycobacteria. Clinically, a brown papule or ulcer with a hemorrhagic base is seen with regional lymphadenopathy 3 to 6 weeks after inoculation. Most ulcers heal spontaneously, albeit slowly. Rarely, the chancre may proceed to lupus vulgaris or miliary tuberculosis. The adenopathy eventually resolves, although it may calcify 2 to 3 years later.

Warty Tuberculosis (Tuberculosis Verrucosa Cutis)

This results from the inoculation of *M. tuberculosis* in a person who has been previously sensitized to the organism. A minor wound is often the site of entry. Many cases occur in pathologists and postmortem attendants—hence the expression ''prosector's warts.'' Inoculation can, however, occur from a patient's own sputum. Clinically, there is usually a single, slow-growing hyperkeratotic plaque or nodule. These lesions tend to occur on the hands of European adults and on the lower extremities of Asian children.

Cutaneous Tuberculosis from an Endogenous Source

Scrofuloderma

Scrofuloderma occurs when there is contiguous spread from an endogenous source (e.g., lymph node, especially cervical; bones; joints; epididymis) with breakdown of the overlying skin. All age groups may be affected, but scrofuloderma is more common in children. Lesions develop as subcutaneous bluish-red nodules overlying the infected focus. These nodules then break down and perforate, leaving undermined ulcers and discharging sinuses. Eventually, scarring occurs, which may be extensive, with fibrous masses coexisting with boggy discharging nodules. Tuberculin sensitivity is high.

Oroficial Tuberculosis

Oroficial tuberculosis is a rare condition that describes tuberculosis of the mucous membranes and skin surrounding orifices usually caused by autoinoculation into these areas, in patients with tuberculosis of internal organs (usually of the gastrointestinal tract, lungs, or occasionally the genitourinary tract). The mouth is the most commonly affected site, particularly the tongue and both soft and hard palates. Anal and vulvar lesions can also occur. Lesions characteristically develop as a painful red nodule that ulcerates to form a punched-out ulcer. Most patients show a positive tuberculin reaction, although anergy may develop. The prognosis is poor and these lesions tend to progress.

Hematogenous Tuberculosis

Acute Miliary Tuberculosis of the Skin

This rare skin condition is caused by hematogenous dissemination of mycobacteria and is traditionally described in infants and young children. It may emerge as a problem in immunosuppressed patients. The focus of infection is usually meningeal or pulmonary. The clinical features are variable, with crops of nodules, papules, vesicles, and pustules being described, usually in severely ill patients. Tuberculin test is usually negative. The outlook is usually poor in children, although a good response to chemotherapy has been reported in some adult patients.

Lupus Vulgaris

Lupus vulgaris is a chronic, progressive form of cutaneous tuberculosis occurring in previously sensitized individuals. It occurs almost exclusively on the head and neck. Immunity is thought to be only moderate, since lesions progress steadily and healing without therapy is rare. The pathogenesis of lupus vulgaris is multifactorial. It originates from a tuberculous focus elsewhere and can arise by direct extension from underlying glands, by lymphatic spread from the mucous membranes of the nose or throat, by hematogenous dissemination, or rarely by direct inoculation or BCG vaccination. Pulmonary tuberculosis and cervical adenitis are the most common underlying foci of infection. Clinically, the typical soft, solitary, brown plaques usually start on the nose or cheek and gradually spread. Involvement of the limbs and trunk is much less common. On diascopy, the characteristic "apple jelly" nodules are seen. Variations include ulcerating, vegetating, tumor-like, papular and nodular forms. Mucous membrane involvement of the mouth, nose, and conjunctiva may occur. Progression is inevitable and relentless, and marked disfiguration may occur. Squamous cell carcinomas and occasionally basal cell carcinomas may occur in chronic lesions.

Metastatic Tuberculous Ulcer

Hematogenous dissemination from a primary focus may occur, leading to a distant subcutaneous abscess that may ulcerate.

The Tuberculids

This category includes lichen scrofulosorum, papulonecrotic tuberculid, and erythema induratum of Bazin. The association of these entities with *M. tuberculosis* infection has been debated. Many now agree that the tuberculids occur as the result of hematogenous dissemination of the tubercle bacilli in patients with a high degree of immunity. With the polymerase chain reaction, mycobacterial DNA has been demonstrated in papulonecrotic tuberculid and erythema induratum of Bazin. The underlying focus of infection is, however, not always apparent clinically.

Lichen Scrofulosorum

Lichen scrofulosorum is a rare eruption of asymptomatic, flat-topped, yellow to pink papules occurring most often on the skin of the trunk of patients with tuberculosis in lymph nodes and/or bone. These lesions can develop into discoid plaques that may last for months but eventually resolve slowly.

Papulonecrotic Tuberculid

Papulonecrotic tuberculid is characterized by asymptomatic, symmetrical, necrotic papules that occur in showers over the extremities of young adults. Occasionally, they may form chronic, ulcerating lesions that may persist for several months.

Erythema Induratum of Bazin

The typical clinical features of this tuberculid include dusky-red tender nodules on the lower legs in middle-aged women. These nodules tend to be persistent or recurrent and heal with scarring. Ulceration is not uncommon. Patients usually have a strong positive tuberculin test; however, few have a history of active tuberculosis. A latent tuberculous focus is thought to be the cause of these skin lesions, possibly as a T-cell–mediated immune response to a tuberculous antigen.

Diagnosis and Differential Diagnosis

Perhaps the most important facet to making a diagnosis of cutaneous tuberculosis is a high index of clinical suspicion. This can be particularly important with the tuberculids, where active tuberculosis elsewhere may not be obvious.

The tuberculin test is used to detect those persons previously infected with tubercle bacilli either by inoculation or invasion. The tuberculin test, however, is not entirely specific for *M. tuberculosis*. Small, nonspecific reactions may occur, with nontuberculous mycobacterial infections.

Demonstration of acid-fast bacilli in the lesion remains the only available way to confirm the diagnosis with certainty. This can be achieved by the following:

1. Microscopy. Skin sections can be stained by the Ziehl-Neelsen or auramine methods and examined for acid-fast bacilli.

2. Culture. Skin biopsy specimens should always be cultured for a definitive diagnosis (if positive) and for drug sensitivity. Culture may take up to 8 weeks.

3. Polymerase chain reaction. This technique may be useful in patients with long-standing lupus vulgaris, scrofuloderma, and the tuberculids.

The histopathology of cutaneous tuberculosis varies depending on the classification and the balance between infection and immunologic response. In the tuberculous chancre an acute necrotic neutrophilic reaction changes to a mononuclear infiltrate and, after 4 to 6 weeks, into typical tubercles (epithelioid cells surrounded by mononuclear cells) in which bacilli can no longer be identified. The center of the tubercle undergoes caseation necrosis and may calcify. In miliary and orificial forms, the characteristic tubercle does not form or is imperfect. Bacilli are numerous. In scrofuloderma, the skin is destroyed by nonspecific abscess, sinus, and ulcer formation. Typical tubercle formation at the periphery can occur. In verrucous tuberculosis, typical dermal changes are missing and bacilli are scarce, but there is verrucous epidermal hyperplasia and hyperkeratosis. The histopathologic features of lupus vulgaris can be variable. Although typical tubercles are often present, the extent of the mononuclear infiltrate may be extensive, and intense fibrosis may occur with healing.

| TABLE 6-4. Differential Diagnosis of Tuberculosis | |
TYPE OF TUBERCULOSIS	IMPORTANT DIFFERENTIAL DIAGNOSES
Tuberculous chancre	Primary chancre Cat-scratch fever Tularemia Sporotrichosis Actinomycosis
Warty tuberculosis	Warts or keratoses Hypertrophic lichen planus Blastomycosis Chromoblastomycosis
Lupus vulgaris	Discoid lupus erythematosus Sarcoidosis Lymphocytoma Tertiary syphillis Deep mycoses
Scrofuloderma	Syphilitic gumma Sporotrichosis Actinomycosis Severe acne conglobata
Orificial tuberculosis	Syphilis Aphthous ulcers Squamous cell carcinoma
Metastatic tuberculous ulcer	Sporotrichosis
Lichen scrofuloderma	Lichen planus Lichen nitidus Micropapular sarcoidosis Eczema
Papulonecrotic tuberculid	Pityriasis lichenoides et varioliformis acuta
Erythema induratum	Nodular vasculitis

Response to antituberculous chemotherapy may also aid in making the diagnosis.

The differential diagnosis of cutaneous tuberculosis is very wide for all types of cutaneous tuberculosis and is summarized in Table 6–4.

Treatment

The standard chemotherapy regimen for tuberculosis is a 2-month regimen of four drugs: isoniazid (300 mg daily), rifampicin (450 to 600 mg daily), pyrazinamide (1.5 to 2.5 g daily), and ethambutol (15 mg/kg daily), followed by rifampicin and isoniazid for an additional 4 months. This regimen should be used for all cases of cutaneous tuberculosis, and in drug-susceptible cases, a cure rate of more than 95% can be expected. Resistant strains of *M. tuberculosis* are emerging. This seems to occur particularly in patients affected with the human immunodeficiency virus and has the ability to spread by nosocomial transmission.

Atypical Mycobacteria

These mycobacteria form a heterogeneous group, and the epidemiology of infections caused by these pathogens is different from that of tuberculosis. They are divided into slow-growing and fast-growing groups. The slow growers are further subdivided according to their ability to form pigment on exposure to light. Cutaneous lesions are usually caused by *M. marinum* and *M. ulcerans.*

Mycobacterium marinum *Infection*

This atypical mycobacterium grows mainly in water that is not often replenished, and therefore human infection usually occurs from swimming pools and fish tanks, (termed *swimming pool granuloma* or *fish tank granuloma).* Clinically, a single nodule or pustule occurs, usually on the hands in fish-keepers and at the sites of trauma in other cases. These nodules may ulcerate and suppurate. Lymphatic spread of the nodules, called sporotrichoid spread, is common. *M marinum* grows best on culture media at low temperature (25°C to 32°C); however, 37°C is the usual temperature used for culturing mycobacteria, leading to a false-negative or delayed diagnosis. Lesions may spontaneously resolve over months. Three drug regimens have proved successful in treatment: (1) rifampicin and ethambutol, (2) tetracyclines, and (3) sulfamethoxazole plus trimethoprim. Many consider minocycline (or doxycycline) 200 mg daily for several weeks as the treatment of choice.

Mycobacterium ulcerans *Infection*

M. ulcerans generally occurs in subequatorial regions, especially in the Nile bed areas of Uganda. It also grows best below body temperature at 32°C to 33°C. Most cases in Africa are in children, in the 5- to 15-year-old age group. Most patients present with a solitary nodule that will ulcerate to form a crater with typical undermined edges. Lesions are usually on the arms and legs. Healing may occur after 6 to 9 months, but some cases may extend widely to involve an entire limb.

M. ulcerans is sensitive to a number of drugs in vitro. Drug therapy, however, remains disappointing, and surgery to excise the diseased tissue is the treatment of choice.

Other Mycobacteria in Skin Disease

Mycobacterium kansasii

This unusual skin pathogen is more commonly associated with pulmonary disease in middle-aged men. The clinical features of *M. kansasii* skin lesions are variable, verrucous nodules with sporotrichoid spread, papulopustules, and crusted ulcerations. Standard antituberculous chemotherapy or minocycline has been used with success.

Mycobacterium avium *Complex*

This organism commonly infects the lungs and lymph nodes, especially in patients with the acquired immunodeficiency syndrome. A variety of cutaneous lesions, including papules and ulcers, can occur secondary to hematogenous dissemination. *M. avium* is not very responsive to chemotherapy.

Mycobacterium fortuitum *Complex*

This complex includes *M. chelonei*. Organisms are both widely distributed and rapid growers. Typical lesions show a red, painful node with subsequent abscess formation at sites of injections or surgery. Standard antituberculous chemotherapy is not helpful. Amikacin or doxycycline may be used in either infections, and while erythromycin and tobramycin are more useful in *M. chelonei* infections, *M. fortuitum* responds better to ciprofloxacin or sulfamethoxazole.

Acquired Immunodeficiency Syndrome and Mycobacterial Infections

Patients with the acquired immunodeficiency syndrome have a high incidence of mycobacterial infections, most of which are due to *M. avium* complex. Infections with *M. tuberculosis*, *M. kansasii*, and *M. scrofulosorum* are also seen. Many of these patients have disseminated disease, and bacilli are generally abundant in the cutaneous lesions.

LEPROSY

(CM&S Chapter 112)

Definition

Leprosy, or Hansen's disease, is a chronic infection of slow onset caused by the acid-fast bacillus *Mycobacterium leprae*, whose medical sequelae are primarily determined by the unique tropism of the causative organism, among bacteria, for invasion and consequent pathology of the peripheral nervous system and the host's specific immunologic response. *M. leprae* invades the cooler tissues of the body, namely, the skin, peripheral nerves, upper respiratory tract, anterior chamber of the eyes, and testes, resulting in clinical signs and symptoms that are largely confined to these tissues. Depending on host cellular immunity, the disease may be benign or malignant, with its course further being complicated by intercurrent immune-mediated reactional states. Because antimicrobial therapy can arrest and even at times cure the disease, early diagnosis and therapy are critical in preventing severe debilitating deformity.

Clinical Description

Epidemiology

The majority of the 5.5 million affected persons reside in the tropics and subtropics, with prevalence being generally inversely proportional to a nation's per capita income. Unlike tuberculosis, leprosy is more a rural than an urban disease. Leprosy is endemic in Asia, Africa, the Pacific Basin, and Latin America. Eighty percent of worldwide cases are found in five countries: India (accounting for 60% of cases worldwide), Myanmar, Indonesia, Brazil, and Nigeria. Leprosy affects all races and age groups, with a peak incidence of onset in the second and third decades of life.

Most persons are immune to leprosy, with subclinical infection believed to be common in endemic areas and only a minority of exposed individuals progressing to actual disease. Owing to *M. leprae*'s uniquely long generation time, the incubation period ranges from 2 to 30 or more years, with an average of 5 years. Children appear more susceptible to disease, and adults are relatively resistant, as suggested by only a 5% incidence of conjugal leprosy. It is unclear whether the disease arises from primary infection or reactivation. Only lepromatous leprosy (multibacillary disease) is considered infectious. Tuberculoid leprosy (paucibacillary disease—no bacilli demonstrable in the dermis) is noninfectious. Although it was long held that close prolonged contact with a highly bacilliferous lepromatous case is the primary mode of transmission, more than 50% of patients with leprosy have no known history of contact with another known patient with leprosy. Intact skin-to-skin transmission has been generally discounted; however, ulcerated lesions or denuded skin may serve as a potential source of infection. Most authorities favor respiratory transmission from heavily infected nasal droplets as the primary mode of transmission. Other possible modes of transmission include environmental factors such as insect vectors and infected soil. Blood-sucking insects are suspected as vectors of leprosy. Bedbugs and mosquitos found in the vicinity of leprosaria regularly harbor *M. leprae*. *M. leprae* has also been found in soil. It is possible that the preponderantly rural prevalence of leprosy may be the result of contact with infected soil and transcutaneous inoculation from walking barefoot.

The household risk of developing disease in endemic areas from a lepromatous patient is about 10%, and in nonendemic areas it is estimated at 1%. In the United States, affected immigrants with the disease pose no threat to nonhousehold contacts. Casual contacts and medical caregivers are not at risk.

Clinical and Immunologic Features

Classification and Skin Testing (Lepromin)

Based on clinical findings and dermatopathology, the Ridley and Jopling classification places patients accurately on the immunologically determined disease spectrum, and can be extremely useful in predicting outcome, likely complications, and possible reactional states (Table 6–5).

Lepromin is a homogenate of heat-killed *M. leprae* that, injected intradermally, is useful in determining whether cellular immunity to

M. leprae is intact. Skin test site induration at 3 to 4 weeks is the preferred method for evaluation.

Complications

Reactional States. The reactional states which complicate leprosy in up to 50% of patients after the initiation of therapy may cause considerable morbidity and be a source of confusion to the patient, whose expectation is improvement and not the appearance of new skin lesions or painful neuropathy. Two major types of reaction occur and are different clinically and immunologically.

Reversal and Downgrading Reactions (Lepra Type 1). Lepra type 1 reactions affect individuals with borderline disease. When they occur before the initiation of therapy they are called "downgrading" reactions and represent a shift toward the lepromatous pole. Reactions that occur after the initiation of therapy are clinically indistinguishable. These "reversal" reactions signify a shift toward tuberculoid disease. Reactions are confined only to lesional skin or inapparent foci and nerves where leprosy antigen is present. Lepra type 1 reactions are common and more severe in borderline lepromatous disease, where more antigen is present. Existing lesions become inflamed and tender. New inflammatory "satellite" lesions may appear for the first time. Reversal reactions can present as acute painful nerve-trunk palsies within 24 to 36 hours. On examination, involved nerves are typically enlarged and tender. Many patients also experience "silent" neuritides that occur slowly and painlessly.

Erythema Nodosum Leprosum (Lepra Type 2). Erythema nodosum leprosum occurs in half of patients with borderline lepromatous and lepromatous leprosy. Although erythema nodosum leprosum may be seen on initial presentation and be a precipitating cause for a patient to seek medical attention, it most often develops within the first few years after therapy has begun, and episodes of the disease resolve spontaneously generally after about 5 years of treatment. The most common clinical manifestation is crops of erythematous, painful nodules of the skin and subcutaneous tissues. If the disease is severe, pustules develop, which can ulcerate and result in suppurative wounds and subsequent scarring. Erythema nodosum leprosum is not limited to the lower extremities, being found virtually anywhere, but most often on the extensor surface of the forearms, medial thighs, and occasionally the face. Individual lesions last only a few days. It is a systemic disorder at times associated with fever, malaise, anorexia, leukocytosis, and anemia. Erythema nodosum leprosum may also result in synovitis, nephritis, neuritis, iritis, lymphadenitis, and epididymo-orchitis.

Diagnosis and Differential Diagnosis

Although the variable skin lesions of leprosy may mimic innumerable other dermatologic diseases, including sarcoidosis, pityriasis alba, vitiligo, psoriasis, granuloma annulare, lupus vulgaris, tinea, dermal leishmaniasis, lymphoma, and syphilis, the combination of skin and nerve involvement in a patient from a known leprosy-endemic area should clearly raise suspicion for leprosy.

TABLE 6-5. Some Clinical and Histologic Features of the Ridley-Jopling Classification of Leprosy

CLINICAL AND HISTOLOGIC FEATURES	TUBERCULOID (TT)	BORDERLINE TUBERCULOID (BT)	BORDERLINE (BB)	BORDERLINE LEPROMATOUS (BL)	LEPROMATOUS (LL)
Skin lesions	Up to three; sharply defined asymmetrical plaques with tendency for central clearing and elevated borders, hypopigmented depressed center	Smaller or larger than TT; potentially more numerous than lesions of TT; usually annular lesions with sharp margination on exterior and interior borders. Borders not as elevated as in TT	Dimorphic lesions intermediate between BT and BL	Few or many LL-type lesions; ill-defined plaques with an occasional sharp margin; shiny appearance	Symmetrical; poorly marginated, multiple infiltrated nodules and plaques or diffuse infiltration; xanthoma-like or dermatofibroma papules; leonine facies and eyebrow alopecia
Nerve lesions	Skin lesions anesthetic early; nerve near lesion may be enlarged	Skin lesions anesthetic early. Nerve trunk palsies asymmetrical. Nerve abscesses most common in BT	Anesthetic skin lesions and nerve trunk palsies	Skin lesions usually hypesthetic; may be anesthetic; nerve trunk palsies common and frequently symmetrical	Hyperesthesia or *late* sign; nerve palsies variable; acral, distal, symmetrical anesthesia common

Lepromin skin test	Positive	Usually positive (80% to 90%)	Negative	Negative	Negative
Lymphocytes	Dense peripheral infiltration about epithelioid tubercle; infiltration into epidermis well developed	Less numerous than TT; peripheral infiltration about granuloma; variable epidermal infiltration usually focal	Lymphopenic	Moderately dense and in the same distribution as macrophages	Scant; diffuse or focal in distribution
Langerhans giant cells	Present, well developed	May be present; usually few in number	Absent	Absent	Absent
Acid-fast bacilli	Rare, less than 1 per 100 oil immersion fields (i.e., bacteriologic index (BI) of zero (paucibacillary))	Rare, usually BI of zero (paucibacillary)	1–10 per oil immersion field or BI of 3 to 4	10–100 per oil immersion field or BI of 4 to 5	100–1000 per oil immersion field or BI of 4 to 6
Immune status	Intact cell-mediated immunity				Specific cell-mediated anergy to M. leprae

From Rea TH, Modlin RL. Leprosy. In: Demis DJ, ed. Clinical Dermatology, 19th revision, vol 3, unit 16–29. Philadelphia: JB Lippincott, 1992.

Treatment

Regimens to Treat Leprosy

There are two important issues affecting the appropriate selection of treatment regimens for the different polar ends of the leprosy spectrum: the number of bacilli and the presence or absence of specific cellular immunity. It naturally follows that in multibacillary disease, more intensive drug regimens for a greater duration are required.

Chemotherapy in leprosy rapidly renders the patient noninfectious to others, probably within the first few weeks of therapy. Viable drug-sensitive bacterial persistence, despite prolonged multidrug regimens including rifampin treatment, threatens our ability to cure lepromatous leprosy. For multibacillary leprosy the WHO recommends daily dapsone, 100 mg, plus clofazimine, 50 mg, and monthly (supervised) rifampin, 600 mg, plus clofazimine, 300 mg, for at least 2 years or until smear-negativity. For paucibacillary leprosy the WHO recommends dapsone, 100 mg daily, plus monthly (supervised) rifampin, 600 mg, for a total duration of 6 months. The rationale behind these regimens was that multidrug chemotherapy rapidly eradicates contagion, can be inexpensive, prevents drug resistance, and that a limited or short course will improve compliance and is operationally more feasible. Unfortunately, these recommendations antedated supportive clinical trials, and, furthermore, the tremendous bacillary load of lepromatous leprosy in these *M. leprae*–anergic hosts, the long time to relapse after discontinuation of rifampin-containing regimens (averaging 7 years), and the affordability of available chemotherapy caused some leprologists to resist these recommendations. Ten years after the discontinuation of therapy relapse rates in multibacillary disease have been at the unacceptably high rate of 20%.

Many experts, therefore, use more conservative regimens. They treat multibacillary leprosy with dapsone, 100 mg, daily for a lifetime and rifampin, 600 mg, daily for the initial 3 years or until skin smears for acid-fast bacilli are negative. For paucibacillary leprosy, they recommend dapsone, 100 mg daily, alone for a total of 5 years.

Monitoring Therapy

Slit-skin smears obtained by scraping the dermis with a scalpel or razor blade are useful in determining the efficacy of treatment as well as in establishing an initial baseline of disease severity. The skin smears are taken from six different skin sites: the earlobes, posterior elbows, and anterior knees, and are examined microscopically for (1) density of organisms (bacteriologic index) and (2) percentage of bacilli that stain uniformly and correlate with actual *M. leprae* viability (morphologic index). In lepromatous leprosy, initial skin smears typically have a bacteriologic index of 4 to 6+, which falls by 1+ per year with effective therapy, becoming 0 usually at about 5 years. The morphologic index falls to 0 rapidly within days to weeks of therapy.

Treatment of Complications

Erythema Nodosum Leprosum. If mild, skin lesions of erythema nodosum leprosum can be treated symptomatically with aspirin or other nonsteroidal anti-inflammatory agents. However, if episodes are severe with multiple skin lesions and systemic symptoms, prednisone is indicated with initial doses of 40 to 60 mg daily, discontinued abruptly in 1 week. If erythema nodosum leprosum occurs repeatedly, thalidomide 100 to 300 mg per night can be used for long-term control.

Reversal Reactions. Corticosteroids for a few months are the only reliably effective treatment for reversal reactions. Hence, minor skin inflammation should be tolerated. Therapy is required for neuritis, lesions that threaten to ulcerate, and those at cosmetically important places such as the face. An initial dose of 40 to 60 mg of prednisone per day is usually adequate, tapered over 2 to 3 months after control has been achieved.

Prophylaxis

It is advised that all household contacts of lepromatous patients, especially children, should be examined annually by experienced personnel for a period of 5 years after the diagnosis of the index case. Dapsone prophylaxis of household contacts of lepromatous patients is no longer advocated since it does not prevent the development of lepromatous leprosy and only partially reduces the subsequent prevalence of tuberculoid leprosy.

NOCARDIOSIS AND ACTINOMYCOSIS

(CM&S Chapter 113)

Nocardiosis

Definition

Nocardiosis refers to the spectrum of disease caused by filamentous bacteria of the genus *Nocardia*. In humans, nocardiosis is caused predominantly by *N. asteroides* and *N. brasiliensis*. Infection may be initiated by inhalation or traumatic inoculation, with possible dissemination. Cutaneous manifestations have been categorized as mycetoma and lymphocutaneous, cervicofacial, superficial, and disseminated infections.

Clinical Description

N. asteroides is isolated from soil in temperate areas. *N. brasiliensis* is endemic in regions of Mexico and Central and South America; it is also occasionally found in the United States. The incidence of infection is highest from ages 20 to 50 years. Approximately 85% of cases are pulmonary or systemic infections and 15% are localized to the skin and soft tissue. *N. asteroides* accounts for the majority of pulmonary and systemic infections, often occurring opportunistically, whereas *N. brasiliensis* usually infects the skin and soft tissue in immunocompetent patients.

Systemic dissemination occurs most frequently in patients with pulmonary infection; however, it may follow primary cutaneous infection. After the central nervous system, the skin and soft tissues are the second most common sites of dissemination. Nodules, pustules, and abscesses occur and may become ulcerated.

The most common manifestation worldwide of primary skin and soft tissue infection is mycetoma. A mycetoma is a chronic infection that usually occurs on the lower extremity as a painless, firm swelling with multiple sinus tracts draining purulent material. Underlying bone is often involved. Mycetomas may be caused by *Nocardia* and other actinomycetes (actinomycetoma) or by true fungi (eumycetoma). Primary cutaneous infection alternatively may occur as pustules, abscesses, ulcers, or cellulitis, all of which may mimic infection caused by more common gram-positive bacteria. A sporotrichoid pattern of linear erythematous nodules can also be seen along an extremity and a cervicofacial variant has occurred in children, who have an erythematous papule or pustule on the face, submandibular lymphadenopathy, and fever.

Diagnosis and Differential Diagnosis

Gram and modified acid-fast stains and culture of clinical specimens (sputum, pus, tissue) establish the diagnosis. *Nocardia* species are aerobic, weakly gram-positive, variably acid-fast, filamentous bacteria. Growth of *Nocardia* organisms may take a week or more on Sabouraud's glucose agar. Serologic tests are unreliable because of cross reactivity with tuberculosis and leprosy.

Since the clinical presentation of nocardiosis is pleomorphic, so is the differential diagnosis, which includes other infectious and granulomatous diseases, as well as tumors.

Treatment and Prognosis

Antimicrobial chemotherapy is administered for prolonged periods, often in combination with surgery to drain abscesses, excise small mycetomas, or debulk larger mycetomas. Sulfonamides, particularly sulfanilamide and trimethoprim-sulfamethoxazole, are the most effective antibiotic agents; however, primary resistance and late relapse are problematic. In serious infections, parenteral amikacin is indicated, often accompanied or followed by another agent, such as a third generation cephalosporin or imipenem.

Actinomycosis

Definition

Actinomycosis is a chronic, suppurative, granulomatous, and fibrosing infection that most often involves the cervicofacial, thoracic, and abdominal areas. It is caused primarily by the endogenous oral bacterium *Actinomyces israelii*. Infection frequently spreads to adjacent tissues, forming cutaneous sinus tracts that discharge ''sulfur granules,'' which are colonies of the causative organism.

Clinical Description

Actinomycosis occurs worldwide with a higher incidence in rural areas. Seen most commonly in the 30- to 60-year age group, cervicofacial infection is the most common.

Patients with actinomycosis, regardless of site, may complain of localized pain and can have a low-grade fever and a normal or mildly elevated white blood cell count. Cervicofacial actinomycosis, or "lumpy jaw," is believed to begin as a periodontal abscess that forms in the mandible or maxilla after dental extraction, oral surgery, or other trauma in the setting of poor oral hygiene. The infection then characteristically spreads (acutely or chronically) to adjacent tissues, forming sinuses to the skin or mouth that drain purulent material, sometimes containing granules. Bone and CNS involvement may occur from direct spread of infection.

Thoracic actinomycosis most frequently occurs after aspiration from the oral cavity. The lung parenchyma (typically basilar), pleura, mediastinum, and chest wall may all be involved. Roentgenographic features include (1) penetration of a pulmonary focus of infection through the chest wall; (2) destruction of adjacent ribs; (3) spread of infection across interlobar fissures; and (4) erosion of the vertebral body and processes.

Diagnosis and Differential Diagnosis

The presence of yellow "sulfur granules," 0.25 to 2.0 mm in diameter, suggests the diagnosis. Their presence is not, however, pathognomonic because similar granules can be seen in mycetomas (caused by fungi, *Nocardia*, *Streptomyces*, or *Actinomadura*) and in staphylococcal botryomycosis. The granules of actinomycosis can be distinguished from the granules of other infections on pathologic examination. Clinically, other infectious agents and tumors must be excluded. The definitive diagnosis of actinomycosis is made by identifying the gram-positive, non–acid-fast, branching, long, slender, filamentous bacteria in culture.

Treatment

Actinomycosis is treated with a combination of long-term (weeks to months) high-dose penicillin and surgical debridement of abscesses and fibrotic tissue.

ROCKY MOUNTAIN SPOTTED FEVER AND OTHER RICKETTSIAL DISEASES

(CM&S Chapter 114)

Rickettsial infections are caused by obligate intracellular bacterial organisms belonging to the family Rickettsiaceae. This family subsumes the genera *Rickettsia, Coxiella,* and *Ehrlichia,* which are responsible for the spotted fever/typhus illnesses, Q fever, and ehrlichiosis, respectively. All have the capacity to produce febrile infectious syndromes, and the spotted fever/typhus group of illnesses have the most distinctive cutaneous manifestations. These diseases are zoonotic infections that are transmitted to humans by arthropod vectors or by aerosol (e.g., Q fever).

Rocky Mountain Spotted Fever

Clinical Description

Rocky Mountain spotted fever (RMSF) is caused by *Rickettsia rickettsii* and is transmitted to humans by the bite of a tick. In the western United States, the primary vector is the wood tick, *Dermacentor andersoni*; the dog tick, *Dermacentor variabilis,* is the principal vector in the eastern and southern states. The reservoirs of the organism are primarily small rodents, but ticks may infect their own offspring. The peak incidence of disease is in the late spring and early summer when nymphs molt to become adults. The highest incidence of disease now occurs in the South Atlantic states of North and South Carolina extending to Texas. Children have the highest incidence of disease.

The incubation period ranges from 2 to 14 days with an average of 7 days. The onset of symptoms is more often abrupt but may be insidious. Early symptoms are usually nonspecific and include fever (100 to 104° F), headache (often severe), myalgias, arthralgias, and malaise. The classic triad of fever, rash, and headache or history of tick exposure may occur infrequently in the first 3 days of illness but is reported in 50% to 60% of confirmed cases.

Rash is the most helpful sign in making the correct diagnosis. It occurs within 1 to 14 days (mean 3 or 4 days); however, it may not develop at all or it may develop too late, delaying diagnosis and resulting in death. The eruption is initially characterized by blanching pink macules beginning on the wrists, ankles, palms, and soles. Application of a warm compress to the extremity or a fever in the early stages may accentuate the rash. Centripetal spread to axillae, buttocks, trunk, and face is characteristic. The color of lesions deepens, and papules evolve 2 to 3 days after onset. In approximately 4 days, petechiae usually develop and may coalesce to form large ecchymotic lesions. The severity of the eruption often correlates with the severity of the illness. Patients with prolonged hypotension with or without evidence of disseminated intravascular coagulation may develop confluent ecchymoses and gangrene of fingers, toes, penis, and/or scrotum.

R. rickettsii infection is a multisystem disease reflecting a widespread infectious vasculitic process. While a petechial eruption is the hallmark of disease, a variety of symptoms reflect systemic involvement. These include gastrointestinal manifestations (in 30% to 50%), pneumonitis, pulmonary edema due to leakage from vasculitis, myocarditis with cardiac dysfunction, skeletal muscle necrosis (manifested by severe myalgias and rises in creatine kinase and aldolase levels), azotemia secondary to volume depletion, interstitial nephritis, and neurologic manifestations such as headache (most frequent complaint), meningismus, seizures, coma, focal deficits, hearing loss, papilledema, and ataxia. Other less common manifestations of disease include conjunctivitis, retinitis, parotitis, and orchitis.

Pathology

A widespread small vessel thrombotic vasculitis is the pathologic hallmark of many forms of rickettsial disease, especially with *R. rickettsii* infections.

Diagnosis and Differential Diagnosis

Diagnosis is most commonly confirmed by acute and chronic serology together with clinical and epidemiologic data. The most sensitive and specific serologic tests are the indirect hemagglutination (IHA) and indirect fluorescent antibody (IFA) tests. Less sensitive tests include latex agglutination, complement fixation, and the Weil-Felix reaction (based on the cross-reactive agglutination of *Proteus* strains OX-19 and OX-2). An acute diagnosis can only be achieved with identification of rickettsiae in skin specimens by immunofluorescence staining of the organism in the blood vessel walls or by immunoperoxidase methods.

The differential diagnosis for RMSF is broad. The most important potentially fatal disease to rule out is meningococcemia (this rash occurs earlier, and the organism can be demonstrated with a Gram stain). The differential also includes an enteroviral infection, measles or atypical measles, rubella, infectious mononucleosis, hepatitis, typhoid fever, leptospirosis, relapsing fever, secondary syphilis, gonococcemia, and noninfectious vasculitides.

Treatment

Without treatment, mortality from RMSF approaches 70%. Appropriate early antibiotic and supportive therapy reduces mortality to less than 10%.

The recommended treatment includes doxycycline, 200 mg per day orally in divided doses; or tetracycline hydrochloride, 25 to 30 mg/kg per day orally in four divided doses; or chloramphenicol sodium succinate, 50 mg/kg loading dose, followed by 50 mg/kg per day orally in divided doses. Patients severely ill or unable to take oral medication should be treated with intravenous medications in the following doses: doxycycline, 4.4 mg/kg per day up to 200 mg per day in divided doses every 12 hours; tetracycline, 15 mg/kg loading dose followed by 15 mg/kg per day in divided doses every 6 hours; or chloramphenicol, 15 to 20 mg/kg loading dose followed by 30 to 50 mg/kg per day in divided doses every 6 hours. Defervescence is usually prompt within 24 to 72 hours, with improvement of general well-being. Treatment is continued until the patient has been afebrile for at least 2 to 3 days.

Supportive therapy with volume replacement including intravenous fluids or blood products may be necessary for the critically ill patient. Corticosteroids may have a role in the treatment of critically ill patients with diffuse vasculitis and shock secondary to increased capillary permeability.

Careful epidemiologic history, detailed physical examination, and a high index of suspicion are necessary for successful early intervention in this disease. RMSF is a disease for which empiric therapy is indicated.

Other Rickettsial Diseases

Rickettsialpox

R. akari is the cause of rickettsialpox and is transmitted to humans by the bite of a mouse mite. The disease is most commonly seen in urban areas. This self-limited spotted fever illness is characterized by a primary lesion at the site of the mite bite commencing as an erythematous papule in which a central vesicle develops. The vesicle eventually dries, leaving a brown or black eschar on a large indurated base. Nonspecific symptoms of fever, headache, myalgias, and malaise develop after an incubation period of 9 to 14 days. Regional lymphadenitis often develops near the site of the eschar, and the appearance of a generalized eruption of erythematous papules with central vesicles, sparing the palms and soles, occurs within 3 days (range, 1 to 4 days) of the onset of systemic symptoms. Diagnosis is made serologically by IFA; the Weil-Felix reaction is negative. The differential diagnosis of rickettsialpox includes other rickettsioses such as spotted fevers and scrub typhus. Nonrickettsial infections in the differential diagnosis include varicella, enteroviruses, and eczema herpeticum. Tetracycline or chloramphenicol is an effective therapy, although untreated cases usually resolve without relapse.

Typhus Fever Group

Epidemic (Louse-Borne) Typhus

Epidemic (louse-borne) typhus is caused by *R. prowazekii* and is transmitted to its human reservoir by the body louse, *Pediculus humanus corporis*. Flying squirrels are also reservoirs for the organism. Epidemics occur, especially with human conditions promoting malnutrition, poor hygiene, and overcrowding. Typhus is most common in colder months. During a blood meal, the infected louse defecates and deposits infected feces onto the skin of the human, inoculating the site of the bite. After replication at the site of entry, the organisms disseminate and infect endothelial cells, causing their proliferation and infiltration of mononuclear cells resulting in diffuse vasculitis.

The incubation period averages 10 days. Abrupt onset of fever, severe headache, myalgias, and arthralgias is the usual presentation. Fever and headache are unremitting, and the patient quickly becomes prostrate. Cutaneous eruption develops 4 to 7 days after the onset of systemic symptoms and is characterized by blanching erythematous macules beginning in the axillary folds and spreading to the trunk and extremities. Palms and soles are spared, except in severe cases, where generalized petechiae and purpuric lesions may develop that may lead to necrosis, especially over bony prominences. Eschars do not occur. The rash is absent in 10% to 50% of patients. Neurologic complications including coma may develop. Other signs and symptoms include conjunctival suffusion, relative bradycardia in the early stages, dry cough, constipation, and abdominal pain. Disease severity correlates with age. Severe vasculitis may predispose the patient to cerebral thrombosis or symmetrical gangrene of the distal digits.

Diagnosis is best made serologically. The Weil-Felix reaction is positive with cross-reactive antibodies to *Proteus* OX-19. Other illnesses presenting with fever and rash are usually distinguished from epidemic typhus by the character and mode of spread of the rash and by the epidemiologic setting in which the illness occurs. If the illness suggests RMSF but the season is autumn or winter, louse-borne typhus should be suspected.

Prompt improvement of symptoms occurs with treatment. Tetracyclines or chloramphenicol is the recommended treatment and is continued until 2 or 3 days after defervescence. A single dose of 100 mg or 200 mg of doxycycline may be effective. Early treatment may be associated with relapse as a result of an ineffective immune response and incomplete eradication of the organism.

Endemic (Murine) Typhus

Endemic (murine) typhus is a worldwide disease caused by *R. typhi*, which is transmitted to humans from its unaffected rat host by the rat flea, *Xenopsylla cheopis*. Man is a dead-end host for the organism. In the United States, the southern Gulf states, particularly southern Texas, have the highest incidence of reported disease. Persons working in areas of food storage are at an increased risk of infection. The organism is transmitted when the flea defecates after its blood meal and infected feces are rubbed into the abraded skin.

After an incubation period of 6 to 14 days, a prodrome of mild headache, malaise, nausea, cough, chest pain, coryza, and myalgias may develop, followed by abrupt onset of fever, chills, more severe headache, and intense myalgias. Rash occurs in 50% to 65% by the fifth or sixth day of symptoms. Pink, blanching macules, originating on the trunk and spreading to the extremities sparing palms and soles, are the characteristic early exanthems. Papular lesions that may become petechial and, rarely, hemorrhagic develop as the rash ages. The rash is less severe than classic epidemic typhus and usually fades in 2 to 9 days. In severe cases, thrombosis of large vessels can occur. Other common symptoms and signs include mental status changes, cranial neuropathies (especially neurosensory deafness), pulmonary infiltrates on chest x-ray, hypotension, and vomiting.

The Weil-Felix reaction is positive with *Proteus* OX-19 agglutination, but this does not distinguish between RMSF and the typhus fever group. Specific diagnosis is confirmed with IFA. The differential diagnosis is similar to that of RMSF.

Treatment with tetracycline, doxycycline, or chloramphenicol is usually successful; efficacy of ciprofloxacin has also been demonstrated. Mortality is generally low. Sulfa drugs may exacerbate the disease.

Scrub Typhus

Scrub typhus is caused by *R. tsutsugamushi* and is transmitted to humans by the bite of the larval form (chigger) of a mite. The disease is endemic to the Far East. The name "scrub" reflects the low vegetation harboring chiggers that carry the organism. *R. tsutsugamushi* is the one rickettsial organism with multiple serotypes; therefore, infection with one does not confer immunity against others.

Chiggers bite with a predilection for pressure points (boot tops, waist line), inoculating organisms into the skin. Local replication followed by dissemination occurs. At the site of the bite, an erythematous papule develops that progresses to a small bulla, to a shallow ulcer, to necrosis with an eschar on a raised erythematous base. After an incubation period of 6 to 21 days, a prodrome of headache, chills, and anorexia develops. Unremitting fever, headaches, and myalgias are the rule and may be accompanied by a dry cough.

The cutaneous eruption occurs in approximately 30% to 35% of cases by the fifth day (range, 3 to 8 days) and is characterized by a self-limited erythematous maculopapular rash beginning on the trunk, spreading centrifugally, and sparing palms and soles. Purpuric lesions are noted in a minority of patients, and larger vessel thrombosis rarely occurs.

The most common physical sign is generalized lymphadenopathy. Other findings include splenomegaly, conjunctivitis, retinal vein engorgement, and papilledema. Diagnosis is most accurately made with IFA or indirect immunoperoxidase testing; the Weil-Felix OX-K test is less specific. If an eschar is not present, the differential diagnosis includes leptospirosis, brucellosis, typhoid fever, viral infectious mononucleosis syndromes, toxoplasmosis, and endemic viral diseases such as dengue fever. Treatment with tetracycline or chloramphenicol reduces the length of illness, but relapses can occur. Mortality is generally low in this disease.

Q Fever

Q fever is the one rickettsial disease that is not usually transmitted by a vector but rather is acquired through inhalation of aerosolized excreta or rarely through ingestion. The illness is caused by *Coxiella burnetii*, which primarily infects cattle, sheep, and goats. Acute onset of systemic symptoms of fever, headache, chills, and anorexia occurs. Pneumonitis is common, and hepatitis may develop. Radiographic findings suggest atypical pneumonia. Endocarditis, osteomyelitis, meningoencephalitis, or granulomatous hepatitis may also occur. A rash is unusual in this disease. It appears as discrete erythematous macules that begin on the trunk and may spread centrifugally. The histopathology is unique among rickettsial diseases. Granulomas with central clearing surrounded by inflammatory cells and a fibrin ring (doughnut lesion) are the distinguishing features. Serologic diagnosis is made with complement-fixation antibody titers or with IFA. Early in the illness, the differential diagnosis includes entities causing systemic illness such as salmonellosis, brucellosis, leptospirosis, viral mononucleosis syndromes, and viral hepatitis. Treatment with tetracycline is effective; ciprofloxacin may also be successful.

Ehrlichiosis

Human ehrlichiosis is a rickettsial disease caused by *Ehrlichia chaffeensis*, which is probably transmitted to humans by a tick bite. Unlike other rickettsial organisms, *Ehrlichia* species invade leukocytes and replicate within intracytoplasmic membrane bound vacuoles until cell lysis occurs.

The endemic focus in the United States appears to be primarily in the south central and southeastern states. The peak incidence is from April to June. The clinical manifestations of the illness are similar to those of other rickettsial diseases except that the eruption rarely involves the palms and soles. Pulmonary and central nervous system complications are not uncommon. In general, the disease is milder than RMSF and may be subclinical in some patients. Patients may present with leukopenia and/or thrombocytopenia, and inclusion bodies may be seen in leukocytes on the peripheral smear. Diagnosis may be made by IFA serology. The differential diagnosis is similar to that of other rickettsial diseases and includes early Lyme disease, babesiosis, and Colorado tick fever as well. Chloramphenicol and tetracycline appear to be equally effective treatments.

BACILLARY ANGIOMATOSIS AND CAT-SCRATCH DISEASE

(CM&S Chapter 115)

Definition

The causative agents of these two zoonoses—bacillary angiomatosis and cat-scratch disease—are closely related alpha-proteobacteria. The diseases may share overlapping epidemiologic and clinical characteristics. These include transmission of infection to humans by an arthropod vector, resulting in a febrile illness accompanied by cutaneous lesions, or lymphadenopathy, or both (Table 6–6).

Although five immunocompetent patients with bacillary angiomatosis have been reported, the disease has been described predominantly in immunocompromised, HIV-infected men or in other immunosuppressed patients. In the United States, cat-scratch disease peaks seasonally during the fall and winter. The disease affects an estimated 22,000 persons and accounts for roughly 2000 hospitalizations each year. Cat-scratch disease occurs predominantly in children and young adults under 18 years of age.

Patients with cat-scratch disease and those with bacillary angiomatosis are more likely than controls to have at least one kitten and to have had recent traumatic contact (bite or scratch) with a kitten.

The pet cat, *Felis domesticus*, is a reservoir for *B. henselae* infection, and the cat flea, *Ctenocephalides felis*, a possible vector for transmission of infection to humans. The reservoir(s) for the second causative agent of bacillary angiomatosis (*B. quintana*) remains unknown.

Clinical Findings

Bacillary Angiomatosis. The clinical spectrum of bacillary angiomatosis has been expanded in the past decade to include patients with single or multiple vascular lesions affecting virtually every organ; however, skin lesions remain the most easily recognized and frequently reported clinical manifestation of the disease. Cutaneous lesions of bacillary angiomatosis, which develop in HIV-infected individuals late in the course of disease, can be easily mistaken for Kaposi's sarcoma.

There are three types of skin lesion. Cutaneous lesions of bacillary angiomatosis begin as small, erythematous vascular papules, which may enlarge to form exophytic, friable nodules surrounded by a collarette of scale with or without erythema. Subcutaneous lesions of bacillary angiomatosis have the appearance of flesh-colored cystic nodules or epidermal inclusion cysts. They can also develop more deeply, presenting as soft tissue masses with or without overlying eruptive vascular lesions of cutaneous bacillary angiomatosis.

TABLE 6-6. Characteristic Features of Patients with Bacillary Angiomatosis and Cat-Scratch Disease

CHARACTERISTIC	BACILLARY ANGIOMATOSIS	CAT-SCRATCH DISEASE
Age of onset	Children and adults	≥ 55% under 18 years
Sex	Male > female	Male = female
Geographic setting	Worldwide	Worldwide
Risk factors	Cat bite/cat scratch Immunodeficiency	Cat bite/cat scratch
Causative bacteria	B. henselae B. quintana	B. henselae
Potential vector(s)	Cat flea, human body louse	Cat flea
Known reservoirs	Domestic cat	Domestic cat
Prominent clinical features	Vascular lesions (skin, liver/spleen, lymph nodes, and bone)	Lymphadenopathy, inoculation papule
Treatment	Erythromycin or doxycycline	Usually self-limited

Cat-Scratch Disease. Cat-scratch disease, typically a benign and self-limited illness lasting 6 to 12 weeks, presents with regional lymphadenopathy. Affected nodes are often tender and occasionally suppurate. The skin lesions typically develop 3 to 10 days after primary cutaneous inoculation and precede the onset of lymphadenopathy by 1 to 2 weeks. Fever, malaise, and constitutional symptoms accompany lymphadenopathy in up to 50% of patients.

Pathology

Bacillary Angiomatosis. There are characteristic lobular proliferations of small, capillary-sized blood vessels with protuberant endothelial cells surrounded by a mixed inflammatory infiltrate. The diagnostic feature seen in no other cutaneous vascular lesion, except verruga peruana, is purple granular material, revealing clumps of tangled bacteria with Warthin-Starry silver staining, scattered between vessels.

Cat-Scratch Disease. The primary inoculation lesion of cat-scratch disease reveals small areas of necrosis and suppuration surrounded by concentric layers of histiocytes, giant cells, and lymphocytes.

Differential Diagnosis

Bacillary Angiomatosis

The differential diagnosis includes other vascular proliferative disorders, mostly Kaposi's sarcoma and pyogenic granuloma. The finding of bacteria surrounding the epithelioid vascular proliferations histologically confirms the diagnosis.

Cat-Scratch Disease

The differential diagnosis includes many diseases associated with lymphadenopathy, including infections such as syphilis, tuberculosis, and lymphogranuloma venereum; granulomatous disorders, such as sarcoidosis; and benign and malignant tumors.

Treatment

Bacillary Angiomatosis. Erythromycin and doxycycline are the agents of first choice. In general, patients with cutaneous bacillary angiomatosis in the absence of osseous and parenchymal disease or bacteremia have responded well to 8 to 12 weeks of oral antimicrobial therapy with one of these two agents (erythromycin, 500mg four times per day or doxycycline, 100 mg twice a day).

Cat-Scratch Disease. For the vast majority of cat-scratch disease patients, no antimicrobial therapy is required because the adenopathy and associated symptoms will resolve without sequelae within 2 to 4 months.

THE ZOONOSES

(CM&S Chapter 116)

Zoonotic infections encompass a large group of bacterial, viral, rickettsial, fungal, and parasitic diseases that are transmitted from animals to humans. A small group of uncommon, but clinically relevant, zoonotic bacterial infections that have a wide variety of dermatologic manifestations (not covered elsewhere), including anthrax, brucellosis, plague, and tularemia, are representative of the many ways humans can acquire zoonotic infections.

Anthrax

Definition

Anthrax is an uncommon bacterial disease of wild and domestic animals caused by *Bacillus anthracis* that is transmitted to humans by inoculation, inhalation, or ingestion.

Clinical Description

The route of infection is cutaneous in 95% of the cases seen in the United States. Inhalation accounts for another 5%, and in other parts of the world gastrointestinal infection has been documented. Although rare in the United States, worldwide it continues to be an important disease and at times can be epidemic. Frequent sources of infection in humans are the hides, bristles, meat, and bones (bone meal fertilizer) of diseased wild and domestic herbivores, including cattle, goats, sheep, and horses.

After an incubation period of 2 to 5 days, the first symptom is pruritus at the site of a small erythematous papule, which soon vesiculates and becomes covered with an eschar. Occasionally, multiple vesicles coalesce into a larger bulla called a malignant pustule, which then forms a shallow crater and eventually heals with a scar. The lesions may be surrounded by nonpitting edema and may be accompanied by some discomfort and regional lymphadenopathy. There may be systemic manifestations, including fever, malaise, and, rarely, toxemia. The location of the lesions is generally on exposed skin, with the arms, face, and trunk involved in that order.

Inhalation anthrax (woolsorters' disease) starts with a vague, nonspecific, systemic reaction 1 to 5 days after exposure with progression to severe respiratory distress. Massive edema of the head and neck may also develop, associated with mediastinal widening and pleural effusions with a nonspecific parenchymal infiltrate on x-ray.

Pathology

Anthrax causes hemorrhagic necrosis of the epidermis and superficial dermis, leading to ulceration with a variable neutrophilic dermal infiltrate. Bacilli can be demonstrated by tissue Gram stain.

Pathogenesis and Etiology

B. anthracis is a large, gram-positive, nonmotile, spore-forming, capsulated bacillus that occurs singly or in short chains in clinical specimens. Spores are resistant to heat and can remain viable for years in dry soil. Cutaneous anthrax results from introduction of spores through an arthropod bite, abrasion of the skin, or scratching. The spores germinate, multiply, and produce a complex toxin.

Diagnosis and Differential Diagnosis

The rapidly evolving ulcer and failure to respond to initial antibiotic therapy are highly suggestive of cutaneous anthrax, especially in patients with a history of industrial or agricultural exposure to the organism.

Laboratory diagnosis is dependent on Gram stain and culture of blood, tissue, cerebrospinal fluid, or sputum. The presence of large gram-positive rods on Gram stain is presumptive evidence of infection, and the definitive diagnosis is made by culture on nutrient agar. A direct immunofluorescence antibody test is useful in making an early specific laboratory diagnosis. Serologic tests are retrospective and confirmatory of infection. The enzyme-linked immunosorbent assay (ELISA), which detects anticapsule antibodies, and the electrophoretic immunotransblot (EITB), which detects lethal factor and protective antigen antibodies, are both sensitive and specific.

The differential diagnosis of cutaneous anthrax includes any disease process that causes a slowly developing ulcer that forms as a vesicle and heals with a scar, including leishmaniasis, orf, staphylococcus abscess, brown recluse spider bite, and tularemia.

Treatment

Untreated cutaneous anthrax can lead to serious complications and death in up to 20% of cases. Gastrointestinal and inhalation anthrax may be fatal even with antibiotic therapy. Mild cutaneous disease can be treated with potassium penicillin V, 30 mg/kg per day orally in four divided doses for 5 to 7 days. Systemic disease requires procaine penicillin G, 20 to 30 mg/kg per day, intramuscularly in two equal doses for 5 to 7 days. Penicillin-allergic patients can be treated with tetracycline, 15 to 20 mg/kg per day, orally in four divided doses. Other forms of anthrax have been treated with massive doses of penicillin and streptomycin. Specific antitoxin is unavailable in the United States. Incision and drainage or excision of cutaneous lesions is specifically contraindicated because of the risk of dissemination of the infection.

Brucellosis

Definition and Clinical Definition

Brucellosis is a zoonotic infection caused by *Brucella* species, usually acquired from infected goats, cattle, pigs, or dogs. Dairy workers, shepherds, abattoir workers, meat packers, microbiologists, and veterinarians are especially at risk for infection. Milk and milk products have been increasingly important sources of infection. Open wounds are portals of entry for the organisms, but aerosols from infected material can invade through mucosal surfaces. Contamination of the environment may be a source of infection as well because *Brucella* can survive for up to 20 weeks in fetal organs left on the soil. Blood transfusion and sexual transmission are also sources of infection. Worldwide, the disease is common, although in the United States, the annual incidence of this disease is only several hundred.

The incubation period of brucellosis can be a few days but most commonly is from 3 to 4 weeks. In its acute form, the disease causes fever, sweats, chills, myalgia, lethargy, and headaches. Lymphadenopathy, splenomegaly, and skeletal problems are common. Other systems may also be affected. Cutaneous manifestations of brucellosis, seen in up to two thirds of affected individuals, include primary (abscesses and *Brucella* dermatitis), disseminated, and secondary (nonspecific) findings. Widespread erythematous to violaceous papules and nodules, particularly on the lower extremities, are the most typical and frequent cutaneous manifestations of brucellosis. However, a wide variety of secondary skin changes, including urticarial, eczematous, psoriasiform, or erythema nodosum, thought to be hypersensitivity reactions, have been associated with this infection.

Pathogenesis and Etiology

There are four species of gram-negative, small, aerobic, nonmotile, intracellular coccobacilli without spores or capsules that are capable of infecting humans: *B. melitensis, B. suis, B. abortus,* and the least common, *B. canis. Brucella* organisms appear in peripheral blood within hours and are engulfed by polymorphonuclear leukocytes and monocytes, eventually being carried to lymph nodes, liver, spleen, and bone marrow.

Diagnosis and Differential Diagnosis

History of exposure to contaminated animals, unpasteurized milk, dairy products, or travel to areas endemic for brucellosis can usually raise the suspicion of infection. Blood culture is most commonly used to isolate this slow-growing organism, which can take up to 6 weeks to be recovered. The differential diagnosis includes typhoid fever, tuberculosis, Q-fever, influenza, tularemia, mononucleosis, and malaria.

Treatment

Tetracycline, either alone or in combination with streptomycin or rifampin, is used for periods of 3 to 6 weeks for acute and chronic infections, respectively. Rifampin is used in pregnant women and trimethoprim-sulfamethoxazole in children.

Plague

Definition

Plague is a gram-negative bacterial infection caused by *Yersinia pestis* that is endemic in wild rodents and is transmitted to humans by fleas. Once established in humans, additional disease transmission can occur through the respiratory route.

Clinical Description

The three clinical forms of plague are bubonic, septicemic, and pneumonic. Bubonic plague is by far the most common form and results from direct contact with infected rodents or most frequently from the bite of fleas infesting infected animals. After an incubation period of 2 to 8 days there is fever, regional lymphadenopathy (bubo) and tenderness. The lymphadenopathy is rapidly progressive and exquisitely tender, quickly followed by systemic symptoms and, if untreated, death. Although skin lesions are inconspicuous, up to one quarter demonstrate pustules, vesicles, eschars, or papules near the bubo or flea bite. Late in the course of infection, purpura and gangrene, which occur as a result of endotoxin and probably account for the name ''black death,'' are seen. The septicemic phase, which may occur without adenopathy, is characterized by fever, chills, prostration, shock, and coma. Pneumonic plague results from secondary hematogenous spread from infected buboes but can also occur directly by aerosol.

Plague has a worldwide distribution in temperate climates. In the United States it is especially established west of the line drawn south from North Dakota to Texas.

Pathogenesis and Etiology

Y. pestis is a gram-negative, aerobic, nonmotile, pleomorphic, slow-growing bacillus that elaborates both endotoxins and exotoxins. Once the bacillus is ingested by the proper vector species of flea, the organisms multiply and eventually block the upper digestive tract of the flea, causing the insect to repeatedly bite its host. When the bacillus is introduced into humans by bite, contact, or inhalation, the organism is phagocytosed and destroyed by polymorphonuclear cells. However, macrophages may engulf bacilli, leading to resistant organisms that ultimately cause septicemia with or without lymphadenopathy.

Diagnosis and Differential Diagnosis

The presenting signs and symptoms of classic bubonic plague are sufficiently dramatic to strongly suggest a diagnosis, particularly in endemic areas. However, atypical syndromes and septicemic plague can often be misdiagnosed.

Treatment

The use of an appropriate antibiotic—streptomycin in two divided I/M doses totaling 30 mg/kg for 10 days—is critical. The best alternate choice is tetracycline 2–4 g/day in four daily doses for 10 days.

Tularemia

Definition and Clinical Description

Tularemia is an uncommon zoonotic infection caused by *Francisella tularensis*. It has six clinical patterns: ulceroglandular, glandular, oculoglandular, oropharyngeal, typhoidal, and pneumonic. The clinical presentation depends on the route of exposure, with the ulceroglandular variety occurring in over 80% of the cases. It is characterized by a small, pruritic, erythematous papule that proceeds to ulcerate, usually with an associated tender, regional lymphadenopathy which may suppurate and drain. Fever, chills, and myalgias are commonly seen in infections of all types.

Skin ulcers my be solitary or multiple and range from several millimeters to several centimeters in diameter. The margins of the ulcer tend to be raised and chancre-like and ultimately form an eschar. Ulcers are most commonly found on the upper extremities when the patient has been exposed to infected animals or on the back, abdomen, and head when infected by arthropod bite. Other cutaneous manifestations are unusual but include erythema nodosum, erythema multiforme, and rarely a diffuse, erythematous macular and papular rash.

The other, less common five types are without cutaneous lesions. Glandular tularemia is identical to ulceroglandular disease, except for this absence. Typhoidal tularemia, which accounts for 15% of cases and may be difficult to differentiate from ulceroglandular tularemia until the latter stages of infection, presents with fever, chills, and sore throat with or without abdominal symptoms. Patients are generally extremely ill, and the infection is probably acquired by inhalation of organisms during the ingestion of contaminated meat.

Epidemiology

Tularemia has been reported most frequently from North America, the Middle East, and Japan. Most of the 200 cases reported per year in the United States occur in Arkansas, Illinois, Missouri, Texas, Virginia, and Tennessee. Wild rabbits are the major source of infections acquired from animals. Two genera of ticks, *Amblyomma* and *Dermacentor*, are the chief vectors of tularemia. Ticks are considered responsible for nearly 90% of human infections in North America.

Pathogenesis and Etiology

F. tularensis is a small pleomorphic gram-negative facultative aerobic coccobacillus. As few as 10 organisms injected subcutaneously or 10 to 50 organisms given by aerosol can cause infection in humans. After the pathogen is introduced through arthropod bite or break in the skin, it is ingested by polymorphonuclear cells and macrophages. It then multiplies intracellularly and spreads to regional lymph nodes, distant lymph nodes, and ultimately liver, spleen, and lungs. Granulomatous inflammation and focal necrosis can occur in these organs and may result in septic shock and death.

Diagnosis and Differential Diagnosis

Gram stain of infected material is rarely useful in the diagnosis of tularemia and culture requires appropriate selective media and a great deal of caution because of the infectivity of the organisms. Diagnosis is generally made with serologic tests, especially serum agglutination (a titer greater than 1 : 160 or a fourfold increase).

The differential diagnosis for a cutaneous ulcer with associated lymphadenopathy is broad and includes anthrax, pyogenic infections, plague, sporotrichosis, cat-scratch fever, and lymphogranuloma venereum.

Treatment

Streptomycin, 7.5 mg/kg given intramuscularly every 12 hours for 10 days, remains the treatment of choice and is considered to be curative in the early stages of disease. Tetracycline and chloramphenicol are as effective as streptomycin, but relapses are more likely.

COMMON SUPERFICIAL MYCOSES

(CM&S Chapter 117)

Pityriasis Versicolor

Definition and Clinical Description

Pityriasis versicolor is a superficial fungal infection caused by the polymorphous endogenous yeast *Malassezia furfur* (*Pityrosporum ovale*, *P. orbiculare*). Pityriasis versicolor generally presents as asymptomatic, slightly scaly, hypopigmented and/or hyperpigmented, erythematous, fawn- or salmon-colored patches on the trunk and upper arms. The most common areas of involvement are the trunk and proximal upper extremities. Except in young children, the face is seldom involved. Lesions are initially discrete, scaly macules that coalesce into large patches. Most patients are asymptomatic and present because of cosmetic reasons. Pruritus is occasionally encountered and is especially pronounced with sweating.

Pityriasis versicolor typically involves postpubertal, otherwise healthy persons of both sexes and occurs worldwide. The highest incidence of infection occurs in warm climates. Most patients develop the disease during the summer months. If untreated, pityriasis versicolor tends to be chronic with periodic exacerbations or remissions often occurring with changes in climate.

Pathogenesis and Etiology

M. furfur is a member of the normal skin flora. Under certain conditions, such as tropical ambient temperatures and increased humidity, the fungus changes from the yeast form to the mycelial form and clinical disease ensues. Other factors that predispose to infection include hyperhidrosis, systemic corticosteroid therapy, Cushing's syndrome, immunodeficiency, malnutrition, and pregnancy.

Diagnosis and Differential Diagnosis

The diagnosis of pityriasis versicolor is based on cutaneous changes and is confirmed by KOH preparation. Direct microscopy reveals short hyphae and yeast cells.

The differential diagnosis includes pityriasis alba, vitiligo, seborrheic dermatitis, and postinflammatory hyperpigmentation or hypopigmentation.

Treatment

Pityriasis versicolor is generally treated topically. In severe or extensive cases, and in patients who do not respond to topical medications, systemic therapy can be considered. A variety of topical medications are effective against *M. furfur*, including selenium sulfide, azole antifungals (e.g., clotrimazole), and allylamine antifungals (e.g., naftifine). It is important to treat the entire trunk, upper extremities to the wrists, and lower extremities to the knees for the highest cure rate. Frequently, a prophylactic regimen is necessary to avoid recurrence of disease.

Oral medications effective against *M. furfur* include amidazole ketoconazole (200 mg/day for 5 to 10 days or 400 mg initially, repeated in 7 days) and the triazoles (fluconazole and itraconazole). Terbinafine is effective when used topically but is ineffective if given orally. Studies are needed to confirm the dosage requirements with the newer triazoles.

"Pityrosporum" Folliculitis

Definition and Clinical Description

"*Pityrosporum*" folliculitis, a folliculitis caused by the yeast *M. furfur*, is named after the prior designation of the organism, *Pityrosporum ovale*. *Pityrosporum* folliculitis may be more common in patients with seborrheic dermatitis, pregnant patients, in patients receiving antibiotics, in immunocompromised patients such as recipients of bone marrow transplants, and in individuals with diabetes mellitus and Hodgkin's disease. It occurs in the same regions as does pityriasis versicolor. The upper back, chest, and lateral upper arms develop an acneiform eruption that may be associated with pruritus. Typically, the patient presents with a history of nonresponsiveness to systemic antibiotic therapy or with an incorrect diagnosis of acne vulgaris. *Pityrosporum* folliculitis can be differentiated from acne vulgaris by the lack of comedones.

Diagnosis and Differential Diagnosis

The diagnosis is based on the clinical picture of a pruritic papular or pustular eruption on the trunk or proximal extremities and can be confirmed by histopathology. Since *M. furfur* is not routinely cultured in the laboratory, the diagnosis of *Pityrosporum* folliculitis is confirmed by histopathology. Large numbers of yeasts, and sometimes hyphae, are seen in dilated hair follicles, which occasionally can rupture. The differential diagnosis includes bacterial or irritant folliculitis, acne vulgaris, and papular urticaria.

Treatment

Treatment is similar to that used for pityriasis versicolor.

THE DERMATOPHYTOSES

(CM&S Chapter 118)

Definition

The dermatophytic fungi are a closely related group of molds that invade the stratum corneum of the epidermis and its keratinized appendages — the nail and hair. Dermatophytes belong to three genera: *Epidermophyton*, *Microsporum*, and *Trichophyton*. Species in all genera are similar in physiology, morphology, and pathogenicity. Although there are over 40 known dermatophyte species, only about 10 are commonly encountered worldwide (Table 6–7).

Dermatophytoses are infections caused by dermatophytes. Infection can be transmitted from human to human (anthropophilic), animal to human (zoophilic), or soil to human (geophilic). The prevalence of organisms varies from country to country. However, the majority of infections worldwide are anthropophilic and caused by *T. rubrum* (see Table 6–7).

Tinea Corporis

Tinea corporis, dermatophytosis of the trunk and extremities, can be caused by all species of dermatophytes. Infection can be spread human to human, animal to human, and rarely from soil to human. The disease occurs worldwide and is generally more prevalent in tropical climates. *T. rubrum* is the most commonly encountered pathogen. In general, tinea corporis caused by zoophilic dermatophytes such as *M. canis* is more inflammatory and more symptomatic than infections caused by anthropophilic dermatophytes.

The archetypical lesion of tinea corporis is an annular scaly patch with a distinctive border, which may be single or multiple. Follicular accentuation is common, and often follicular pustules occur. In zoophilic tinea corporis, pustules and even vesicles often occur, while with anthropophilic fungi, slightly scaly, large patches with minimal erythema are typical.

Risk factors for infection include exposure to infected animals, persons, and soil. Those at risk include athletes, veterinarians, animal handlers, and anyone who works outdoors. Cushing's syndrome, diabetes mellitus, atopy, and most immunodeficiency conditions predispose to infection.

Tinea Capitis

Tinea capitis, dermatophytosis of the hair follicles of the scalp, is caused by dermatophytes in the genera *Microsporum* and *Trichophyton*. Most cases occur in children. The causative pathogens vary among countries. In the United States *T. tonsurans* predominates, in Europe the most common organism is *M. canis*, in parts of Africa, *T. violaceum* and *T. soudanense* are common, whereas *M. ferrugineum* is prevalent in southeast Asia.

There are three patterns of dermatophytic scalp infections: ectothrix, endothrix, and favus. Classification is based on the pattern of arthroconidia (spore) location in relation to the hair shaft. In ectothrix invasion, arthroconidia form both inside and outside the hair shaft with the cuticle being destroyed. In endothrix invasion,

TABLE 6-7. Common Dermatophytes and Prevalence

SPECIES	PREVALENCE AND REGION OR COUNTRY	ECOLOGY	PREDOMINANT INFECTION
Microsporum Genus			
*M. audouinii	Rare in North America	Anthropophilic	T. capitis
M. canis	Worldwide	Zoophilic	T. capitis
M. ferrugineum	Africa, Eastern Europe, Asia	Anthropophilic	T. capitis
M. gypseum	Worldwide	Geophilic	T. corporis
Trichophyton Genus			
T. mentagrophytes var. mentagrophytes	Worldwide	Zoophilic	T. barbae and T. pedis
T. mentagrophytes var. interdigitale	Worldwide	Anthropophilic	T. pedis
T. rubrum	Worldwide	Anthropophilic	T. pedis, unguium, cruris, and corporis
T. tonsurans	United States, Mexico, South America, Canada	Anthropophilic	T. capitis
T. violaceum	South America, Central America, Asia, Africa	Anthropophilic	T. capitis
T. verrucosum	Worldwide	Zoophilic	T. corporis and barbae
*T. schoenleinii	Eurasia, Africa, Eastern Europe	Anthropophilic	Favus
Epidermophyton Genus			
*E. floccosum	Worldwide, India, Southeast Asia	Anthropophilic	

*Uncommon dermatophytes.

arthroconidia formation occurs within the hair shaft and the cuticle remains intact. In favus, fragmented hyphae and air spaces occur within the hair shaft. The clinical presentation also varies among these patterns. In general, in endothrix invasion, hair breakage occurs at the scalp level, resulting in "black dots." Infection may be inflammatory or noninflammatory. Black children with endothrix *T. tonsurans* tinea capitis often present with prominent kerion, which is an exuberant inflammatory response to the dermatophyte and may resemble bacterial furunculosis. With ectothrix tinea capitis, hair generally breaks 1 to 2 mm above the scalp level and erythema and scale also occur. This is the presentation typically produced by the cat and dog dermatophyte *M. canis*. Kerion reaction may also occur.

In favus, caused by *T. schoenleinii*, extensive crusts, often intertwined with matted hair, are typical of infection. Scarring alopecia is a common sequelae.

The diagnosis of tinea capitis can often be made by shining a filtered ultraviolet light (Wood's light) on the lesions, because certain species in the genus *Microsporum* fluoresce a yellow-green.

Tinea Pedis and Tinea Manuum

Tinea pedis, a dermatophytic infection of the plantar surface and toe webs, is the most common dermatophyte infection. Tinea manuum is a similar process infecting the palm and interdigital spaces. Tinea pedis is generally caused by anthropophilic fungi. The most common organism is *T. rubrum*, followed by *T. mentagrophytes* and *E. floccosum*.

There are three common presentations of tinea pedis: moccasin, interdigital, and inflammatory. In the interdigital variety, scale, crusting and maceration develop in the interdigital spaces and predominantly in the fourth and fifth spaces. Bacteria and the yeast *Candida* may be secondary invaders and produce moist, erosive, and often odoriferous infections. In moccasin tinea pedis, one or both plantar surfaces develop erythema, scale, and crusting. Inflammatory tinea pedis is generally caused by zoophilic strains of *T. mentagrophytes*. Vesicles and bullous lesions generally develop on the medial aspect of the plantar surface.

Tinea manuum generally occurs in association with tinea pedis. One hand and both feet are often involved.

Tinea Unguium (Onychomycosis)

Tinea unguium (onychomycosis) is mycotic infection of the nail unit. Tinea unguium is generally caused by members in the genera *Trichophyton* and *Epidermophyton* and is most common in adults. *T. rubrum* causes the majority of infection.

Onychomycosis causes about 50% of dystrophic nails, accounts for 30% of all mycotic skin infections, and occurs in about 3% of the population. Predisposing factors include tinea pedis, communal bathing, hyperhidrosis, trauma, diabetes, advancing age, poor peripheral circulation, and immunodeficiency. Most disease occurs in men, and toenails are affected four times as often as fingernails. *C. albicans* usually invades the nail unit as a result of a paronychial infection and is generally more common on the fingernails of women.

Dermatophytes generally invade the nail plate from the nail bed.

There are three patterns of onychomycosis. In distal subungual ony-chomycosis, the distal and lateral margins of the nail bed develop hyperkeratosis, which eventuates in onycholysis, thickening, and discoloration of the nail plate. In proximal white subungual onycho-mycosis, generally cuased by *T. rubrum,* most common in persons infected with human immunodeficiency virus, infection begins in the proximal nail fold, and the organism invades under the cuticle and first infects the proximal nail bed. A white color develops in the proximal nail plate, which may extend distally. In white superficial onychomycosis, caused most often by the dermatophyte *T. menta-grophytes,* these fungi bore holes in the nail plate, resulting in the nail plate becoming white and rough.

Tinea Cruris

Tinea cruris, dermatophytosis of the groin, caused predominantly by *T. rubrum* and *E. floccosum,* typically occurs in men. Erythema and scale develops in the proximal medial thighs and generally occurs bilaterally. A raised, often noninflammatory, erythematous advancing edge occurs. The scrotal skin appears immune to infec-tion. This finding helps to differentiate it from candidal infection, which often presents as a scrotal dermatosis.

Tinea Facei and Tinea Barbae

Tinea facei refers to dermatophytosis of the face other than the beard area, and tinea barbae to infection in the beard area and neck. Both are most frequently caused by zoophilic fungi.

Diagnosis and Differential Diagnosis

The diagnosis of dermatophytic infection can be confirmed by direct microscopic examination of skin scales and by fungal culture. Direct microscopy is usually performed with a keratin clearing agent, such as potassium hydroxide. Septate, nondistinct hyphae that are 2 to 3 μm in diameter are visualized microscopically. Pre-cise identification of a genus and species, which requires consider-able expertise, can be accomplished by a fungal culture by looking at colony morphology and its microscopic appearance. Identifica-tion of the causative pathogen is important to determine the pattern of spread (anthropophilic, zoophilic, and geophilic). For differential diagnoses see Table 6–8.

Treatment

Antifungal drugs target the unique presence of the membrane sterol ergosterol in fungal cells in a variety of ways. Dermatophytes infect the stratum corneum and its keratinized appendages. In choosing an antifungal agent, the serum concentration is of little relevance to treatment outcome and the primary determinant of therapeutic success is the level in the stratum corneum. Drugs topi-cally delivered can reach the stratum corneum in adequate concen-tration and, providing they persist for sufficient time to inhibit the target pathogen, are generally satisfactory. Oral agents useful for

TABLE 6-8. Differential Diagnosis of Dermatophytoses	
DISORDER	**DIFFERENTIAL DIAGNOSIS**
Tinea corporis	Psoriasis, pityriasis rosacea, annular erythemas, eczema, and folliculitis
Tinea capitis	Noninflammatory disease; seborrheic dermatitis, psoriasis, alopecia areata, and trichotillomania
	Inflammatory disease; bacterial furunculosis
Tinea pedis	Interdigital: erythrasma, bacterial infection, and candidiasis
	Moccasin: psoriasis, pityriasis rubra pilaris, keratoderma, and eczema
	Inflammatory: dyshidrosis
Tinea unguium	Psoriasis
Tinea cruris	Candidiasis, erythrasma, eczema, and psoriasis

dermatophytic infection include griseofulvin, the azole family (ketoconazole, itraconazole, and fluconazole), and the allylamine terbinafine.

Management of Specific Dermatophytic Infection

Topical versus Systemic Therapy

Topical therapy is generally effective for uncomplicated tinea corporis, tinea cruris, and tinea pedis. It is ineffective as sole therapy in tinea capitis and tinea unguium. Additionally, in extensive dermatophytosis, in tinea folliculitis, in moccasin tinea pedis, and in immunocompromised patients, systemic therapy is indicated. Most patients with uncomplicated tinea corporis and tinea cruris experience clearance of their lesions within 2 weeks. However, therapy should be continued until the patient is clinically and mycologically clear of infection. An exception is topical terbinafine, which is effective after 1 week of usage probably because of its fungicidal action.

Oral Therapy

Griseofulvin. Griseofulvin has been extensively used over almost 40 years to treat dermatophytosis of the skin, hair, and nails. The ultramicrosize and microsize forms are absorbed best, and a fatty meal may enhance absorption. A dosage of 10 to 15 mg/kg is required until the patient is clinically and mycologically cured. Griseofulvin is highly effective for *M. canis* infection. It is disappointing for *T. rubrum* infection; cure rate for tinea unguium is about 25% after 1 year of therapy for toenail disease. The allylamine terbinafine and the triazole itraconazole are significantly more effective than griseofulvin in vitro against *T. rubrum* and *T. tonsurans* and may usurp the usage of griseofulvin in the near future.

Ketoconazole. Ketoconazole is the first oral broad-spectrum antifungal. Effective for dermatophytic infections, it must be administered until the patient is clinically and mycologically normal. In patients allergic, intolerant, or nonresponsive to griseofulvin, ketoconazole may be an excellent alternative. Dosages of 200 mg daily are generally required. Use of this agent is limited by hepatotoxicity, which occurs in 1 in 10,000 patients.

Fluconazole. This triazole is indicated for candidiasis and cryptococcosis. It appears effective for dermatophytic nail disease. Dosages of 50 to 100 mg daily may be required, although pulse dosages of 150 mg per week to 450 mg per week (administered as a single dose) appear useful in tinea unguium of both fingernails and toenails. This drug has an excellent safety profile, is well tolerated, and may prove to be an excellent alternative to griseofulvin.

Itraconazole. This triazole is specifically indicated in therapy for blastomycosis and histoplasmosis. It appears to be an excellent alternative to griseofulvin in most dermatophytic infections. In patients with recalcitrant tinea pedis, a 1-week course of 200 mg twice daily is very effective. Additionally, a 30-day course of 100 mg daily in *T. tonsurans* tinea capitis is effective. For nail infections, two possible regimens are under investigation. The pulse dosage of 400 mg daily for 1 week, given 1 week per month for 3 to 4 months, has an 80% cure rate after 1 year of therapy. The alternative regimen has a similar cure rate and is given at a dosage of 200 mg daily for 12 weeks.

Terbinafine. The allylamine terbinafine is the only orally active fungicidal agent for dermatophytic infections, which may account for a very low relapse rate. This agent is under investigation in the United States. A dose of 250 mg daily is generally adequate. Six weeks of therapy is required for fingernail infections, and 12 weeks is needed for toenail infections. Two weeks of therapy is adequate for extensive tinea corporis and cruris, and 2 to 4 weeks is needed for tinea capitis.

CUTANEOUS CANDIDIASIS

(CM&S Chapter 119)

Definition

Members of the genus *Candida* are unicellular, unencapsulated, budding fungi capable of forming germ tubes in serum at 37° C and of producing skin and mucous membrane infections. In this genus, the prototypical species, *C. albicans*, is by far the most common cause of human disease.

Clinical Description

The morphologic characteristics of candidiasis vary according to the affected anatomical area. On keratinized surfaces, candidiasis appears as a pustular, red, scaling eruption that may be well marginated. On mucous membranes, these infections produce a white, cheesy adherent mass surrounded by erythema.

Pathogenesis and Etiology

C. albicans is a normal commensal colonizing the mouth, gastrointestinal tract, and vaginal mucosa. About 25% of the normal adult population carry *Candida* orally, and about 20% of healthy women carry this yeast on their vaginal mucosa. A variety of factors may perturb the local microenvironment to encourage the proliferation of *C. albicans* sufficient to produce a clinical infection. These include infancy, old age, pregnancy, local occlusion, epithelial destruction, diabetes mellitus, antibiotic or hormonal therapy, and immunosuppression.

Diagnosis and Differential Diagnosis

If pustules are a component of any cutaneous eruption, the diagnosis of candidiasis should be suspected. The differential diagnosis of cutaneous candidiasis and of nail disease caused by *C. albicans* includes pyogenic bacterial infection, dermatophytosis, intertrigo, and seborrheic dermatitis. Mucous membrane candidiasis can resemble lichen planus, leukoplakia, or benign hyperkeratosis.

The diagnosis of cutaneous and mucous membrane candidiasis can be considered if scrapings reveal hyphae when examined by light microscopy after potassium hydroxide digestion. However, because yeast forms are difficult to visualize under these conditions, it is rarely possible to differentiate such findings from those seen in dermatophyte infections. In an exudate prepared using Gram stain, the presence of yeast forms producing germ tubes is confirmatory of the diagnosis of candidiasis. The cultural isolation of *C. albicans* must be interpreted with some caution because this yeast can be part of the normal flora. *Candida* can also be visualized in routine histopathologic specimens.

Treatment

Effective treatment of cutaneous candidiasis often requires simple changes in the local microenvironment. Replacement of poorly fitted dentures can result in the resolution of oral candidiasis. Control of the blood glucose level in diabetic patients can enhance their recovery from balanitis and vaginitis caused by *C. albicans*. Ending antibiotic or oral contraceptive therapy may be all that is needed to control candidiasis in certain patients. Diaper dermatitis caused by *Candida* can be prevented by the application of thick layers of zinc oxide paste to the perineal and perianal regions. Enhancing evaporation of water and sweat can aid the resolution of paronychia and truncal candidiasis.

Drugs useful in treating candidiasis belong to two chemical groups: the polyenes and the azoles. Nystatin and amphotericin B are polyenes. Ketoconazole and clotrimazole are members of the azole group. Typically, an azole is applied to the affected area twice a day until clearing.

DEEP FUNGAL AND OPPORTUNISTIC MYCOSES

(CM&S Chapter 120)

Cryptococcosis

Definition and Clinical Description

Cryptococcosis is primarily an opportunistic systemic disease that affects the central nervous system (CNS). The causative agent is a yeast, *Cryptococcus neoformans*. Persons between the ages of 30 and 60 years are most often affected. Isolated from soil and abundant in pigeon droppings, the organism has an affinity for the immunocompromised host.

The organism, acquired by the respiratory route, can produce disseminated disease. The initial pulmonary infection is usually asymptomatic and self-limited. Disseminated disease typically involves the CNS, usually in the form of meningitis. Headache, malaise, and fever are the most common symptoms of meningeal infection, although patients with AIDS may have few or no symptoms suggestive of meningitis. Skin findings are varied and include papules, pustules, vegetative and infiltrated plaques, nodules, subcutaneous swellings and abscesses, cellulitis, acneiform eruptions, ulcers, granulomas, and palpable purpura. Disease is usually painless. In patients with AIDS, skin disease may resemble molluscum contagiosum, herpes infection, and Kaposi's sarcoma. Disseminated cryptococcosis is a sign of AIDS in the presence of laboratory evidence of HIV infection. Even with seemingly isolated skin involvement, evaluation for systemic disease is necessary. Skin disease can precede CNS infection by 2 to 8 months.

Pathology

In the gelatinous reaction, the inflammatory infiltrate is minimal and numerous organisms (4–12 μm in diameter) are encased by wide gelatinous capsules. In the granulomatous reaction, the yeast (2–4 μm) is primarily located within giant cells and histiocytes.

Diagnosis

India ink examination of cerebrospinal fluid, pus, skin lesions, and other fluids may reveal the yeast. Culture is necessary for confirmation. The cryptococcal latex agglutination test can detect capsular antigen in cerebrospinal fluid and/or blood; the test is positive in cerebrospinal fluid in more than 90% of patients with cryptococcal meningitis.

Treatment

Amphotericin B, with or without flucytosine, is the treatment of choice for cryptococcosis. Amphotericin B has been used in doses of 0.3 to 1.0 mg/kg per day intravenously for 6 weeks for a total dose of 1.5 to 3.0 g. Side effects of amphotericin B include fever, chills, and, most important, nephrotoxicity. Oral doses of flucytosine have ranged from 75 to 150 mg/kg per day. The use of flucytosine in patients with AIDS is still controversial; concerns regarding its benefit and toxicity (particularly bone marrow toxicity) in this setting exist. Fluconazole and itraconazole, both triazole compounds, have been useful agents for systemic cryptococcosis. Fluconazole (100–400 mg per day orally) is the agent of choice for chronic suppressive therapy in patients with AIDS. In selected patients, primary cutaneous cryptococcosis has responded to the use of fluconazole alone.

Sporotrichosis

Definition and Clinical Description

Sporotrichosis is a chronic subcutaneous infection arising from the traumatic inoculation of the dimorphic fungus *Sporothrix schenckii*. *S. schenckii* exists worldwide, especially in temperate and tropical regions. This yeast resides in soil, plants, and decaying vegetation; sources include rose thorns, sphagnum moss, and hay.

Clinically, sporotrichosis has cutaneous and extracutaneous forms. The cutaneous form has three types: lymphocutaneous, fixed cutaneous, and disseminated cutaneous. Lymphocutaneous sporotrichosis is the classic presentation and accounts for up to 80% of cases, with the dominant upper extremity most often affected. At the site of inoculation a painless, indurated nodule develops, which may ulcerate to form a sporotrichoid chancre; other asymptomatic nodules along the draining lymphatics and regional adenopathy may follow. This combination is known as sporotrichoid spread—a characteristic of sporotrichosis, although not unique. The fixed cutaneous form occurs more often in endemic areas. Children commonly have this form, usually on the face, with asymptomatic papules, ulcers, or verrucous plaques commonly localized to the site of inoculation. Disseminated cutaneous sporotrichosis is rare and may result from either hematogenous spread or autoinoculation. Extracutaneous sporotrichosis encompasses primary pulmonary sporotrichosis and systemic sporotrichosis; both are rare. Skin findings, usually absent in the former, include multiple papules, nodules, ulcers, or plaques. Disease can involve any organ in systemic sporotrichosis, with skin, bone and joints, and muscle most commonly affected; meningitis is uncommon. Disseminated disease has occurred in HIV-infected patients.

Pathology

Early lesions show a nonspecific mixed inflammation; later, granulomas, giant cells, and dermal and intraepidermal abscesses appear. The lymphatic nodules of lymphocutaneous sporotrichosis and the nodules of systemic sporotrichosis reveal a suppurative and granulomatous dermatitis. In the localized form, there is often pseudocarcinomatous hyperplasia overlying the infiltrates. In most biopsy specimens (except in systemic sporotrichosis) organisms are absent or sparse. In tissue, the yeast (4–6 μm in size) is cigar shaped with single, and occasionally multiple, buds. Hyphae are rare. The asteroid body, a central oval basophilic spore surrounded by radiating eosinophilic material, may be present in the centers of suppurative foci; the entire body may be 25 μm in diameter.

Diagnosis and Differential Diagnosis

Direct fluorescent antibody techniques help to identify the organism in histologic sections. Serial sections stained with PAS-D or methenamine silver can also be used to detect organisms in cases in which the initial sections do not show them. Culture of the organism confirms the diagnosis. The fungus grows within 3 to 5 days on most fungal media and exhibits thermal dimorphism. Serologic tests may be helpful, primarily in extracutaneous disease. Meningitis warrants a search for antibodies to *S. schenckii* within the cerebrospinal fluid. The differential diagnosis includes atypical mycobacterioses, tuberculosis, furunculosis, anthrax, tularemia, deep fungal infections, cat-scratch disease, syphilis, foreign body granuloma, sarcoidosis, and pyoderma gangrenosum.

Treatment

For the cutaneous forms, saturated solution of potassium iodide is the agent of choice. It is given orally, usually beginning at a low dose (5 drops three times a day) and gradually increasing by 3 to 5 drops per day as tolerated to a maximum dose of 30 to 50 drops three times a day. The medication is given in water or juice, with treatment continued for 1 month beyond apparent clinical resolution. Locally applied heat may be helpful as adjunctive therapy. Ketoconazole, terbinafine, and itraconazole have been used with success in cutaneous sporotrichosis.

For extracutaneous disease, amphotericin B is usually necessary. In primary pulmonary sporotrichosis, complete surgical resection of localized diseased tissue, coupled with either perioperative saturated solution of potassium iodide or amphotericin B, may be necessary; itraconazole has been effective therapy as well. Amphotericin B, 0.4 to 1.0 mg/kg per day given intravenously for 2 to 3 months, is necessary for disseminated disease, either cutaneous or systemic. Treatment of sporotrichosis in patients with AIDS has involved multiple agents, including ketoconazole, amphotericin B, flucytosine, and fluconazole; all have only limited success.

Coccidioidomycosis

Definition and Clinical Description

Coccidioidomycosis is a systemic mycosis acquired by inhalation of the fungus *Coccidioides immitis*. It is usually a self-limited pulmonary infection but can occasionally disseminate hematogenously.

C. immitis, a dimorphic fungus found in soil, is endemic to the desert regions of the southwestern United States, Mexico, and Central and South America. Disease in nonendemic areas may result from travel, past residence in endemic regions, or exposure to contaminated fomites (i.e., packing materials) from these places. Risk factors for dissemination include male sex, pregnancy, race (blacks, Filipinos, Hispanics), and immunosuppression (i.e., iatrogenic, AIDS). Reactivation of arrested disease may occur, particularly in immunosuppressed patients.

Coccidioidomycosis may appear as primary pulmonary disease (most common), disseminated disease, or, rarely, primary cutaneous disease. Primary pulmonary disease is asymptomatic in 60% of cases; in the remainder, symptoms are usually mild and flu-like. Skin findings of primary pulmonary infection include a generalized morbilliform eruption, erythema nodosum, and erythema multiforme. Valley fever is the combination of erythema nodosum or erythema multiforme, arthritis, and ocular symptoms (i.e., episcleritis) in the setting of primary pulmonary infection. Coccidioidomycosis is the main cause of erythema nodosum in endemic regions. The initial pulmonary infection is usually self-limited but may progress to chronic pulmonary or disseminated disease. Dissemination is rare (less than 1% of all cases). Common sites for dissemination are the skin, bones and joints, and meninges. Skin findings consist of verrucous papules and nodules, pustules, subcutaneous abscesses, ulcers, and sinuses, with a predilection for the face, especially the nasolabial fold. HIV-associated infection is usually disseminated and associated with low CD4 counts. In HIV-infected patients, skin findings may resemble molluscum contagiosum or acne. Such patients may have a diffuse reticulonodular pattern on chest radiography. In a patient with HIV infection, the presence of disseminated coccidioidomycosis establishes the diagnosis of AIDS.

Pathology

Histopathologic examination reveals a suppurative and granulomatous inflammatory infiltrate, within which are the tissue phase of the organism, termed *spherules*. Spherules can be recognized in hematoxylin and eosin–stained sections. They have a refractile capsule and often contain many endospores. They measure from 40 to 60 μm in diameter and can be found within giant cells and free in the dermis. Special stains, such as digested PAS and methenamine silver, may help to demonstrate the spherules.

Diagnosis and Differential Diagnosis

Potassium hydroxide preparations of sputum, pus, and other body fluids may reveal the characteristic spherules. Cultures are highly infective. Serologic testing is helpful for diagnosis. Precipitin antibodies (IgM) form early in the course of disease. Complement fixation antibodies of the IgG class appear slowly during infection. Complement fixation antibody quantitation has prognostic implications; a rising titer indicates a poor prognosis and probable dissemination. The presence of complement fixation antibodies in cerebrospinal fluid supports the diagnosis of coccidioidal meningitis. Skin test reactivity simply indicates exposure to the fungus, not necessarily active disease. Cutaneous anergy in the setting of known coccidioidomycosis is a poor prognostic sign. The differential diagnosis of skin disease includes other infections (deep fungal, bacterial, mycobacterial, viral) verrucae, prurigo nodularis, keratoacanthoma, halogenoderma, and rosacea.

Treatment

Primary pulmonary infection is usually self-limited; bed rest, supportive therapy, and close follow-up are required. Disseminated disease or severe pulmonary disease or disease in pregnant women, in persons with an increased likelihood of dissemination, or in patients with diabetes, cancer, or other pulmonary disease deserves treatment, as does primary cutaneous coccidioidomycosis in children. The mainstay of therapy is amphotericin B (0.5–1.0 mg/kg per day given intravenously; total dose, 1.0–3.0 g). Ketoconazole (400 mg per day orally) has shown mixed results. Fluconazole (200–400 mg per day orally) has been effective for both meningeal and nonmeningeal disease. More recently, itraconazole (100–400 mg per day orally) has shown efficacy. Relapse is common. Surgical therapy may be helpful in some cases of pulmonary and joint disease.

Histoplasmosis

Definition and Clinical Description

Histoplasmosis is a systemic fungal disease, primarily involving the reticuloendothelial system. The causative organism is *Histoplasma capsulatum*. Its main endemic area is the Ohio and Mississippi River valleys of the United States, where up to 80% of the residents may have positive histoplasmin skin tests. Immunosuppression predisposes to disseminated infection. The organism lives in the soil, particularly in association with bird droppings and bat guano.

The symptomatic forms of histoplasmosis include acute pulmonary histoplasmosis, disseminated histoplasmosis, chronic pulmonary histoplasmosis, and the rare primary cutaneous histoplasmosis. In most patients, primary pulmonary infection is asymptomatic and skin test conversion confirms exposure. Symptomatic acute pulmonary histoplasmosis exhibits flu-like symptoms and retrosternal or pleuritic chest pain; chest radiography may reveal hilar or mediastinal lymphadenopathy. Skin findings consist of erythema nodosum or erythema multiforme. Disseminated histoplasmosis is rare. With dissemination, mucosal disease is more common than skin disease; common sites are the tongue, palate, buccal mucosa, and pharynx. Skin findings include erythematous macules, papules, nodules, pustules, petechiae, purpura, exfoliative erythroderma, granulomatous ulcerations, abscesses, cellulitis, and panniculitis. Adrenal gland involvement can result in Addison's disease. In patients with AIDS, histoplasmosis tends to be disseminated, with fever and weight loss the most common signs of disease. A septic shock–like picture may occur in such patients, with multiorgan failure and a fulminant course. Disseminated histoplasmosis is an AIDS-defining infection. Chronic pulmonary histoplasmosis mimics tuberculosis and usually arises in the setting of emphysema.

Pathology

"Parasitized macrophages" arranged as nodular or diffuse dermal infiltrates are characteristic of histoplasmosis. Such macrophages have cytoplasm embedded with many round-to-oval 2- to 4-μm spores, with a surrounding clear space around the spores; in the past, this space was mistakenly thought to be a capsule. The organism is visible with hematoxylin and eosin stain but is more apparent with the methenamine silver or Giemsa stain.

Diagnosis and Differential Diagnosis

Examination of tissue, especially bone marrow or peripheral blood, with a silver stain may reveal the organism. Radiographs can detect calcified granulomas of resolved disease in affected organs. Culture of the fungus (i.e., from bone marrow) confirms the diagnosis, although growth may take 6 weeks. Incubation at room temperature yields a white colony, and microscopic examination reveals the diagnostic tuberculate macroconidia of *H. capsulatum*. The culture is highly infectious. Serologic testing is useful, specifically the use of complement fixation antibodies and immunodiffusion tests for H and M precipitins. A complement fixation antibody titer of 1 : 32 or higher suggests recent or current infection. Rapid diagnosis of histoplasmosis is possible with the detection of *H. capsulatum* polysaccharide antigen in urine, blood, and other body fluids.

Cutaneous disease is varied, and the differential diagnosis includes other infections (deep fungal, mycobacterial, leishmaniasis) and lymphomas.

Treatment

Generally, only bed rest and symptomatic treatment are needed for treatment of acute pulmonary histoplasmosis. For severe acute pulmonary disease and disseminated disease amphotericin B (0.5–0.6 mg/kg per day intravenously; total dose 2.0–2.5 g), ketoconazole (400–800 mg per day orally), or itraconazole (200–400 mg per day orally) would be appropriate. Ketoconazole has been effective for some cases of chronic pulmonary histoplasmosis, although many cases are difficult to treat and fail to respond to ketoconazole. Some cases of chronic pulmonary histoplasmosis have responded to therapy with itraconazole. Determination of the role of fluconazole awaits further studies. In the immunosuppressed patient, amphotericin B is the drug of choice for induction therapy. Suppressive maintenance therapy requires amphotericin B, ketoconazole, or itraconazole. In this setting, amphotericin B is given intravenously as weekly doses of 0.5 to 1.5 mg/kg per dose.

Blastomycosis

Definition and Clinical Description

Blastomycosis is a systemic mycosis caused by the dimorphic fungus *Blastomyces dermatitidis,* which primarily infects the lungs and occasionally the skin, bone, and genitourinary tract. Most cases have occurred in the areas bordering the Ohio and Mississippi Rivers, Great Lakes, and the southeastern states. Soil is the organism's likely habitat, but recovery of the organism has been difficult. Exposure to soil and water probably predisposes to infection. Both humans and animals (especially dogs) can acquire the disease, and sexual transmission has been reported. There is no increased incidence of disease in immunosuppressed patients, including patients with HIV infection.

Blastomycosis primarily infects the lungs, less so the skin, bone, and other organs. The initial pulmonary infection may be asymptomatic, but self-limited flu-like symptoms can occur. Pulmonary disease can become chronic, with signs and symptoms mimicking tuberculosis or malignancy. The skin is the most common extrapulmonary site of involvement with exposed areas and mucous membranes. Annular verrucous plaques studded with peripheral microabscesses are the hallmark of skin disease. The plaques heal centrally with atrophic scarring and may ulcerate; the active pustular border continues to advance. Asymptomatic bone and joint involvement occurs in approximately half of patients, characterized by well-circumscribed osteolytic lesions on radiography. Genitourinary disease occurs in approximately 25% of men but rarely in women. CNS disease, usually meningitis and/or brain abscess, occurs in 5% to 10% of patients with disseminated disease. In the few patients with AIDS and blastomycosis, both localized pulmonary disease and disseminated disease have occurred. With disseminated disease, there is a much higher incidence of CNS involvement (40% in one study) compared with the immunocompetent population of patients. The rare self-limited primary inoculation blastomycosis consists of a nodule at the site of inoculation and regional lymphadenopathy.

Pathology

Histology reveals marked pseudoepitheliomatous hyperplasia with scattered intraepidermal microabscesses and a mixed neutrophilic and granulomatous infiltrate in the dermis. Yeast organisms (8–15 μm in diameter) may lie either free in tissue or within giant cells; they have a double-contoured refractile wall and exhibit characteristic broad-based single budding. A silver or PAS-D stain facilitates visualization of the organism.

Diagnosis and Differential Diagnosis

Potassium hydroxide examination of pus, sputum, and tissue may reveal the yeast. Culture of the organism at 30°C on routine fungal media yields a cottony white mold, and microscopic examination reveals round to pear-shaped conidia. Serologic tests are limited by low sensitivity and specificity. Skin testing has questionable value.

The differential diagnosis includes other infectious and noninfectious disorders such as verrucae, tuberculosis, leprosy, nocardiosis, actinomycosis, mycetoma, ecthyma, tertiary syphilis, granuloma inguinale, leishmaniasis, squamous cell carcinoma and halogenoderma.

Treatment

Until recently, amphotericin B (0.3–0.6 mg/kg per day intravenously; total dose, 2.0 g) was the preferred treatment for blastomycosis. Now, ketoconazole (400 mg per day orally) and itraconazole (200–400 mg per day orally) have proven to be effective agents for mild to moderate nonmeningeal blastomycosis in immunocompetent patients. Therapy should last for at least 6 months. For life-threatening or CNS disease and for disease in immunosuppressed patients, amphotericin B remains the preferred therapy. Chronic administration of one of the oral azoles or amphotericin B is warranted in patients with AIDS.

Chromoblastomycosis

Definition and Clinical Description

Chromoblastomycosis is a chronic dermal or subcutaneous infection characterized by the presence of pigmented sclerotic bodies in affected tissue. It occurs worldwide, with the highest incidence in the tropics and subtropics. The causative organisms are saprophytes that are found in soil and decaying vegetation. Several dermatiaceous fungi can produce chromoblastomycosis: *Fonsecaea compactum*, *F. pedrosoi*, *Phialophora verrucosa*, *Cladosporium carrionii*, and *Rhinocladiella aquaspersa*. Infection can occur in animals and humans (mainly men aged 30 to 40 years old involved in farm work). There is no evidence for human-to-human transmission.

Chromoblastomycosis primarily causes disease at the site of inoculation and differs from mycetoma, which is more invasive locally, often affecting underlying bone. Initially, a small scaly papule, usually on the exposed leg or foot, develops, which over time enlarges as satellite papules appear. Through coalescence, multilobulated, verrucous or smooth plaques develop, which can be pruritic and painful; plaques are often covered with "black dots" of purulent discharge. Secondary bacterial infection is common. Lymphatic obstruction can occur, sometimes followed by elephantiasis. Disease can remain indolent over many years. Dissemination and CNS disease are rare.

Pathology

Biopsy usually reveals pseudoepitheliomatous hyperplasia and suppurative and granulomatous dermal infiltrates. Organisms appear in tissue as characteristic sclerotic bodies (Medlar bodies, "copper pennies")—dark brown, round, thick-walled structures, 6 to 12 μm in diameter, usually found singly or in clusters, either free in tissue or within giant cells. Morphologically, the "black dots" are sites of transepidermal elimination of necrotic debris and sclerotic bodies.

Diagnosis and Differential Diagnosis

Both a potassium hydroxide examination of scrapings from "black dot" areas and a biopsy specimen will reveal characteristic sclerotic bodies. A culture of pus or tissue is essential for diagnosis. The colonies are green-black with a velvety surface. Precipitating and complement-fixing antibodies may be helpful in following the course of the disease. Skin testing is not helpful. The differential diagnosis includes blastomycosis, yaws, and leprosy.

Treatment

Both surgical and nonsurgical modalities have been useful. For localized disease, wide surgical excision is warranted. Both cryosurgery and local heat therapy can be effective physical modalities. Chemotherapy should begin with flucytosine (100–200 mg/kg per day orally) either alone or in combination with other agents. Other effective drugs include amphotericin B, ketoconazole (200–400 mg per day orally), thiabendazole, and, most recently, the newer triazoles itraconazole (200–400 mg per day given orally) and saperconazole. As a rule, prolonged administration of the medications is necessary.

Mycetoma

Definition and Clinical Description

Mycetoma is a chronic infection of subcutaneous tissue characterized by tumefaction, sinus tract formation, and the presence of grains.

Mycetoma occurs worldwide, most commonly in tropical and subtropical regions, where etiologic agents reside in soil. Men between the ages of 20 and 40 years old are most frequently affected, and occupational exposure to soil predisposes to infection. Etiologically, mycetoma is either actinomycetoma, caused by the filamentous actinomycete bacteria, or eumycetoma, caused by true fungi. In the United States, mycetoma is uncommon; when it occurs, *Pseudoallescheria boydii* is the most frequently isolated organism. In Mexico and Central and South America, *Nocardia brasiliensis* accounts for almost 90% of cases. *Madurella mycetomi* and *Streptomyces somaliensis* predominate in Africa, and *M. mycetomi* and *N. madurae* are common in India.

The triad of tumefaction, sinus tracts, and grains is characteristic of mycetoma. After traumatic inoculation, a nodule slowly develops, enlarges, and may discharge serosanguineous or purulent material. Other nodules appear in contiguous fashion. Sinus tracts form and often interconnect. Grains, actually colonies of the causative organism, are hard concretions readily visible within drainage sites and affected tissue. Infection may spread to fascia, muscle, and bone. The repeated swelling, drainage, and subsequent fibrosis lead to enlargement and deformity of the affected site, usually an extremity. Mycetoma is generally painless; systemic symptoms usually occur only with secondary bacterial infection. The most common site of involvement is the dorsal foot. Mycetoma follows a chronic progressive course over years.

Pathology

Biopsy reveals suppurative granulomas and grains. The grains vary in size from 0.2 to 5 mm and are visible within abscesses. Eosinophilic ''clubs,'' known as the Splendore-Hoeppli phenomenon, may surround the grains. The material in the clubs is derived in part from the granules of eosinophils. A Brown-Brenn, PAS-D, or silver stain provides better visualization of the organisms within the granules. True fungi appear as 3- to-5-μm-wide septate hyphae. Actinomycetes appear as 1- to 2-μm-wide branching filaments.

Diagnosis and Differential Diagnosis

The clinical triad establishes the diagnosis. Grain color, size, and shape help to identify an etiologic agent. Radiography to evaluate bone involvement should be performed. Culture of pus, grains, or tissue helps to identify organisms. The true fungi grow on Sabouraud's medium with antibiotics; actinomycetes grown on Sabouraud's medium or brain-heart infusion agar without antibiotics. The differential diagnosis includes botryomycosis, actinomycosis, cutaneous tuberculosis, leprosy, sporotrichosis, deep fungal infections, syphilis, yaws, leishmaniasis, neoplasms, foreign body granuloma, and Kaposi's sarcoma.

Treatment

The treatment of mycetoma is inexact and often problematic. In general, therapy is more successful for actinomycetoma than for eumycetoma. Surgery can be helpful, either through surgical excision of small nodules or through debridement of sinus tracts and diseased tissue in larger nodules and plaques. Chemotherapy can be the main modality or adjunctive therapy with surgery. For actinomycetoma, streptomycin plus dapsone or trimethoprim-sulfamethoxazole (TMP-SMZ) has been effective therapy. Doses used have included streptomycin, 1 g per day intramuscularly; dapsone, 200 mg per day orally; or TMP-SMZ (80 mg/400 mg), one to two tablets twice daily orally. Other sulfonamides, tetracycline, erythromycin, rifampin, and amikacin have also been effective singly and in combination. Penicillin is the drug of choice for disease caused by *A. israelii.* For eumycetoma, griseofulvin, amphotericin B, flucytosine, miconazole, and oral azoles have yielded variable success.

Other Opportunistic Mycoses

Aspergillosis

Aspergillosis is primarily a pulmonary infection of immunocompromised or chronically debilitated patients; with dissemination, skin disease can occur. Predisposing factors include neutropenia, hematologic malignancy, immunodeficiency (e.g., AIDS, organ transplantation), and corticosteroid or cytotoxic therapy. *Aspergillus fumigatus* is the most common human pathogen. Skin disease usually implies dissemination but may occur as a primary event in healthy or ill patients. Patients with disseminated disease may develop reddened macules, papules, pustules, nodules, or granulomas; cellulitis, purpura, and ulceration are less common. In primary aspergillosis, indurated purple plaques and nodules, hemorrhagic bullae, or cellulitis usually follows trauma; ulceration with a black eschar may develop. Skin biopsy, with special staining (e.g., methenamine silver) to identify septated, branching hyphae, is necessary to establish diagnosis. Cultures, which are often negative, help to confirm the diagnosis.

Zygomycosis

Zygomycosis represents a severe, often lethal, infection with a fungus from the genera *Absidia, Mucor, Rhizopus,* or *Cunninghamella*—"bread molds" of the class Zygomycetes that are ubiquitous. Infections, usually with a *Rhizopus* species, are most common in patients with diabetes, leukemia, and lymphoma; disease rarely occurs in healthy persons. Rhinocerebral disease is the most common presentation and occurs most often in patients with diabetic ketoacidosis. Disease is invariably severe and fulminant.

Patients have facial edema; often unilateral, bloody nasal discharge; ulcers of the septum and palate, usually with adherent, necrotic tissue; headache; and altered mental status. Infection can extend rapidly to produce ophthalmoplegia, orbital apex syndrome, thrombosis of the cavernous sinus and carotid artery, and brain abscess. Skin disease can be a primary event, usually as a secondary infection of burns. With infection, healthy persons usually, after trauma or fracture, have superficial disease manifested by vesicles, pustules, or plaques. Compromised patients usually have gangrenous disease with purple-red plaques or indurated, dusky nodules that may be painful. The pathologic hallmark of infection is hyphal invasion of blood vessels that yields thrombus formation, infarction of surrounding tissues, and necrotic black debris.

HERPESVIRUS INFECTIONS

(CM&S Chapter 121)

Herpes Simplex Virus

Definition

There are seven closely related human herpesviruses: herpes simplex virus (HSV) 1 and 2, varicella zoster virus (VZV), Epstein-Barr virus (EBV), cytomegalovirus (CMV), human herpesvirus 6 (HHV 6), and human herpesvirus 7 (HHV 7).

HSV is subdivided into two closely related types: HSV 1 and HSV 2. Oral-labial HSV, most commonly caused by HSV 1, affects an estimated one third of the population of the United States; however subclinical infection is common.

An estimated 25 million American adults have serologic evidence of exposure to HSV 2, the most common cause of genital herpes. It has been associated with acquiring HIV infection in both heterosexual and homosexual groups.

Primary herpes infection is defined as the first viral exposure in a seronegative individual. Most often, this involves direct mucocutaneous contact between uninfected and infected individuals. After primary infection, HSV establishes a latent infection in the nerve root ganglion and then may reactivate to cause disease recurrences.

Primary oral-labial herpes presents as an acute pharyngitis in college students. Primary genital herpes occurs 3 days to 2 weeks after exposure to an infected sexual partner, who often sheds virus asymptomatically. Acute genital herpes manifests as a group of painful vesicles on an erythematous base that progress to ulcers over several days. Primary disease is typically severe, with large, multiple ulcerations and tender inguinal lymphadenopathy.

Up to 20% of patients with acute genital herpes have dysuria and urinary retention. The formation of the new lesions and active viral shedding continue for 7 to 10 days, with compete resolution of lesions by about 3 weeks. HSV 1 produces the same acute clinical syndrome but is associated with fewer recurrences.

Neonatal HSV develops most frequently after exposure to infected maternal vaginal secretions during delivery, and, untreated, is associated with a significant mortality rate. The risk to the newborn is highest when the mother acquires a primary genital herpes infection during pregnancy. Most mothers of these infants do not have a history of genital herpes and are unaware of prior exposure.

Recurrent herpes infections occur when latent virus is reactivated, and precipitating factors include sunlight exposure, fatigue, menstruation, stress, trauma, and surgical manipulation. They are less severe than primary disease.

Recurrent orofacial HSV ("cold sores") occurs an average of three or four times a year. Local dysesthesias precede a cluster of small papulovesicles that quickly ulcerate, often at the border of the lip. Crusting occurs in a few days, and viral shedding ceases. Complete healing of lesions occurs within about 10 days.

Recurrent genital herpes typically occurs within a year of primary infection with three, four, or more recurrent outbreaks a year. Prodromal symptoms of burning or tingling at the site of the outbreak often precede a cluster of painful vesicles, which progress to crusted ulcers. The lesions are typically fewer in number and smaller than in primary disease. and there are milder constitutional symptoms. Many cases of erythema multiforme follow recurrent cutaneous herpes simplex.

Herpetic whitlow seen in health care workers refers to herpetic infection of the fingers or hands from direct manual contact with oral or genital lesions. Latex gloves used when contacting oral or genital lesions or saliva should prevent such infections. HSV rarely causes noncutaneous systemic diseases. Patients with atopic dermatitis and Darier's disease are at risk to develop widespread HSV infection. This is known as Kaposi's varicelliform eruption or eczema herpeticum. It may resemble impetigo.

Pathology

Similar histopathologic findings are seen in cutaneous lesions of herpes simplex and herpes zoster. Initially, the nuclei of keratinocytes develop a homogeneous "steel gray" appearance, eosinophilic intranuclear inclusions, and multinucleation. There is often an interface dermatitis, which can resemble that of erythema multiforme, adjacent to the lesion. As papulovesicles develop, intracytoplasmic edema (ballooning), enlarged keratinocytes with pallid cytoplasm, acantholysis, membrane rupture, and reticular degeneration of the epidermis ensues, with strands of cytoplasmic membranes that are still interconnected occur. Such intraepidermal vesiculation is usually present, although some herpetic vesicles are subepidermal. In late lesions, many neutrophils are present within blister cavities. Secondary vasculitis is sometimes present.

Diagnosis and Differential Diagnosis

Herpes infection is suspected when a patient presents with a cluster of small vesicles or erosions on an erythematous mucocutaneous surface. A positive Tzanck smear, indicated by the presence of multinucleated keratinocytic giant cells, signifies the presence of either HSV or varicella-zoster virus. To perform a Tzanck smear, one unroofs an active vesicular lesion, takes a sample of cells from the base or roof of the vesicle, and transfers it to a glass slide. The slide is stained with a Wright-Giemsa stain.

The gold standard for diagnosis of HSV infections is viral culture of vesicular fluid or skin biopsy material, which is positive 90% of the time. The differential diagnosis of HSV infections includes aphthous ulcers, enterovirus infection, erythema multiforme, pemphigus, and, for genital herpes, trauma or any sexually transmitted disease that causes ulcers or erosions.

Treatment

Acyclovir is the treatment of choice for HSV infections. As an analog of guanosine, it is specifically taken up by virally infected cells and subsequently phosphorylated to its monophosphate form by viral-specific thymidine kinase. Host cell enzymes produce acyclovir triphosphate, which both inhibits the viral DNA polymerase and functions as a viral DNA chain terminator. Due to its specific uptake and viral enzyme inhibition, acyclovir remains a remarkably safe and active drug with low toxicity. For primary genital herpes, oral acyclovir at a dose of 200 mg five times daily for a total of 10 days decreases viral shedding, pain, and the development of new lesions with more rapid healing. Topical acyclovir is less effective than the oral preparation. For recurrent genital herpes, acyclovir therapy is most effective when initiated within 48 hours of prodromal symptoms. In immunocompromised hosts with orofacial herpes, both topical and parenteral acyclovir therapy are beneficial.

For prevention, a dose of 400 mg of oral acyclovir twice daily markedly reduces recurrent episodes.

With the widespread use of repeated courses of acyclovir in immunocompromised hosts (with typically large viral loads), the development of acyclovir-resistant HSV disease, most commonly due to altered viral thymidine kinase activity, has occurred. Current alternative drugs include intravenous foscarnet and topical trifluridine.

Varicella-Zoster Virus

Definition

Varicella zoster virus (VZV) is a member of the human herpesvirus family. Primary infection with VZV occurs in the nasopharynx via the respiratory route, resulting in viremia, with subsequent dissemination to the skin and viscera, causing the primary VZV disease, varicella (chickenpox). The sensory nerve ganglia become the site of latent VZV infection. At some point, the virus becomes reactivated, and manifests as secondary VZV disease, herpes zoster (shingles).

Clinical Description

In the United States, primary VZV infection, varicella, is primarily a disease of children. VZV is highly infectious and infection is endemic in the population, with localized epidemics occurring in the winter and early spring in the United States. More than 90% of American adults show serologic evidence of previous VZV infection. Zoster affects over 10% of the total population over their lifetimes. Reactivated VZV infection, herpes zoster, occurs at all ages, though uncommonly under the age of 50. Patients with immune compromise have significantly higher rates of herpes zoster infection. In a cohort of gay men, the age-adjusted relative risk of developing zoster was 17 times higher in HIV-infected men than in their seronegative counterparts. The occurrence of herpes zoster in populations at risk for HIV infection is highly predictive of HIV seropositivity. It is reasonable to suggest HIV testing in such patients.

Clinical Findings

Primary VZV infection manifests about 2 weeks after exposure to an infectious individual (range 10 to 20 days).There may be a prodrome of fever, chills, malaise, myalgias, and arthralgias for a day or two followed by erythematous maculopapules that rapidly progress to vesicles ("dew drops on a rose petal"). Initially, lesions appear on the head or trunk, and extend centripetally in crops over 2 to 4 days to involve the extremities, including the palms and soles and, less commonly, the oral and genital mucosa. The vesicles progress from clear to cloudy fluid as inflammatory cells appear and then begin to crust over, signaling the end of viral shedding and infectivity. Lesions at all stages of disease occur simultaneously. Constitutional symptoms are common. Crusted lesions ultimately resolve over 1 to 2 weeks.

The most common complication of varicella is secondary bacterial infection, most often with streptococcal or staphylococcal species, often prompted by excoriation. Immunocompromised hosts may have more severe disease, with greater numbers of lesions, prolonged healing time, visceral complications, and an increased mortality. Visceral complications include neurologic complications, pneumonitis, and Reye's syndrome.

Neonatal varicella results when maternal varicella occurs from 5 days before to 2 days after delivery and is associated with visceral disease and significant mortality. Maternal varicella occurring at 8 to 20 weeks of gestation causes the fetal varicella syndrome, characterized by prematurity, low birth weight, hypoplasia, and ocular and neurologic abnormalities.

Zoster presents with local radicular pain 2 to 3 days before the eruption occurs, involving one to three contiguous dermatomes. The thoracic dermatomes are most frequently involved, followed by the lumbar, trigeminal, cervical, and sacral dermatomes. Several vesicles may be found outside such dermatomes. The lesions evolve similarly to primary VZV infections.

Widespread lesions (disseminated) are found most commonly in immunocompromised patients or in the aged.

Herpes zoster ophthalmicus is zoster localized in the ophthalmic (V1) branch of the trigeminal nerve. Lesions on the tip of the nose reflect the V1 nerve distribution and often indicate ocular involvement. Inflammation of the conjunctiva and cornea may lead to scarring and visual loss.

Postherpetic neuralgia is defined as debilitating pain at the site of previous zoster that persists more than 1 month and affects up to one half of patients over age 50, especially after trigeminal nerve zoster. Herpes zoster may disseminate and/or involve extracutaneous sites.

Immunocompromised hosts have more severe herpes zoster. Atypical chronic herpes zoster occurs in HIV-infected patients receiving chronic acyclovir therapy. The lesions are verrucous, hyperkeratotic, ecthymatous, or pox-like papules, nodules, or ulcerations with or without an eschar and are acyclovir resistant.

Pathology

Vesicles of varicella or herpes zoster show histopathologic changes similar to those of herpes simplex. Verrucous lesions harboring cells with viral inclusions are found in immunosuppressed patients.

Diagnosis and Differential Diagnosis

Both varicella and herpes zoster are most commonly diagnosed clinically on the basis of a compatible history and physical examination. A Tzanck smear is often positive, as in HSV infections; however, viral culture is less helpful, as the VZV is difficult to isolate.

Serology may document acute or previous exposure. Vesicular cells or tissue biopsy specimens may be directly stained for the VZV antigen. The differential diagnosis of VZV infection includes HSV atypical measles, and enteroviral infections. Early zoster can simulate erysipelas and cellulitis.

Treatment

Acyclovir is the antiviral of choice for VZV infection when necessary. The mechanism of action of the drug against VZV is identical to that for HSV, as discussed previously. The 50% inhibitory concentration of acyclovir in vitro is three to six times higher for VZV than for HSV, and treatment doses must be increased accordingly.

Uncomplicated varicella in children should be managed with supportive care: bathing, cutting fingernails short to prevent excoriation, and the use of antipruritics and antipyretics. Salicylates should not be given because of the risk of Reye's syndrome. There may be clinical benefits from the use of acyclovir in healthy children if started within 24 hours of the onset of rash, at a dose of 20 mg/kg, four times a day. Similarly, the use of oral acyclovir at a dose of 800 mg five times daily for 7 days in immunocompetent adults with varicella within 24 hours of rash onset was associated with a reduction in the number and healing time of lesions and the duration of fever and other symptoms. Acyclovir is the treatment of choice for immunocompromised hosts with varicella, at a dose of 500 mg/m^2 (or 10 mg/kg) intravenously every 8 hours for 10 days.

Acyclovir at an oral dose of 800 mg five times daily or an intravenous dose of 10 mg/kg every 8 hours to 7 to 10 days is effective for herpes zoster in immunocompetent hosts.

There is the suggestion that acyclovir prevents the development of postherpetic neuralgia. Adding steroids offers little further benefit. Famciclovir, 500 mg three times daily, may be used. Acute neuritis and postherpetic neuralgia may be managed with traditional analgesics, or combinations of amitriptyline and perphenazine, topical capsaicin, or regional nerve blocks.

Acyclovir is the treatment of choice for herpes zoster in immunosuppressed hosts. AIDS patients with resistant VZV infection may benefit from a 10-day course of foscarnet at a dose of 40 mg/kg every 8 hours. A vaccine for varicella has recently been released in the United States.

Epstein-Barr Virus

Definition

The Epstein-Barr virus (EBV), the fourth human herpesvirus, is morphologically indistinguishable from the other herpesviruses. The virus is tropic for B lymphocytes and nasopharyngeal and salivary gland epithelial cells.

Whereas the other herpesviruses produce cytopathic changes, EBV establishes a latent state in infected B lymphocytes and subsequently synthesizes viral proteins (Epstein-Barr nuclear antigens) that promote cellular proliferation and transform affected cells, conferring immortality. This property likely gives EBV its oncogenic potential.

Clinical Description

Over 90% of adults will have a positive EBV serology, and once infection is established, it is lifelong. Primary infection with EBV occurs in two distinct age groups: young children and young adults. Reactivation infection occurs primarily in immunocompromised patients. Primary infection occurs most often with oral contact. Asymptomatic shedding may occur up to 18 months after complete recovery from the acute syndrome.

Clinical Findings

Primary infection with EBV occurring in young children is often subclinical or nonspecific, with low-grade fever and pharyngitis.

Papular acrodermatitis of childhood or infantile papular acrodermatitis (Gianotti-Crosti syndrome) has been associated with EBV. It presents acutely as symmetrical flat, 2-mm papules localized to the face and extremities with sparing of the trunk. The lesions may be skin colored or erythematous and are nonpruritic. Generalized lymphadenopathy is often present. The syndrome lasts about 3 weeks.

Primary infection with EBV in young adults (age 15 to 25) manifests clinically as infectious mononucleosis (glandular fever) with pharyngitis, fever, and cervical lymphadenopathy. Skin eruptions are rare and present as generalized macular erythema, urticaria, or scarlatiniform eruptions, with upper eyelid edema or a petechial palatal enanthem. Symptoms last weeks to a few months.

Long-term complications include chronic active mononucleosis syndromes, erythema multiforme, and possibly chronic fatigue syndrome.

Inadvertent treatment of acute EBV mononucleosis with antibiotics, such as ampicillin, often results in a hypersensitivity eruption with extensive pruritic maculopapular lesions and fever.

Burkitt's (B-cell) and other B- and T-cell lymphomas and nasopharyngeal (epithelial cell) carcinoma occur in the setting of immune compromise and may reflect reactivation or secondary EBV infection. HIV-infected patients may develop EBV-related oral hairy leukoplakia, raised, striated white areas on the sides of the tongue or on the buccal mucosa.

Pathology

The pathology of EBV-related lesions is nonspecific, showing spongiotic dermatitis in the Gianotti-Crosti syndrome and a mild superficial perivascular dermatitis with slight spongiosis and/or vacuolar change in mononucleosis.

Diagnosis and Differential Diagnosis

The diagnosis of the disease syndromes of primary or reactivation of EBV infection is often made clinically. The typical clinical syndrome of infectious mononucleosis occurring in the setting of a more than 50% lymphocytosis with more than 10% atypical (large, activated) lymphocytes and a positive serum heterophile antibody test establishes the diagnosis.

In children younger than 5 years, fewer than 50% will develop a positive test. The positive serology will persist as long as 6 to 9 months after illness. False-positive tests occur with hepatitis and hematologic malignancies.

The differential diagnosis of EBV-related mononucleosis infection includes cytomegalovirus mononucleosis, viral hepatitis, toxoplasmosis, and streptococcal pharyngitis. Oral hairy leukoplakia should be differentiated between thrush, lichen planus, and geographic tongue.

Treatment

EBV disease in the immunocompetent host is most often self-limited, and specific treatment is not required. Limitation of exertion is warranted to avoid splenic rupture as a complication of acute mononucleosis.

Steroids may help with certain complications of mononucleosis: severe pharyngitis with airway edema or immune cytopenias.

Acyclovir, ganciclovir, zidovudine (AZT), and topical application of podophyllin have been shown to cause regression of oral hairy leukopenia.

Cytomegalovirus

Definition

Like the other herpesviruses, cytomegalovirus (CMV) is a double-stranded DNA virus that causes a primary infection, then establishes clinical latency, and subsequently may reactivate to cause secondary infection, particularly with immunosuppression.

Clinical Description

Between 40% and 100% of adults are seropositive for CMV antibody. Transmission occurs in three distinct periods of life: perinatally from infected mother to child; in young childhood from other children in families or day care settings; and in the reproductive years from sexual contact. CMV transmission also occurs with blood transfusion or tissue donation.

CMV infection is most often clinically inapparent. Distinct clinical entities include congenital CMV infection, CMV mononucleosis in the normal host, and reactivation of CMV causing disseminated or visceral disease in the immunocompromised host. Dermatologic manifestations of CMV are uncommon and nonspecific. CMV is the most common congenital viral infection. Some may develop the TORCH (toxoplasma, other [bacterial sepsis, syphilis, etc.], rubella, cytomegalovirus, and HSV) syndrome, consisting of hepatosplenomegaly, neurologic abnormalities, ophthalmologic disease, and typical cutaneous lesions. The classic dermatologic findings in congenital CMV disease are purple-red papules or nodules, "blueberry muffin" lesions. These are sites of extramedullary hematopoiesis in the dermis, and lesions may last from 4 to 6 weeks. Petechiae, purpura, or jaundice may occur.

CMV mononucleosis is a disease of young adults (average age, 28 years) and presents with fever lasting up to 2 weeks, myalgias, malaise, pharyngitis, and headache. Splenomegaly, pharyngeal erythema, and lymphadenopathy occur in about one third of patients. Laboratory studies reveal atypical lymphocytosis and elevations in liver enzymes.

A rash similar to EBV mononucleosis occurs after ampicillin. Systemic complications occur infrequently. Other rashes are rubelliform-like, scarlatiniform, maculopapular, follicular, or urticarial, both generalized and localized to the lower extremities.

Immunocompromised patients are at high risk for reactivation of latent CMV infection, causing pneumonitis, hepatitis, colitis, retinitis, encephalitis, or adrenalitis. Dermatologic manifestations of CMV disease are uncommon and occur in two patterns: localized ulcerative lesions of the perianal or genital areas or extremities, and disseminated purpuric macules.

Pathology

The hallmark of cutaneous infection with CMV is enlargement of the nuclei of venular endothelial cells, which can contain either intranuclear or intracytoplasmic inclusions, or both.

Diagnosis and Differential Diagnosis

The diagnosis of CMV infection is made by histopathologic demonstration of characteristic CMV viral inclusion bodies in tissue biopsy specimens. Body fluid viral cultures are often unreliable. The differential diagnosis of CMV disease in immunocompromised hosts includes disseminated fungal and mycobacterial disease, drug reactions, HSV, and VZV. The differential diagnosis of mononucleosis is similar to that of EBV mononucleosis.

Treatment

CMV disease in the normal host is most often a self-limited disease. In the immunocompromised host, ganciclovir or foscarnet is used. The role of therapy for isolated cutaneous CMV disease in the immunocompromised host is unclear.

Human Herpesvirus 6

Definition

The sixth human herpesvirus, human herpesvirus 6 (HHV 6), is tropic for T lymphocytes and has morphological and biologic similarities to the other human herpesviruses. HHV 6 has two closely related strains or genotypes, designated types A and B.

Clinical Description

Exposure to HHV 6 is ubiquitous and occurs worldwide, most frequently at an early age. Primary infection with HHV 6 in children causes exanthem subitum (roseola infantum, sixth disease), a common childhood illness, characterized by acute fever without localizing signs and the subsequent development of an erythematous macular rash as the fever subsides. HHV 6 is an important cause of acute febrile childhood illness and is not always associated with the typical exanthum subitum rash. Primary infection with HHV 6 in immunocompetent adults produces a mononucleosis-like syndrome.

After primary infection, HHV 6 presumably remains latent in the body. It may be isolated from the saliva and salivary gland tissue, lymph nodes, and monocytes and macrophages. Reactivation of HHV 6 infection has been reported in organ transplant patients, causing fever, rash, interstitial pneumonitis, bone marrow suppression, and possibly transplant rejection.

Diagnosis and Differential Diagnosis

Serologic confirmation of seroconversion supports the clinical diagnosis. The differential diagnosis of HHV 6 infection includes other causes of mononucleosis, rubella, measles, erythema infections and other viral exanthens, scarlet fever, and drug eruption.

Pathology

There are no specific histologic changes associated with HHV 6 infection.

Treatment

There is no specific treatment for primary HHV 6 infection in children or adults because this is in general a benign, self-limited viral illness.

POXVIRUSES

(CM&S Chapter 122)

Viruses of the family Poxviridae are large, ovoid, or brick-shaped particles containing a double-stranded DNA genome. Smallpox, the most significant of the poxviruses, was eradicated in the past century.

Vaccinia

Clinical Description

Abnormal reactions to smallpox vaccination could be either local or generalized. Bacterial superinfection and accidental inoculation of virus to other body sites or individuals were the main local complications. Although these were generally trivial and avoidable, inoculation of vaccinia to certain sites (e.g., the eye) or individuals (e.g., the immunosuppressed) could be dangerous. Eczema vaccinatum occurred in children with a history of atopic dermatitis and was acquired either through primary vaccination or by contact with a vaccinee. Lesions appeared at sites that were or had been involved by eczema. For this reason, atopic dermatitis was regarded as a contraindication to vaccination. Progressive vaccinia occurred in immunodeficient patients and resulted in progressive enlargement of the inflammatory lesion at the vaccination site. Sometimes the entire upper arm and shoulder were involved, and distant secondary lesions developed. The disease was usually fatal.

Generalized reactions could be relatively benign or severe. Erythema multiforme could be associated with vaccination, and in generalized vaccinia a widespread eruption developed 6 to 9 days after vaccination. Both of these eruptions had a benign prognosis. Vaccinial encephalitis and congenital vaccinia, in which virus was disseminated to the fetus from the mother, could be fatal.

Pathology

The histopathologic features of vaccinia include an intraepidermal vesicle with ballooning of keratinocytes leading to reticular alteration of the epidermis. Intracytoplasmic inclusions are the hallmark of disease.

Diagnosis

The diagnosis of vaccinia should be confirmed by virologic studies (culture, electron microscopy, and serology), and investigations to identify immunologic defects should be performed in persons with reactions other than simple secondary infection or autoinocculation. Human immunodeficiency virus has been associated with severe vaccination reactions.

Treatment

Prevention of reactions by appropriate clinical screening for immunodeficiency and eczema was important, as was advice on appropriate care of the vaccination site. Those with severe reactions could be treated with hyperimmune globulin (VIG, vaccinia immune globulin) together with antiviral agents such as vidarabine or interferon.

Cowpox

Definition

Cowpox is an uncommon poxvirus zoonosis circulating in Europe that occasionally affects humans, generally causing a localized self-limiting inflammatory reaction.

Clinical Description

Although initially isolated from cows and farm workers, and hence named cowpox, this disease is rare in cattle. Its natural reservoir remains unknown but has been suggested to be a small mammal, and infection of domestic cats is not uncommon. Human infections occur at the site of minor trauma and are generally limited to the hands. The lesion starts as an inflammatory papule with associated erythema and hemorrhage and may ulcerate. Sporotrichoid spread has been reported. Local lymph node enlargement and fever occur often, sometimes necessitating admission to hospital. The lesion resolves in 4 to 6 weeks and may be complicated by secondary bacterial infection or, very rarely, encephalitis.

Pathology

Like smallpox, early cowpox lesions show prominent reticular degeneration, and eosinophilic cytoplasmic inclusions are often present.

Diagnosis and Differential Diagnosis

In the context of contact with an infected animal, clinical diagnosis is not difficult. However, in the absence of this history other diagnoses must be considered, including orf, milker's nodule, and anthrax.

Treatment

Because of the self-limiting and mild nature of the disease, no treatment is generally necessary. In severe cases, however, human cowpox should respond to vaccinia immune globulin. Patients with infection should be warned about transferring it to other sites or persons.

Orf and Milker's Nodule

Definition

Orf and milker's nodule are caused by closely related parapoxviruses and are discussed here together because of their clinical, pathologic, and virologic similarities. The human diseases can generally be distinguished only by history, with orf resulting from contact with sheep and milker's nodule occurring in persons in contact with cattle. The collective term *farmyard pox* has been proposed.

Clinical Description

These diseases are found in persons who have contact with sheep and cattle, on farms, or in the meat trade. The virus is resistant to drying: infection may therefore be acquired indirectly from contaminated structures on farms. Infection occurs through small cuts and abrasions, and the site depends on local practice in handling animals. Lesions are generally solitary, although multiple lesions can occur and are found predominantly on the extremities. Lesions start as an erythematous papule that subsequently develops a white halo, becomes nodular, and may ulcerate. Most cases resolve in about 6 weeks. Lesions average 1 to 2 cm in diameter, although giant orf has been reported in immunosuppressed individuals. Systemic upset is uncommon, but erythema multiforme has been associated.

Pathology

Orf and milker's nodule both begin with ballooning of keratinocytes, spongiosis, and epidermal hyperplasia. Small round eosinophilic viral inclusions are present in the cytoplasm of infected keratinocytes. Intraepidermal vesiculation, necrosis, and ulceration occur in later lesions, accompanied by dense dermal infiltrates of lymphocytes and plasma cells.

Diagnosis and Differential Diagnosis

The diagnosis of orf and milker's nodule is generally a clinical one and is often suggested by the patient. However, in the absence of a history, diagnoses such as cowpox, herpetic whitlow, atypical mycobacterial infection, and pyogenic granuloma must be considered.

Treatment

Generally no treatment is required since both conditions are self-limiting. Correct diagnosis is important to avoid mutilating surgery on the assumption that the lesion represents a rapidly growing malignant tumor. Attention should be paid to the avoidance of secondary infection.

Molluscum Contagiosum

Definition

Molluscum contagiosum is a common poxvirus infection of the skin and mucous membranes characterized by pearly umbilicated papules.

Clinical Description

Although it may occur at any age, the majority of cases occur in childhood, with boys being more frequently affected than girls. Transmission is thought to be by person-to-person spread, and genital lesions in adults are probably transmitted sexually. The disease is more severe in the immunosuppressed, and giant lesions are a feature of human immunodeficiency virus infection. Infection is more common in children with atopic eczema. Lesions may occur at any site and start as grouped, flesh-colored, or pearly papules a few millimeters in diameter. As they progress, they develop a distinct central depression (umbilication), and a white, curd-like core may easily be expressed. The lesions are generally asymptomatic, but occasionally there is surrounding eczematization and pruritus may then be a feature. Like virus warts, molluscum contagiosum exhibits the Koebner phenomenon. Individual lesions last about 2 months and resolve either spontaneously or after minor trauma, but the eruption as a whole frequently persists longer than this.

Pathology

Molluscum contagiosum appears to infect follicular epithelium, because its viral inclusions are found within endophytic, bulbous lobules of keratinocytes attached to the epidermis, and not within the interfollicular epidermis itself. The distinctive large, round molluscum bodies that are the hallmark of the condition form above the basal layer and are initially eosinophilic. They consist of masses of brick-shaped viral particles.

Diagnosis and Differential Diagnosis

The clinical appearance is generally characteristic, but in cases of doubt, histologic examination should be diagnostic. In human immunodeficiency virus infection, molluscum contagiosum must be distinguished from cutaneous cryptococcal infection.

Treatment

Because the lesions are self-limiting, heal without scarring, and tend to occur in childhood, treatment is generally not required. However, if considered necessary, gentle manual expression of the central core or pricking with a sterile needle is effective. There is also some evidence that simple painting with iodine solutions is helpful. In adults, cryotherapy with liquid nitrogen using a cotton-wool bud or spray gun is the mainstay of treatment, although several sessions of therapy may be required to eradicate the numerous lesions.

HUMAN PAPILLOMAVIRUSES

(CM&S Chapter 123)

Definition

The papillomaviruses cause a spectrum of epithelial diseases, ranging from cutaneous and genital warts to papillomas of the mucosal epithelium of the larynx and cervix. All papillomaviruses are DNA viruses that differ in the specific order of their nucleotides. These human papillomavirus (HPV) types are referred to as genotypes. Nearly 70 have been isolated. These differences in DNA sequence are responsible for their varying pathogenic outcomes. Specific HPV types have been strongly associated with the development of epithelial cancers.

The HPV genotypes have preferred sites of infection and lesion morphology (Table 6–9).

Clinical Description

Warts occur most frequently on the hands, feet, face, legs, and external genital area. They are often classified based on anatomic distribution (face, hands, periungual, plantar, or genital). Morphologically, cutaneous warts are of two major types: common warts and flat warts. Common warts, or verruca vulgaris, are hard papules

TABLE 6-9. Human Papillomavirus Genotypes and Their Most Common Clinical Manifestations

CLINICAL LESIONS	HPV GENOTYPES
Cutaneous warts, including plantar, palmar, and flat	1-4, 10, 28, 29, 37, 41, 48, 60, 63, 65
Epidermodysplasia verruciformis; immunosuppression	5, 8, 9, 12, 14, 15, 17, 19-27, 36, 46, 47, 49, 50
Mucosal ("low risk"): Anogenital and cervical papillomas; oropharynx and respiratory tract papillomas	6, 11, 30, 34, 40, 42-44, 55, 57-59
Mucosal ("high risk"): Anogenital and cervical papillomas; bowenoid papulosis; cervical dysplasia; oropharynx, anogenital cancers including cervical	16, 18, 31, 33, 35, 39, 45, 51, 52, 56

HPV, human papillomavirus.

or plaques often with an irregular, spiked, scaly surface. Flat warts, or verruca plana, are small, 2- to 4-mm, slightly raised, slightly scaly papules.

The diagnosis of warts is based primarily on clinical morphology. On the soles of the feet, there is difficulty distinguishing solitary plantar warts from a clavus or corn. Viral warts lack dermatoglyphics and have small thrombosed capillaries that appear as punctate, blue-black stippling, whereas a clavus has dermatoglyphics but not the stippling.

In the genital area, differences in keratinization and hair-bearing qualities influence wart morphology. Condyloma acuminata are pedunculated cauliflower-like verrucous papules and nodules seen primarily on moist, non–hair-bearing, incompletely keratinized surfaces such as the vulvar labia, under the foreskin of the penis, and the perianal area. Condyloma lata of secondary syphilis can be mistaken for condyloma acuminata. Smooth papular and keratotic genital warts occur more commonly on keratinized genital skin. In the genital area, HPV DNA has also been found in lesions clinically consistent with seborrheic keratosis. Perianal genital warts occur, but intra-anal warts occur in patients who have had receptive anal intercourse.

Application of dilute acetic acid or vinegar to genital mucosa may bring out *subclinical (acetowhite)* warts. This significance is unclear because not all genital warts will whiten, and any condition that disrupts the mucosa may whiten.

Warts can also occur on nasal, conjunctival, oral, and laryngeal epithelial surfaces. Respiratory papillomatosis can lead to obstruction of the airway. In the oral cavity, HPV has also been associated with focal epithelial hyperplasia, which is a non–sexually transmitted oral infection with HPV consisting of multiple smooth, soft, whitish papules and small plaques on the oral mucosa.

Common genital warts are most commonly types 6 and 11. On the external genital area, the high-risk HPV types have been associated with bowenoid papulosis or squamous cell carcinoma in situ, which present as small, 1- to 4-mm, dome-shaped papules or, at times, velvety, sometimes bluish patches or plaques. It is currently believed that squamous cell carcinoma in situ of the external genitalia rarely results in invasive squamous cell carcinoma of the external genitalia, which is relatively uncommon. However, women with vulvar bowenoid papulosis, or female partners of men with bowenoid papulosis, need to be monitored closely for cervical cancer because the risk of transition to cancer is much higher in the cervix than in the genital skin. The smooth papular genital warts may, on biopsy, actually prove to be squamous cell carcinomas in situ or bowenoid papulosis. For this reason, one should biopsy genital warts that are refractory to treatment.

The most frequent site of HPV-related oncogenicity is the transformation zone of the uterine cervix. A majority of woman with external genital warts have vaginal or cervical HPV infection, and should have a complete gynecologic examination. Because genital warts in adults are predominantly a sexually transmitted disease, sexual partners should be examined. This is complicated by the fact that incubation time from infection to clinical manifestation can range from months to years. After successful treatment of visible warts, it is not known whether a patient is rendered noninfectious. Immunosuppressed patients should be carefully examined for the presence of perianal and intra-anal warts and need to be monitored for the development of anal carcinoma.

Verrucous carcinoma is a locally invasive, cytologically bland form of squamous cell carcinoma that does not metastasize unless transformation to high-grade carcinoma occurs. Early lesions may simulate a wart. There have been reports of verrucous carcinoma on fingers, toes, and genitalia, where it has been called "giant condyloma of Bushke and Lowenstein." Genital verrucous carcinoma usually contains low-risk HPV, such as type 6 or 11.

Immunocompetent Patients

Common and plantar warts are the most frequently occurring warts. Filiform, periungual, plaque, and mosaic plantar warts are less common. A combination of common warts is sometimes seen. Nearly any age group can be affected; however, children are most frequently affected.

Environmental factors associated with acquisition of warts include frequent wet work involving the hands, hyperhidrosis of the feet, and butchers and slaughterhouse workers. The number of warts increases with duration of infection.

Immunocompromised Patients

HPV infection and HPV-associated carcinoma are common complications of chronic immunosuppression. Immunocompromised patients are infected by the same HPV types as seen in immunocompetent patients as well as by HPV types usually seen in patients with epidermodysplasia verruciformis (EV). Immunosuppressed patients also demonstrate an accelerated course from wart to carcinoma. Caution is necessary in the clinical evaluation of warts in these patients. Although in immunocompetent patients, the histology of common warts is quite predictable, this is not so in renal allograft recipients. Biopsy specimens that clinically appear to be common warts often squamous cell carcinomas or dysplasia.

An increased incidence of warts has also been noted in patients with malignancy. Patients with HIV infection have been noted to have macular lesions similar to those noted in EV.

Epidermodysplasia Verruciformis

EV is a rare disease characterized by chronic, extensive HPV-induced warts (most typically types 5 and 8), that frequently progress to squamous carcinoma. In EV, the clinical morphology can be that of reddish, scaly papules that resemble other flat warts or scaly macules that have a striking resemblance to tinea versicolor. Approximately 25% of cases are familial. Autosomal recessive inheritance appears to be the predominant mode. The development of skin cancer, usually occurs during the second decade of life or 2 to 20 years after the onset of warts. The reported incidence of skin cancer ranges from 30% to 100% and tends to occur on sun-exposed areas.

Genital Human Papillomavirus Infections

Genital warts as a manifestation of HPV infection are very common in the sexually active population. Asymptomatic infection appears to be far more common than symptomatic infection. It has been estimated that 1% of all sexually active adults in the United States have visible genital warts at any given time. Another 2% of the population have warts that can be detected after soaking with acetic acid, and 20% to 50% have infection of the genital tract based on detection of HPV DNA.

Juvenile Laryngeal Papillomatosis

Juvenile laryngeal or respiratory papillomatosis is an HPV infection of the larynx, usually seen in young children. It is thought to be transmitted through an infected birth canal. These laryngeal papillomas are almost uniformly associated with low-risk mucosal HPV types such as 6 and 11.

Genital Human Papillomavirus Infection in Children

The exact route of transmission of genital papillomas in children is not certain. While some have acquired these via sexual abuse, most probably have acquired the infection via other routes. The papillomavirus is relatively resistant to physical and chemical destruction and may remain infectious for weeks or months at room temperature or be transmitted by fomites such as clothing, washcloths, and towels. Evaluation for sexual abuse should be considered in children with genital warts.

Pathology

A verruca vulgaris is characterized by digitated epidermal hyperplasia with papillations that radiate outward, inwardly bowed rete ridges, compact orthokeratosis with tiers of parakeratosis at the tips of digitations, and dilated, tortuous capillaries within dermal papillae. In warts that still harbor HPV, the granular layer in the dells between papillations contain cells with coarse keratohyaline granules, and vacuoles surround the wrinkled-appearing nuclei of these keratinocytes.

Flat warts, or verrucae planae, have features that resemble those of verrucae vulgares but are muted in comparison and have prominent perinuclear halos around nuclei of cells in the granular layer (owl's eye cells).

Condyloma acuminatum demonstrates gently papillated epithelial hyperplasia, with thick, rounded rete ridges and occasional horn pseudocysts.

Bowenoid papulosis often resembles condyloma acuminatum but differs in that there is cytologic atypia.

Verrucous carcinoma typically is a vertically oriented, exoendophytic, slightly papillated proliferation of cytologically bland keratinocytes in which bulbous rete ridges can penetrate deeply within the dermis. Furrows containing necrotic debris are often present between papillations. Atypical keratinocytes are in the basal layer of the thick, blunt-ended rete ridges.

Diagnosis and Differential Diagnosis

The differential diagnosis of warts includes molluscum contagiosum, seborrheic keratosis, squamous cell carcinoma, and actinic keratosis. Flat warts can look like lichen planus or freckles. Condyloma lata, lichen planus, skin tags, Tyson's glands, and pearly penile papules can simulate genital warts.

Treatment

The mainstay of treatments of nongenital warts are cryotherapy and topical keratolytics. Paring and use of salicylic acid plasters or topical liquids containing salicylic acid and lactic acid (Duofilm, Duoplant) are popular, often effective, nontraumatic therapies that can be administered at home by the patient. Other treatments include cantharidin, oral cimetidine, hypnosis, electrodesiccation and curettage, laser surgery, and intralesional bleomycin. Patients with frequent recurrences need to be seen and treated promptly. Treatment of genital warts and bowenoid papulosis includes caustic agents (trichloro- or bichloro-acetic acid) cryotherapy, 5-fluorouracil, interferons, podophyllin, podofilox, retinoids, and surgery (laser, cold steel, or electrosurgery).

All current treatments have about a 50% complete response rate and a 25% to 50% recurrence rate. Screening for other sexually transmitted diseases is an important part of the management of genital warts, as is addressing any emotional issues that may result from this condition.

VIRAL EXANTHEMS

(CM&S Chapter 124)

Viral exanthems are acute, generalized cutaneous eruptions due to viral infection. They may result from either direct viral invasion of the skin or host immune response to viral assault. Because patterns of cutaneous response to viral and other systemic infections are limited, totally unrelated infectious agents may cause similar exanthems. Conversely, identical agents may cause eruptions with different appearances, depending on the patient's age or duration of infection. Exanthems from bacterial and rickettsial infections, as well as drug eruptions, may mimic viral rashes. This makes the evaluation of the patient with a possible viral exanthem a formidable task (Table 6–10).

Measles (Rubeola)

Measles is a common childhood exanthem caused by a paramyxovirus that is closely related to the canine distemper virus. There is only one antigenic type, and humans are the natural hosts and only reservoir of the infection.

Epidemiology

Most cases in the United States occur in infants younger than 15 months of age, with a second peak in incidence in adolescence. Measles has continued to be a major health problem in many developing countries. The disease is most prevalent in winter and spring. It is spread by droplets from respiratory secretions. The incubation period is from 9 to 12 days from the time of exposure to the onset of symptoms.

Clinical Description

The prodrome of measles lasts from 2 to 4 days. Fever as high as 38.5°C to 40°C, nasal congestion, sneezing, rhinitis, conjunctivitis, and cough are nearly always present. A transitory macular or urticarial rash has been described early in the prodrome. Koplik spots, which are pathognomonic of measles, develop during the prodrome, consisting of tiny white or bluish-gray specks approximately 1 mm in size, superimposed on an erythematous, granular base, beginning on the buccal mucosa, opposite the lower molars, and then spreading to involve other parts of the buccal mucosa and the palate. The pharynx is frequently infected.

The exanthem begins behind the ears and at the hairline and spreads centrifugally from head to foot, so that by the third day of the rash the whole body is involved. Lesions begin as discrete, erythematous papules, which gradually coalesce. They are occasionally

TABLE 6-10. Exanthems		
DISEASE (ETIOLOGY)	**USUAL AGE**	**SEASON**
Viral Causes		
Measles (rubeola virus)	Infants to young adults	Winter/spring
Rubella (rubella virus)	Adolescents/young adults	Spring
Erythema infectiosum (parvovirus B19)	5–15 y	Winter/spring
Roseola (herpesvirus 6)	6 mo–3 y	Spring/fall
Human immunodeficiency virus	Adults	Any season
Chickenpox (varicella-zoster virus)	1–14 y	Late fall/ winter/spring
Enteroviral exanthems (coxsackleviruses, echoviruses, other enteroviruses)	Young children	Summer/fall
Epstein-Barr exanthems (Epstein-Barr virus)	Young children/ adolescents	Any season
Gianotti-Crosti syndrome (Hepatitis B, coxsackievirus infection, Epstein-Barr virus)	1–6 y	Any season
Bacterial and Rickettsial Causes		
Staphylococcal scalded skin syndrome (*S. aureus*/ epidermolytic toxin)	Neonates and infants	Any season
Toxic shock syndrome (staphylococcal toxin)	Adolescents/young adults	Any season
Scarlet fever (β-*Streptococcus*)	School-age children	Fall to spring
Meningococcemia (meningococcus)	<2 y	Winter/spring
Rocky Mountain spotted fever (*Rickettsia rickettsii* carried by ticks)	Any age	Summer
Unknown Cause		
Kawasaki disease (etiology unknown)	6 mo–6 y	Winter/spring

TABLE 6-10. Exanthems	
PRODROME	**MORPHOLOGY**
High fever, signs and symptoms of upper respiratory tract infection, conjunctivitis	Erythematous macules and papules become confluent
Absent or low-grade fever, malaise	Rose-pink papules that are not confluent
Usually none	Slapped cheeks: reticulate erythema or maculopapular
High fever for 3-5 days	Maculopapular rash appears after fever declines
Fever, malaise, sore throat, diarrhea	Roseola-like hemorrhagic macules
Usually none	Macules, papules rapidly become vesicles on erythematous base, then crusts
Fever (occasional)	Extremely variable; maculopapular, petechial, purpura, vesicular
Fever, adenopathy, sore throat	Maculopapular or morbilliform
Usually absent	Papules/papulovesicles; may become confluent
None	Abrupt onset, tender erythroderma
None	Macular erythroderma
Acute onset with fever, sore throat	Diffuse erythema with sandpaper texture
Malaise, fever, upper respiratory tract infection symptoms	Papules, petechiae, purpura
Fever, malaise	Maculopapular/petechial rash
Irritability	Polymorphous-papular morbilliform, erythema with desquamation

Continued

TABLE 6-10. Exanthems (Continued)		
DISEASE (ETIOLOGY)	**DISTRIBUTION**	**ASSOCIATED FINDINGS**
Viral Causes		
Measles	Begins on face and moves downward over whole body	Koplik's spots, toxic appearance, photophobia, cough, adenopathy, fever
Rubella	Begins on face and moves downward	Postauricular and occipital adenopathy; headache, malaise
Erythema infectiosum	Usually arms/legs; may be generalized	Rash waxes/wanes several weeks; occasional arthritis, headache, malaise
Roseola	Trunk, neck; may be generalized; lasts hours to days	Cervical and postauricular adenopathy
Human immunodeficiency virus	Upper body predominates, palms, soles	Adenopathy
Chickenpox	Often begins on scalp/face; more profuse on trunk than extremities	Pruritus, fever, oral
Enteroviral exanthems	Usually generalized, may be acral	Low-grade fever; occasional myocarditis, aseptic meningitis, pleurodynia, malaise
Epstein-Barr exanthems	Trunk, extremities	Cervical adenopathy Liver/spleen enlarged
Gianotti-Crosti syndrome	Face, arms, legs, buttocks; spares torso	Occasional lymphadenopathy, hepatomegaly, splenomegaly
Bacterial and Rickettsial Causes		
Staphylococcal scalded skin syndrome	Diffuse with perioral, perinasal scaling	Fever, conjunctivitis, rhinitis
Toxic shock syndrome	Generalized	Hypotension; fever, myalgias, diarrhea/ vomiting
Scarlet fever	Facial flushing with circumoral pallor, linear erythema in skin folds	Exudative pharyngitis, palatal petechiae, abdominal pain
Meningococcemia	Trunk, extremities, palms, soles	Temp > 40°C Meningismus, circulatory collapse
Rocky Mountain spotted fever	Wrists, ankles, palms, soles; trunk later	Central nervous system, pulmonary, cardiac lesions
Unknown Cause		
Kawasaki disease	Generalized, often with perineal accentuation	Conjunctivitis, cheilitis, glossitis, peripheral edema, adenopathy

TABLE 6-10. Exanthems (Continued)

DIAGNOSIS	SPECIAL MANAGEMENT
Clinical; acute/convalescent hemagglutinin serology	Report to public health; oral vitamin A therapy
Rubella IgM or acute/ convalescent hemagglutinin serology	Report to public health; check for exposure to pregnant women
Usually clinical; acute/ convalescent serology	
Usually clinical	
Acute and convalescent HIV-1 serologies	Counseling, referral for consideration of antiviral therapy and follow-up
Usually clinical; Tzanck prep, direct immunofluorescence or viral culture	Antihistamines for itching; aspirin contraindicated (Reye's syndrome); acyclovir
Usually clinical; viral culture from throat, rectal swabs in selected cases	If petechiae or purpura, must consider meningococcemia
Monospot; Epstein-Barr nuclear antigen acute/convalescent; IgG-viral capsize antigen	
Clinical; hepatitis B and Epstein-Barr serologies	
Clinical; culture of *S. aureus* from systemic site (not skin)	Neonate: if blistering present, hospitalize for intravenous nafcillin and fluid/electrolyte therapy
Clinical case definition criteria; isolation *S. aureus* cervix, etc.	Treatment of hypotension, admit to hospital; antibiotics to eradicate *S. aureus*
Throat culture	Penicillin, intramuscularly or orally
Clinical blood culture, spinal tap	Immediate intravenous penicillin in emergency department; treatment for shock, if present
Serology	Treat on presumptive clinical grounds
Clinical	Admit to hospital for intravenous gamma globulin, salicylates

Adapted from Williams ML, Frieden IJ. Dermatologic disorders. In: Grossman M, Dieckman RA, eds. Pediatric Emergency Medicine: A Clinician's Reference. Philadelphia: JB Lippincott, 1991.

purpuric, but pruritus is uncommon. The rash fades after 3 to 4 days but may persist for 6 to 7 days.

Most children with typical measles appear ill. Complications include pneumonia, otitis media, laryngotracheobronchitis, encephalitis, myocarditis, and pericarditis. Infection during pregnancy is associated with a high incidence of fetal wastage and in some cases congenital malformations.

A milder form of measles, "modified measles," usually occurs in partially immune hosts, such as infants younger than 9 months of age and in cases in which partial vaccine failure has occurred. The prodrome may be shortened, and cough, congestion, and fever may be less severe. The presence of Koplik spots is variable. The skin eruption is usually less confluent. "Atypical measles," due to infection with wild-type virus after vaccination with killed virus vaccine, is extremely rare. Its main characteristics are fever, onset of an acrally located hemorrhagic rash, and pneumonia.

Pathology

The pathologic findings in measles are characterized by the presence of multinucleated giant cells. Biopsy specimens of lesional skin show a slight spongiotic, psoriasiform dermatitis with occasional dyskeratotic cells and parakeratosis. The epidermis also contains syncytial keratinocytic giant cells. Nuclear and cytoplasmic inclusions are often present.

Diagnosis and Differential Diagnosis

Virus may be isolated from the blood, respiratory tract, skin, and other organs, but acute and convalescent serologic samples for hemagglutination inhibition or measles IgM are reliable and usually more practical. Typical measles may be confused with drug eruptions and other exanthems, particularly Kawasaki disease.

Treatment

High oral doses of vitamin A significantly decrease morbidity and mortality in hospitalized children with measles. Vitamin A can be given as retinyl palmitate in two doses of 200,000 IU each separated by 24 hours. No specific antiviral therapy is available.

Rubella

Rubella, an RNA virus and member of the Togaviridae, generally produces a mild exanthematous illness except when it is transmitted in utero when it may result in severe congenital infection.

Epidemiology

Rubella was once a common exanthematous disease of childhood, but after the use of vaccine the number of cases has dropped precipitously. Epidemics of rubella occasionally occur in developed countries, and rubella infection continues to be common in countries where vaccinations are not widely available.

Most cases occur in the spring. The incubation period ranges from 12 to 23 days but is between 15 and 21 days in most cases. The period of communicability is from 5 to 7 days before the appearance of the rash until 3 to 5 days after its appearance. Spread is probably through the respiratory route.

Clinical Description

Inapparent infection is common and may represent 50% to 80% of actual infections. A prodrome of malaise, cough, sore throat, eye pain, headache, swollen glands, red eyes, runny nose, fever, aches, chills, anorexia, and nausea may be present for 1 to 5 days before onset of rash. Pain on lateral and upward eye movement is a common and at times distressing symptom.

The progression, extent, and duration of the exanthem are variable. The rash, consisting of discrete pink macules and papules, begins on the face and progresses downward to the trunk, then to the extremities. In typical cases, the rash covers the entire body in the first 24 hours, then fades on the face on the second day, and disappears entirely by the end of the third day, but it may last less than 24 hours. An enanthem consisting of pinhead-sized, rose-red macules or petechiae on the soft palate and uvula is seen occasionally.

Suboccipital and posterior auricular adenopathy occurs in the majority of patients with rash. Generalized adenopathy may also occur. Arthritis and arthralgia are well-described complications of rubella, and their incidence increases with age.

Diagnosis and Differential Diagnosis

Virus may be isolated from the throat, urine, and other body fluids, but the availability of specific serologic tests usually makes this unnecessary. Rubella-specific IgM or acute and convalescent hemagglutination inhibition titers are helpful in determining prior exposure (particularly in pregnant women).

The exanthem of rubella is not specific and may resemble viral exanthems produced by many other viruses (including enteroviruses, reoviruses, adenoviruses, rubeola) as well as streptococcal scarlet fever.

Treatment

There is no specific treatment, but live viral vaccine is now widely administered to prevent disease. The disease should be reported to the local public health department. Hospitalized patients should be placed in respiratory isolation. All hospital personnel who may come in contact with pregnant patients with rubella should be screened for immunity to rubella.

Erythema Infectiosum

Erythema infectiosum (fifth disease) is caused by parvovirus B19, a single-stranded encapsulated DNA virus. In addition to rashes, the virus causes several other forms of clinical illness, including acute arthritis in adults, aplastic crises in patients with hereditary hemolytic anemias, chronic anemia in immunodeficient hosts, and hydrops fetalis or fetal death in some women infected during pregnancy.

Epidemiology

Infection is year-round and may be sporadic or occur in large outbreaks. The exanthem is most common in school-aged children. The virus is spread through respiratory secretions, usually through close contact. The incubation period is usually between 4 and 14 days.

Clinical Description

The primary manifestation of erythema infectiosum is its distinctive exanthem. Prodromal symptoms such as low-grade fever, malaise, and headache may be present for 1 or 2 days before the exanthem. Typically, the exanthem has three stages. First, a fiery red, macular erythema appears on the cheeks. Within days, discrete erythematous macules and papules appear on the proximal extremities, sometimes involving the trunk as well. The eruption may evolve into a characteristic lacy or reticulate pattern. The third stage of the exanthem, a waxing and waning of the eruption, varies in duration from one to several weeks, brought about by changes in environmental temperature, exposure to sunlight, exercise, crying, and emotional factors. Pruritus is occasionally present.

Most children with erythema infectiosum appear well. Headache, fever, sore throat, coryza, sore eyes, abdominal pain, anorexia, and joint pain may occur but are more common in adults. Encephalitis is extremely rare.

Multiple cases of intrauterine infection with acute maternal parvovirus B19 infection, resulting in hydrops fetalis and fetal death, have been described. The risk of developing hydrops is greatest if infection occurs in the first trimester, with fetal wastage as high as 19%. The risk in the second half of pregnancy is considerably lower.

Diagnosis and Differential Diagnosis

Laboratory tests are rarely necessary in typical cases of erythema infectiosum, but diagnosis of acute parvovirus B19 infection can be confirmed by the presence of specific IgM antibodies or seroconversion with specific IgG antibodies. The reticulocyte count may be low even in patients without anemia due to the effect of the virus on erythroid precursors. The leukocyte count is usually normal. Mild eosinophilia may be present.

When the typical exanthem is present, the findings are usually distinct enough to establish a diagnosis. Other diagnostic considerations include juvenile rheumatoid arthritis.

Treatment

No specific treatment is available. Patients with the rash can return to school, since viral shedding is generally over at the time of appearance of rash. Patients with aplastic crises or chronic B19 infection should have respiratory isolation and not be cared for by pregnant women. Exposed pregnant women may have serologic testing and if found to be infected can be evaluated with ultrasound, α-fetoprotein levels (which may be elevated in infection), and other diagnostic tests.

Roseola

Roseola (exanthema subitum) is a common, self-limited illness of infancy characterized by 3 to 5 days of high fever followed by an exanthem. The etiologic agent, human herpesvirus 6 (HHV 6), is a member of the Herpesviridae, and like other herpesviruses it is an enveloped, double-stranded DNA virus. It is similar to cytomegalovirus in its morphology and DNA sequences.

Epidemiology

Most newborns have transplacental maternal antibody that wanes by 5 to 6 months of age. The exact mode of spread is not yet known, but acquisition from asymptomatic adults with salivary shedding is suspected.

After initial infection, the virus may persist in a latent state in salivary glands or in blood monocytes or tissue macrophages. Thus, HHV 6 may be reactivated later and be shed or produce disease, especially in the setting of immune deficiency.

Clinical Description

Roseola typically begins with the sudden onset of high fever (up to 40°C) in children 6 months to 3 years of age. The fever persists for 3 to 5 days, usually with no other symptoms, although occipital adenopathy and/or mild pharyngitis may be present. Many infants with roseola appear happy and well. The rash, characterized by discrete, irregular, 2- to 5-mm, rose-pink macules and papules appearing on the trunk and neck, typically develops after defervescence, either on the same day or 1 to 2 days later. It fades completely within hours or days without desquamation.

The rash may develop without fever, fever may occur without the rash, and asymptomatic infection can occur. HHV 6 has also been implicated in a wide range of diseases other than roseola, including a mononucleosis-like illness, pneumonitis, and a fatal disseminated infection. Although most cases have a benign course, neurologic complications include febrile seizures, a relatively common problem, and encephalitis, a rare one. Other rare complications include hemophagocytic syndrome and immune thrombocytopenic purpura.

Diagnosis and Differential Diagnosis

In most cases of self-limited roseola, a clinical diagnosis based on a typical clinical picture is sufficient. Complete blood cell count will show a relative neutropenia and lymphocytosis. Acute and convalescent titers of HHV 6 can be measured by immunofluorescent antibody test, enzyme-linked immunosorbent assay, and neutralizing antibody test; the latter two are more sensitive. Polymerase chain reaction has been used to detect HHV 6 in peripheral blood mononuclear cells from patients with exanthema subitum. Viral culture from peripheral blood mononuclear cells is most sensitive during the febrile part of the illness.

The differential diagnosis of roseola includes other viral exanthems, especially enteroviruses, rubella, and measles. In young infants presenting with high fever and no obvious source, pursuit of a possible bacterial infection is warranted.

Treatment

Treatment is usually limited to supportive measures, such as control of fever with acetaminophen.

Varicella

Varicella (chickenpox) is one of the most common childhood exanthems. It is caused by the varicella-zoster virus, a double-stranded DNA virus that is a member of the Herpesviridae.

Varicella is a highly contagious disease. Both airborne and direct person-to-person contact can result in infection. The average incubation period is 14 to 16 days. Although later winter and early spring peaks of infection are common, the disease can occur at any time of the year.

Clinical Description

A mild prodrome of fever and malaise may occur 1 to 2 days before onset of the rash. A transient maculopapular or urticarial phase before vesicular eruption has also been reported. Typically, the exanthem begins on the scalp or trunk. Lesions occur in crops as erythematous macules and papules that rapidly evolve into vesicles, said to resemble "a dew-drop on a rose petal." They spread to involve nearly any part of the body, usually with centrifugal spread, and may be accentuated in areas of friction or previous skin injury such as a sunburn. Younger children generally have milder disease than adolescents and adults. As the lesions evolve they form crusts and then generally begin to heal. Pruritus is variable but can be severe. The rash usually resolves over 4 to 6 days. Patients are considered infectious until all lesions have crusted over.

In some patients, particularly immunocompromised hosts, skin lesions may be bullous and/or hemorrhagic, with less rapid crusting, resulting in a more monomorphous appearance of the rash. Mucous membrane lesions are common, typically involving the palate and uvula, but may also occur on the conjunctiva, vulva, and other sites.

Complications of varicella occur in a small percentage of cases, the most common being secondary bacterial skin infections and scarring. Others include otitis media, pneumonia, hepatitis, purpura fulminans, carditis, encephalitis, and Reye's syndrome. Severe, life-threatening varicella has been well documented in immunocompromised hosts but can occur in others, particularly those receiving systemic corticosteroids, even only briefly.

Pathology

Skin biopsy of primary varicella is rarely performed; but if it is done, the specimen shows features indistinguishable from those of vesicular lesions of herpes zoster or those caused by herpes simplex.

Diagnosis and Differential Diagnosis

The diagnosis of varicella is usually made clinically. Further documentation can be obtained by viral culture by Tzanck preparation, by demonstrating multinucleated giant cells, or by fluorescent or immunoperoxidase antibody slide tests, which are both sensitive and specific in early lesions.

The differential diagnosis includes other vesicular viral exanthems, particularly those caused by enteroviruses, herpes simplex infection, insect bite reactions, pityriasis lichenoides et varioliformis acuta, and autoimmune blistering diseases, such as chronic bullous dermatosis of childhood. Recurrent varicella-zoster virus infection in apparently immunocompetent children has been reported, so previous history of varicella does not exclude the diagnosis.

Treatment

Oral acyclovir (20 mg/kg given four times per day; up to 800 mg qid) has been demonstrated to be moderately effective in decreasing time to new lesion formation and total number of skin lesions if given within 24 hours of the onset of rash. It should probably be used in adolescents and adults, in whom varicella is known to be more severe, but its routine use in otherwise healthy children is controversial. Intravenous acyclovir is the treatment of choice for immunocompromised hosts, although in some cases with relatively mild immune deficit, oral therapy may be employed.

Oral antihistamines may be helpful in patients with severe pruritus. Bland shake lotions such as calamine may also help, but those with topical diphenhydramine should be avoided.

Enteroviral Infection

Enteroviruses are the most common cause of viral exanthems in the summer and fall in temperate climates. Members of the Picornaviridae, they are single-stranded, unenveloped RNA viruses.

Epidemiology

Infection is spread by the fecal-oral and, more rarely, the respiratory route. The incubation period is 4 to 7 days, and the majority of infections are asymptomatic. When symptoms are present, they are highly variable, depending on the host and the serotype of enterovirus.

Clinical Description

Enteroviruses can cause virtually any type of exanthem, but the hand-foot-and-mouth syndrome is the most distinctive of these. After 1 or 2 days of fever, small vesicles develop on the gingivae and lingual and buccal mucous membranes. The cutaneous lesions then appear as multiple, 3- to 7-mm usually oval vesicles. They develop on the dorsa and, less commonly, on volar hands and feet. Buttock lesions also occur in younger children. The exanthem resolves spontaneously within days. Coxsackievirus A16 is the most common cause of hand-foot-and-mouth disease, but many other enteroviruses have been implicated.

Enteroviruses can also cause macular, papular, morbilliform, vesicular, urticarial, petechial, rubelliform, and roseola-like eruptions. Echoviruses 25 and 32 have caused hemangioma-like lesions, which are small papules with a dilated vessel in the center that blanch with pressure and have surrounding white halos. These papules resolve spontaneously within days. Echovirus 16 causes outbreaks of an acute febrile illness with a roseola-like exanthem known as Boston exanthem. Other eruptions caused by enteroviruses include Kaposi's varicelliform eruption in patients with preexisting skin disease (e.g., atopic dermatitis or Darier's disease) and a zosteriform eruption. A fatal dermatomyositis-like syndrome caused by echovirus 24 has been described in a patient with hypogammaglobulinemia. Herpangina, an enanthem characterized by small papulovesicles on the soft palate, uvula, and tonsils, is caused by several different enteroviruses.

Systemic involvement in enteroviral infection may include mild fever, vomiting and diarrhea, and respiratory symptoms. Myocarditis and aseptic meningitis are less common complications.

Diagnosis and Differential Diagnosis

Enteroviral exanthems are usually diagnosed clinically, based on morphology and the time of year; but when a specific diagnosis is required, viral cultures from rectum, eye, nose, and oropharynx may be obtained. The results of serologic tests are usually not helpful, owing to the large number of enteroviral serotypes. Because enteroviral infections are frequently diagnosed clinically, skin biopsy is only performed if other conditions are suspected. The blisters show intraepidermal vesiculation secondary to ballooning and reticular degeneration of the epidermis, along with superficial perivascular lymphocytic infiltrates and papillary dermal edema. Inclusions and giant cells are absent.

The differential diagnosis is broad and, depending on the presentation, includes herpes stomatitis, varicella-zoster infection, aphthous stomatitis, roseola, group A streptococcal infection, and meningococcemia.

Treatment

There is no specific antiviral therapy for enteroviral infections. Supportive measures, such as administration of acetaminophen for fever and fluids to prevent dehydration, are indicated. Local measures, such as rinsing the mouth with antacids, may alleviate discomfort associated with oral lesions.

Epstein-Barr Virus

Epstein-Barr virus (EBV) is a double-stranded DNA virus and a member of the Herpesviridae. Its clinical manifestations are protean and depend on the age of the patient at the time of infection. EBV causes infectious mononucleosis in adolescents, but it causes rash and upper respiratory tract symptoms with only mild adenopathy in young children. Infection is spread by close interpersonal contact.

Clinical Description

Young adults with primary EBV infection present with an acute illness consisting of fever, sore throat, and fatigue known as infectious mononucleosis. A striking, frequently exudative, tonsillopharyngitis is seen, often with a characteristic petechial enanthem at the junction of the hard and soft palate. Adenopathy (particularly posterior cervical), hepatosplenomegaly, and jaundice are not uncommon. Periorbital edema has been reported and may be the presenting symptom. Rash occurs in a minority of patients in this age group. However, if amoxicillin is given, a morbilliform exanthem may develop. This resolves within 5 days and does not represent a true drug allergy.

Children younger than 5 years old may present with an acute illness similar to infectious mononucleosis, with fever, malaise, pharyngitis, and cervical adenopathy. In addition, many of these younger patients have prominent upper respiratory tract symptoms, such as runny nose, cough, and otitis media. Younger children are more likely to have rash, which may be maculopapular, petechial, papulovesicular, or erythema multiforme–like. EBV may also cause Gianotti-Crosti syndrome.

Complications of acute EBV infection include upper airway obstruction due to markedly swollen lymphoid tissue, co-infection with group A *Streptococcus,* and pneumonia. Neurologic disturbances (seizures, encephalitis) and hematologic abnormalities (thrombocytopenia with bleeding) occur occasionally. Most patients recover without treatment within a month, although it may be several months before they feel normal.

Pathology

Although the common exanthem of mononucleosis shows only sparse lymphocytic infiltrates, minimal vacuolar change, and papillary dermal edema, a severe eruption due to EBV has been described in immunosuppressed patients, in whom an interface reaction with many necrotic keratinocytes and parakeratosis can occur. EBV can be demonstrated in the nuclei of lesional keratinocytes in this eruption.

Diagnosis and Differential Diagnosis

Routine laboratory assessment of patients with infectious mononucleosis will show absolute lymphocytosis, prominent atypical lymphocytes, mild thrombocytopenia, and mildly to moderately elevated results of liver function tests. In adolescents and young adults, heterophil antibody tests are usually positive, but they are often negative in younger children. Measurement of acute and convalescent titers to the Epstein-Barr nuclear antigen (EBNA) may also be helpful. The differential diagnosis of adolescents with infectious mononucleosis includes adenoviral infection, rubella, cytomegalovirus infection, acute toxoplasmosis, streptococcal pharyngitis, and scarlet fever. An infectious mononucleosis–like illness due to HHV 6 has been described. EBV infection in young children is difficult to diagnose since nonspecific cold symptoms and exanthems can be caused by a variety of viruses that affect the respiratory tract.

Treatment

Treatment of acute EBV infection is supportive. Patients with upper airway obstruction may be helped by administration of prednisone. Antibiotics should be reserved for those patients with proven bacterial superinfection, such as streptococcal pharyngitis. There are no specific antiviral drugs clinically proven effective in EBV infection, although high doses of acyclovir have been used in immunosuppressed patients with some effect.

Gianotti-Crosti Syndrome

In 1955, Gianotti and Crosti described a distinctive eruption characterized by the presence of multiple, discrete, nonpruritic, erythematous papules located exclusively on the face, neck, and extremities. The rash, called "papular acrodermatitis of childhood," was later found to be caused by hepatitis B. The forms caused by other agents have sometimes been called "papulovesicular acrolocated syndrome" to distinguish them from the hepatitis B–associated exanthem.

The age of affected children varies from 3 months to 15 years, with a peak incidence at 2 to 5 years of age. Both sexes are affected equally. Most cases associated with hepatitis B infection are due to the ayw subtype. Most children in the United States do not have hepatitis B infection. Epstein-Barr virus and enteroviruses are the most common causes, but cases have been reported due to poliovaccine virus, cytomegalovirus, hepatitis A, and parainfluenza virus.

Clinical Description

The distribution of Gianotti-Crosti syndrome is distinctive and usually the first clue to diagnosis. Whereas most exanthems have significant involvement of the torso, this syndrome spares the torso, with most lesions being noted on the face and extremities with occasional involvement of the buttocks. Lesions may vary from flat-topped papules to "juicy," papulovesicular lesions resembling insect bites. Pruritus is variable. Hepatomegaly and lymphadenopathy may be present, depending on the etiology. The rash persists longer than most exanthems, often lasting from 2 to 4 weeks.

Diagnosis and Differential Diagnosis

Evaluation of children with papular acral eruptions should include a history of exposure to hepatitis and other infectious illnesses. Evaluation should include a careful examination for lymphadenopathy, hepatomegaly, and splenomegaly. If an exposure history suggests the possibility of hepatitis B infection, laboratory evaluation including a complete blood cell count, liver function tests, and hepatitis B surface antigen should be obtained. Because hepatitis B is quite rare in the United States, such serologic testing is probably not necessary in all cases.

The differential diagnosis includes papular urticaria, erythema multiforme, and lichenoid dermatitis.

Pathology

The cutaneous lesions of Gianotti-Crosti syndrome are produced by spongiotic dermatitis, sometimes accompanied by superficial and deep lymphocytic infiltrates. Fully developed lesions can show marked edema of the papillary dermis and psoriasiform epidermal hyperplasia.

Treatment

There is no specific treatment. Oral antihistamines are occasionally necessary. The prognosis is generally good, although some children with hepatitis B–associated disease go on to develop chronic hepatitis.

HUMAN IMMUNODEFICIENCY VIRUS INFECTION AND THE CUTANEOUS COMPLICATIONS OF IMMUNOSUPPRESSION

(CM&S Chapter 125)

Human Immunodeficiency Virus Infection and Its Cutaneous Complications

Clinical Description

Human immunodeficiency virus (HIV) is spread by exchange of body fluids. The most common modes of transmission are sexual contact, intravenous drug use, blood or blood product transfusion, and spread from mother to child during birth (perinatal transmission). Since HIV-infected persons are frequently asymptomatic but infectious for many years before they develop clinical disease, large numbers of persons may become infected before the presence of an epidemic is recognized.

Human immunodeficiency virus type 1 (HIV-1) infects cells that bear surface CD4 receptors: helper T cells and members of the monocyte/macrophage system. HIV binds to CD4 receptors through its surface glycoprotein, gp 120.

During initial infection, there is transient viremia, during which time CD4 cells fall abruptly, but HIV is rapidly cleared from the circulation by the immune response. This phase is called primary HIV disease. After the primary stage, the immune system appears to largely contain the virus within the reticuloendothelial system, primarily in lymph nodes. Virema is no longer detectable, and the helper T cells initially return to normal levels. This second phase is called the asymptomatic stage because the infected person usually has no symptoms (except perhaps generalized lymphadenopathy). There is a gradual depletion of helper T cells in most persons, while HIV proliferates within lymph nodes. Symptomatic HIV disease (the third phase of infection) begins on the average about 10 years after infection and is often manifested by fever, night sweats, diarrhea, or weight loss. Helper T-cell counts are variable but usually less than 400 cells/mm^3. Everyone who develops symptomatic HIV disease progresses to acquired immunodeficiency syndrome (AIDS), the fourth stage of infection. AIDS is diagnosed by the presence of certain neoplastic, infectious, or laboratory (a helper T-cell count < 200 cells/mm^3) complications of infection. Once the infected person develops AIDS, there is a gradual deterioration of his or her health as a result of recurrent infections and/or neurologic complications. The final stage of HIV infection occurs at a helper T-cell count less than 50 cells/mm^3 (advanced AIDS). At this stage, certain chronic infections reactivate, therapy for infections becomes more difficult, and death supervenes.

More than 90% of persons who seroconvert for HIV suffer an acute mononucleosis-like illness. The incubation period range is approximately 2 weeks. The most characteristic symptoms are fever, sore throat, malaise, myalgias, and headache. Enlarged lymph nodes are found in 50% to 90% of patients, as well as an inflamed throat. A cutaneous eruption occurs in 25% to 75% of patients and consists of either a diffuse morbilliform or papular exanthem or 5- to 10-mm oval, papulosquamous, maculopapular lesions sometimes with central (petechiae) predominantly over the upper trunk. The palms and soles may be involved. Skin biopsy specimens show a sparse mononuclear cell upper dermal infiltrate with slight exocytosis and occasionally hemorrhage.

An enanthem is seen in about one third of patients with primary HIV disease. Oral candidiasis may be present. Oral, genital, anal, and esophageal ulcerations are frequent, and odynophagia and/or retrosternal pain may occur. HIV has been identified in these ulcerations. The acute illness lasts 1 to 2 weeks. Most patients recover within 4 weeks, but lymphadenopathy and lethargy may persist. Acute hepatitis may occur. Neurologic disease in the form of encephalitis, neuritis, or myelitis may develop 2 to 3 weeks after the acute illness and in persons at risk is highly suggestive of acute HIV infection.

The diagnosis of group I, or primary, HIV disease is confirmed by detecting HIV seroconversion, an IgM antibody response in the second to tenth week, and isolation in the blood of HIV virus or antigens during the acute episode. IgG antibodies detected by Western blot analysis may be present at the onset of the illness although enzyme-linked immunosorbent assays are negative. There is a reversal of the helper/suppressor T-cell ratio, which is normally 2:1.

Bacterial Infections

The nasal carriage rate of *Staphylococcus aureus* is approximately 50% in HIV-infected persons of all stages of disease, and staphylococcal pyodermas are very common. Staphylococcal infections manifest as folliculitis, ecthyma, abscess, or tender boggy plaques. Treatment of staphylococcal pyoderma is with oral antibiotics, and prolonged courses may be required. Ablation of nasal carriage with topical mupirocin or oral rifampin may benefit patients with recurrent episodes.

Viral Infections

Molluscum Contagiosum

Clinical Description

Molluscum contagiosum affects between 10% and 20% of patients with AIDS. Eighty percent of patients with molluscum contagiosum have a helper T-cell count (CD4) below 200 cells/mm^3. Patients with extensive molluscum usually have fewer than 50 helper T cells/mm^3.

Molluscum contagiosum preferentially affects the genital area and face, especially around the eyes. In the beard area, lesions begin at the follicular opening as barely visible skin-colored papules. A large solitary lesion may simulate a basal cell carcinoma. Disseminated fungal infections, especially cryptococcosis, may mimic molluscum contagiosum, but in these cases the onset is usually more rapid, and the lesions tend to be of a uniform size.

Treatment

Cryotherapy is the usual method of treatment. Alternative methods of therapy include gentle electrosurgery, cantharidin, and removal by curette. Recurrence is almost universal. Shaving with razor blades should be stopped if lesions are in the beard area. The nightly application of topical retinoic acid at the highest strength tolerated appears to reduce the rate of appearance and size of new lesions.

Herpes Simplex Virus Infection

Clinical Description

Early in the course of HIV disease herpes simplex virus (HSV) infection is often a self-limited disorder. Once significant immunosuppression occurs, however, lesions persist. The presence of mucocutaneous HSV infection for more than 1 month is an indicator disease for AIDS. Tender, often painful, ulcerative lesions of the penis, perianal area, and lip are the hallmark. Less commonly, periungual lesions (herpetic whitlow) or follicular facial lesions (herpetic folliculitis) occur. Multiple scattered lesions in one area are not uncommon, but widespread dissemination of HSV even in AIDS is unusual. *Any ulcerative or erosive lesion in a patient with HIV disease should be considered HSV until proven otherwise.*

The diagnosis of HSV infection is by Tzanck smear, viral culture, and/or direct fluorescent antibody staining of scrapings from lesions or skin biopsy. It is not uncommon to find evidence of cytomegalovirus (CMV) expression in chronic perianal ulcerative (and occasionally oral) lesions in patients with advanced HIV disease.

Treatment

For active mucocutaneous lesions, therapy consists of 200 to 400 mg of acyclovir five times daily until the lesions have healed. If ineffective, increased oral doses (up to 800 mg five times daily) or intravenous acyclovir (5 mg/kg three times daily) may be used. Since the likelihood of recurrence is high, chronic suppressive acyclovir (400 mg twice daily) is given indefinitely, once lesions have healed.

The therapy for acyclovir-resistant HSV infection is with trisodium phosphonoformate (foscarnet). Once lesions heal, acyclovir suppression may be reinstituted, although suppressive foscarnet may be required.

Varicella-Zoster Virus

Clinical Description

Many HIV-infected persons develop zoster before they have other symptoms of HIV disease. Zoster has also been reported to follow rapidly primary varicella in HIV-infected children.

HIV-infected persons when exposed to VZV for the first time may develop varicella. Although varicella may follow a benign course, resolving without therapy, pulmonary involvement and fatal disease may occur, even in patients with asymptomatic HIV infection. Complications appear to be more common in HIV-positive children than in adults.

In the HIV-infected patient with few or no HIV-related symptoms, herpes zoster usually follows a course similar to that seen in healthy persons. Severe ulceration with pain and post-herpetic neuralgia are not uncommon, however. Disseminated zoster is uncommon and usually seen in HIV-infected persons with advanced disease. Because in HIV disease disseminated VZV is much more common than disseminated HSV, patients with disseminated herpetic lesions must be assumed to have VZV and treated appropriately.

In addition to the typical vesiculobullous lesions commonly seen with disseminated VZV, patients with AIDS develop two unusual clinical patterns: ecthymatous, crusted, punched-out ulcerations or true verrucous lesions that may be seen alone or in association with vesicular or ecthymatous lesions. These patterns may be associated with acyclovir resistance.

The diagnosis of varicella or herpes zoster is made in a similar manner as HSV infection.

Treatment

HIV-infected persons with varicella, either as a primary infection, a second episode, or a reactivation, should be evaluated carefully for evidence of systemic involvement. If evidence of pulmonary, hepatic, or other systemic disease is found, intravenous acyclovir at a dosage of 10 mg/kg every 8 hours, adjusted for renal function, should be given. Oral acyclovir at a dosage of 800 mg every 4 hours may be used in persons without evidence of visceral disease, but these patients should be followed carefully, and if evidence of visceral disease occurs, intravenous acyclovir therapy should be instituted.

The management of herpes zoster is determined by two factors: (1) the overall immune status of the patient and (2) the location of the VZV infection. First and foremost, since herpes zoster is a common presenting sign in HIV disease, all persons with herpes zoster should be questioned about HIV risk factors and examined for other manifestations of HIV disease. HIV serologic testing should be considered. Oral acyclovir in the dose of 800 mg five times daily for 7 to 10 days is recommended. All HIV-infected persons with herpes zoster ophthalmicus should be given intravenous acyclovir, in a dosage of 10 mg/kg three times daily, adjusted for renal function. Other indications for intravenous acyclovir are uncontrollable pain, Ramsay Hunt syndrome, dissemination, visceral disease, and failure of oral treatment.

As with HSV, acyclovir-resistant isolates of VZV are deficient in thymidine kinase and foscarnet in a dosage of 40 mg/kg every 8 hours is recommended.

Systemic Fungal Infections

Cryptococcosis

Clinical Description

Virtually all infections with *Cryptococcus neoformans* involve the central nervous system, with meningitis the most frequent manifestation. The disease is subacute, and often mild headache, fever, and malaise are the predominant features. Lesions outside the central nervous system occur in about half of patients with AIDS with cryptococcosis.

Cutaneous cryptococcosis in HIV infection usually presents as 0.2- to 1-cm papules with a central umbilication or crust and have been described as resembling molluscum contagiosum or herpes simplex. The face is most often involved. Tumors and ulcerative lesions of the skin or mucous membranes are also seen. In the setting of renal transplantation and other forms of immunosuppression, cutaneous cryptococcosis may present as a cellulitis. Biopsy specimens usually show the gelatinous rather than the granulomatous pattern of infection.

Treatment

Amphotericin B or fluconazole is the initial therapy. Lifelong maintenance therapy, usually with fluconazole, is required. In the setting of cryptococcal cellulitis the diagnosis is confirmed by skin biopsy. Visceral disease may not be present in HIV-seronegative immunosuppressed patients.

Histoplasmosis

Clinical Description

In the central United States, disseminated histoplasmosis is a common opportunistic infection of patients with AIDS. Cutaneous histoplasmosis may present as many different types of lesions. Papular and papulonecrotic skin lesions appear to be most common. Other morphologies include exanthematous, scaling maculopapular lesions resembling a dermatitis, cup-shaped papules, vegetative plaques, and diffuse purpura. Diffuse purpura may be associated with disseminated intravascular coagulopathy and is usually fatal. Oral ulcerations may also be seen. Biopsy of skin lesions confirms the diagnosis in more than 80% of cases. Amphotericin B is the treatment of choice, and maintenance therapy, usually with fluconazole or itraconazole, is required.

Sporotrichosis

In patients with AIDS, characteristic skin lesions of sporotrichosis are chronic ulcerations with crusting. Multiple visceral organ involvement may occur, characteristically including septic arthritis. Amphotericin B or itraconazole, not potassium iodide, should be used for treatment in immunosuppressed patients with sporotrichosis.

Cutaneous Mycobacterial Infection

Infections with *Mycobacterium avium-intracellulare* and *M. tuberculosis* are frequent in patients with HIV disease. These infections may be disseminated, unusual, and severe. Cutaneous lesions are unusual and present as chronic sinuses over involved lymph nodes, chronic ulcerations, or hemorrhagic macules.

In most cases the presence of acid-fast bacilli in skin lesions indicates disseminated mycobacterial disease, usually from *M. avium-intracellulare*. Treatment with effective antimycobacterial agents may result in cure in HIV-infected patients with localized disease.

Scabies

Clinical Description

Most cases of scabies are associated with close personal contact, including sexual exposure. In the setting of advanced HIV infection, however, a source of infection is frequently not found. Virtually all patients with a helper T-cell count of more than 200 cells/mm³ have typical scabies and a normal response to therapy; unusual manifestations and treatment failures are seen in patients with fewer than 200 CD4-positive cells/mm³.

Atypical variants of scabies include bullous scabies, exaggerated scabies, papular scabies, and crusted scabies. Crusted scabies is usually nonpruritic and is characterized by sand-like, thick, tan crusts that flake off, revealing underlying normal skin. Lesions are usually generalized. Fissures may be the source of fatal septic events. Crusted scabies appears to be associated with HIV-neuropathy or dementia. Patients with crusted scabies may be the source of epidemics of scabies in hospices and nursing homes.

Treatment

Virtually all patients with a CD4-positive count of more than 200 cells/mm³ will respond to standard therapy with lindane. Treatment failure appears to be related to immunosuppression, high mite burden, and, perhaps, associated central nervous system disease. For AIDS patients with scabies, permethrin 5% lotion is initial therapy. Patients may require multiple treatments. Crusted scabies is extremely difficult to eradicate and may require repeated applications of scabicides for weeks to months. Ivermectin, given as a single dose, has recently been reported to be highly effective treatment for crusted scabies.

Superficial Fungal Infections (Tinea and Candidiasis)

Clinical Description

Trichophyton rubrum causes almost all dermatophytoses in HIV-infected persons. Tinea pedis is the most common pattern in patients with asymptomatic HIV disease, usually manifested by the typical interdigital maceration and scale and by hyperkeratosis diffusely of the sole. Bullous lesions, two foot–one hand involvement, or onychomycosis is sometimes also seen. The rate of dermatophytosis is not increased in this group over control groups of athletes.

Once patients develop AIDS the pattern of dermatophytosis appears to change. Dystrophy of a few or many toenails frequently occurs. Proximal subungual onychomycosis represents 90% of onychomycosis in patients with AIDS. Patients with toenail onychomycosis may not have evidence of tinea elsewhere on the feet. Fingernail onychomycosis is one tenth as frequent as toenail involvement and is virtually always limited to, begins, or is worse on one hand. *Candida albicans* alone may be the cause of onychomycosis of the fingernails and should be suspected if "two feet-one hand" dermatophytosis is not seen.

Tinea cruris follows tinea pedis and onychomycosis in frequency presenting as an expanding scaling plaque of the upper thighs, with central clearing and a red, elevated border. Tinea corporis in the setting of HIV disease virtually always represents tinea cruris that has extended beyond the groin onto the trunk. In severely immunosuppressed patients with AIDS, lesions may have little inflammation and often lack the elevated border and central clearing typical of tinea. They are recognized as sharply marginated areas of hyperkeratosis resembling dry skin.

In pediatric HIV infection, candidal diaper dermatitis is frequent. *T. rubrum* may also cause eruptions in the diaper area. Tinea capitis due to *T. tonsurans* is seen in HIV-infected children.

More than 70% of women with AIDS suffer recurrent vaginal candidiasis, and it is the presenting sign in 24% of women. Intermittent or prophylactic therapy is usually required.

Treatment

For uncomplicated tinea pedis, a topical imidazole or allylamine is effective. Tinea corporis, if extensive, often requires systemic therapy with oral griseofulvin, an imidazole, or an allylamine. As in non–HIV-infected persons, fingernail infection can usually be cured with 3 to 6 months of an oral agent. Toenail infection requires longer treatment. Low gastric acidity in patients with AIDS may reduce absorption of ketoconazole, decreasing efficacy. For candidiasis of the intertriginous areas, drying the skin is most important. Topical nystatin or imidazoles are effective. In women, vaginal candidiasis is usually the source of groin candidiasis.

Inflammatory Cutaneous Complications of HIV Infection

Eosinophilic Folliculitis

Most patients with AIDS with a chronic, pruritic, follicular eruption of the central trunk or face have eosinophilic folliculitis. The primary lesion is an edematous, almost urticarial, follicular papule often *without* a central pustule. The most common areas of involvement are the forehead, cheeks, central back, and chest. The eruption classically waxes and wanes independent of treatment. The pathogenesis of eosinophilic folliculitis is unknown. *Demodex* is found in some lesions and may be pathogenically related. The diagnosis is established by skin biopsy, which shows in early lesions perifollicular inflammation with eosinophils at the level of the sebaceous glands extending into the surrounding dermis and in late lesions an intrafollicular abscess with many eosinophils. Treatment options include class I topical corticosteroids, antihistamines, ultraviolet B (UVB) light or psoralens and ultraviolet A light (PUVA) phototherapy, and itraconazole. Many patients require maintenance therapy.

Insect Bite Reactions

Hypersensitivity to insect bites is extremely common in HIV disease. Patients note exaggerated and persistent lesions after bites of potentially sensitizing insects. Treatment consists of the extermination of biting insects from the patient's environment, insect repellents and clothing to deter the insects, topical corticosteroids to the individual lesions, and chronic potent antihistamines to reduce the hypersensitivity. Intralesional triamcinolone may be used in persistent lesions.

Other Diseases

Granuloma annulare, anetoderma, and papular mucinosis are not uncommon findings in HIV-infected persons at all stages of HIV disease, early in HIV disease, and in advanced disease, respectively.

Drug Reactions

Clinical Description

The frequency of drug reactions is increased in HIV-infected patients, especially to certain medications: trimethoprim-sulfamethoxazole (37–45%), antituberculosis regimens (10%), and amoxicillin-clavulanate. Patients with AIDS have more frequent reactions if their CD4 count is less than 200 cells/mm^3.

Most adverse reactions in HIV disease occur to antibiotics, especially sulfonamides. The patterns of cutaneous reactions to medications that are increased in HIV-infected persons are morbilliform reactions, fixed drug reactions, erythema multiforme major (Stevens-Johnson syndrome), and toxic epidermal necrolysis. Morbilliform drug reactions usually begin during the second week of treatment. No maculopapular drug reaction has converted to a more severe form *during the same course of treatment*. Rechallenge with the drug at a later date may, however, result in a more severe reaction (e.g., Stevens-Johnson syndrome). Desensitization can be considered if the medication is required.

Fixed drug reactions are most frequently seen with trimethoprim-sulfamethoxazole and can be in response to either component. Most HIV-infected patients with Stevens-Johnson syndrome or toxic epidermal necrolysis have AIDS. Long-acting sulfonamides are the most common cause.

Foscarnet causes penile ulcerations, most commonly in uncircumcised patients. It appears to be a direct toxic effect of the medication. Zidovudine causes pigmentation of the nails and oral mucosa, especially in pigmented races. The nail pigmentation appears as blue lunulae, as longitudinal pigmented bands, or as diffuse blue or black pigmentation. It is dose dependent and resolves with discontinuation of the medication. The oral mucosa is pigmented on the lateral tongue most commonly, but the buccal mucosa is also pigmented. Similar oral hyperpigmentation may be seen in the setting of HIV infection without zidovudine administration. In all cases the pigment is due to increased melanin deposition.

Eczematous Eruptions

Dry skin is extremely common in HIV disease, especially AIDS. The cause is unknown. Dry skin frequently accompanies or is the basis for eczematous eruptions. In addition, in AIDS patients, any pruritic eruption may induce scratching and secondary eczematous eruptions of the skin, so eczematous plaques may accompany scabies, staphylococcal folliculitis, or eosinophilic folliculitis.

Atopic Dermatitis

Atopic eczema is common in children with HIV disease. In addition, in HIV-infected adults atopic dermatitis may appear in those with a prior history of atopy (allergic rhinitis, asthma).

Asteatotic Eczema (Dry Skin Eczema, Winter Itch)

The underlying xerosis of HIV disease is a major cause of pruritus as it is in the geriatric population. The skin is slightly scaly and shiny with little erythema. Small fissures filled with fine crusts may be seen on the most severely affected areas. These fissures characteristically form small (0.5 – 1.0 cm) circles. Untreated xerotic eczema may progress to nummular dermatitis.

Nummular Dermatitis

In HIV disease, nummular dermatitis is usually a consequence of atopic dermatitis, xerotic eczema, or seborrheic dermatitis and appears similar in HIV infection as in the normal population. Secondary infection with *S. aureus* is often present.

Photosensitivity

HIV-infected patients may develop dermatitis from ultraviolet light exposure due to medications (drug-induced photosensitivity) or as polymorphous light eruption or actinic prurigo (with prurigo nodularis). Chronic actinic dermatitis may develop. Histologically, most patients with photosensitivity have features of chronic spongiotic dermatitis or polymorphous light eruption. The most frequent offending medications are sulfonamides and nonsteroidal anti-inflammatory agents. Many patients are sensitive only to UVB, but some also have UVA sensitivity and require more broad sun protection. Black men with CD4 counts of less than 50 cells/mm^3 are at particular risk for chronic actinic dermatitis.

Papulosquamous Eruptions

Seborrheic Dermatitis

Seborrhea usually affects hair-bearing areas, especially the scalp, eyebrows, moustache, and beard, as well as the nasolabial fold and behind and in the ears. Involvement of the axillae and groin is not uncommon. Red, nonscaling patches with no central clearing and involvement of the scrotum and penis are characteristic. Lesions may extend from the scalp onto the central back and mid chest. Pruritus is variable; it is usually absent or mild, but it occasionally is severe on the scalp. Standard therapy is usually effective.

Psoriasis

Psoriasis is seen in HIV-infected persons with at least as great a frequency as the general population. HIV-infected persons with psoriasis often have either HLA-B27. All clinical patterns of psoriasis may be seen in HIV-infected persons, but axillary and groin involvement (inverse pattern) and palm and sole involvement (similar to Reiter's syndrome) appear to be especially common.

HIV-associated psoriasis is clinically similar to psoriasis seen in uninfected persons. Factors that exacerbate common psoriasis may flare HIV-associated psoriasis as well (i.e., streptococcal colonization or infection of the throat and certain medications, such as lithium and beta-blockers). HIV-associated psoriasis may flare severely in association with staphylococcal sepsis, and in any HIV-infected person with sudden worsening of psoriasis this must be considered, even if the patient does not appear severely ill.

Psoriasis may appear at any stage of HIV disease and may worsen as HIV disease progresses. The arthritis seen in HIV-infected patients with psoriasis is similar to the joint disease seen in psoriasis unassociated with HIV disease.

Treatment of psoriasis in patients with HIV disease uses standard modalities. Zidovudine, but not didanosine or zalcitabine (DDI or DDC), improves psoriasis and may be added or increased as a part of psoriasis treatment. Etretinate is safe and effective. When topical measures fail, UVB alone or in combination with tar (Goeckermann regimen) or PUVA is useful. Light therapy has not appeared to enhance HIV expression in HIV-infected persons. Immunosuppressive agents such as methotrexate and cyclosporine must be considered experimental in the setting of HIV disease and are of potentially high risk.

Reiter's syndrome and pityriasis rubra pilaris are also seen in HIV-infected individuals.

Oral Manifestations of HIV Disease

Oral Candidiasis

Thrush affects most HIV-infected persons at some time during the course of their disease. The most common pattern is the pseudo-membranous type. The erythematous or atrophic type appearing as denuded red areas may be seen alone or in combination with the more common pattern. Angular cheilitis (perlèche) often accompanies oral thrush. Candidiasis may extend into the posterior pharynx and down the esophagus. Candidal esophagitis is the most common cause of dysphagia in HIV disease and is an AIDS-defining illness.

Treatment options for oropharyngeal candidiasis include clotrimazole troches or vaginal suppositories; nystatin suspension, lozenges, or vaginal pastilles; and systemic imidazoles. Higher-dose products are better for active disease. Recurrence within 3 months is universal in all patients with CD4 counts of less than 200 cells/mm^3. Prophylaxis with topical or systemic agents may be required.

Oral Hairy Leukoplakia

Oral hairy leukoplakia is caused by Epstein-Barr virus infection of the oral epithelium. It presents as adherent corrugated white plaques on the lateral aspects of the tongue. Lesions may extend onto the dorsum or ventral surface of the tongue and less commonly on other mucosal surfaces. Lesions are usually asymptomatic and do not require therapy. A single application of 25% podophyllin for 30 seconds to 1 minute, topical retinoic acid twice daily, and high doses of oral acyclovir are effective treatments. Recurrence is expected.

Recurrent Aphthous Ulceration

HIV-infected persons may develop recurrent aphthous ulceration at any stage of HIV disease. Lesions may be of the minor, major, or herpetiform types. Involvement of the posterior pharynx and esophagus may cause dysphagia. In most cases, the clinical morphology is typical and lesions are smaller than infectious ulcerations. Larger lesions should be cultured for herpes simplex; if lesions persist or are atypical, they should be sampled. Potent topical corticosteroid ointments, intralesional corticosteroids, steroid oral suspension (dexamethasone), and systemic steroids are effective. These therapies should be accompanied by good oral hygiene and anticandidal prophylaxis.

Neoplastic Complications of HIV Disease

Skin Cancer

Basal cell carcinomas are extremely common in HIV-infected white men. They are most frequently located on the trunk and are commonly of the superficial type. Treatment is by standard modalities with similar cure rates. Squamous cell carcinomas in sun-exposed sites are seen in the setting of HIV disease. Patients with squamous cell carcinomas in general have had greater sun exposure than those with basal cell carcinomas. Unlike renal transplant patients, the ratio of squamous cell carcinoma to basal cell carcinoma is not reversed in most HIV-infected persons.

Genital squamous cell carcinomas of the rectum in homosexual men and of the cervix in women who are HIV infected are increased. These are related to human papillomavirus infection, analogous to cervical cancer in the immunocompetent population. In the setting of HIV infection, however, the progression from human papillomavirus infection to dysplasia and then to carcinoma appears to be accelerated.

Melanoma may have a worse prognosis in the setting of HIV disease. The sudden onset of atypical nevi has been reported in HIV infection, but it has not been associated with the development of melanoma.

Kaposi's Sarcoma

Kaposi's sarcoma occurs in four relatively distinct populations. Classic Kaposi's sarcoma is primarily a skin disease of the lower extremities affecting predominantly elderly men of Mediterranean, East European, or Jewish heritage. The disease course is typically indolent, with patients surviving an average of 10 to 15 years before dying of unrelated causes; secondary malignancies (primarily lymphomas) develop in more than one third of cases. African-endemic Kaposi's sarcoma has been described in two age groups: (1) young adults with generally benign cutaneous nodular disease but sometimes aggressive or florid disease fatal within 5 to 8 years and (2) young children with fulminant lymphadenopathic disease, typically fatal within 2 to 3 years. Iatrogenic, immunosuppressive drug-associated Kaposi's sarcoma is frequently seen among organ transplant recipients. Spontaneous remission after discontinuation of immunosuppressive therapy may occur. Kaposi's sarcoma associated with AIDS occurs predominantly among homosexual men.

Early in the AIDS epidemic, as many as 60% of homosexual men with AIDS developed Kaposi's sarcoma, and this population is still the most likely to develop AIDS-associated Kaposi's sarcoma. AIDS-associated Kaposi's sarcoma is associated with an increased number of sex partners, a prior history of oropharyngeal gonorrhea, and increasing contact with a sex partner's feces through oral-anal contact.

Since the onset of the AIDS epidemic, there has been a gradual decline in the proportion of HIV-infected homosexual men presenting with AIDS-associated Kaposi's sarcoma, suggesting that changes in sexual behavior and sexual practices may have reduced the risk of Kaposi's sarcoma for men not already infected with both HIV and the proposed Kaposi's sarcoma agent. Nevertheless, Kaposi's sarcoma remains a major clinical manifestation of AIDS in the United States, accounting for more than 15% of all AIDS diagnoses reported.

A causative agent of Kaposi's sarcoma has not been identified, although it is thought most likely to be of infectious etiology. Recent evidence implicates HHV-8 in the pathogenesis of Kaposi's sarcoma.

Clinical Description

Although Kaposi's sarcoma may first appear at any stage of HIV disease, most patients with AIDS-associated Kaposi's sarcoma have CD4 counts of less than 500 cells/mm^3. Common cutaneous sites include the oral cavity, face, trunk, penis, and the lower extremities. Half of patients with cutaneous lesions will develop lymph node disease.

Cutaneous lesions may be single or grouped. New lesions may develop rapidly over a few days, frequently in a symmetrical distribution. The progression of each individual lesion is unpredictable, and lesions in one area may involute while similar lesions at more distant sites may enlarge. The progression of the disorder roughly correlates with the overall activity of the patient's HIV disease.

Macular, Papular, and Nodular Lesions. Macular lesions are faint, are red to purple, and vary from several millimeters to several centimeters. These lesions are usually asymptomatic and are frequently seen on the soles of the feet, the hard palate, and the tip of the nose. Macular lesions are rarely accompanied by edema. Papular lesions of the face are usually oval and less than 1 cm in size; papular lesions on the nose may expand, forming large plaques covering the entire nasal bridge. Lesions on the neck, trunk, and lower extremities are typically papular and oblong, following skin tension lines.

Lesions of the gums, hard palate, and distal extremities may progress from macules and papules to form exophytic friable nodules. Confluence of leg lesions frequently results in painful, edematous, ulcerative disease. Pseudomonas and anaerobic bacteria may colonize chronically ulcerated lesions. Penile lesions are characterized by papules and nodules often accompanied by edema. Trauma or prior cutaneous disease may give rise to Kaposi's sarcoma (Koebner's phenomenon).

Plaques and Lymphatic Disease. AIDS-associated Kaposi's sarcoma of the distal extremities may present as grouped papules expanding peripherally and forming large plaques. Lymphatic involvement may occur at any site but is most commonly seen in the inguinal region, giving the skin a doughy or woody texture, with or without overlying cutaneous lesions. Extensive lymphatic infiltration may lead to severe cutaneous and subcutaneous complications, including severe pain, maceration, and ulceration. Even without extensive lymphatic infiltration, lymph node involvement may cause edema of the genitalia and intermittent or chronic edema of the lower extremities.

Mucocutaneous and Ocular Lesions. Oral lesions are frequent. The palate is the most common site for oral disease, which occurs in about 50% of patients. Kaposi's sarcoma involving ocular adnexal structures is reported to occur in up to 20% of patients; benign lesions of the conjunctiva are the most common site of ocular involvement. Periorbital edema may be present in conjunction with periocular lesions.

Visceral Lesions. Visceral lesions are extremely common among patients with AIDS-associated Kaposi's sarcoma. Although usually asymptomatic, common sites of visceral involvement include the lungs, bowel, liver, spleen, pharynx, heart, bone marrow, genitourinary tract, brain, kidney, and adrenal glands. Death can be attributed to visceral disease in 10% to 20% of patients with AIDS-associated Kaposi's sarcoma.

Pathology

The three histologic stages of Kaposi's sarcoma are patch, plaque, and nodular disease and correlate with the clinical appearance of lesions. In patch-stage disease, there is proliferation of small, irregular, and jagged endothelium-lined spaces lined by cytologically bland spindled cells surrounding normal dermal vessels and adnexal structures. A normal vessel or adnexal structure protruding into an ectatic vascular space (promontory sign) is a hallmark for patch-stage disease. Plaque-stage disease is a spindle-celled vascular process that permeates dermal collagen bundles, forming irregular, cleft-like, angulated vascular channels containing erythrocytes. Nodular-stage lesions are composed of sheets and fascicles of spindled cells with mild to moderate cytologic atypia, single cell necrosis, and trapped erythrocytes within an extensive network of slit-like vascular spaces. All three patterns are usually accompanied by an inflammatory lymphocytic infiltrate with or without plasma cells. The cell of origin of Kaposi's sarcoma is unknown.

Differential Diagnosis

Clinical lesions that can mimic AIDS-associated Kaposi's sarcoma include dermatofibroma, hemangioma, scar, bacillary angiomatosis, acroangiodermatitis, pyogenic granuloma, ruptured epidermoid cysts, post-inflammatory hyperpigmentation, prurigo nodularis, blue nevi, malignant melanoma, and cutaneous lymphoma. These lesions are easily distinguished histopathologically.

Treatment

No cure for AIDS-associated Kaposi's sarcoma exists, and palliative therapy, either alone or in combination with zidovudine antiviral therapy, has not been shown to prolong survival. The majority of patients with AIDS-associated Kaposi's sarcoma die of opportunistic infection rather than from Kaposi's sarcoma. Therefore, the primary goal of treatment is to provide safe and effective palliation. Indications for treatment include cosmetic control of disfiguring Kaposi's sarcoma lesions, shrinkage of problematic oral lesions, abatement of pain and edema associated with lymphadenopathy or extensive cutaneous disease, and alleviation of symptomatic visceral disease.

Cryotherapy. Among patients with limited numbers of macular and papular lesions, liquid nitrogen cryotherapy has demonstrated an 85% complete or partial clinical response rate following an average of three treatments. Cosmetic improvement is a direct consequence of acceptable superficial scarring that camouflages persistent Kaposi's sarcoma in the reticular dermis.

Intralesional Therapy. Intralesional antineoplastic chemotherapy of cutaneous Kaposi's sarcoma with vinblastine or vincristine has demonstrated complete or partial clinical response rates of up to 88%. Visibly recurrent disease is seen in approximately 40% of lesions within 6 months after therapy. Advantages of intralesional chemotherapy over cryotherapy include higher response rates for papulonodular lesions greater than 1 cm in diameter and the ability to treat symptomatic oral lesions to reduce pain and to prevent ulceration and bleeding.

Approximately 85% of nodular intraoral lesions will also respond to intralesional sclerotherapy with 3% sodium tetradecyl sulfate. Intralesional interferon alfa has demonstrated similar results. Intralesional therapy with tumor necrosis factor–α and recombinant granulocyte-macrophage colony stimulating factor is also effective; however, the former is associated with significant local and systemic side effects, and the latter has not been systematically evaluated.

Radiation Therapy. Radiation therapy appears best suited for symptoms due to mass effects, including large intraoral lesions and localized disease resulting in pain, extensive lymphadenopathy, or lymphedema of the extremities and penis.

Laser and Surgical Treatment. Carbon dioxide and argon lasers and photodynamic therapy have been used successfully to treat large oral lesions. Pulsed-dye laser therapy is effective for cutaneous macular lesions, but lesions typically recur within 12 weeks. Local excision can be beneficial for troublesome lesions at selected sites.

Systemic Treatment. Patients with disease that is not easily managed with local treatment frequently respond to systemic therapy, despite the increased risk of significant side effects. Systemic treatment can be divided into limited intervention (interferon $\pm$ zidovudine) and aggressive intervention (chemotherapy $\pm$ zidovudine). In general, pretreatment CD4 counts appear to be the best independent predictor of response. Patients with CD4 counts of more than 400 cells/mm^3, 200 to 400 cells/mm^3, and less than 200 cells/mm^3 have objective response rates of 40% to 50%, 30%, and 10%, respectively.

Systemic Chemotherapy. For AIDS-associated disease, single-agent regimens for patients with minimal disease and extensive disease have demonstrated response rates of about 40% and 80%, respectively. Because these patients frequently develop cytotoxic drug toxicity at dosages required for clinical response when administered as single agents, multiagent cytotoxic regimens that reduce the cumulative toxicities of drugs administered as single agents are generally preferred. Frequently used multidrug regimens include combinations of *Vinca* alkaloids (vincristine and vinblastine) or a *Vinca* alkaloid combined with one or more of the following: bleomycin, an anthracycline, or etoposide. These regimens have shown promising results in patients with extensive cutaneous and visceral disease, and even in patients with severely compromised immune function.

Systemic Treatment in Combination with Zidovudine. Several clinical studies have evaluated the synergistic antiviral effect of combination zidovudine with interferon alfa demonstrated in vitro. In general, clinical response rates range from 30% to 60%, and antiviral effects can be demonstrated by peripheral blood HIV cultures and tests for HIV p24 antigen.

Cutaneous Complications of Immunosuppression

Neoplastic Complications

Neoplasia is an important complication of the immunosuppression of congenital immunodeficiency states (primary immunodeficiency), of immunosuppressive agents for organ transplantation or other diseases, or in the setting of HIV infection. Three classes of tumors are especially increased in the setting of immunosuppression: lymphoreticular malignancies, Kaposi's sarcoma (not in primary immunodeficiency states), and squamous cell carcinomas of the skin and genital tract.

Non-Hodgkin's lymphoma is the lymphoreticular malignancy most frequently reported in the setting of immune suppression, although Hodgkin's disease is also seen. It is characterized by extranodal location (especially central nervous system), by high grade, and by presentation at an advanced stage. These tumors are primarily of the B-cell type, monoclonal or polyclonal, but T-cell lymphomas also occur (including cutaneous T-cell lymphoma).

In organ transplant recipients, nonmelanoma skin cancers represent between 38% and 77% of the cancers that develop in these patients. These tumors occur primarily on sun-exposed skin, although genital squamous cell carcinomas are also increased. Squamous cell carcinomas are the most frequent tumor, occurring 3 to 15 times more frequently than basal cell carcinomas. These actinic lesions can be aggressive; they metastasize in 5% to 12% of patients and cause death in as many as 5%. Cutaneous squamous cell carcinoma represents 82% of skin cancer metastases and 64% of skin cancer deaths in organ transplant patients. The incidence of malignant melanoma is also increased.

Human Papillomavirus Infection

Epidemiology

Immunosuppressed patients have greater numbers of warts than the general population, and many demonstrate multiple DNA types. The most common human papillomavirus (HPV) types are 16, 18, and 33 through 35 with cervical, anal, penile, and subungual squamous cell carcinoma. Anal squamous cell carcinoma is more common in homosexual men.

Cervical dysplasia/neoplasia related to HPV infection is more common in women who are immunosuppressed as a result of organ transplantation, lymphoreticular malignancy (especially Hodgkin's disease), and HIV disease. Cervical carcinoma is an index AIDS diagnosis. Genital warts and cervical dysplasia/neoplasia increase in frequency and severity with advancing immunosuppression. Noncervical cancers of the anogenital area are also increased in immunosuppressed transplant patients.

Patients receiving immunosuppressive therapy to prevent organ transplant rejection are at high risk of developing nongenital warts. Both the prevalence of wart infection and the number of warts increase with length of immunosuppression. HIV infection also predisposes patients to cutaneous warts. Most nongenital warts in the setting of immunosuppression are of the common "benign" types.

Some patients are infected with epidermodysplasia verruciformis "specific" HPV types. As in classic epidermodysplasia verruciformis, immunosuppressed patients with warts are at increased risk of developing cutaneous squamous cell carcinomas, especially on sun-exposed skin. These carcinomas have been shown to contain the DNA of epidermodysplasia verruciformis "specific" HPV types.

Clinical Description

Multiple, large, and treatment-resistant warts are the hallmark of symptomatic HIV infection, especially in patients with AIDS. Flat warts of the beard area may also be seen. In the anogenital area, typical condylomata to large vegetating masses occur, especially if there is a history of receptive anal intercourse. Lesions may extend into the anal canal, requiring anoscopy to evaluate the full extent of the infection.

Flat lesions of HPV infection (often hyperpigmented) may histologically demonstrate features similar or identical to squamous cell carcinoma in situ (bowenoid papulosis). In HIV infection, these hyperpigmented plaques may involve substantial portions of the genital area. Although the natural history of such lesions is unknown, it is hypothesized that the associated immunosuppression may lead to more frequent development of genital squamous cell carcinoma. The transition zones of the cervix and anus are at highest risk for malignancy.

Treatment

Treatment of warts is difficult, and recurrence is to be anticipated. The management of common and plantar warts is by the usual methods. Flat warts of the beard area may respond to topical 13-*cis*-retinoic acid or 5-fluorouracil. Shaving using razor blades should be discontinued until the beard area is free of lesions.

The most effective treatment of condylomata appears to be frequent (weekly) destructive therapy with liquid nitrogen, trichloroacetic acid, podophyllin, or electrocautery. 5-Fluorouracil can be used topically to treat bowenoid dysplasia of the genitalia and to reduce recurrence of treated lesions. Refractory lesions should be sampled. Due to the high risk of cervical dysplasia in immunosuppressed women, annual Papanicolaou smears are recommended. Once cervical dysplasia is detected or the patient develops AIDS, the frequency of Papanicolaou smears should increase to every 3 or 6 months, respectively.

Herpes Simplex Infection

Suppression of cell-mediated immunity with organ transplantation, bone marrow transplantation, hematologic malignancy, or the immunosuppressive agents used to treat these conditions frequently leads to reactivation of herpes simplex. The degree of immunosuppression correlates with the likelihood of reactivation. Since the seroprevalence for HSV type 1 is higher than HSV type 2, most reactivations are in the orolabial area. Clinically, they present as erosions or ulcerations that may be extensive, destructive, and persistent. Acyclovir is effective in both prevention and treatment.

Varicella-Zoster Virus

Varicella is substantially more severe in immunosuppressed persons, especially those in whom the cell-mediated immune system is impaired by malignancy or chemotherapy, including corticosteroids alone. The rash is more extensive and lasts longer, and visceral disease and death are much more common. Lymphopenia (< 500 lymphocytes) is the major risk factor for dissemination and death. Varicella pneumonia is the most common complication, but encephalitis, hepatitis, and purpura fulminans can also occur. The most effective management strategy is to prevent or attenuate disease with the appropriate use of varicella-zoster immune globulin and varicella vaccination in at-risk persons. Acyclovir given intravenously at a dose of 500 mg/m^2 every 8 hours is effective treatment, especially if instituted in the first 72 hours.

Recurrence of varicella-zoster virus in the form of herpes zoster is a common complication of immunosuppression, especially in hematologic malignancies and particularly Hodgkin's disease. In the immunosuppressed person, herpes zoster tends to last longer and be more painful, is frequently hemorrhagic, and often scars. Dissemination is common. Fatal complications include pneumonitis, encephalitis, and hepatitis.

Uncomplicated herpes zoster in the immunocompromised host should be treated with acyclovir. Intravenous acyclovir (10 mg/kg every 8 hours) is the treatment of choice for patients with severe immunosuppression. Mildly immunosuppressed patients may be managed with oral acyclovir (800 mg orally five times daily) if there is no evidence of dissemination and if they are observed closely. Dissemination, ophthalmic involvement, Ramsay Hunt syndrome, and failure of oral acyclovir are all indications for intravenous use of acyclovir. Zoster immune globulin prevents dissemination. After bone marrow transplantation, prophylactic acyclovir may be used to prevent herpes zoster.

Pseudomonas *Infection*

Pseudomonas aeruginosa rarely causes systemic infection in the immunocompetent host. Immunosuppression, especially neutropenia, is associated with the development of life-threatening infection with this organism. Ecthyma gangrenosum is the most common cutaneous manifestation of *Pseudomonas* infection. It may be associated with *Pseudomonas* sepsis or may be seen in neutropenic patients without sepsis. Lesions usually occur in the groin as red plaques that develop a pseudobullous violaceous center and eventually ulcerate. A rarer cutaneous manifestation of *Pseudomonas* sepsis is red subcutaneous nodules.

Fungal Infections

Candidiasis is the most common fungal infection complicating immunosuppression. It usually presents as oral, vaginal, or intertriginous lesions. The combination of impaired mucosal barriers in the mouth and gastrointestinal tract plus neutropenia may be associated with candidal septicemia. *Candida albicans* is the most common cause, but *C. krusei, C. tropicalis,* and others are also pathogenic in this setting. Skin lesions present as 0.5- to 1.0-cm erythematous, sometimes purpuric papules with central pallor or pustulation. Less commonly, necrotic skin lesions are seen. Histologically, the dermal infiltrate may be scarce, but yeast forms and pseudohyphae are abundant. Increasing imidazole resistance by non–*C. albicans* species is being noted in immunosuppressed persons.

Aspergillus species are the most common cause of noncandidal fungal infections in the immunosuppressed patient. *Aspergillus* is most frequently a pulmonary pathogen that disseminates hematogenously. Metastatic skin lesions are seen in fewer than 5% of patients with disseminated aspergillosis. Primary cutaneous aspergillosis is also seen. Lesions occur at the sites of intravenous catheters or more commonly at sites of minor trauma around catheters, such as tape or armboard erosions. *A. niger, A. flavus,* and *A. fumigatus* have all been implicated. These organisms have occasionally been cultured from tape and armboard material. Most patients are leukopenic and on broad-spectrum antibiotic therapy. Erythema, induration and pustulation, or hemorrhagic bullae progressing rapidly to necrosis are characteristic. The diagnosis may be established by identifying hyphae on potassium hydroxide preparations or by skin biopsy. Disease may remain limited to the skin or may disseminate. Treatment optimally involves the reversal of leukopenia, amphotericin B (or possibly itraconazole), and local care.

LEISHMANIASIS

(CM&S Chapter 126)

Definition

Leishmaniasis is a protozoal disease whose diverse clinical manifestations are dependent both on the infecting species of *Leishmania* and the immune response of the host. Transmission of the disease occurs by the bite of the female sandfly infected with Leishmania parasites. Infection may be restricted to the skin in cutaneous leishmaniasis (CL), limited to the mucous membranes in mucosal leishmaniasis (ML), or spread throughout the reticuloendothelial system in visceral leishmaniasis (VL) or kala-azar. Three rare clinical variants of cutaneous leishmaniasis include diffuse cutaneous leishmaniasis (DCL), leishmaniasis recidivans, and post–kala-azar dermal leishmaniasis (PKADL).

Clinical Description

Leishmaniasis is present on all continents except Australia and Antarctica. Localized cutaneous leishmaniasis (LCL) is widespread throughout the Old World and is primarily caused by the organism *L. major.* New World LCL is endemic in Central and South America. Two independent species or ''complexes'' of parasites are responsible for New World LCL, including *L. braziliensis* and *L. mexicana.*

LCL usually affects unclothed parts of the body easily bitten by the sand fly vector, including the face, neck, and arms. New World leishmaniasis commonly presents as a solitary primary lesion, while multiple primary lesions are often found in Old World disease. After an incubation period of 1 week to 3 months, a red papule appears that enlarges to a plaque or nodule. The lesion often develops into an ulcer with a granular-appearing crusted base, which is well circumscribed with a violaceous raised border. Lymphangitic spread leads to painless rubbery subcutaneous nodules or cords around the ulcer and lymph node enlargement. Inflammatory satellite papules and subcutaneous induration may develop around the primary lesion representing a reaction to local dissemination of the parasite or its antigenic products. A generalized papular eruption may also develop, representing a hypersensitivity reaction. Itching and pain are mild, if present. After 6 to 12 months the ulcer spontaneously regresses leaving a scar with hypo- or hyperpigmentation. Immunity is not always complete, and secondary infection may occur in up to 10% of individuals.

Diffuse cutaneous leishmaniasis (DCL) is an anergic variant of LCL in which lesions are disseminated, resembling lepromatous lepropsy, but without nerve involvement. Infection is primarily caused by *L. aethiopica* in the Old World and *L. amazonensis* in Central and South America. The disease usually begins with an initial primary lesion and then disseminates to involve other areas of the skin. The lesions are nonulcerative nodules that are often scattered over the limbs, buttocks, and face. The disease responds partially to treatment and often relapses, becoming chronic.

Leishmaniasis recidivans or "recurrent leishmaniasis" refers to the development of new lesions in the center or periphery of a scar of a healed acute lesion of leishmaniasis, which presents as scaly, erythematous papules within scars of healed lesions. The active disease is confined to the scar and immediate contiguous area. The causative organism is usually *L. tropica* in the Middle East and less commonly *L. braziliensis* in South America. Lesions tend to resist treatment and become chronic. Fifty percent of the recurrent strains differed from the initial strain, suggesting exogenous reinfection as a mechanism in many of the cases rather than reactivation.

Post–kala-azar dermal leishmaniasis (PKADL) generally occurs 1 to 3 years after recovery from visceral leishmaniasis. This disease is primarily caused by *L. donovani* and is endemic in India and Bangladesh. Dermatologic manifestations of PKADL consist of hypopigmented macules which never completely depigment, erythematous macules, and nodules. Cases of PKADL are more resistant to treatment, requiring higher doses of systemic medication. Hypopigmented areas almost never completely repigment.

Mucocutaneous leishmaniasis (MCL) is most commonly reported in the New World. *L. braziliensis braziliensis* is the most common etiologic agent, although cases due to other *Leishmania* subspecies have been reported. The disease usually presents 2 years to decades after the initial cutaneous lesions. In MCL, which typically affects a small percentage of individuals previously infected with *L. braziliensis* subspecies, mucous membrane involvement probably develops due to hematogenous or lymphatic dissemination or occasionally from direct extension of nearby skin lesions. The disease often begins in the nasal septum, which becomes inflamed and infiltrated and subsequently perforates. MCL has a predilection for the distal cartilagenous part of the nose, resulting in a "parrot's beak" deformation. Mutilation of the nasal septum, palate, pharynx, tonsils, gums, and/or lip may ensue, whereas bony structures remain intact. Malnutrition and acute respiratory pneumonia, a result of invasion of the respiratory tract, are the leading causes of death in patients with MCL.

Kala-azar or visceral leishmaniasis (VL) is a systemic disease caused by the dissemination of *L. donovani* throughout the reticuloendothelial system. Characteristic signs and symptoms include fever, splenomegaly, emaciation, pancytopenia, and hyperglobulinemia. The primary lesion of VL is a small erythematous papule usually seen on the legs, sometimes referred to as a "leishmanioma." During the active period of VL, a patchy blackening of the skin secondary to increased melanocytic activity as well as an enhancement of the natural skin color due to xerosis appears that is the origin of the name *kala-azar*, meaning "black fever." VL runs an insidious chronic course until treatment , which is successful in 95% to 98% of cases.

Pathology

The histopathologic findings in leishmaniasis reflect the immunity of the host, the stage of the infection, and, to a lesser extent, the infecting species. During active, acute infection, Leishman-Donovan bodies, the amastigotes, are found within macrophages. Leishman-Donovan bodies are faintly visible in hematoxylin and eosin–stained sections, but their appearance is enhanced by the Giemsa stain.

Diagnosis and Differential Diagnosis

The differential diagnosis for leishmaniasis is extensive, including other infections, such as bacterial, fungal, and parasitic infections; inflammatory diseases such as psoriasis; and neoplasms such as CTCL. The diagnosis is often made on clinical grounds alone, especially in endemic areas. Diagnostic techniques include skin biopsy, a touch prep, fine-needle aspiration of a lesion culture, and examination for antileishmania antibodies in blood.

Because the identification of the specific species of parasite responsible for infection is important for the diagnosis of disease, evaluation of therapy, and prognosis, a number of laboratory techniques have been developed designed for species-specific identification of parasites within the genus *Leishmania*, including monoclonal antibodies to parasite surface antigens and the use of molecular biology techniques, which can be performed on miniscule amounts of material, such as tissue sections or touch preparations, rather than on the cultured organisms needed for the other analyses. Other methods of characterization involve molecular analysis of kinetoplast DNA (kDNA), by determination of the buoyant density of kDNA, DNA hybridization, polymerase chain reaction, and restriction endonuclease digestion of kDNA.

Treatment

The natural history of leishmaniasis must be considered when evaluating therapeutic agents. Lesions of cutaneous leishmaniasis heal spontaneously over 1 month to 3 years, while lesions of mucocutaneous and visceral disease rarely, if ever, heal without treatment. Consequently, all cases of MCL and VL require treatment, but therapy is not always essential in LCL. Patients with LCL should, however, be treated in two situations. Patients with lesions on the face or other cosmetically important area should be treated to reduce the size of the resultant scar. In addition, the species of parasite should be identified so that infection with *L. braziliensis braziliensis* and *L. braziliensis panamensis* can be treated to reduce the risk of development of mucocutaneous disease.

The pentavalent ammonial compound sodium stiboglucanate (Pentostam) is the conventional therapeutic agent. The accepted dose for the treatment of leishmaniasis is 20 mg/kg given intravenously or intramuscularly daily, without an upper limit on the daily dose. Cutaneous disease is treated for 20 days, and visceral and mucosal disease is treated for 28 days. Side effects include arthralgias, myalgias, abdominal discomfort, reversible elevations of hepatocellular enzymes, electrocardiographic abnormalities, and occasional anemia, leukopenia, or thrombocytopenia.

A wide variety of alternative systemic and topical treatments have been used to treat leishmaniasis. Both pentamidine. and amphotericin B have been used successfully as second-line agents for VL and New World CL, and amphotericin B has some effectiveness in mucosal disease. Allopurinol and ketoconazole may have some effectiveness against VL and New and Old World CL. Immunotherapy consisting of three vaccinations of live bacille Calmette Guérin (BCG) with killed *Leishmania* promastigotes appears as effective as pentostam in Venezuelan LCL. Topical paromomycin ointment is effective in the treatment of Old World LCL.

Methods of prevention or control of leishmaniasis have included eradication of the vector or its habitat, destruction of animal reservoirs, treatment of human reservoirs, and vaccination. Control and prevention of leishmaniasis in the future depends on the development of more efficacious vaccines and convenient, nontoxic therapeutic agents.

PARASITIC DISEASES

(CM&S Chapter 127)

Protozoan Infections

Amebiasis

Amebiasis is a cosmopolitan gastrointestinal infection caused by *Entamoeba histolytica*. These parasitic protozoans have pseudopods that provide motility and enable them to capture food. *E. histolytica* has the unique capability of erythrophagocytosis; ingested red blood cells in the trophozoites often aid in diagnosis. Although approximately 90% of those infected are asymptomatic, invasive intestinal and extraintestinal disease may occur. Humans are the reservoir, with asymptomatic carriers sporadically excreting up to 45 million cysts in a day. Cyst-contaminated hands, water, drinks, or food, and oral-anal sex may be sources of transmission. The hardy ingested (10–20 μm) cysts survive gastric digestion, multiplying and dwelling in the cecum and colon as trophozoites. These may be seen in watery stools; however, it is usually only the cyst form, which the trophozoites produce by binary fission, that is excreted. High-risk groups include the institutionalized, mentally retarded, promiscuous male homosexuals (''gay bowel syndrome''), acquired immune deficiency syndrome and other immunocompromised individuals, and immigrants from endemic areas, such as Mexico, South America, Africa, and South Asia. Symptomatic infection typically presents as colitis, abdominal pain, bloody diarrhea, and mucosal ulcerations. Extraintestinal complications of hepatic abscess, empyema, pericardial effusion, ameboma, and cutaneous disease are rare. The skin of the anus, buttocks, and perineum is involved by direct extension from the rectum. Draining abscesses, fistulae, and abdominal surgery may result in skin disease elsewhere. Ill-defined erythematous, raised, or overhanging borders surround painful ulcers, which are covered in exudate. Tissue destruction may advance rapidly postoperatively, simulating synergistic gangrene of Meleney and provoking extensive surgical debridement in place of appropriate therapy.

Diagnosis may be made upon identifying cysts or trophozoites in freshly passed stools. On histologic examination, biopsy specimens from the rectum or perianal skin are often flanked by pseudocarcinomatous epidermal hyperplasia and have bases of granulation tissue above which is a neutrophilic infiltrate containing trophozoites. The organisms range from 12 to 20 μm in diameter. The abundant cytoplasm of trophozoites sometimes contains phagocytized erythrocytes, highlighted in periodic acid–Schiff–stained sections. The cutaneous differential diagnosis includes herpes simplex, tuberculosis, atypical mycobacteria, syphilis, chancroid, ecthyma, squamous cell carcinoma, and metastases.

Therapy for invasive disease is metronidazole, 750 mg, or diloxanide, 500 mg three times per day for 10 days; tinidazole, 2 g once a day for 2 days for adults and 50 to 60 mg/kg per day in a single dose for children; or alternatively emetine hydrochloride, 1 to 1.5 mg/kg per day (maximum 90 mg per day), subcutaneously or intramuscularly for 5 to 10 days. To eradicate cyst carriage, any of the above regimens should be followed by iodoquinol, 650 mg three times per day for 20 days, or paromomycin, 25 to 30 mg/kg per day in three doses for 7 days.

American Trypanosomiasis

American trypanosomiasis, commonly termed Chagas' disease, occurs only in the Western hemisphere and is caused by the protozoan *Trypanosoma cruzi (Schizotrypanum cruzi)*, which infects large, bloodsucking insects of the family Reduviidae. Humans and animals are reservoirs for *T. cruzi*. Transmission may occur by intrauterine infections, transfusions, or triatomine insect species.

The disease usually occurs in three phases. The *acute* or *primary stage* is characterized by the ''chagoma of inoculation,'' a boardlike induration with edema, erythema, and tenderness at the bite site. This often occurs at an early age when the reduviid bugs, attracted to CO_2, bite sleeping children on the face, hence the term *kissing bugs*. The infected bug feces are scratched or rubbed into the bite or skin wound, conjunctiva, lips, or mucous membranes. The resulting chagoma appears within 5 to 14 days and is usually accompanied by regional adenopathy. Romana's sign (oculoglandular syndrome) is a unilateral bipalpebral edema and is often accompanied by preauricular adenopathy. Malaise, variable fever, and lymphadenopathy are common in the primary stage; however, a macular rash, hepatosplenomegaly, thrombocytosis, leukocytosis, and eosinophilia may also be present. Many infected individuals are asymptomatic. The acute symptoms and chagoma usually last 2 months and may result in a hyperpigmented and depressed area at the bite site. In most cases the patient recovers, but myocarditis and meningoencephalitis are life-threatening complications that may require pacemaker insertion. In the *intermediate phase*, the patient is clinically symptom-free, but serologically positive. *T. cruzi*, measuring 20 μm long, is found in the blood in early stages of the disease but does not divide there. Instead the trypanosomes penetrate into the cells of heart and other voluntary muscles where they lose their flagellae and become *amastigotes*. These multiply by binary fission while destroying organ tissue, with each producing a flagellum and transforming into *epimastigotes*. These give rise to *trypomastigotes*, which enter the blood, and the cycle continues over and over. Years to decades may pass before the *third-stage* clinical symptoms appear. The most common sequela of chronic Chagas' disease is cardiac damage. Cardiac failure, sudden cardiac death, heart block, arrhythmias, embolic phenomena, and intestinal tract involvement with megaesophagus and megacolon may occur.

Diagnosis in the acute stage is made by detection of trypanosomes in blood either from a fresh smear or after hemoconcentration, culture, or PCR.

Treatment is useful only in the acute stage and consists of oral therapy using nifurtimox, 8 to 10 mg/kg per day in four doses for 60 to 120 days, or benznidazole, 5 to 7 mg/kg per day for 30 to 120 days. Both drugs have serious side effects and are of little or no value in the chronic stage. Transfusion acute disease can be prevented by better screening techniques such as PCR or by treating blood with gentian violet (1 : 4000) for 24 hours.

African Trypanosomiasis

African trypanosomiasis, commonly called African sleeping sickness, is a systemic protozoan disease transmitted by an infected tsetse fly. This disease is endemic in a belt running through tropical Africa where the vector, the tsetse fly, is prevalent.

Trypanosoma brucei gambiense are elongated parasites 10 to 30 μm in length and 1.5 to 3.5 μm in width, each containing a nucleus and kinetoplast. Their body is like a curved, flattened blade with a single flagellum projecting from the posterior end of the body and running along the undulating membrane to the anterior end, often extending beyond this point as a "free flagellum." They always swim in the direction of the anterior end. It is impossible to differentiate the two subspecies morphologically. When a tsetse fly bites a patient with parasitemia, trypanosomes are sucked into the gut of the fly with the bloodmeal, reaching the salivary glands, where they develop into "metacyclic" infective forms within 2 to 5 weeks. The *first stage* occurs when the fly's saliva, containing infected trypanosomes, is injected into the subcutaneous tissues of the host, usually resulting in local inflammation, with a "chancre" appearing at the bite site within 4 to 10 days. The chancre spontaneously resolves in about 2 weeks, and the *second stage* soon follows, with the trypanosomes invading the peripheral blood, resulting in irregular fevers and symmetrical adenopathy. Possible cutaneous symptoms include edema of the hands, feet, or eyelids, erythema nodosum, and annular or serpiginous erythemas that often resemble erythema multiforme. Nonspecific neurologic manifestations, such as headache, insomnia, and a delayed deep hyperesthesia, may occur at this stage. The *third stage* of African sleeping sickness consists of progressive deterioration due to central nervous system (CNS) involvement. Symptoms associated with CNS invasion by the protozoans are paresis, seizures, ataxia, and personality changes. Blindness, myocarditis, and heart failure may occur. Rarely are cutaneous signs present, but xerosis and pruritus may be present. The disease is lethal within a few weeks to 9 months. The Gambian form may exist as a chronic condition for years before the parasites enter the CNS. Other modes of transmission include direct inoculation with infected material, blood transfusions, and intrauterine infection. Both forms of African trypanosomiasis are fatal without treatment.

Diagnosis is made by finding trypanosomes in blood, lymph or cerebral spinal fluid, or Giemsa-stained smears made from the exudates of chancres. PCR has been successfully used to detect *Trypanosoma brucei* subspecies.

Because treatment depends on the stage of the disease, the cerebral spinal fluid should be examined prior to treatment. If there is any abnormality, the patient is treated as having advanced disease.

Suramin is the drug of choice for the early stages of either form of African trypanosomiasis. The treatment regimen consists of 20 mg/kg intravenously to a 1-g maximum single dose on days 1, 3, 7, 14, and 21. Close supervision is necessary when using this toxic drug, whose most significant side effect is kidney damage. Pentamidine, 3 to 4 mg/kg intramuscularly for 10 days or every other day for a 10-dose total, is the alternative therapy. Melarsoprol, given intravenously at 3.6 mg/kg per day for four injections over 1 week, is highly effective for either type and all stages of African sleeping sickness, even in cases of treatment failure with suramin or pentamidine. Eflornithine, an ornithine decarboxylase inhibitor, is effective and possibly the preferable drug of choice for Gambian disease with CNS involvement.

All patients, regardless of the type of therapy or disease form, should be seen at 3, 6, 12, and 24 months after treatment to check the possibility of relapsed infections.

Toxoplasmosis

Humans acquire infection with the obligate intracellular protozoan *Toxoplasma gondii*, congenitally or at any age, by ingesting oocysts shed in cat feces or tissue cysts in undercooked meat. Iatrogenic infection may result from transfusion, transplantation, or laboratory inoculation. Acute infection in the immunocompetent human is underdiagnosed because it is of short duration and may be asymptomatic or nonspecific in presentation. Infection persists, latently, as cysts in tissue, kept in check by both humoral and cellular immunity, but can reactivate if the host becomes immunocompromised.

Congenital infection occurs only if the mother becomes infected during pregnancy and has not been previously exposed. Although the risk of fetal transmission increases during the pregnancy, the severity of infection decreases after the first trimester. Affected neonates may suffer from chorioretinitis, microphthalmia, blindness, seizures, microcephaly, hydrocephalus, intracerebral calcifications, encephalitis, mental retardation, lymphadenopathy, hepatosplenomegaly, myocarditis, and interstitial pneumonitis. The skin findings are nonspecific, and include jaundice, petechiae, ecchymoses, and the bluish macules or plaques of dermoerythropoiesis. "Blueberry muffin" lesions are also seen in congenital cytomegalovirus and rubella infections, and in leukemia. Diagnosis depends upon clinical presentation and the presence of specific IgM antibodies directed against *Toxoplasma*. Serial titers at 3 weeks are helpful.

Skin lesions in children and adults are very uncommon in acquired toxoplasmosis, and are pleomorphic. They have been described as resembling erythema multiforme or roseola, or as telangiectatic or hemorrhagic macules, lichenoid or erythematous papules, pustules, vesicles, or purpuric nodules. Lymphadenopathy, especially of the head and neck, fever, headache, malaise, arthralgia, and bone pain may be present. Patients immunocompromised by steroids, cytotoxic agents, or acquired immunodeficiency syndrome are highly susceptible to toxoplasmosis, probably by reactivation more often than acute infection. Encephalitis and chorioretinitis are the most common manifestations, but the skin may be rarely involved in disseminated disease. The histology of the lesion depends upon the clinical nature, and organisms are rarely found. When present, organisms are seen as pseudocysts within the cytoplasms of macrophages that comprise sparsely cellular dermal infiltrates. They can also lie freely within the dermis as 3- to 4-mm oval to cigar-shaped trophozoites. Organisms stain with periodic acid–Schiff and Giemsa, and pseudocysts must be differentiated from other intracellular parasites.

Combined therapy with sulfadiazine, 1 to 2 g per day, and pyrimethamine, 25 to 100 mg per day, with folinic acid for 3 to 4 weeks is standard. Spiramycin, 3 to 4 g per day, is less active but also less toxic and has been used effectively in pregnant women and infants.

Early therapy may prevent late sequelae. Steroids are indicated for inflammatory eye disease. Instruct pregnant women to eat well-cooked meats, and to avoid kittens and any contact with cat feces, such as changing litter boxes; frequent handwashing helps to prevent infections.

Trichomoniasis

Trichomonas vaginalis, a common sexually transmitted disease, produces a genitourinary infection of both sexes, which may or may not be symptomatic. Trichomoniasis is one of the most common sexually transmitted diseases, estimated to have a prevalence of 180 million cases per year worldwide. Infection may rarely be transmitted perinatally.

The most common clinical complaint by women is of vaginal discharge, which is typically malodorous, frothy, and yellow-green. Pruritus and irritation are also common, followed by dysuria and dyspareunia; infection may be asymptomatic. Other findings include vulvar or vaginal erythema. Visualization reveals a "strawberry" cervix, but its detection may require colposcopic examination. Infected males complain of a clear urethral discharge. Persistent infection has been associated with infertility, preterm labor, premature rupture of membranes, low birth weight, increased postsurgical infection of the reproductive tract, urethritis, epididymitis, and prostatitis. Infection in men may spontaneously clear by 2 weeks after exposure.

The causative agent is a motile, 10- to 20-μm, oval protozoan. Its movement is readily detected in saline wet mounts of vaginal or urethral discharge. Potassium hydroxide examination is often performed concurrently in the evaluation of vaginal discharge, and a characteristic odor may be associated with trichomonas-positive samples. Culture of vaginal or urethral discharge is the most accurate method of diagnosis, when available. Differential diagnosis includes bacterial and candidal vaginoses.

Treatment with metronidazole, 2 g orally once, or in a split dose the same day, is effective in the majority of cases. Dosing with 250 mg three times daily for 7 days is an alternative. Sexual partners need to be treated concurrently, as recurrent infection is common. Other nitroimidazoles are also effective: tinidazole 2 g orally once, or nimorazole, 2 g per day orally for 2 days. Local agents are used in pregnancy, such as tinidazole vaginal suppositories, metronidazole gel, or nonoxynol-9; however, they are less effective. Condom use is preventative.

Tissue Nematode Infections

Onchocerciasis

Onchocerciasis, due to infection by *Onchocerca volvulus*, is an important parasitic infection that primarily involves the skin. It is the second leading cause of infectious blindness globally. The bulk of disease is found in equatorial Africa. Transmission occurs from the bite of the female black fly of *Simulium* species within a few kilometers of river banks, where breeding occurs. Prolonged exposure with repeated bites of infected flies is required to produce clinical disease, unlike leishmaniasis. Eye disease is more prevalent in savannah compared with forest areas, due to parasite strain differences.

The hematophagous black fly vector ingests microfilariae present in the upper dermis of infected humans, the reservoir. Maturation into infective larvae occurs within the fly over 6 to 8 days. When the fly next feeds, these are passed to another person. The larvae molt twice to become adults during a 9- to 18-month period. Adults are usually localized in small groupings within a fibrotic capsule (onchocercoma), releasing large numbers of microfilariae into the surrounding skin. It is the microfilariae, not the adults, that lead to clinical disease. The immune response of the individual determines the extent of the disease. Those with mild disease tend to be hyporesponsive to parasite antigens. Hyperreactive individuals may have severe dermatitis and pruritus.

Pruritus is the most common skin manifestation. An acute papular to nearly vesicular eruption may be scattered on the upper body or in patches. This type of reaction can follow use of diethylcarbamazine as a treatment or as a provocative diagnostic test. Other early changes are urticarial, eczematous, or lichenified. Localized limb swelling with tender adenopathy may rarely occur. More specific but subtle fullness may be seen on the upper chest and back, appearing shiny, ''plump and juicy,'' or even sclerodermatous. The nonpitting interfollicular turgidity produces a peau d'orange texture, which over time regresses to leave patulous follicles and interfollicular sag. *Erisipela de la costa* refers to edematous erythema of the face with fever, photophobia, and headache. Thickening of the ears and facial skin results in leonine facies. *Mal de morado* describes lichen planus–like plaques.

Chronic onchodermatitis develops after years of disease, and may manifest as lizard skin, crushed tissue paper skin, atrophy, pachydermia, leopard skin, pigmentary changes, and doughy abdomen. Milder hypopigmentation and hyperpigmentation are common as well. *Sowda* (Arabic for black) is a form of onchocerciasis with intense pruritus, lichenification, and hyperpigmentation. The affected limb may be swollen, with reactive adenopathy.

Onchocercomas are asymptomatic, rubbery subcutaneous nodules, usually felt over bony prominences. In Africa, they localize to the sacrum, coccyx, iliac crest, and greater trochanter. Nontender, fibrotic adenopathy is typical. Adenocele formation follows; folds of skin may droop in the groin and genital area as an end stage called *hanging groin*. Hernias are common. Back, joint, and muscle pains are frequent systemic complaints.

Both anterior and posterior segments of the eye can eventually be affected by onchocerciasis. Corneal opacities are initially punctate, termed *fluffy* or *snowflake*. These can resolve without scarring. Anterior uveitis, iridocyclitis, sclerosing keratitis, optic atrophy, and chorioretinitis are common eye findings that may result in blindness.

The skin histopathology consists of a sparse perivascular infiltrate of lymphocytes and eosinophils. Less commonly, granuloma formation occurs. In severe end-stage atrophy, there is a marked loss of elastic fibers. Onchocercomas reveal multiple cross sections of the tightly coiled worms within a sclerotic capsule. Microfilariae may be seen in the upper dermis between collagen fibers.

Diagnosis is typically made by skin snips. These can be obtained by tenting the skin with a needle and slicing off a 2-mm section through the dermal papillae. The best sites are over the scapulae, the posterior iliac crests, the calves, and over any nodules. Each skin snip is placed on a glass slide or in a microtiter well with 0.1 mL saline. Microfilariae will leave the skin within a few hours, but samples should be allowed to sit at room temperature for 24 hours before discarding as negative. *Mansonella streptocerca*, which also produces a pruritic eruption due to migration of microfilariae through the skin, must be distinguished morphologically. An eye examination is essential in evaluating the possibility of onchocerciasis. Ultrasound has been helpful at localizing deeper nodules.

Oral ivermectin, 150 to 200 μg/kg, is the treatment of choice, given every 6 months. It is microfilaricidal only, so therapy may need to be given as long as the adult worms survive. Side effects are less severe than with DEC, but hypotension, although rare, may occur. DEC, 6 mg/kg, for 11 days following an initial dose of 3 mg/kg per day, is reserved for situations in which ivermectin cannot be given, such as meningitis, pregnancy, the first month of breast feeding, drug allergy, or age younger than 5 years, because toddlers cannot successfully swallow the pills. Nodulectomy is reasonable for accessible onchocercomas, especially in the head region. Disease prevention for the traveler includes protective clothing, insect repellent, and avoidance of the vector habitat, if possible.

Filariasis

Filariasis is a nematode infection caused by infestation with *Wuchereria bancrofti, Brugia malayi,* or *B. timori. Wuchereria bancrofti* is found in Africa, Asia, Oceania, Latin America, and the Caribbean. *Brugia malayi* is found in Southeast Asia, India, and Indonesia, and is the only form that also has a zoonotic component, with a reservoir in monkeys, macaques, and felines. *Brugia timori* is found in foci of Indonesia. Mosquitoes are the vectors, ingesting the L_1 microfilariae in the blood meal from an infected human host. The larvae develop through the L_2 stage into infective larvae, L_3, during 1 to 3 weeks. The L_3 are passed with subsequent feedings into a new human host, where they develop into L_4 and adult forms over a period of 4 to 6 months. The adults dwell within the lymphatics adjacent to lymph nodes and genitalia, shedding microfilariae into the peripheral blood. Although the presence of the adults results in lymphatic dilation and thickening of the walls, obstruction occurs primarily due to the host's immune reaction to dead worms, with inflammation, granuloma formation, and fibrosis.

Most individuals in filarial-endemic regions are asymptomatic and microfilaremic, and are considered to be immunologically tolerant or hyporesponsive. Responders have eventual disease manifestations such as elephantiasis and hydrocele, despite often being amicrofilaremic. Acute attacks of retrograde lymphangitis, fever, and malaise lasting 3 to 15 days are irregularly recurrent. Lymphadenitis affects the groin or axilla, and may suppurate. Recurrent orchitis and epididymitis may lead to hydrocele. Eosinophilia and high levels of IgE are found. Reversible pitting edema of the legs, scrotum, or arms results from acute attacks, becoming eventually nonpitting and persistent. The breast, penis, and labia are involved less frequently. Progression of disease appears to be more rapid in nonendemic individuals. Cutaneous changes of elephantiasis are secondary to the chronic lymphedema, with thickening of the skin that can be smooth or verrucous and nodular over many years. Transverse skin folds are typical between the foot and ankle. Infections, fissures, and ulcers may develop in the fibrotic skin. Elephantiasis due to *Brugia* is softer, producing a "water bag" deformity of the lower legs. Rarely, individuals develop a hyper-responsive state manifest as tropical pulmonary eosinophilia, which is more common in young men, with asthma-like wheezing, adenopathy, and marked eosinophilia.

Diagnosis depends upon epidemiology, the clinical picture, and, if possible, the demonstration of the microfilaria in the peripheral blood. Serial blood samples for concentration (1 to 10 mL anticoagulated blood) should be obtained around midnight to identify the nocturnally periodic *W. bancrofti.* Parasites are susceptible to jet lag as are humans and may delay during travel in establishing their characteristic periodicity. Microfilariae found in the blood should be stained with Giemsa or hematoxylin to identify the morphologic features that allow differentiation of the various blood-dwelling filariae.

Standard therapy for filariasis is with oral microfilaricidal DEC, 6 mg/kg for 12 days, preceded by a single dose of 3 mg/kg. The Mazzotti reaction does not occur in filariasis as in onchocerciasis, and the drug is well tolerated. Mass treatment with a single yearly dose appears to be efficacious in reducing transmission. Aggressive repeated therapy with DEC is macrofilaricidal to *W. bancrofti*. Iver-mectin, 200 to 400 μg/kg in a single oral dose, is microfilaricidal and has similar efficacy to DEC with fewer side effects. Surgery is indicated in moderate to advanced cases of elephantiasis, by lymph nodovenous shunt or an excisional operation.

Trichinosis

Humans become accidentally infected with *Trichinella spiralis* by ingesting raw or insufficiently cooked meat, usually from wild carnivores or swine. Trichinosis is found worldwide, except for Australia and some Pacific islands. Formerly, pigs had been the main source of infection, however, this has changed in the United States with improved meat inspections and the regulation to boil any garbage or food scraps fed to pigs. Infections are most likely to come from eating undercooked or microwaved bear, wild boar, bush pig, wart hog, polar bear, walrus, or homemade sausage of wild animal meat or noncommercial pork. Raw horse meat has been a source in France, presumably through contamination of the feed. Carnivores eat the muscles of infected animals, and the larvae ex-cyst in the stomach and mature into adults in the small intestine epithelium. Mating of adult worms results in discharge of live larvae within a week. The larvae migrate into the circulation and invade striated skeletal muscle. Within the muscle cell, the larvae coil and a cyst forms around them by 3 weeks after infection. The encysted larvae may survive for years in this state, although calcification can eventually occur.

Gastrointestinal complaints are predominant during the first week, followed by the classic features associated with encystment of the larvae: fever, myalgia, periorbital edema, and eosinophilia. A macular or petechial rash may also occur, simulating a viral ex-anthem. Subungual or retinal splinter hemorrhages and subconjunc-tival hemorrhage and chemosis can sometimes be seen.

Diagnosis is made from the clinical picture with a history of questionable meat ingestion. Pronounced eosinophilia is typical be-ginning the tenth day, and muscle enzymes may be elevated. Anti-bodies develop by 4 weeks, and acute and convalescent titers may help distinguish new from old infection. Analysis of a muscle biopsy specimen from a tender swollen muscle may reveal coiled larvae within the fiber, surrounded by eosinophils and lymphocytes. The differential diagnosis includes viral infections, dermatomyosi-tis, and typhoid.

Treatment is suboptimal. Thiabendazole, 25 mg/kg/day for 1 week, is larvicidal if started within 24 hours of ingesting contami-nated meat. Thereafter, mebendazole, 200 to 400 mg three times daily for 3 days, followed by 400 to 500 mg three times daily for 10 days, may be used in conjunction with prednisone, 40 to 60 mg/day, especially if symptoms are severe. Disease is self-limited. Preven-tion is easy by heating meat to 77° C or freezing for 3 weeks.

Loiasis

Loa loa is a filarial nematode infecting humans in equatorial rain forests of West and Central Africa. Transmission from infected human to human is mediated by female tabanid fly vectors of the genus *Chrysops*, which bite during the day, ingesting the diurnal microfilariae from the bloodstream. Infective filariform larvae develop in 10 to 12 days and are released from the proboscis in subsequent feedings. Maturation results in adult worms, surviving up to 17 years and producing sheathed microfilariae that circulate in the peripheral blood by 1 year after infection. The microfilariae are not considered to be pathogenic, except following treatment with DEC, when large numbers may die and block cerebral vessels. Clinical manifestations relate to movement of the adults through the subcutaneous tissues and subconjunctivae. Recurrent subcutaneous swellings 10 to 20 cm in diameter, termed *Calabar swellings*, are most common on the forearms, wrists, ankle, and face. The Calabar swellings are the result of allergenic response to the worm's by-products released into the dermis, and may last for hours or days, recurring at irregular intervals of weeks or months for up to 15 years. Although *Loa loa* usually does not cause serious harm, the lumps can be painful, erythematous, and pruritic.

DEC is effective against developing larvae, microfilariae, and adult worms and should be administered at the same doses recommended for filariasis. Repeated courses may be necessary. In severe cases, 1 mg/kg of prednisone for the first week to 10 days with DEC has been advised. A single dose of oral ivermectin, 300 to 400 μg/kg, has been shown to be effective for 3 months in the treatment of loiasis and has fewer and less severe side effects than DEC. Because ivermectin kills only the microfilariae and not the adult worm, further dosing regimens need to be investigated.

Dirofilariasis

Zoonotic infection of man with *Dirofilaria* species is usually manifest by pulmonary or subcutaneous lesions. Cases are described worldwide, wherever people live in proximity to the definitive hosts: dogs, coyotes, wolves, cats, foxes, raccoons, opossums, bears, and otters. Mosquitoes are the vector and intermediate host. Blood containing microfilaria is ingested from an infected animal. Infective third-stage larvae develop in the mosquito over a 2-week period, and are deposited with subsequent feedings on the animal or human host. In animals, the microfilaria mature over several months, migrating through venous channels to lodge and reproduce in the right ventricle. The gravid female produces several thousand microfilaria per day, and eventually the animal succumbs to right-sided heart failure.

In humans, maturation and propagation do not occur, and the microfilaria die. Prior to death, the microfilaria may migrate through subcutaneous tissues, provoking a local reaction anywhere in the body, or into the venous system, where embolization to the lungs may be detected as a "coin" lesion on chest roentgenogram. This event may be asymptomatic or accompanied by cough, hemoptysis, or pleuritic pain and is usually due to infection with *D. immitis*, the dog heartworm. Other species may produce subcutaneous masses, which may be asymptomatic, firm, and cystic, or migratory, erythematous, and pruritic. The breast, head, neck, and eye are common sites of involvement. *D. tenuis* (*D. conjunctivae*) (raccoon) and *D. ursi* (bear) are the agents most often encountered in the United States, whereas *D. repens* (dog or cat) is found in Europe. Eosinophilia, if present, is mild. Diagnosis is usually made upon identifying the nematode in the dermis or subcutaneous tissues, often surrounded by a granulomatous reaction. The differential diagnosis is primary or metastatic cancer, cutaneous cysts, and other skin tumors. The diagnosis is rarely entertained prior to biopsy. Specific therapy in humans is seldom necessary; DEC and ivermectin have been used anecdotally.

Intestinal Nematode Infections

Cutaneous Larva Migrans

Cutaneous larva migrans (CLM), also known as creeping eruption or sandworm disease, is a self-limited cutaneous eruption caused by larvae of roundworms that do not normally parasitize humans. *Ancylostoma braziliense*, the dog and cat hookworm, is the most common agent. Larvae of several other nematode species may also cause creeping eruption, but are less common. *Strongyloides stercoralis* can produce CLM, although it is usually associated with larva currens, a more rapidly migratory condition. Larvae of *Necator americanus* and *A. duodenale*, human hookworm, can cause abortive forms of creeping eruption. CLM has a worldwide distribution, including the Caribbean, the southeastern United States, Central and South America, Africa, and Southeast Asia. CLM is found in the coastal areas of the United States from New Jersey to Texas, with a high incidence in Florida. Beaches tend to be the most common reservoir of CLM, although it may result from contact with sand in children's sandboxes or in construction sites. To limit transmission, dogs are prohibited from roaming on many beaches in Florida.

Nematode eggs are passed in the feces of infected animals, which hatch into filariform larvae in soil or sand. Humans become accidentally infected upon exposure to the larvae, capable of quickly penetrating skin. Patients recall a tingling or stinging sensation upon initial penetration of the larvae, and an erythematous papule or nonspecific dermatitis may develop within hours. Migration of larvae usually occurs within a week, although it can be delayed for several weeks or months. As the larvae migrate in human skin, they produce an intensely pruritic, 2- to 4-mm wide, erythematous, slightly elevated, vesicular, serpiginous track. The larvae are restricted to the epidermis, where they wander aimlessly, unable to penetrate the basement membrane or complete their life cycle. The larva is found in normal skin 1 to 2 cm beyond the track, which marks the host's allergic reaction to the larva or its products. The larvae travel at a rate of several millimeters to 2 cm per day. Untreated, lesions spontaneously resolve within weeks to months, following the eventual death of the larvae. The feet are the most common site for CLM, followed by the hands, arms, and buttocks. Diagnosis is based upon clinical findings with an appropriate history. Secondary bacterial infection, usually yielding *Streptococcus pyogenes*, may result in cellulitis and edema, making the tracks difficult to see, and may lead to the misdiagnosis of acute or secondarily infected tinea pedis.

Oral thiabendazole at 25 mg/kg twice a day for 2 days is usually effective but has a high incidence of side effects including nausea, vomiting, and diarrhea. Topical thiabendazole liquid at 10% to 15% applied topically two to four times daily for a week is a safe and highly effective therapy for CLM. Oral albendazole, 400 mg a day for 3 days, is effective and side effects are rare. Ivermectin in a single dose of 200 μg/kg appears to be well tolerated and effective.

Strongyloidiasis

Larva currens, or "running larva," is the cutaneous manifestation of intestinal infection and autoinfection with the human nematode *Strongyloides stercoralis*, and rarely, *S. fulleborni*. It is found in feces-contaminated, moist, tropical and subtropical soil, where it may be free-living. Infection follows skin penetration by filariform larvae measuring 500 $\times$ 16 μm. These larvae enter the bloodstream and exit via the lungs, to ascend to the glottis and be swallowed. Maturation and reproduction occur in the upper small bowel. This organism is unusual in that rhabditiform (noninfective) larvae hatch from ova within the gastrointestinal tract. These larvae may transform into infectious filariform larvae, which reinfect the host by penetrating the intestinal mucosa (internal autoinfection) or the skin of the perianal and perineal areas, and occasionally the buttocks, abdomen, and thighs (external autoinfection). Chronic steroid use, immunodepressed states, achlorhydria, nephrosis, burns, leprosy, and institutionalization predispose to chronic infection and to hyperinfection, where the larvae are widely disseminated.

Reminiscent of CLM, pruritic, erythematous, serpiginous tracks migrate through the skin, but at the alarming rate of up to 10 cm per hour. Nonspecific rash, urticaria, papules, and vesicles can also be seen; individual lesions persist only about 48 hours. Cutaneous lesions are more widespread in hyperinfection, and may be petechial or purpuric in a reticulated pattern, especially in the periumbilical area. Gram-negative bacteremia is common. Mortality is high in these patients. Löffler's syndrome, shortness of breath with wheezing, transient pulmonary infiltrates, fever, and eosinophilia, may accompany the migration of larvae through the lungs.

Except in the extreme immunocompromised patient, eosinophilia is common, in association with gastrointestinal complaints. Diagnosis is made upon identification of *S. stercoralis* ova or larvae in the stool. Since excretion of larvae is sporadic, multiple samples should be obtained and examined after Baermann-type concentration. Worms may also be recovered by oral passage and recovery of a string attached to a gelatin capsule. Immunofluorescent antibody assay and ELISA may be useful in nonendemic settings. A biopsy is likely to be diagnostic only in hyperinfection, where larvae are numerous.

Oral thiabendazole, 25 mg/kg twice daily for 2 to 5 days, is the drug of choice; a 2-day course may be repeated 1 week later. Mebendazole, 100 mg twice daily for 4 days, is an alternative, but may be poorly absorbed. Albendazole, 400 mg daily for 3 days, and ivermectin, 200 μg/kg daily for 1 to 2 days, have also been used. Eradication of infection may be extremely difficult in immunocompromised individuals, in whom prolonged therapy is recommended.

Toxocariasis

Visceral larva migrans is caused by the migration of zoonotic helminth larvae, most commonly the dog and cat ascarids, *Toxocara canis* and *T. cati*, in human eyes or tissues other than the skin.

Infection occurs following ingestion of embryonated eggs from contaminated soil or hands. Cutaneous manifestations include generalized pruritus, urticaria, or urticarial papules of the trunk and extremities. A panniculitis consisting of firm, tender, subcutaneous nodules lasting 1 to 2 weeks and resembling erythema nodosum has been reported. Eosinophilia is typical; ELISA can be diagnostic. Infection is self-limited, usually running a chronic benign course for up to 18 months. The treatments of choice are DEC, 2 mg/kg three times a day for 7 to 10 days; thiabendazole, 25 mg/kg twice daily for 5 days; or mebendazole, 100 to 200 mg twice daily for 5 days. Visceral larva migrans will spontaneously remit without therapy; however, the duration of the disease may last up to 18 months.

Enterobiasis

Enterobiasis is the most common helminth infection in the United States and Western Europe, especially among school-age children. It occurs worldwide, and humans are the only host. Adult pinworms attach to the mucosa of the cecum, appendix, and nearby bowel, living up to 13 weeks. The females, 8 to 13 mm in length, migrate nightly to the anus and perineum for oviposition. The eggs are ovoid, 55×25 μm, flattened on one side, and embryonate in 6 hours. Transmission is usually from the hands of infected individuals, but may be from fomites. After ova are ingested, the larvae hatch in the duodenum and develop through two molts into adults by 1 to 2 months.

Pruritus ani, especially at night, is the most common clinical presentation. Although frequently asymptomatic, anorexia, abdominal pain, irritability, restlessness, insomnia, dysuria, and enuresis have been attributed to infection. Rarely, ectopic infection results in vaginitis, endometritis, salpingitis, epididymitis, urethritis, or pyelitis.

Diagnosis is made by applying adhesive tape to the anal area in the early morning, and affixing this to a microscope slide to identify the ova; sensitivity increases up to five examinations. Ova or larvae may rarely be detected in urine. Eosinophilia occurs only in invasive disease. The differential diagnosis includes idiopathic pruritus ani and localized disease as suggested by physical examination.

Therapy is effective with mebendazole, 100 mg, pyrantel pamoate, 11 mg/kg (maximum 1 g), and albendazole, 400 mg. All are given as a single oral dose, best repeated in 2 weeks. Reinfection is frequent; treatment of the entire household is often indicated.

Trematode Infection

Schistosomiasis

Human schistosomiasis is caused by blood flukes of the superfamily Schistosomatoidea. They differ from the other trematodes that infect man, because the sexes are separate and the adults inhabit the blood, being parasitic in the portal system. The three schistosomes that cause disease in humans are *Schistosoma haematobium* (prevalent from Africa to Iran), *S. mansoni* (found in Africa and South America), and *S. japonicum* (which occurs in the Far East). Humans and animals are the definitive hosts of schistosomes, with a variety of snail genera as intermediate hosts. Schistosomiasis has also been termed *bilharziasis*.

The fork-tailed cercaria (immature form), which are found in fresh water contaminated with snails, penetrate exposed skin or mucous membranes. They enter the lymphatics and the blood-stream, reaching the liver, which is the site of maturation and sexual differentiation. The adult parasites move to various sites. *S. haematobium* migrates down the portal vein and mesenteric branches to the rectal plexus, which communicates freely with the vesical plexus and the prostatic or interovaginal plexi. *S. mansoni* and *S. japonicum* migrate via the portal vein down to the ileocolic and colic branches of the superior and inferior mesenteric veins. The eggs of *S. haematobium* are spindle-shaped, large (140×50 μm), with a short terminal spine, and contain highly organized miracidium. The eggs of *S. haematobium* do not hatch in the urine, nor do *S. mansoni* or *S. japonicum* hatch in human feces; instead the eggs rupture when exposed to fresh water, releasing ciliated miracidium. Humans become infected from drinking, swimming, bathing, or wading in cercaria-infested water. If the cercaria are unable to find a human host in 2 to 3 days, they die. In *S. mansoni*, the eggs are 150×60 μm and have a lateral spine, with the adult male measuring 1 cm and the female 1.4 cm. The eggs of *S. japonicum* are considerably smaller than the other two species (90×50 μm) with a small knob on the side and near the pole. After the embryo has matured, an enzyme is secreted from the egg, resulting in necrosis of blood vessels and tissue. If the ovum does not find its way outside the body, the embryo inside becomes calcified and the tissues react to it as a foreign body.

Symptomatology is related to the location and number of eggs in the host. *S. haematobium* produces urinary tract manifestations, such as dysuria, hematuria, and urinary frequency. *S. mansoni* and *S. japonicum* produce intestinal and hepatic symptoms, which include abdominal pain, hepatosplenomegaly, and diarrhea.

Cutaneous manifestations of schistosomiasis can be divided into four types depending upon the stage of development of the parasite and the chronicity of the systemic disease: (1) *Dermatitis schistosomica* is caused by skin penetration by cercaria; (2) *bilharzides* represent the allergic anaphylactoid reactions that occur when large quantities of eggs (new antigenic material) are released and antibodies cross-react; (3) *bilharziasis cutanea tarda* is the specific schistosomal skin lesion caused by the deposit of eggs in the dermis; (4) lesions are related to complications of schistosomiasis. *Schistosomal dermatitis* refers to exposure to human blood flukes cercariae. The first exposure may go unnoticed; however, the host becomes more sensitized with repeated encounters, resulting in pruritic papules to hive-like swellings. *S. haematobium* reactions are less severe than those of *S. mansoni* or *S. japonicum*. *Bilharzides* may develop early in the invasive and development stage, or late in oviposition, when tissue reaction to eggs occurs. This syndrome is termed *Yangtze River fever* in China and *Katayama fever* in Japan. Clinical findings consist of fever, transient edema (face, trunk, limbs, or genitals), chills, joint pain, malaise, diarrhea, abdominal cramps, bronchitis, and pneumonitis. Hepatomegaly, splenomegaly, and lymphadenitis may occur, and there is leukocytosis, eosinophilia, and an elevated sedimentation rate. *Bilharziasis cutanea tarda* is usually manifested by granulomatous anogenital lesions. Extragenital or papular ectopic lesions are less common and are found on the trunk and umbilical area, often in a zosteriform distribution. Primary lesions are 2- to 3-mm flesh-colored, asymptomatic, firm papules that develop into irregular plaques, that may darken, become scaly, and occasionally ulcerate. The eggs, not the adult worms, cause the pathologic changes associated with schistosomiasis.

With respect to systemic manifestations, visceral *S. haematobium* infection is characterized by terminal hematuria, bladder papilloma, and ulceration. Intestinal schistosomiasis, caused by *S. mansoni* or *S. japonicum*, produces dysenteric symptoms and leads to cirrhosis of the liver, ascites, and splenomegaly.

Diagnosis of *S. haematobium* infection is made by identifying eggs in centrifuged urine. In suspected cases with negative urine samples, rectal biopsies are highly diagnostic. For diagnosis of *S. mansoni* and *S. japonicum*, fecal samples should be examined for eggs using either a direct smear procedure or the Kato thick smear technique. Among serologic tests, the complement fixation fluorescence test is the most sensitive and has the advantage of early detection and the disadvantage of being impractical for field use. PCR has also been used in *S. mansoni* infections.

The treatment of choice for schistosomiasis is praziquantel administered in the following dose regimens: for *S. haematobium* and *S. mansoni*, 40 mg/kg per day in two doses × 1 day; for *S. japonicum*, 60 mg/kg per day in three doses × 1 day.

Cercarial Dermatitis

Cercarial dermatitis, commonly known as swimmer's itch, is a distinctive papular eruption caused by penetration of the skin by cercariae of nonhuman schistosomes. This cutaneous schistosomiasis is usually limited to the exposed areas of the body. It is associated with freshwater lakes, although "clam digger's itch" has been reported from the saltwater tributaries of Long Island Sound, New York. The cercariae responsible infect birds, rodents, or ungulates, and belong to the species *Schistosoma, Ornithobilharzia, Gigantobilharzia, Austrobilharzia, Trichobilharzia,* and *Orientobilharzia.* Cercarial dermatitis is a potential hazard worldwide, wherever people share an aquatic environment with vertebrates and mollusks harboring schistosomes.

These blood flukes require an intermediate snail host and a definitive vertebrate host to complete the life cycle. Inasmuch as man is an accidental host, development cannot proceed, and clinical manifestations of cercarial penetration resolve spontaneously within a week. A prickling sensation lasting minutes to an hour results from exposure to cercariae-infested water. Pruritic erythematous macules, papules, and occasionally, papulovesicles and wheals can be seen soon thereafter. Postinflammatory hyperpigmentation is a common sequela. Edema, lymphangitis, and regional adenopathy develop in some individuals, as may eosinophilia and systemic symptoms of generalized urticaria, nausea, and vomiting. Repeated exposures produce more severe insect bite reaction, with perivascular lymphocytes, histiocytes, and eosinophils.

Treatment is oriented toward the relief of symptoms. Oral antihistamines, topical steroids, and topical antipruritic agents may be helpful. The rash may be prevented by toweling off vigorously and showering promptly after freshwater bathing.

Seabather's Eruption

Seabather's eruption is a highly pruritic cutaneous eruption that occurs primarily under swimwear after bathing in the ocean. It is caused by the stinging nematocysts of the larvae of the phylum Cnidaria (formerly Coelenterata), which includes jellyfish, Portuguese man-of-war, sea anemones, hydroids, and fire coral. These pinhead-sized larvae become trapped between the skin and bathing apparel. Pressure or exposure to freshwater elicits the release of the coiled nematocysts, which fire irritating toxins into the skin. The larva of *Edwardsiella lineata*, a sea anemone, is the probable cause of seabather's eruption in the North Atlantic coastal states and occurs from August through October. The larva of *Linuche unguiculata*, the thimble jellyfish, is the cause on the southern Atlantic coast, especially Florida and the Caribbean, and has been reported from March to August, usually peaking in late May. Seabather's eruption is often inappropriately termed *sea lice*. "Sea lice" refer to metazoan parasites of fish and do not affect humans.

Lesions appear within a few hours of exposure and consist of pruritic erythematous papules and wheals, often developing into pustules or vesicles. Although lesions usually resolve in a few days, some patients have a delayed hypersensitivity that occurs about 10 days after the initial exposure and is often more severe, extending to exposed areas of the body, which were not previously affected. Fever (101° F to 104° F), nausea, vomiting, and diarrhea may occur, with frequency and severity more common in children. Recent history of ocean exposure is the most important diagnostic aid. Oral antihistamines, systemic and medium to high-strength topical corticosteroids, and antipruritic agents are effective in most cases. Bathing suits should be washed in fresh water and detergent and dried prior to reuse.

Larval Cestode Infection

Cysticercosis

Humans are the definitive host for gastrointestinal infection with the adult pork tapeworm, *Taenia solium*. Cysticercosis, however, is caused by infection with the larval stage, cysticercus cellulosae, in which humans are an incidental intermediate host, usually transmitted by oral-fecal contamination or by eating inadequately cooked "measly pork." Ingested eggs hatch in the stomach, penetrating the intestinal wall and developing into oncospheres, then infective larval cysts. Cysts are viable up to 5 years, and elicit little reaction until death and subsequent calcification. Cysticercosis is encountered most often in Mexico, South America, and parts of Europe, Asia, and Africa.

Cysticercus cysts may develop anywhere in the body, but show predilection for the brain, meninges, eyes, muscle, heart, liver, lungs, oral cavity, and skin. Clinical disease usually relates to the central nervous system involvement. Subcutaneous nodules are round, rubbery, and asymptomatic, reaching 1- to 2-cm size, and eventually calcifying. Diagnosis is made after excision or roentgenogram, with confirmatory serology. Treatment has been surgical, but can be accomplished with praziquantel, 50 mg/kg per day in three divided doses for 2 weeks, or alternatively albendazole, 15 mg/kg per day in three divided doses for 8 days. Seizure control and steroids may be required concurrently.

BODY LICE, HEAD LICE, PUBIC LICE, AND SCABIES

(CM&S Chapter 128)

Pediculosis Corporis (Body Lice)

Definition and Clinical Description

Body lice is caused by *Pediculus humanus corporis*. Body lice occur in epidemics during times of social unrest, poverty, and war, as a result of humans living in overcrowded conditions. Infestations are passed from person to person through direct physical contact or through fomites such as blankets, pillows, and sleeping bags. The organism feeds on the body but lives on clothes and lays its eggs near the seams. The body louse is anatomically indistinguishable from the head louse. In most instances fewer than 10 adult organisms are present, but this number may range up to 200 or more. The lice move freely about on the body and are blood-sucking insects, which gives rise to the clinical features of pruritus and excoriations.

Differential Diagnosis

The differential diagnosis consists of entities that make the back itch, such as Grover's disease, acne, xerosis, dermatitis herpetiformis, and delusions of parasitosis.

Pediculosis Capitis (Head Lice)

Definition and Clinical Description

Pediculosis capitis is caused by the louse *Pediculus humanus capitis*. Infestation with head lice is quite common in school-aged children in the United States of all socioeconomic classes, except in blacks. The disease is spread from person to person through direct physical contact or through the use of fomites such as combs or other toilet articles, hats, scarves, and towels. Adult lice live for 1 to 2 months, and the female deposits four to six eggs per day on the most proximal part of the hair shaft, cementing them at an oblique angle with chitin in egg sacks referred to as nits. Pruritus is the first clinical symptom. The pruritus increases and is often accompanied by excoriations and secondary infection. More advanced cases feature lesions over the neck, ears, and upper back with associated local adenopathy. Chronic scratching as well as serous exudate often produces matted clumps of hair that are difficult to untangle.

Diagnosis and Differential Diagnosis

The diagnosis is confirmed by finding nits or adult mites. Confusing artifacts consist of hair spray, hair scale, and trichorrhexis nodosa. Important considerations in the differential diagnosis are conditions that produce an itchy scalp or impetiginization of the ears, neck, and shoulders such as seborrheic dermatitis, psoriasis, atopic eczema, and delusions of parasitosis.

Treatment

The standard of care involves eradication of all live lice, destroying the incubating larvae, nit removal, and treatment of secondary infection. Pyrethrins and synthetically related compounds are the mainstays in the treatment of head and body lice. Sold without prescription, these preparations (e.g., RID) require a second application approximately a week after the first, since they are not ovicidal.

Pyrethroids, synthetic derivatives of pyrethrins (e.g., permethrin [Nix]), have residual activity of 7 to 10 days and are also ovicidal. Thus they can be used as a single 10-minute treatment application.

Lindane (Kwell) is effective against adults but not against the nits, and therefore requires a second application after a week's interval. Combs are effective at removing the majority of nits.

All family members must be treated even if they do not exhibit signs or symptoms of the disease. All of the patient's household personal use items and bedding must be deloused. Combs, brushes, caps, scarves, and sheets, pillow cases, and other bedding should be thoroughly washed in hot water. However, it is not necessary to disinfect the entire house. Articles of personal hygiene can be soaked in rubbing alcohol or may be washed in a kitchen dishwasher.

Pediculosis Pubis (Pubic Lice)

Definition

Pediculosis pubis is a condition of infestation of the pubic hair with *Phthirus pubis* that is spread by sexual contact.

Clinical Description

Phthirus pubis, commonly called the pubic or crab louse, is morphologically distinct from the somewhat cylindrically shaped head and body lice. It is shorter and more rounded, has the compact shape of a crab, and has legs developed into heavy pinchers.

The disease is usually self-diagnosed because of the pruritus in the genital area and a sensation of insects crawling over the skin. There are usually many organisms and nits present that are often easy to see. In children who have been exposed to affected adults, the organisms will frequently take up residence in the eyelashes if the patient lacks appropriate pubic hair, producing itching and discharge from the eyes.

Pubic lice are not known to transmit any serious diseases, although impetigo normally accompanies their infestation.

Differential Diagnosis

The differential diagnosis includes other pruritic conditions of the groin, including tinea cruris, candidiasis, and simple intertrigo.

Treatment

The choice of agents is similar to that listed in the section for head lice and, as in that condition, repeated treatment is recommended.

Scabies

Definition and Clinical Description

Scabies is infestation with the human itch mite *Sarcoptes scabiei*, which is spread primarily by person-to-person contact, with fomites playing a lesser role. The adult female mite becomes fertilized on the surface of the skin, and then burrows into the stratum corneum at the rate of 2 to 4 mm per day, laying 2 to 3 eggs per day for a total 10 to 25 eggs. The larvae emerge after 3 to 4 days, going through several moltings and maturing in approximately 2 weeks. The adult female is an oval, whitish arthropod with four pairs of stubby legs.

The clinical manifestations begin several weeks after infestation, in part because it takes the host this long to become sensitized to the mite's excreta and saliva and because it also takes the mites a significant period of time to reach a noticeable population. The chief clinical symptom is notorious pruritus, which can occur on any part of the body but most commonly occurs on the hands, waist, and genital area. Repeated scratching produces widespread weeping eczematous patches that are frequently secondarily infected. Red-brown hyperkeratotic scaling nodules commonly develop near the axilla, on the genitalia, and on the trunk.

In infants, lesions may be distributed on all body parts, but in those older than age 3 or 4 years, lesions are usually confined from the neck to the toes.

Patients who are immunologically suppressed or who have a variety of neurologic disorders such as Down syndrome or severe depression often develop crusted (Norwegian) scabies with tremendous numbers of mites that live in a honeycomb of crust, serum, and debris.

Pathology

In a classic case, mites will be found from the stratum corneum throughout the upper layers of the epidermis in their burrows with an accompanying inflammatory response that usually features superficial and deep perivascular and interstitial collections of lymphocytes, histiocytes, eosinophils, and plasma cells.

Diagnosis and Differential Diagnosis

Scabies should be suspected in every patient who presents to the physician's office with a complaint of itching. Although the most diagnostic lesions are the burrows, a careful search may be necessary to identify them. Burrows are small, crooked lines 4 to 6 mm in length that are most common in the web spaces of the fingers, sides of the hands, flexor surfaces of the wrist, and (especially in the children) the lateral and medial surfaces of the foot nearest the heel. After a burrow is identified (which is easier with the aid of magnification), the lesion should be moistened, then scraped vigorously until it is deroofed. After each scraping the material is transferred to a slide, which is then covered with potassium hydroxide and then examined under low power. Diagnostic findings are of the mite itself, legs, eggs, egg cases, or the golden-brown fecal pellets. In cases where the scraping is negative, treatment should be instituted without proof of the existence of the mite.

The differential diagnosis consists of other pruritic diseases such as atopic dermatitis, insect bites, nummular eczema, psoriasis, prurigo nodularis, and delusions of parasitosis.

Treatment

Treatment is divided into four areas: (1) eradication of the mites on the patient; (2) treatment of associated problems such as pruritus, scabietic nodules, and impetigo; (3) treatment of personal contacts; and (4) destruction of the mite in the patient's surroundings.

Permethrin 5% (Elimite) and lindane (Kwell) are the mainstays of therapy. Ivermectin, given as a single oral dose, has recently been reported to be effective treatment for crusted scabies. Self-treatment should be performed from the neck to the toes; with particular attention to the crusted areas and around the fingernails. Applications should remain on 8 to 12 hours and then rinsed off. This treatment should be repeated in a week in all patients who have itching and visible lesions. Exposed but asymptomatic patients should be treated only once. Intermediate-potency topical steroids help decrease pruritus and should be used in most cases after the first application of a scabicide. The itching may continue for a period of weeks and occasionally months but this rarely indicates the presence of active scabies.

Used properly, both permethrin and lindane are safe, but lindane has the greatest potential for adverse reaction if it is misused (e.g., used on a daily basis, used two or three times a day). Toxicity from lindane poisoning usually takes the form of seizures. Consequently, patients who are prone to seizures should not be treated with this agent. Neither of these agents is proven safe in the treatment of pregnant women, but there have been no reported adverse fetal effects in widespread laboratory investigation and in clinical use.

Children may continue to develop small vesicles and pustules on the sides of the hands and feet without burrows that are repeatedly negative on scraping and do not respond to further treatment with scabicides of lindane or permethrin.

Since the scabies mite is not very mobile, it is not necessary to fumigate the entire house. Routine cleaning of the bedding, clothes, and personal articles using hot water washing cycles is probably all that is required.

chapter 7

What Diseases Alter Skin Color?

VITILIGO

(CM&S Chapter 130)

Definition and Clinical Description

Vitiligo is an acquired disorder of depigmentation characterized by loss of melanocytes from the epidermis, the mucous membranes, and other tissues.

A lesion of vitiligo typically presents as either a hypopigmented or snow-white well-circumscribed macule or patch, which is most easily noticed in dark-skinned and/or tanned individuals. In fair-skinned individuals, the sharp border of the lesions becomes apparent with Wood's light examination. The borders of the lesion can be trichrome in which almost the entire lesion or a narrow peripheral area within its margin may be light brown or tan or, less frequently, exhibits erythema, suggesting an inflammatory process.

In three fourths of cases a single lesion is initially noticed, whereas in the remaining cases multiple initial lesions that are bilateral and often remarkably symmetrical are observed. While vitiligo can affect any site, the face, joints, hands, and legs are most commonly affected. The progression of the disease is variable. New lesions can develop immediately after the initial macule, or there may be an extended period of time—up to years—before additional lesions develop. Lesions progress in size and number, sometimes at a slow rate and in some patients very rapidly. Adjacent lesions will frequently coalesce. In the course of the disease, periods of slow or rapid enlargement of the lesion, arrest in depigmentation, and spontaneous or partial repigmentation can occur. Eventually the number and size of vitiligo lesions on a patient become extremely heterogeneous. Vitiligo can be classified as focal, segmental, generalized, or universal based on the extent and distribution of cutaneous depigmentation.

Although the cutaneous depigmentation is almost always the primary and initial symptom in vitiligo, other symptoms and medical problems may be associated with this disease. The ocular and auditory changes observed in patients with vitiligo suggest that extracutaneous melanocytes may also be affected. In the eye, there are neural crest–derived melanocytes within the uveal tract and retinal pigment epithelium. Uveitis, chorioretinal depigmentation, iris and conjunctival depigmentation, and retinitis pigmentosa frequently occur in patients with vitiligo. Melanocytes exist within the stria vascularis of the cochlea in the inner ear and may contribute to the developmental or functional role of hearing. Partial sensorineural hearing loss and bilateral and unilateral hypoacusis in patients with vitiligo can occur.

Thyroid diseases (both hypothyroidism and hyperthyroidism as well as Graves' disease), diabetes mellitus, pernicious anemia, Addison's disease, multiglandular insufficiency syndrome, and alopecia areata all occur in patients with vitiligo. Vitiligo has also been reported in patients with Hodgkin's disease, multiple myeloma, dysgammaglobulinemia, cutaneous T-cell lymphoma, thymoma, and immune deficiency diseases such as AIDS.

Pathology

Vitiligo is caused by a loss of melanin from the epidermis, coupled with a decrease in the numbers of melanocytes in affected areas.

Pathogenesis and Etiology

The etiology of vitiligo is unknown. There appears to be a complex inheritance pattern that predisposes one to vitiligo. Current hypotheses for the pathogenesis of vitiligo have been classified into two broad categories that include intrinsic melanocyte dysfunction and/or death and an autoimmune-mediated destruction.

Differential Diagnosis

The differential diagnosis of vitiligo and other diseases of depigmentation/hypopigmentation is listed in Table 7–1.

TABLE 7–1. Differential Diagnosis of Vitiligo

CUTANEOUS DISORDERS WITH DEPIGMENTATION OR HYPOPIGMENTATION

Piebaldism
Lupus erythematosus
Tinea versicolor
Pityriasis alba
Lichen sclerosus et atrophicus
Cutaneous T-cell lymphoma
Sarcoidosis
Scleroderma
Nevus anemicus
Postinflammatory hypopigmentation
Idiopathic guttate hypomelanosis
Pityriasis lichenoides chronica
Chédiak-Higashi syndrome
Tuberous sclerosis
Hypomelanosis of Ito
Nevus depigmentosus

Treatment

Therapy can be divided into two general types: medical and surgical. Medical therapies include topical steroids and phototherapy. Surgical treatments include various forms of melanocyte grafts and tattooing.

Medical Therapies

Topical Steroids. Steroids have been used for years to treat vitiligo. Because treatment must be continued for many months, systemic steroids are not considered appropriate because of the numerous side effects. Topically applied steroids avoid systemic toxicity.

Topical steroids can be useful in children under the age of 10 years or for those with limited depigmentation. A low-potency (class 4 or 5) preparation applied only once daily for several months or longer is the optimal therapy. If repigmentation is not observed within 3 months, the applications should be discontinued and tried again 6 months later or another treatment tried.

Phototherapy. Psoralens and exposure to ultraviolet light in the 320- to 400-nm spectrum (PUVA) is the most common treatment for vitiligo. It can be employed on individuals aged 10 years or older. Generally the psoralens are taken by mouth, although topical psoralens are also used by some practitioners.

Topical PUVA. For topical use, 8-methoxypsoralen (8-MOP) or trimethylpsoralen (TMP) is dissolved at least 1:10 or preferably 1:100 in petrolatum or ethanol. Thirty minutes later, the treated skin is exposed to UVA beginning at 0.12 joule (J). Treatments are repeated twice weekly but never on consecutive days. The dose of UVA is increased 0.12 J per session until a slight erythema is produced. Treatment is continued for 3 months after the erythema dose is reached. If no evidence of repigmentation is observed by this time, treatment should be discontinued and tried again 6 months later.

Topical psoralens should never be used with direct sunlight because small errors produce severe second-degree burns. The patient must apply a UVA sunscreen immediately after treatment is complete and avoid all sun exposure for the remainder of the day, including that obtained through the windows of an office or car.

Systemic PUVA. Psoralens taken by mouth have a wider margin of safety, although they can produce severe burns or even death if not used with caution. The source of UVA is a medical phototherapy unit. The standard recommendation is for the patient to take 0.25 to 0.4 mg/kg of 8-MOP 1 hour before exposure to 1 to 2 J of UVA. The dose of UVA is increased by 1 J at each treatment until erythema is noted.

Systemic therapy is continued for 3 to 4 months. If no response is noted, treatment should be stopped and tried again in 6 months. It is continued as long as repigmentation is observed. Generally, 100 treatments given two to three times per week (never on consecutive days) are required. PUVA will not repigment glabrous skin or skin with white terminal hair.

Depigmentation. Depigmentation that involves more than half of the integument responds poorly to both medical and surgical therapies. For such individuals, total permanent depigmentation should be considered. Monobenzone is applied to the pigmented skin twice daily. The residual pigment disappears gradually, leaving the individual with an excellent outcome.

Surgical Therapies

Patients with small, stable areas of vitiligo are good candidates for surgical therapy, which is transplantation of autologous melanocytes into an area that has no pigment cells and cannot be repigmented by medical therapies. Surgical therapies include punch grafts, minigrafts, suction blisters, autologous cultures, and autologous melanocyte grafts. Repigmentation and spread of color begin about 4 to 6 weeks after the graft. Complications of surgical therapy include irregular pigmentation, depigmentation of the donor site, infection, scarring, and graft failure.

ALBINISM AND OTHER DISORDERS OF HYPOPIGMENTATION

(CM&S Chapter 131)

An absence of melanocytes, a decrease in the number of melanocytes, and a decrease in the function of melanocytes are three major explanations for observed decreases (hypopigmentation) or absence (depigmentation) of pigment.

Oculocutaneous and Ocular Albinism

In oculocutaneous albinism (OCA), an autosomal recessive condition, reduced or absent melanin production leads to pigmentary dilution of the eyes, hair, and skin. The degree of diffuse hypopigmentation that is observed is dependent on the specific type of OCA as well as the racial background of the patient. In the past, OCA was divided into two major clinical categories: tyrosinase-negative and tyrosinase-positive. This distinction was based on the presence or absence of melanin pigment and tyrosinase activity in the hair or skin of these patients. Tyrosinase is the major enzyme in the melanin biosynthetic pathway and therefore plays a key role in determining the degree of pigmentation.

At birth, individuals with albinism often have a similar appearance: the hair is white, the eyes are gray to blue, and the skin is pink to white. If the parents and siblings are skin type I or even II, the pigmentary dilution may go unnoticed. Individuals with tyrosinase-positive OCA may have lightly pigmented hair at birth, but as they age there is darkening of hair, eye, and skin color, the degree of which is dependent on racial background and the particular subtype of OCA. For example, a person with OCA and skin type IV or V can develop lentigines and have red to light brown hair and, if seen in the absence of his or her relatives, can be mistaken for an unaffected person with skin type I or II. However, a major clue to the diagnosis of OCA is the presence of ophthalmic abnormalities including nystagmus, decreased visual acuity, monocular vision, and photophobia. The decreased visual acuity is thought to be related to hypoplasia of the fovea (a relatively hyperpigmented portion of the retina), and the monocular vision is a reflection of a decrease in the ipsilateral fibers that run from the temporal retina to the visual cortex through the lateral geniculate body.

With the advent of molecular biology, there have been further refinements in the categorization of patients with OCA. OCA is classified into seven types, depending on the abnormalities in the tyrosinase gene and the classical findings (Table 7-2). One major group is now referred to as type I OCA or tyrosinase-related OCA; the latter name reflects the identification of abnormalities in the tyrosinase gene in these patients. Persons previously referred to as tyrosinase-positive are now categorized primarily as type II OCA. Because it is important to identify those individuals with Hermansky-Pudlak syndrome or Chédiak-Higashi disease, the evaluation of a patient with OCA should include ancestry as well as the possible history of a bleeding diathesis, recurrent infections, or shortness of breath.

Diagnosis and Differential Diagnosis

Diagnosis of OCA at an early age is important so that recommendations can be made regarding daily sunscreen use and limited sun exposure. Referral to an ophthalmologist for longitudinal care is also indicated. For an improved cosmetic appearance, the patient can try creams that contain dihydroxyacetone. As patients enter their 20s, they need to have total-body skin examinations on a regular basis to detect cutaneous malignancies, especially squamous cell carcinoma.

The differential diagnosis includes phenylketonuria, the Prader-Willi syndrome, histidinemia, homocystinuria, Apert's syndrome, copper deficiency, Menkes' kinky hair syndrome, malabsorption secondary to chronic pancreatic disease, selenium deficiency, and kwashiorkor. Generalized vitiligo is distinguished by its progressive nature, lack of eye findings characteristic of OCA, and, if present, prematurely gray (not lightly colored) hair. In addition, biopsy specimens of skin from patients with OCA contain a normal number of melanocytes.

Individuals with ocular albinism (OA) have the same eye findings as in OCA, but pigmentary dilution of the hair and skin is either absent or more subtle.

Piebaldism

In this autosomal dominant disorder, the areas of leukoderma are congenital and, in the majority of cases, stable in relative size and configuration. The cutaneous lesions favor the midforehead, the ventral trunk, and the midportions of the extremities but routinely spare the midline of the back. Within the patches of leukoderma, macules of normal and hyperpigmented skin 1 to 5 cm in diameter are often seen. Poliosis (circumscribed area of white hair) is seen most commonly in the midline of the frontal scalp as a white forelock in 80%–90% of patients. White hairs can also be found in the eyelashes, eyebrows, and areas of hypopigmentation. Multiple café-au-lait spots are often seen in uninvolved skin, and their presence does not require the diagnosis of a second genodermatosis. The majority of investigators have noted an absence of melanocytes or a markedly reduced number of melanocytes in the amelanotic areas. Deletions in the KIT gene (chromosome segment 4q12) have been identified in human piebaldism.

Treatment of piebaldism is difficult; psoralens and ultraviolet A (PUVA) light therapy and grafts of cultured melanocytes do not produce cosmetically significant results. Greater success has been reported with minigrafts of normally pigmented, autologous skin. It is important to screen patients with piebaldism for possible deafness and to be aware, especially in infants, of the association with Hirschsprung's disease (congenital megacolon).

Waardenburg's Syndrome

The classic sextad of Waardenburg's syndrome consists of dystopia canthorum (lateral displacement of the inner canthi), a broad nasal root, confluent eyebrows, iris heterochromia (total or partial), congenital sensorineural hearing loss (unilateral or bilateral), and a white forelock or piebaldism. In addition to the latter cutaneous findings (seen in 15% to 60% of patients depending on the series), premature graying of the hair has also been reported. Although Waardenburg reported an incidence of 99% for dystopia canthorum in his original series, the incidence in subsequent studies was significantly less. These discrepancies have been resolved by dividing Waardenburg's syndrome into three different forms, depending on the combination of physical findings. In the classical form (type I), a mutation in the *Pax-3/HuP2* gene (chromosome 2q37) has been identified. Waardenburg's syndrome, like piebaldism, can be associated with congenital megacolon (Hirschsprung's disease).

Nevus Depigmentosus

Nevus depigmentosus is a common birthmark, occurring in approximately 1 in 125 neonates. There is usually a single, well-demarcated hypomelanotic patch ranging in size from 0.5 to 10 cm. Less often, the distribution will be segmental or systematized (multiple streaks along the lines of Blaschko). It is fairly simple to distinguish nevus depigmentosus from nevus anemicus because the boundary of the former does not disappear with diascopy. However, the ash-leaf spot of tuberous sclerosis can have the same clinical and histologic appearance as nevus depigmentosus with partial loss of pigment and a decreased to normal number of melanocytes. If there is a single lesion and the child is asymptomatic, longitudinal observation is indicated; if there are multiple lesions or additional signs or symptoms suggestive of tuberous sclerosis, then diagnostic imaging can be performed.

Hypomelanosis of Ito

Patients with hypomelanosis of Ito have multiple streaks of hypopigmentation in addition to systemic abnormalities, especially neurologic, musculoskeletal, and ocular. Associated findings include mental retardation, seizures, craniofacial dysmorphism, triphalan-

Text continued on page 480

TABLE 7-2. Clinical Characteristics of the Different Forms of Oculocutaneous Albinism

CHARACTERISTIC	TYPE IA, TY-NEG	TYPE IB, YM	TYPE I, TS
Hair	White throughout life	White at birth; yellow-red by 6 months	White at birth; develops slight yellow tint (scalp); lower leg hair dark brown
Skin color	Pink to red	White at birth; cream, slight tan on exposed skin	Creamy white; slight tan
Pigmented nevi and freckles	Absent (nevi are nonpigmented)	Present	Present
Susceptibility to skin neoplasia	++++	++	
Eye color	Gray to blue	Blue in infancy; darkens with age	Blue
Red reflex	Present	Present	Present
	0	Present	0
Fundal pigment	++++	+ to +++	++++
Nystagmus	++++	+ to ++	++++
Photophobia			++++
Visual acuity	Majority legally blind; constant or worsens with age; 20/200 to 20/400+	20/90 to 20/400	20/200

474

Melanosomes in hair bulbs	Stages I and II only	To stage III pheomelanosomes	Stages I, II (scalp hair): stages, I, III, IV (leg hair)
Incubation of hair bulbs in tryosine Gene mutations	No pigmentation Tyrosinase gene (>35 different mutations lead to absence of enzymatic activity) (t^-/t^-)	None to questionable Tyrosinase gene (1 allele as in IA and 1 allele decreased enzyme activity vs two alleles decreased enzyme activity) (t^-/y vs y/y)	None (scalp hair) Tyrosinase gene (1 allele as in IA and 1 allele enzyme less active at higher temperatures)
Other	Heterozygotes have near zero tyrosinase activity; prenatal diagnosis possible by biopsy of scalp	Hair bulb test shows increased red or yellow with tyrosine-cysteine incubation	Hair bulb tyrosinase assay; loss of activity above 35° C–37° C; temperature-sensitive mutation

Continued

TABLE 7-2. Clinical Characteristics of the Different Forms of Oculocutaneous Albinism (*Continued*)

CHARACTERISTICS	TYPE I, MINIMAL PIGMENT	TYPE II, TY-POS	TYPE IV, BROWN OCA	TYPE V, RUFOUS OCA
Hair	White at birth to white or very slight yellow in adults	White, yellow tan; darkens with age	Beige to light brown in Africans	Mahogany red to deep red
Skin color	Pink-white, no tan	Pink-white to cream, lentigines but no tan	Cream to light tan on exposed skin; tans lightly	Reddish brown
Pigmented nevi and freckles	Absent	May be present and numerous	Uncommon	May be present
Susceptibility to skin neoplasia	Unknown, probably ++++	++++	Similar to whites in Africa+	Low
Eye color	Gray to blue	Blue, yellow-brown; age and race dependent	Hazel to light tan	Reddish brown to brown
Red reflex	Present	May be absent in darker-race adults	Present in children; may be absent in adults	Unknown

Fundal pigment	0 to ? in adults	0 to + in adults	+ to +++ in adults	+ to +++
Nystagmus	++++	++ to +++	+ to ++	0 to ++
Photophobia	++++	++ to +++	+ to ++	0 to ++
Visual acuity	20/160 to 20/200	Children, severe defect; adults, same or better; 20/200 to 20/400+	20/30 to 20/150	Normal to 20/100, most 20/30
Melanosomes in hair bulbs	Late stage II, some with melanin	To stage III, eumelanosomes	Stage I to Stage II, some lightly pigmented stage IV	Unknown
Incubation of hair bulbs in tryosine	Unknown	Pigmentation marked	Slight to no pigment increase	Pigmentation
Gene mutations	Tyrosinase gene (1 allele as in IA and 1 allele decreased enzyme activity)	P gene (chromosome 15q)	Unknown	Unknown
Other	Heterozygotes have zero to normal tyrosinase activity	Tyrosinase assay suggests heterogeneity	Tyrosinase activity normal; seen in New Guineans, Africans, and black Americans	Seen in New Guineans and Africans

Continued

TABLE 7-2. Clinical Characteristics of the Different Forms of Oculocutaneous Albinism (*Continued*)

CHARACTERISTICS	TYPE VIA, HPS	TYPE VIB, CHS	TYPE VII, AUTOSOMAL DOMINANT OCA
Hair	White, red, brown	Blond to dark brown; steel-gray tint	White to cream with reddish tint
Skin color	Cream-gray to light normal	Pink to pink-white	White to cream
Pigmented nevi and freckles	Present	Present	May be present
Susceptibility to skin neoplasia	+++	++	Unknown
Eye color	Blue-gray to brown; age and race dependent	Blue to dark brown	Gray to blue
Red reflex	Present in fair-skinned individuals; not in dark races	Present, less after 5 years	Present in children
Fundal pigment	0 to + in adults	+ to +++	0 to +

Nystagmus	+ to +++	+ to ++	++ to +++
Photophobia	+ to +++++	+ to ++	++ to +++
Visual acuity	20/70 to 20/400	Normal to moderate decrease	20/70 to 20/200
Melanosomes in hair bulbs	To stage III, pheomelanosomes and eumelanosomes	Macromelanosomes and normal to stage IV	Stage I to early stage III; no structural abnormality
Incubation of hair bulbs in tryosine	Pigmentation, slight increase	Pigmentation	Pigmentation; increased tyrosinase activity in Golgi bodies
Gene mutations	? Pallid gene	Unknown	Unknown
Other	Lysosomal disease, platelet-dense granules absent; ceroid storage (symptomatic in lungs and gastrointestinal tract)	Lysosomal disease; susceptibility to infection; giant lysosomal granules; platelet-dense granules can be absent; lymphoreticular malignancy	

Ym, yellow mutant; Ts, temperature sensitive; ty-neg, tyrosine negative; ty-pos, tyrosine positive; HPS, Hermansky-Pudlak syndrome; CHS, Chédiak-Higashi syndrome.

geal thumbs, and hypertelorism. The streaks of hypopigmentation can be unilateral or bilateral; and although the majority follow Blaschko's lines, lesions can also be patchy. The lesions are usually present at birth but may appear in early childhood; an increase in the extent of lesions during infancy can be followed by spontaneous repigmentation at a later age. Pathologic findings are not diagnostic. There is a reduction in the melanin content of the basal layer of the epidermis in association with either a normal or a decreased number of melanocytes. In contrast to incontinentia pigmenti, no dermal melanophages are seen, and this is one of the reasons that the name hypomelanosis of Ito is favored over that of incontinentia pigmenti achromians.

In the differential diagnosis, the major consideration is systematized nevus depigmentosus, and the distinction is made by the lack of associated systemic abnormalities. Other differential diagnoses include focal dermal hypoplasia (Goltz's syndrome), lichen striatus, segmental vitiligo, and late stage incontinentia pigmenti.

Idiopathic Guttate Hypomelanosis

Idiopathic guttate hypomelanosis affects approximately 50% of individuals in their 40s and more than 70% of those in their 60s. The lesions are well demarcated, range in size from 2 to 6 mm, and favor the extensor surfaces of the upper and lower extremities.

Treatment options are limited but ironically, successful results have been reported after a light freeze with liquid nitrogen. The major differential diagnosis is the confetti-like lesions of tuberous sclerosis, although nondermatologists often confuse the disease with vitiligo.

Hypopigmentation Secondary to Inflammation or Neoplasms

Several common inflammatory disorders such as psoriasis and atopic dermatitis can resolve, leaving areas of postinflammation hypopigmentation. There are several disorders that can present as just hypopigmentation in the absence of classic primary lesions, including atopic dermatitis (pityriasis alba), sarcoidosis, mycosis fungoides, pityriasis lichenoides chronica, lichen sclerosus et atrophicus, and alopecia mucinosa.

Pityriasis alba is a common disorder in children that favors the face. One theory for the associated hypopigmentation in pityriasis alba is a block in the transfer of melanosomes from melanocytes to keratinocytes as a result of inflammation and edema. Treatment options include mild topical corticosteroids, emollients, or PUVA therapy for extensive disease.

Hypopigmentation Secondary to Infectious Diseases

Hypopigmentation of the skin is associated with several infectious agents, including the bacteria *Treponema pertenue*, *Trep-*

onema carateum, and *Mycobacterium leprae*; the yeast *Pityrosporum orbiculare*; the protozoan *Leishmania donovani*; and the helminth *Onchocerca volvulus*.

MELASMA AND OTHER DISORDERS OF HYPERPIGMENTATION

(CM&S Chapter 132)

Disorders of hyperpigmentation have common clinical, histopathologic, and etiologic factors (Table 7–3). There are two patterns of hyperpigmentation. Brown hyperpigmentation or hypermelanosis results from increased melanin in the basal layer melanocytes and keratinocytes. Some hypermelanosis may be associated with dermal macrophages containing melanin. Slate-gray to blue pigmentation of the skin results from the Tyndall effect on pigment deposits in the dermis.

Melasma

Definition

Melasma is an acquired, brown hypermelanosis of the face that develops slowly and symmetrically. Although it has been associated with multiple etiologic factors (pregnancy and genetic, racial, and endocrine factors), sunlight appears to be one of the primary causes of its exacerbation.

Clinical Description

Melasma is more common in women and persons of Latino origin living in tropical areas. It has been reported in ½ to ¾ of pregnant women and in up to ⅓ of nonpregnant women taking birth control pills. Pregnancy- and contraceptive-related melasma are more common during the summer and in southern latitudes, probably secondary to sunlight exposure. Melasma in men shares the same clinicopathologic characteristics as in women, but hormonal factors do not seem to play a significant role.

Melasma presents as a symmetrical, irregular, light to dark brown hyperpigmentation of the face with three different clinical patterns: centrofacial (the most common, affected almost ⅔ of patients), malar, and mandibular. Melasma can be also classified on the basis of Wood's light (320–400 nm) examination. The three major types are (1) an epidermal type, which shows enhancement of the pigmentation; (2) a dermal type, with no enhancement of color; and (3) a mixed type that shows no or slight enhancement. These types correlate with the histologic deposition of melanin: epidermal, dermal, and epidermal and dermal, respectively. The epidermal type is the most common, occurring in 70% of patients, and the most amenable to treatment. The pigmentation in melasma is secondary to an increase in the number and activity of melanocytes, which appear highly dendritic with highly melanized melanosomes (mostly at stage IV).

TABLE 7-3. Disorders of Hyperpigmentation

HEREDITARY OR DEVELOPMENTAL DISORDERS

Incontinentia pigmenti
Dyskeratosis congenita
Poikiloderma congenitale (Rothmund-Thomson syndrome)
Acromelanosis progressiva
Dermal melanocytosis
  Nevus of Ota
  Nevus of Ito
  Mongolian spot

METABOLIC DISORDERS

Hemochromatosis
Niemann-Pick disease
Gaucher's disease
Macular and lichenoid amyloidosis
Ochronosis (endogenous)
Porphyria cutanea tarda
Wilson's disease

ENDOCRINE DISORDERS

Melasma (and other facial melanoses)
Addison's disease
MSH-producing neoplasm
Exogenous ACTH therapy

INFLAMMATORY DISORDERS

Erythema dyschromicum perstans
Lichen planus and variants
Lupus erythematosus
Pigmented contact dermatitis
Fixed drug eruption
Postinflammatory hyperpigmentation

CHEMICALLY INDUCED DISORDERS

Antimalarial agents
Tetracyclines
Heavy metals
Chemotherapeutic agents
Corticosteroids
Phenothiazides
Tar melanosis
Arsenic intoxication
Exogenous ochronosis
Berloque dermatitis
Amiodarone

NUTRITIONAL DISORDERS

Pellagra
Vitamin B_{12} deficiency
Kwashiorkor

NEOPLASTIC DISORDERS

Metastatic melanoma
Mastocytosis

Diagnosis and Differential Diagnosis

The diagnosis of melasma is usually made clinically. The differential diagnosis includes Riehl's melanosis, poikiloderma of Civatte, berloque dermatitis, postinflammatory hyperpigmentation, drug-induced hyperpigmentation, actinic lichen planus, exogenous ochronosis, and pigmented contact dermatitis.

Poikiloderma of Civatte refers to a sun-induced, reticulated, brownish pigmentation with telangiectases limited to sun-exposed areas such as the face, the sides of the neck, and the ''V'' of the chest.

Exogenous ochronosis refers to the pigmentary changes that occur after prolonged topical application of hydroquinones, phenol, or resorcinol. A blue-black pigmentation develops on the face, sides and back of the neck, upper aspects of the chest, and the extensor aspect of the extremities. The histopathologic changes are characteristic and consist of yellow-brown, bizarre-shaped collagen bundles with jagged, sharp edges that result from pigment deposits within the bundles. These findings mimic those seen in ochronosis, hence the name *exogenous ochronosis*.

Treatment

Therapy for melasma should begin with the identification and elimination of causative factors such as oral contraceptives and other hormone-containing drugs, photosensitizing drugs and cosmetics, and sunlight.

Broad-spectrum sunscreens with ultraviolet A (UVA) and ultraviolet B (UVB) light protection, sun protection with head wear, and sun avoidance are essential to treatment success.

Twice daily application of hydroquinone, an inhibitor of tyrosinase, used alone or in combination with topical steroids and retinoic acid, is the most commonly used agent in the treatment of melasma.

Results of treatment may be predictable from Wood's light testing. Epidermal pigment responds much more favorably to the other two patterns. Other potentially effective treatments include combining hydroquinone 5% with retinoic acid 0.1% and triamcinolone 0.1% (Kligman's formula), azaleic acid, chemical peel, and short-pulsed lasers such as the Q-switched ruby laser.

Chemically Induced Hyperpigmentation

Definition

The pigmentation from chemical exposure (see Table 7–3) may be induced by direct deposition of the chemical, stimulation of melanin formation, binding to melanin, and production of metabolites or nonmelanin pigments. Exposure to ultraviolet light seems to enhance hyperpigmentation in some of the cases. Offending agents include antimalarial agents, antibiotics, heavy metals, cancer chemotherapeutic agents, and topical preparations such as tar-containing compounds.

Clinical Description

The clinical presentation of chemically induced hyperpigmentation is highly variable. The pigmentation may be localized or diffuse; may involve hair, nails, and mucosa; and may vary from red or bright yellow to brown, blue-gray, or black.

The antimalarial agents, including chloroquine, hydroxychloroquine, and quinacrine, cause bluish black to slate-gray pigmentation of the face, extremities, oral mucosa, and nails. Those changes may be limited to the cartilaginous structures (pseudo-ochronosis). Mepacrine produces a yellowish discoloration of the skin.

Pigmentary change, which is rare, is a side effect of prolonged high-dose administration. The pigmentation may involve the skin, nails, bones, teeth, aorta, endocardium, and sclerae. These pigmentary changes may occur in three different forms: (1) blue-black pigmentation in the areas of previous inflammatory lesions, such as acne lesions; (2) involvement of the sun-exposed areas; and (3) diffuse ''muddy brown'' pigmentation that can affect the entire skin.

Heavy metals, such as gold, silver, and mercury, may cause skin pigmentation. Gold produces a characteristic slate-gray pigmentation in sun-exposed skin, while silver-induced pigmentation affects both sun-exposed and nonexposed areas, including sclerae, nails, and mucous membranes. Mercury-induced pigmentation usually involves the skin folds.

Cancer chemotherapeutic agents, particularly alkylating agents and antibiotics, are well recognized as a cause of hyperpigmentation. Of the alkylating agents, cyclophosphamide produces transverse or longitudinal brown to black pigmentation of the nails and teeth and busulfan may cause a dusky pigmentation of the face, forearms, chest, and abdomen, without a predilection for sun-exposed areas.

Of the chemotherapeutic antibiotics that may cause hyperpigmentation, bleomycin causes the characteristic linear or ''flagellate'' hyperpigmentation in areas of trauma, daunorubicin may produce a brown-black transverse hyperpigmentation of the fingernails and toenails, and doxorubicin may cause mucosal hyperpigmentation.

Prolonged use of phenothiazines, particularly chlorpromazine, may cause purplish skin hyperpigmentation that most commonly involves the sun-exposed areas, not dissimilar in appearance to amiodarone pigmentation.

Clofazimine, a commonly used antileprosy agent, usually causes a generalized redness that is followed by a dark-brown pigmentation.

Pathology and Pathogenesis

The pathology and pathogenesis of chemically induced hyperpigmentation depend on the etiologic agent. For example, the hyperpigmentation caused by antimalarial agents appears in the dermis as a dense amorphous material, probably composed of melanin and hemosiderin, while minocycline pigmentation may be a combination of minocycline, melanin, and hemosiderin; and the pigment in heavy metal pigmentation is the chemical itself.

Diagnosis

The diagnosis of chemically induced hyperpigmentation is often difficult to make. A thorough history and physical examination, and possibly a skin biopsy, may aid in making a correct diagnosis.

Treatment

Chemical-induced hyperpigmentation is often persistent. The most effective treatment is stopping the offending drug.

Erythema Dyschromicum Perstans (Ashy Dermatosis)

Definition and Clinical Description

Erythema dyschromicum perstans is a cutaneous disorder seen most commonly in people of Spanish or Indian descent. It has an unknown etiology characterized by widespread blue-gray-brown pigmented macules and patches that have an erythematous, raised border in the early stages. The most common locations are the face, neck, trunk, and upper limbs. In the late stage, the patches are gray-blue-brown with an ill-defined border. The lesions are usually asymptomatic, and the disease has a chronic, insidious course.

Pathology

Histopathologic examination of the active red border reveals vacuolar alteration of the basal layer, necrotic keratinocytes in the basal layer, and a sparse superficial perivascular lymphocytic infiltrate with many melanophages.

Pathogenesis and Etiology

The etiology of erythema dyschromicum perstans is unknown. There is controversy as to whether it is a variant of lichen planus, particularly lichen planus pigmentosus. However, on the basis of its unique clinical characteristics in the early stages, the distribution, and the chronic, asymptomatic course, it appears that erythema dyschromicum perstans is not a variant of lichen planus.

Diagnosis and Differential Daignosis

In its early stages, erythema dyschromicum perstans can be accurately diagnosed clinically. In subsequent stages it must be differentiated from lichen planus pigmentosus, postinflammatory hyperpigmentation, and macular amyloidosis.

Treatment

There is no effective treatment for erythema dyschromicum perstans.

Postinflammatory Hyperpigmentation

Definition and Clinical Description

Postinflammatory hyperpigmentation refers to the brown macules and patches that may be seen after any inflammatory condition of the skin, either endogenous or exogenous. Exogenous causes include physical and chemical agents that are used topically or systemically. Endogenous causes include lichen planus, discoid lupus erythematosus, macular amyloidosis, fixed drug eruption, and other primary inflammatory conditions of the skin.

In some cases, as in lichen planus and fixed drug eruption, the pigmentation is so distinctive that a retrospective diagnosis can be made. In most cases, however, the cause of the hyperpigmentation is not known.

Pathology and Pathogenesis

In late stages, postinflammatory hyperpigmentation is characterized histologically by a sparse, superficial perivascular infiltrate with melanophages. In earlier stages, one may find changes suggestive of the etiology. The melanin produced by the melanocytes, which increase in size, number, and activity after being stimulated by chemical irritation, ultraviolet light irradiation, and many diverse inflammatory conditions, is subsequently found in the dermis and is the cause of the hyperpigmentation seen clinically.

Treatment

Treatment of postinflammatory hyperpigmentation is often inadequate. Bleaching creams may be tried in those cases in which the pigment is more superficially located. Topical tretinoin (0.1% retinoic acid cream) is effective in lightening postinflammatory hyperpigmentation from acne in black persons.

Nevus of Ota and of Ito

Definition

Nevus of Ota and nevus of Ito are hamartomas of dermal melanocytes. These lesions may be present at birth or appear during the first year of life or adolescence.

Clinical Description

Nevus of Ota, which is uncommon in Caucasians but which affects one in every 200 Japanese, presents as a unilateral blue-brown speckled patch usually involving the malar region, periorbital area, temple, and forehead, but may also affect the eye, ocular muscles, periosteum, oral and buccal mucosa, and the retrobulbar fat. These lesions enlarge slowly, become deeper in color, and persist throughout life. They are more common in females (80%), and 5% to 10% are bilateral rather than unilateral. Nevus of Ota is benign, but in rare cases melanoma can arise within it.

Nevus of Ito differs from nevus of Ota only by the location in the supraclavicular, side of the neck, shoulder, and scapular areas.

Pathology

Both nevi demonstrate an increased number of elongated, dendritic melanocytes scattered throughout the dermis.

Treatment

The Q-switched ruby laser is effective at lightening most nevi of Ota with a low incidence of scarring.

Mongolian Spot

Definition and Clinical Description

The mongolian spot, most commonly found in Asian and black infants, is a congenital blue-gray patch usually localized in the sacral region. It rarely occurs at other sites such as the middle or upper back or as multiple lesions. Mongolian spots usually disappear spontaneously during childhood, although rarely they persist into adulthood. Dendritic dermal melanocytes scattered between collagen bundles disappear with age.

chapter 8

What Diseases Alter Hair, Nails, and Sweat Glands?

BIOCHEMISTRY AND CONTROL OF HAIR GROWTH AND ANDROGENETIC DISORDERS

(CM&S Chapter 133)

Anatomy

Hair Dynamics

The hair cycle is divided into three cycles; anagen, the active growth phase; catagen, the growth arrest phase; and telogen, the resting phase. The normal duration of anagen in human scalp hairs is genetically determined and ranges from 2 to 8 years, versus 1 to 6 months for body hair (eyelashes, trunk, extremities). The resting, telogen phase lasts approximately 100 days, regardless of their location.

The ratio of anagen to telogen hairs is approximately 90:10, since the percentage of hairs in catagen at any given moment is small. The average number of hairs shed per day is 100. The human scalp has approximately 100,000 follicles, with blondes having more and redheads fewer. Seasonal variation in human scalp hair follicles growth indicates that over 90% of hair follicles are in anagen in the spring, decreasing to about 80% at the end of summer. These are approximate figures representing the dynamics of follicular activity.

Biochemistry and Control of Hair Follicle Growth

Hair Types

In humans, hair follicles are classified into three types: nonsexual hair, ambosexual hair, and male sexual hair. Nonsexual hair is hair that grows independent of the presence of steroid hormones. These follicles are located on eyebrows, eyelashes, occipital scalp, forearms, and lower legs. Ambosexual hair is dependent on female levels of steroid hormones, localized in the lower pubic triangle, axillae, and other parts of the body. Male sexual hair is dependent on androgens and is localized to the beard, ears, nasal tip, pubis, and frontal to vertex scalp.

Hormonal Effects

The effects of hormones on the hair cycles have been studied in both humans and animals. Estrogens retard the rate of growth during anagen, and prolong the duration of anagen, while androgens have "dual" effects of stimulating and inhibiting hair growth; follicles on axillary, pubic, and beard hair grow in response to androgens, yet those on the scalp regress and recede in genetically susceptible men and women. The way that androgens exert their effect on hair growth is still not totally clear. The target tissue androgens testosterone and dihydrotestosterone have an effect on shortening the length of anagen; ironically, in other areas of the body they stimulate hair growth. Follicles as well as sebaceous glands can metabolize weak androgens, such as dehydroepiandrosterone and 4-androstenedione, to testosterone and dihydrotestosterone via enzymes such as 5α-reductase, in the steroid cascade.

Another enzyme in the pathway, aromatase, a cytochrome P-450 enzyme, is found at higher levels in hair follicles from the scalps of women than men. This enzyme is responsible for converting 4-androstenedone and testosterone to estrogens, such as estrone and estradiol, and it has been hypothesized to be important in mediating a balance of androgens in the hair follicle, thus regulating the hair cycle.

Once dihydrotestosterone or testosterone is formed, it binds to a specific intranuclear receptor protein, namely the androgen receptor, which then forms an "activated" hormone-receptor complex.

Thioredoxin, an enzyme system that influences intramolecular disulfide bonding of the androgen receptor, which affects hormone binding to its binding site, is found in high levels in anagen follicles but is diminished in balding areas. The low amounts may be a reflection of the balding process or may represent hair follicles that are in a metabolically resting telogen state.

Androgenetic Disorders

Definition

Androgenetic alopecia is an inherited, androgen-dependent form of hair loss. Synonyms include common baldness, male-pattern baldness, female-pattern baldness, and diffuse alopecia of women.

Clinical Description

The prevalence of androgenetic alopecia has not been accurately recorded in any population. It may approximate 100% in Caucasians, in contrast to other races. Male androgenetic alopecia has been classified by Hamilton into eight types, from Type I (normal scalp before puberty) to Type VIII (extensive baldness). Hamilton found that over one half of men who were 50 years of age and older had Type V to Type VIII, and the extent of baldness was noted to increase with aging.

In male androgenetic alopecia, there is a continuing decrease in the percentage of hairs in the anagen phase, total hair density, and meaningful hair density. A greater than 15% decrease in hair density has to take place before patients became aware of a change in hair density. A large proportion of hairs less than or equal to 40 mm in length with diameters similar to those of longer hair fibers are found.

The "male" pattern of alopecia does occur in women, but a more common presentation is widening of the part width associated with a diffuse pattern of scalp hair loss on the crown and preservation of the frontal hair line. In Ludwig's classification, women with Grade I show perceptible thinning of hair on their crown with no loss of the frontal hairline and a relatively normal part width. Women with Grade II have pronounced thinning of the hair on the crown and an increase in their part width diameter and those with Grade III show extreme baldness on the crown and further widening of their part width. Hamilton found that about 25% of women had Type IV androgenetic alopecia by the age of 50. There is a correlation between decreased circulating estrogen levels and an increased presentation of patterned androgenetic alopecia. Many, if not all women experience a change in their scalp hair pattern after puberty, and classic male-type Hamilton patterns have been frequently noted in women after they experienced menopause.

Men with more extensive balding, younger men, single men, and those with an earlier hair-loss onset have less body image satisfaction, are considerably preoccupied with their hair problem, and have moderate stress compared to nonbalding controls. The presence of androgenetic alopecia is especially stressful for women. Affected women have been shown to have a more negative body image and a pattern of less adaptive functioning than affected men.

The presence of androgenetic alopecia in males has been hypothesized to be a predictor of cardiovascular disease. The risk of myocardial infarction has been found to significantly increase as the degree of vertex baldness increased.

Pathology

The main histopathologic findings in male androgenetic alopecia derive from shortening of the follicular cycle, coupled with incomplete descent of hair bulbs in anagen. With each successive cycle, anagen resumes in follicles whose bulbs are smaller and more superficially situated, producing progressively more narrow hair shafts. In biopsy specimens of evolving andogenetic alopecia, there are increased numbers of catagen and telogen follicles and anagen follicles of intermediate size.

Pathogenesis and Etiology

The genetic inheritance in both men and women is believed to be autosomal dominant with variable penetrance, but a multifactorial inheritance has not been excluded. Androgens are the other major linked factor. When testosterone is administered to males castrated prior to puberty, androgenetic alopecia develops only in those presumed to be genetically predisposed. When administration of the hormone testosterone is discontinued, the balding process does not progress, but it also does not reverse. Levels of circulating free or total androgens are usually normal in individuals predisposed to developing androgenetic alopecia. Individuals with complete androgen insensitivity syndrome also have relatively normal testosterone levels but lack functional androgen receptors. Such individuals exhibit a female phenotype but at adolescence do not develop any terminal body hair or pubic or axillary hair. They also do not develop balding.

In target tissues, testosterone is reduced by the enzyme 5α-reductase to 5α-dihydrotestosterone. Early studies noted that 5α-reductase enzyme activity is increased in hair follicles of balding scalp, but not in nonbalding scalp, but this finding has not been reproducible. 5α-reductase–deficient individuals have less temporal hair regression.

Diagnosis and Differential Diagnosis

Hyperandrogenism implies an elevated androgen concentration or an exaggerated clinical response to androgen action. Clinical features may include any of the following: hirsutism, acne, primary or secondary amenorrhea, increased libido and muscle mass, loss of breast tissue, deepening of the voice, infertility, and clitoral enlargement, as well as androgenetic alopecia. Androgenetic alopecia not associated with an underlying endocrinologic disturbance is considered "idiopathic" and is the main presentation of androgen excess in the majority of women. However, between 30% and 40% of women with androgenetic alopecia will have an underlying adrenal or ovarian disorder to explain their androgenetic alopecia.

The main causes of androgen dysfunction in females include abnormalities in the pituitary/adrenal and pituitary/ovarian axes or abnormal target cell hormone metabolism and utilization. Subtle defects can also exist in the adrenal steroidogenic pathway and these can contribute to androgen-mediated diseases. Abnormalities in the enzyme pathway can be diagnosed only by adrenocorticotropic hormone (ACTH) stimulation tests because basal blood hormone levels do not usually reveal these subtle abnormalities.

The evaluation of the male or female patient who presents with hair loss should include taking a good medical history and a careful assessment of drug use. The appearance of thin, sparse hair on the crown of the head of women has been associated not only with androgen excess but also thyroid disease, particularly hypothyroidism, and abnormal iron metabolism. If indicated, the laboratory evaluation should consist of assessing thyroid function, serum ferritin, and other parameters of iron metabolism, and an assessment of androgen metabolism. The laboratory assessment of women with treatment-resistant acne or hirsutism or alopecia includes assessing DHEA-S, free testosterone, SHBG, and total testosterone. In women with more severe disease, other tests to be performed include an ACTH stimulation test and 17-hydroxyprogesterone. If menstrual dysfunction accompanies the other findings, a prolactin level, luteinizing hormone and follicle-stimulating hormone levels and a serum estradiol level should also be obtained.

Treatment

Treatments for androgenetic alopecia range from nonhormonal therapy with topical minoxidil to the experimental use of antiandrogens and various combinations of medical and surgical treatment. Topical 2% minoxidil (Rogaine) is a piperidinopyrimidine derivative that is effective in the treatment of androgenetic alopecia. Minoxidil has been widely tested in multicenter trials and in the United

States is approved by the Food and Drug Administration for the therapy of androgenetic alopecia in both men and women. Hair growth appears to peak at 1 year, but maintenance of nonvellus hair beyond that seen at baseline can still be found in patients on long-term therapy—up to 5 years. Discontinuing therapy is associated with loss of the hair gained within 4 to 6 months of stopping the drug. The best responders are those in whom the balding process is relatively early, the pretreatment hair density is greater than 20 hairs/cm^2, and the maximum diameter of the bald area is less than 10 cm. The mechanism by which minoxidil induces hair regrowth remains to be elucidated, but may be related to the drug having a direct effect on the proliferation of follicular cells. Side effects are minimal and include local irritation and facial hypertrichosis. Adding topical tretinoin to topical minoxidil therapy may produce an additive effect.

Antiandrogens have been used topically and administered orally or intralesionally to retard the extension of androgenetic alopecia.

The competitive inhibitors—those compounds structurally similar to testosterone or dihydrotestosterone such as progesterone and 17α-hydroxyprogesterone—have been used to treat androgenetic alopecia. However, these antiandrogens also have the potential to provoke the process because of their androgenic potential. No controlled, large-scale studies have been performed to confirm the efficacy of this approach.

When choosing an oral contraceptive, not only the progestational agent needs to be considered but also the estrogen component. The estrogen component decreases ovarian and adrenal androgen production and stimulates SHBG, which binds to free circulating androgens. Although there is evidence that higher dose estrogen pills and mid-potency oral contraceptives are effective in treating hirsutism, there are no well-controlled studies to support one product over another in treating androgenetic alopecia.

In postmenopausal women, estrogen supplementation (without progestin) has been suggested as a useful therapy for androgenetic alopecia as well as acne and hirsutism. Topical estrogen-containing hair preparations have also been used to treat androgenetic alopecia. However, no topical estrogen-containing hair preparations are approved for the treatment of androgenetic alopecia in the United States. In addition, no controlled studies are available on the usefulness of this modality.

The oral administration of finasteride, a 5α-reductase inhibitor, alone or in combination with topical 2% minoxidil is presently undergoing study for the therapy of male androgenetic alopecia.

Other approaches to the management of androgenetic alopecia include wearing creative hairstyles and using correct shampoos and conditioners, mousses, colorants, and styling gels. Surgical treatment of androgenetic alopecia is based on surgical removal of the affected area and replacement with hair-bearing skin. Hair grafting, scalp reduction, scalp lifting, and temporo-parietal flaps are the hair replacement techniques used. The underlying principle of hair replacement surgery is the concept of donor dominance. Donor dominance refers to skin flaps or characteristics regardless of the properties of the recipient site onto which they are placed.

ALOPECIA AREATA AND OTHER NONSCARRING ALOPECIAS

(CM&S Chapter 134)

Alopecia Areata

Definition and Clinical Description

Alopecia areata is clinically recognized as patchy hair loss that may occur in any hair-bearing area on the body surface. The process is mediated by lymphocytic infiltrates in and around hair bulbs. Extensive involvement may result in total scalp hair loss (alopecia totalis), total body hair loss (alopecia universalis), diffuse scalp hair loss (diffuse alopecia areata), or localized hair loss along the scalp margin (ophiasis).

In alopecia areata, extensive body hair loss may be present, sometimes for many years, before the onset of patchy loss of scalp hair. Nail abnormalities, predominantly nail pitting, may precede or occur in conjunction with active alopecia areata.

Itching, tingling, burning, or painful sensations frequently occur at the sites of hair loss. These sensations may begin 1 to 2 weeks before or during the time of active hair shedding; thus, patients can often predict where their next areas of hair loss will occur.

Exclamation point hairs, when present, are diagnostic of alopecia areata. These characteristic hairs fracture at their distal end as they taper and lose pigment proximally toward the scalp, giving them the appearance of an exclamation point. During periods of active disease, telogen hairs are readily pulled from the periphery of patches. In diffuse alopecia areata or disease rapidly progressing to alopecia totalis or universalis, telogen and rarely anagen hairs may be easily pulled anywhere on the scalp surface. The skin surface in involved areas may appear normal, slightly erythematous and/or scaly, slightly hyperpigmented, and rarely depigmented.

Alopecia areata is thought to be an autoimmune disorder. Atopy, thyroid disease, vitiligo, and lupus erythematosus and other autoimmune disorders are more common in patients with alopecia areata. The incidence of alopecia areata is increased in patients with lichen planus and Down syndrome. A positive family history of alopecia areata occurs in about 20% of patients.

The course of alopecia areata is difficult to predict. Some patients have minimal transient hair loss followed by spontaneous regrowth and no further hair loss. Other patients have a few chronic stable patches of hair loss that may last many years. Patients with extensive disease usually have a chronic or chronically recurrent problem with hair loss. The alopecia may be extensive from its onset or may evolve to a more extensive form with repeated flares of hair loss. Pigmented hairs may be shed while white hairs are spared. Regrowing hairs may initially be white and later darken to a normal shade. Regrowing hair is usually but not always of normal texture.

Poor prognosis of alopecia areata is associated with childhood onset of disease, atopy, ophiasis, and/or onychodystrophy.

Pathology

Patches of active alopecia areata show increased numbers of catagen and telogen hairs, with infiltrates of mononuclear cells in and around hair bulbs.

Differential Diagnosis

The differential diagnosis of alopecia areata includes trichotillomania, tinea capitis, syphilis, telogen effluvium, androgenetic alopecia, and loose anagen syndrome.

Treatment

Because of the enormous psychosocial significance of alopecia areata, *key elements to treat it effectively* include (1) helping the patient understand the disease, (2) encouraging the patient to share his or her feelings about the disease, and (3) helping the patient to maintain a sense of hope for future scientific knowledge and treatment of the disease.

Of the large number of treatments tried for severe alopecia areata, none is uniformly effective and some are not safe for long-term use. All topical treatments for alopecia areata must be tried for a minimum of 3 months since early hair regrowth may not occur before that time.

Mild disease, defined as stable patches involving less than 25% of the scalp, can be treated successfully with intralesional or midpotency topical steroids. Daily shampoos are recommended to minimize the potential for folliculitis. If no response is obtained or if the response plateaus, topical anthralin cream 1.0% (Drithocreme) can often be effectively substituted. It is applied for 10 to 20 minutes daily to the patch and 1 cm of adjacent scalp skin and then shampooed off the scalp. Combining steroids and anthralin seems to decrease the efficacy of each of them. Some patients will also respond to topical minoxidil (Rogaine).

Extensive disease, defined as greater than 25% scalp hair loss, can respond to topical steroids or anthralin. Because these patients often develop new patches during treatment, medication should be applied to the entire scalp to maximize the likelihood of cosmetically adequate regrowth. Treatment of only patches often results in "chasing" the disease and is less likely to elicit a cosmetic effect.

Treatment of resistant disease is very difficult. Combination therapies such as topical minoxidil plus topical steroid or topical minoxidil plus topical anthralin appear to offer a therapeutic advantage. It is often a temptation to use systemic steroids or psoralens and ultraviolet A light (PUVA) to treat these patients. If appropriate combinations of topical treatments cannot control a flare of the disease or enhance regrowth, then the patient will often require either lengthy or frequent courses of systemic steroids or PUVA, exposing the patient to the attendant risks of such treatments.

Diffuse Alopecia

Definition and Clinical Description

Excessive telogen (club) hair shedding usually produces a diffuse alopecia that may or may not be clinically obvious. A variety of hormonal (hypothyroidism, hyperthyroidism, pregnancy, and androgenetic alopecia) and nutritional factors (weight loss, protein–calorie malnutrition, iron deficiency, zinc deficiency, and biotin deficiency), ingestion of various drugs (oral contraceptives), exposure to certain chemicals, systemic and local cutaneous disease (fever, chronic systemic illness, and surgery), as well as psychological stress have all been associated with telogen hair shedding. Prognosis for hair regrowth is usually good if the cause can be found and eliminated and if the patient does not have associated androgenetic alopecia.

A decrease of at least 25% of scalp hairs may be necessary for an objective observer to consistently diagnose diffuse alopecia. Examination of scalp and body hair for density and distribution as well as comparative assessment of part width at several sites on the scalp should be done. The parts should be observed from a tangential vantage point for evidence of short hairs of normal texture (regrowing hairs) versus short hairs of visibly diminished shaft diameter (indeterminate hairs of androgenetic alopecia). Evidence of underlying scalp and/or other cutaneous or systemic disease or nail changes should be sought.

The light hair pull test should be performed at several sites on the scalp by pinching approximately 20 hairs between the thumb and index finger and gently pulling. If any anagen hairs are extracted, then further evaluation is definitely warranted. In a normal situation fewer than two telogen (club) hairs are extracted per light pull. If more hairs are pulled, abnormal telogen shedding is likely. The light pull test may be falsely negative if the patient's hair has recently been combed, brushed, or shampooed.

Daily hair collections can be placed into separate envelopes and marked with the date, number of hairs collected, and whether the patient shampooed his or her hair on that day. Normally 50 to 100 telogen hairs are shed per day.

Treatment

Identification and elimination of the etiologic factors responsible for hair loss is the best treatment if possible. Prognosis for hair regrowth is generally good if the cause of the alopecia can be found and eliminated or adequately treated and if the patient does not have associated androgenetic alopecia.

SCARRING ALOPECIA

(CM&S Chapter 135)

Definition

Clinically, scarring alopecias are characterized by permanent hair loss with partial or complete loss of follicular orifices. Scarring alopecias may be either primary or secondary, depending on the pattern of follicular destruction. Primary scarring alopecia is defined as preferential destruction of hair follicles and/or associated adventitial dermis. In primary scarring alopecias, the hair follicle is the primary target of destruction and alteration as the result of inflammation, interface alteration, infection, and/or vesicle formation. The interfollicular epidermis may be affected in some primary scarring alopecias (e.g., discoid lupus erythematosus and lichen planopilaris), but the epidermal changes in and of themselves do not result in follicular destruction.

The destruction of hair follicles in secondary scarring alopecia results from nonfollicular events that impinge on the follicular unit (e.g., alteration of the reticular dermis, epidermis, or subcutis that eventually eradicates the follicle). Examples of pathomechanisms resulting in secondary scarring alopecia include reticular dermal sclerosis, neoplasia, and nonfolliculocentric inflammation (i.e., sarcoidosis).

Permanent "scarring" alopecia may also occur in diseases that have not been traditionally considered cicatricial. This group of alopecias generally results from persistence of abnormalities of follicular dynamics, eventually causing "dropout" of affected follicles. Examples of this type of permanent alopecia include chronic, ongoing traction alopecia and trichotillomania, as well as persistent, nonremitting alopecia areata, androgenetic alopecia, and telogen effluvium. In addition, certain hair shaft abnormalities may result in permanent partial alopecia. Finally, permanent scarring alopecia may be a feature of several inherited genodermatoses.

Primary Scarring Alopecias

Pustulofollicular Primary Scarring Alopecias

The term *pustulofollicular primary scarring alopecias* is used to classify a group of alopecias that have some clinical and microscopic similarities on the basis of clinical and microscopic pustules and purulent follicular infiltrates.

Dissecting Cellulitis of the Scalp (Perifolliculitis Capitis Abscedens et Suffodiens)

Clinical Description. The lesions most commonly begin on the vertex or occiput as relatively painless, deep-seated, firm to fluctuant nodules and abscesses. The nodules and deep abscesses commonly extend to form a complex serpiginous or reticulate pattern of interconnecting sinuses and abscesses filled with purulent, seropurulent, or hemopurulent material. Pressure applied to one nodule or abscess can cause purulent exudate to emerge several centimeters away. The epidermal surface overlying the sinuses and nodules may or may not be erythematous and scaly. Scattered superficial follicular pustules are frequently present on the surface of the nodules. Hypertrophic and keloidal scarring may occur in affected areas.

Dissecting cellulitis of the scalp is more common in young to middle-aged black men. It may occur simultaneously with acne conglobata and hidradenitis suppurativa. This complex is known as the follicular occlusion triad. The pathogenesis of dissecting cellulitis of the scalp is poorly understood.

Pathology. Biopsy specimens from well-developed fluctuant nodules and sinuses reveal large, perifollicular, mid to deep reticular dermal abscesses often rich in plasma cells. Abscesses are located immediately adjacent to follicles, between follicles in the mid and deep reticular dermis, and subjacent to follicles within the superficial subcutis. Dense dermal fibrosis eventually surrounds the sinus tracts and the affected follicles are destroyed by the fibroinflammatory process. Bacteria may be present within dilated follicular infundibula but are not routinely observed within the dermal abscesses.

Differential Diagnosis. The differential diagnosis of dissecting cellulitis of the scalp includes other pustulofollicular alopecias: folliculitis decalvans, acne keloidalis nuchae, and erosive pustular dermatosis of the scalp.

Treatment. A permanent cure is rarely achieved in patients with dissecting cellulitis of the scalp. Initial therapy frequently involves oral antibiotics such as tetracycline (1 to 2 g per day), doxycycline (200 mg per day), and minocycline (50 to 200 mg per day). Combination antibiotic therapy of cephalexin (1 g per day) and rifampin (600 mg per day) have also been helpful. Intralesional corticosteroid injections (triamcinolone acetonide, 40 mg/mL) can be helpful in noninfectious nodules and sinuses. Oral corticosteroids, isotretinoin (1 mg/kg per day), and dapsone have been successfully used. Assessment of glucose-6-phosphate dehydrogenase level and follow-up evaluation for hemolytic anemia and methemoglobinemia are essential in dapsone-treated patients. Oral zinc has also been reported to be effective.

Surgical therapy may be considered in advanced cases but is usually quite deforming. Complete scalp excision, carbon dioxide laser excision, or more conservative local incision and drainage of individual lesions may be considered.

Acne Keloidalis Nuchae

Clinical Description. Acne keloidalis nuchae is a destructive pustulofollicular process of unknown etiology that invariably occurs on the occipital scalp and posterior neck and primarily affects young black men. The lesions begin as discrete follicular pustules and papules but progress to form less discrete, large, exophytic keloidal nodules and plaques largely devoid of hair. The severity of involvement is variable and ranges from few small follicular pustules and papules with minimal alopecia to extensive keloidal plaque formation with prominent patterned alopecia. Similar lesions may occur in the beard area of patients with pseudofolliculitis barbae.

Pathology. Early lesions are characterized by comedonal dilatation of the follicular infundibulum similar to that seen in folliculitis decalvans and dissecting cellulitis of the scalp. The inflammation in older lesions consists of perifollicular and perivascular predominantly lymphoplasmacytic infiltrates with fewer neutrophils. Perifollicular granulomatous inflammation may also be present.

Differential Diagnosis. The typical distribution and morphology of acne keloidalis nuchae readily suggest the correct diagnosis. The differential diagnosis includes bacterial folliculitis, cylindroma, trichilemmal cyst, proliferating pilar tumor, cutaneous metastasis, and other tumors.

Treatment. Long-term oral antibiotics such as tetracycline (1 g per day), doxycycline (200 mg per day), minocycline (50 to 100 mg per day), or erythromycin (1 g per day) are useful in inflammatory pustular lesions. Topical antibiotics in a drying vehicle (2% erythromycin and 1% clindamycin) are also helpful. The combination of oral or topical antibiotics with tretinoin cream or gel is helpful for preventing formation of new lesions and fairly effective for resolution of minimally scarred lesions. Topical benzoyl peroxide and sulfurated solutions may also be used.

Intralesional corticosteroid injections into large and small papules and plaques are helpful in reducing inflammation and size of the lesions. Superpotent corticosteroids may also reduce inflammation but may exacerbate the acneiform component of this disorder.

Large, keloidal nodules and plaques are generally unresponsive to medical therapy and require surgical excision for removal. However, keloid recurrence at the site of excision may recur, and therefore close clinical follow-up and prophylactic intralesional corticosteroid injections into the surgical excision site are recommended.

Folliculitis Decalvans

Clinical Description. Folliculitis decalvans primarily affects the scalp of both sexes and results in patches of patterned alopecia, but involvement of beard, axillary, pubic, and inner thigh hair has also been reported. In classic folliculitis decalvans, well-developed clinical lesions consist of irregular- to oval-shaped atrophic patches of alopecia with small follicular pustules present at the advancing edge of the patch of alopecia. In progressive folliculitis decalvans, the area of scalp affected by the scarring alopecia gradually enlarges and multiple sites of involvement are present. Extensive scarring alopecia may result. Older, inactive patches of folliculitis decalvans in which pustules are not present closely resemble pseudopelade of Brocq. The etiology of folliculitis decalvans is unknown.

Pathology. In early lesions, comedonal follicular infundibular dilatation is present with neutrophillic infiltrates. In more advanced lesions, follicular destruction is evident and large numbers of admixed lymphocytes and plasma cells are present around the affected follicles.

Differential Diagnosis. The differential diagnosis of folliculitis decalvans includes bacterial folliculitis, dermatophytic infection, and pseudopelade.

Treatment. Oral and topical antibiotics are the mainstay of therapy as in dissecting cellulitis of the scalp.

Tinea Capitis, Kerion, Favus

Follicular dermatophyte infections lead to a permanent scarring alopecia. Other scalp infections that may lead to a scarring alopecia such as herpes zoster are not folliculocentric and therefore are considered secondary scarring alopecias.

Uncomplicated tinea capitis is a common childhood infection and does not cause a scarring alopecia. However, two subtypes of tinea capitis—kerion and favus—may result in permanent hair loss. Kerion is a very inflammatory form of tinea capitis that is most commonly caused by a zoophilic or geophilic dermatophyte infection. Kerions are characterized by well-circumscribed, crusted, boggy plaques with decreased follicular density and numerous broken hair shafts. Cervical adenopathy and an accompanying eczematous ''id'' eruption are common.

Favus is an uncommon chronic dermatophyte infection of the scalp seen in rural areas and associated with poor hygiene and poor nutrition. Clinical lesions are characterized by cup-shaped yellow crusts (scutula) that may progress to patches of scarring alopecia. The etiologic agent is usually *Trichophyton schoenleinii.*

Pathology. The follicular infundibula are dilated and filled with keratin and neutrophils. The infundibular epithelium is frequently ruptured and surrounded by dense perifollicular mixed inflammation. Endothrix (hyphae within hair shafts) and ectothrix (hyphae around hair shafts) dermatophyte infections are usually detectable on routine hematoxylin and eosin–stained sections but are best seen in periodic acid–Schiff-stained or silver-impregnated sections.

Treatment. See Chapter 6 in this text (Chapter 118 in CM&S).

Lymphocyte-Associated Primary Scarring Alopecias

Pseudopelade of Brocq

Clinical Description. The alopecia is usually patterned and consists of round to irregularly shaped patches of complete or near-complete alopecia most commonly on the vertex or crown. In classic cases of pseudopelade of Brocq, the skin in the patches of alopecia is smooth, shiny, and atrophic. Scattered isolated hairs may be present in the patches of alopecia. In addition, minimal perifollicular erythema and scale may be present at the periphery of some of the alopecic patches. Onset is usually between 25 and 45 years of age, and there is a female predominance. The etiology of pseudopelade of Brocq is unknown.

Some authors believe that pseudopelade of Brocq is not a distinct clinicopathologic entity but only represents a form of end-stage alopecia caused by other scarring alopecias such as discoid lupus erythematosus, lichen planopilaris, and folliculitis decalvans.

Pathology. Early lesions are characterized by perifollicular and perivascular lymphocytic infiltrates of variable density *without* associated interface alteration. In advanced lesions, the follicular epithelium is entirely destroyed, and only naked hair shafts surrounded by histocytic and foreign body giant cell inflammation remain.

Differential Diagnosis. The combination of clinical and microscopic features of this form of scarring alopecia without preceding cutaneous lupus erythematosus, lichen planus, or folliculitis warrants the designation of a separate scarring alopecia, termed *pseudopelade of Brocq*.

Treatment. Topical corticosteroid cream or solution may be used as a palliative treatment. No effective therapy exists for pseudopelade of Brocq, and irreversible scarring alopecia results.

Lichen Planopilaris (Follicular Lichen Planus)

Clinical Description. Lichen planopilaris is more common in women between 30 and 70 years of age. Early lesions consist of acuminate, spinous, and hyperkeratotic follicular papules with perifollicular erythema. The hair follicles are subsequently destroyed, yielding atrophic, irregular, especially angular or polygonal shaped patches of alopecia with similar follicular papules at the periphery of the patch of alopecia. In addition, similar spinous follicular papules as well as more typical lichen planus lesions are frequently present elsewhere on the body, including mucous membranes and nails. The pathogenesis of lichen planopilaris is unknown.

The clinical triad of classic plaque-type lichen planus, spinous or acuminate lesions, and alopecia of the scalp or other hairy areas has been described as the Graham-Little syndrome. The main symptom is pruritus. Acuminate lesions, the most consistent clinical feature, are dilated hair follicles filled with keratin plugs and perifollicular erythema occurring at any hair-bearing site, including the scalp, chest, back, axillae, and groin. The other manifestations may or may not be present. When scalp involvement occurs, initial perifollicular erythema is often followed by the follicular acuminate papules. The lesions progress to smooth patches of hair loss, and in the scalp, scarring alopecia is a common sequela. End-stage lesions frequently exhibit a permanent loss of pilosebaceous units and may clinically resemble pseudopelade of Brocq.

Pathology. Lichenoid interface alteration of the epidermis and follicular epithelium is characteristic of lichen planopilaris.

Differential Diagnosis. The differential diagnosis of lichen planopilaris includes pseudopilade of Brocq, chronic cutaneous lupus erythematosus, and discord lupus erythematosus.

Treatment. The course of lichen planopilaris usually resembles that of typical lichen planus (see Chapter 2 in this text or Chapter 20 in CM&S) and can last several months to several years.

Therapy is directed at controlling perifollicular inflammation and pruritus. High-potency topical corticosteroids and oral corticosteroids are the most effective therapies in lichen planopilaris.

Discoid Lupus Erythematosus

Clinical Description. Discoid lupus erythematosus is a common form of chronic cutaneous lupus erythematosus (for detailed information, see Chapter 2 in this text or Chapter 24 in CM&S). Lesions are most commonly located on the face, scalp, and inner ear. Approximately 50% of patients have scalp lesions, and in 10% of patients, scalp involvement may be the sole manifestation of discoid lupus.

Early lesions consist of small erythematous papules or irregular small, scaly plaques that expand to form round to irregular shaped atrophic, sclerotic plaques. Thick, adherent scale frequently develops that when removed reveals keratinous plugs on its undersurface. These follicular plugs are the mirror image of dilated follicular orifices. When active, the peripheral borders are erythematous or violaceous and continue to enlarge to involve other areas of the scalp. Active lesions are symptomatic and patients complain of lesional pruritus, burning, and pain. Multifocal involvement is also common. Postinflammatory pigmentary alteration, both hypopigmentation and hyperpigmentation, is frequently seen. Central atrophy and telangiectasia eventually become prominent. Advanced plaques are scarring both clinically and histologically.

Hypertrophic discoid lupus, a less common but very destructive variant of discoid lupus erythematosus, may occur on the scalp. The greatly elevated, verrucous, red-violet plaques with thick adherent scales result in tender inflammatory lesions, severe tissue destruction, and scarring alopecia. Hypertrophic discoid lupus lesions typically occur in patients with a long history of more typical discoid lupus but may present in the scalp as a sole cutaneous manifestation of systemic lupus erythematosus. The epidermis ranges from atrophic to acanthotic (hypertrophic discoid lupus).

Differential Diagnosis. The differential diagnosis of discoid lupus erythematosus includes psoriasis, lichen planopilaris, folliculitis decalvans, and pseudopelade of Brocq.

Treatment. Topical and intralesional corticosteroids are the mainstays of conservative local therapy in patients with relatively limited involvement.

If extensive scalp or cutaneous involvement is present and is not responding to local therapy, consideration may be given to systemic therapy. Effective systemic medications include oral prednisone and the antimalarial drugs: chloroquine diphosphate (Aralen), hydroxychloroquine sulfate (Plaquenil), and quinacrine hydrochloride (Atabrine).

Alopecia Mucinosa (Follicular Mucinosis)

Clinical Description. This clinical syndrome of patches and plaques of alopecia occurs as a result of mucin deposition and subsequent degeneration of hair follicles. Alopecia mucinosa most commonly involves the face, scalp, and neck, but involvement of extremities may also occur. Clinically detectable alopecia is most often present in those lesions involving the scalp and face. Scalp lesions have variable morphology ranging from scaling erythematous infiltrated plaques and nodules to noninflammatory circular patches resembling alopecia areata. Age at onset ranges from 2 to 80 years. Alopecia mucinosa usually does not result in permanent alopecia unless mucin deposition completely destroys the follicular epithelium. The pathogenesis of alopecia mucinosa is unknown.

Two clinically distinct groups of alopecia mucinosa (follicular mucinosis) exist: lymphoma associated and non–lymphoma associated. Mycosis fungoides is the most common lymphoproliferative disorder associated with alopecia mucinosa and follicular mucinosis and usually occurs in patients 30 years of age and older.

The non–lymphoma-associated alopecia mucinosa (follicular mucinosis) frequently occurs in children and young adults and is usually self-limiting without resultant permanent alopecia. In addition, Hodgkin's lymphoma may rarely occur in association with childhood alopecia mucinosa (follicular mucinosis).

Pathology. The earliest findings are mucin deposition within the outer root sheath. Mucin is usually detected in routine hematoxylin and eosin–stained sections but is best appreciated with stains such as colloidal iron and consists primarily of hyaluronic acid.

Differential Diagnosis. Infiltrative erythematous plaques with associated alopecia are clinically suggestive of alopecia mucinosis (follicular mucinosis). Microscopic examination and close clinical follow up are essential given the potential association with cutaneous lymphoma.

Treatment. Non–lymphoma-associated alopecia mucinosa (follicular mucinosis) usually resolves spontaneously. In children and young adults, permanent scarring alopecia is uncommon. Topical and intralesional corticosteroids may be of some therapeutic benefit. The treatment of lymphoma-associated alopecia mucinosis (follicular mucinosis) is that of the underlying cutaneous T-cell lymphoma in general and is discussed in Chapter 10 in this text (Chapter 158 in CM&S).

Vesiculobullous Disease Causing Alopecia

Cicatricial pemphigoid and certain forms of epidermolysis bullosa may cause a primary permanent scarring alopecia. Other bullous diseases, unless complicated by extensive secondary impetiginization, do not typically result in a scarring alopecia.

Secondary Scarring Alopecias

The hair loss of secondary scarring alopecias occurs as a result of nonfolliculocentric skin disease, genetic defect, or external injury and are listed in Table 8–1. Follicular destruction is only incidental in secondary scarring alopecias. The clinical and histologic features of secondary scarring alopecias are typical for the specific disease involved.

Pediatric Scarring Alopecias

There are several scarring alopecias that almost always present in childhood. Many of these latter pediatric scarring alopecias are thought to be due to genetic defects. The etiology of most pediatric scarring alopecias is unknown, but both primary and secondary types of scarring alopecia exist.

Scarring Follicular Keratosis

Clinical Description. Several hereditary syndromes involving follicular dilatation, hyperkeratosis, and ultimate follicular destruction associated with keratosis pilaris have been described. The three major variants of the scarring follicular keratosis are keratosis pilaris decalvans, keratosis pilaris atrophicans (ulerythema ophryogenes), and atrophoderma vermiculata.

Scarring alopecia of the scalp is generally seen only in keratosis pilaris decalvans. In this entity, lesions of keratosis pilaris begin in childhood. Similar dilated hair follicles with hyperkeratosis and focal surrounding erythema occur throughout the scalp and lead to scarring alopecia. Facial involvement with keratosis pilaris–like lesions also frequently occurs. Palmar and plantar hyperkeratosis,

---

TABLE 8–1. Secondary Scarring Alopecia

I. Sclerosing Disorders
   A. Morphea
   B. Sclerodermoid porphyria cutanea tarda
   C. Lichen sclerosus et atrophicus
   D. Parry-Romberg syndrome
II. Physical and Chemical Agents
   A. Mechanical trauma, laceration
   B. Thermal burns
   C. Chemical burns
   D. Radiation dermatitis
III. Dermal Infiltrative Processes
   A. Tumors
      1. Basal cell carcinoma
      2. Squamous cell carcinoma
      3. Metastatic carcinoma
      4. Lymphoma
      5. Adnexal tumors
   B. Granulomatous
      1. Sarcoidosis
      2. Necrobiosis lipoidica
      3. Actinic granuloma
      4. Infections
   C. Amyloidosis

photophobia, keratoconjunctivitis, cataracts, and other corneal abnormalities may also be associated with keratosis pilaris decalvans.

Keratosis pilaris atrophicans begins in childhood with keratosis pilaris–like lesions of the lateral portion of the eyebrow. Follicular destruction with permanent loss of the lateral eyebrows occurs. Similar lesions may also be present to a variable degree on the cheeks. Scarring alopecia of the scalp does not usually occur.

Atrophoderma vermiculata consists of follicular plugging of the cheeks and preauricular area with subsequent follicular destruction and resultant reticulate atrophy. The scalp is generally not involved.

Pathology. The microscopic findings are not specific.

Treatment. There is no effective therapy.

DISORDERS OF NAILS

(CM&S Chapter 136)

Nail Bed Disorders

Nail bed disorders often appear as changes in nail color. *Anemic pallor* is visible as a paleness of the normally pink nail bed. *Cyanosis* is visible as a bluish color of the nail bed. In psoriasis, the *"salmon patch" macule* appears as erythema of the nail bed or as punctuate erythematous dots in the lunula and the *"oil drop" sign* is visible through the nail plate as a yellow "oil drop" on the nail bed surface.

Onycholysis is a common disorder characterized by the formation of a distal or lateral cleft between the nail plate and bed. The affected plate usually appears white but may appear yellow, brown, or green, depending on the degree of subungual hyperkeratosis, inflammation, and secondary bacterial or yeast proliferation. Onycholysis may be caused by overhydration in individuals whose hands are immersed in water throughout the day, from nail enamel use, particularly in women with long or acrylic nails, in dermatophyte infections, as a result of drug ingestion, and in a number of dermatologic disorders including eczema. Systemic diseases or conditions that cause onycholysis include diabetes mellitus, thyroid disease, and impaired circulation.

To treat onycholysis, first identify its cause. Overhydration is best managed by removing the overlying onycholytic nail plate; the patient's exposure to water should be curtailed, and nail enamel use must be stopped. In local infections the overlying plate must be removed and clear tincture of iodine mixed 1:1 with 70% isopropyl alcohol is applied to the nail bed repeatedly throughout the day and at bedtime. Therapy for psoriatic onycholysis, which is usually unrewarding, includes topical corticosteroids; intralesional triamcinolone acetonide, 1.5 mg/mL injected into the nail bed or systemic antipsoriatic agents may be used, if more extensive disease warrants their use.

Splinter hemorrhage and *subungual hematoma* differ in the extent of nail bed hemorrhage. In splinter hemorrhage, blood is confined to thin grooves between the nail bed's longitudinal epidermal ridges. They appear as thin black lines 1 to 2 mm long located in the distal third of the nail bed. Although a sign of subacute bacterial endocarditis, splinter hemorrhage is most frequently caused by trauma, as are subungual hematomas.

Subungual hyperkeratosis results from epidermal hyperplasia of the nail bed and is found most frequently in psoriasis, and onychomycosis. KOH and mycologic cultures should always be performed.

Three distinctive signs of systemic disease are reflected in the nail unit. *Terry's nail*, in which the proximal nail bed is white, the lunula is obscured, and the distal pink nail bed is preserved, is associated with cirrhosis and congestive heart failure and is a normal finding in the elderly. *Muehrcke's lines*, characterized by double, white, translucent bands separated from one another and from the lunula by the normal pink nail bed, are associated with hypoalbuminemia. *Lindsay's half and half nail*, in which the proximal nail bed is dull white and obscures the lunula, is a sign of chronic renal failure.

Periungual fibromas, which develop in 50% of patients with tuberous sclerosis, appear as pink linear lesions with a hyperkeratotic tip that protrudes from the undersurface of the nail fold or plate and displace the nail plate, causing it to groove.

Nail Plate Disorders

Loss of the normal inverted 160-degree angle (Lovibond's angle) between the nail plate and the proximal nail fold defines *clubbing* where the angle is everted and exceeds 180 degrees. Clubbing is most commonly secondary to a number of pulmonary, cardiovascular, gastrointestinal, and endocrinologic disorders as well as with intrathoracic neoplasms.

In *koilonychia* the nails are spoon shaped and concave; the edges evert upward. Koilonychia occurs in normal neonates, is associated with nail thinning in the elderly, but is most frequently associated with iron deficiency anemia, particularly in children. The pathogenesis has not been established.

Anonychia, partial or complete loss of the nail plate, may be congenital or may result from permanent damage to the nail matrix from trauma and from destructive disorders such as lichen planus.

Nail plate thickening must be differentiated from subungual hyperkeratosis, which simulates thickening. It is produced by chronic trauma and typically occurs in onychomycosis, psoriasis, lichen planus, and pachyonychia congenita. *Onychogryphosis*, an extreme form of nail thickening, usually occurs in the great toenails of the elderly and infirm. The hypertrophic nail plate is shaped like a ram's horn. Therapy consists of nail plate trimming, avulsion, total matricectomy for permanent removal, and/or appropriate footwear alterations.

In *pincer nail*, the nail is overly curved transversely, a curve that is accentuated distally. The pincer nail tip may constrict tissues of the distal nail unit, causing intense pain. Pincer nails are most commonly caused by subungual exostoses and pressure from tight shoes.

In *ridging (onychorrhexis)*, thin longitudinal elevations/ridges alternate with depressions or grooves along the nail plate surface. Mild ridging occurs as a normal finding in the elderly. Severe ridging is prototypic of lichen planus.

In destruction of the matrix, which leads to scarring and atrophy seen in lichen planus, adherence of the nail fold to the underlying nail bed produces *dorsal pterygium*.

Median nail dystrophy is characterized by an irregular, often symmetrical, longitudinal depression in the midportion of the nail plate, usually occuring on the thumbs. Typically, the dystrophy is caused by pressure from the index finger nail; the patient has a habit or tic of pressing the sharp end of the index nail into the nail of the thumb at the proximal nail fold margin. By avoiding trauma, the affected nail will return to normal.

Beau's lines are transverse grooves or ridges in the nail plate that traverse the entire width of the nail plate. A transient, diminished production of nail by the matrix during acute illness causes this dystrophy; the width of the depression corresponds precisely to the duration of diminished matrix activity. The distance of the line from the proximal nail fold corresponds to the time when nail production was impaired.

Brittle fingernails are encountered most commonly in the elderly, in individuals who repeatedly immerse their hands in water throughout the day, and in women who continually wear nail enamel or use acrylics, although brittleness may result from fungal infections and from systemic disorders.

Little can be done to clear brittleness in all situations. Liberal application of emollient lotions after hand washing helps keep the nail hydrated. Tretinoin (0.1% cream) applied to the nail folds twice daily is also thought to be helpful. Clipping immediately after bathing when the plate is hydrated and soft is less traumatic to the nail than clipping when it is dry and brittle. Filing rough edges in one direction reduces the likelihood of the edge being caught and tearing the nail further.

In *pitting*, the surface of the nail plate is occupied by cup-shaped depressions that vary in size, number, depth, and pattern. Psoriasis and alopecia areata are the common causes.

Pigmentary Disorders

Longitudinal melanonychia is characterized by a longitudinal band of brown melanin pigment that extends from the cuticle to the distal edge of the nail plate. Increased pigment in longitudinal melanonychia may be due to increased melanin production by normal melanocytes as well as by hyperplasias or proliferations of normal or abnormal melanocytes. Differentiating longitudinal melanonychia from subungual hematomas may be difficult: subungual hematomas usually migrate distally with time; longitudinal melanonychia does not. Differentiating among the various benign and malignant causes of longitudinal melanonychia on clinical grounds alone can be difficult; biopsy is often necessary. Clinical clues that suggest a benign etiology are multiple bands of longitudinal melanonychia as opposed to a single band; very pale tan bands are unlikely to be caused by melanoma, and longitudinal melanonychia arising in children is distinctly unlikely to represent melanoma. Dark-skinned individuals are more likely than fair persons to develop longitudinal melanonychia. Longitudinal melanonychia occurs in essentially all blacks by age 70. *Melanoma* (1) may be associated with periungual pigmentation; (2) usually begins in older persons; (3) is usually subject to clinical change as opposed to being morphologically static; (4) often becomes wider or darker with time; (5) may occur in the presence of a history of trauma; (6) is often characterized by ill-defined, blurred lateral margins; (7) should be suspected if the band is black or variegated in color; (8) may be accompanied by nail dystrophy; and (9) often occurs in the thumb, great toe, or index finger.

Proximal and Lateral Nail Fold Disorders

Within the proximal nail fold, increased numbers of dilated and tortuous *capillary loops* may be found in patients with a variety of connective tissue disorders, including progressive systemic sclerosis, lupus erythematosus, and dermatomyositis.

Paronychia is characterized by erythema, edema, and tenderness of the proximal and lateral nail folds. In acute paronychia, usually caused by bacteria, injury to the cuticle or nail folds enables bacteria to enter the nail unit, proliferate, and produce infection. In chronic paronychia, characterized by erythema and edema as well as by retraction of the proximal nail fold, the onset is much more insidious, and pain tends to appear later in the course of the disease.

In acute paronychia, incision and drainage is recommended. Effective management of chronic paronychia includes limiting as much as possible the cycle of hydration and dehydration in persons who work in a waterborne environment, discovering and treatment of contact dermatitis, frequent application of emollient lotions to hydrate the cuticle, and wearing cotton gloves inside rubber gloves to offer important protection for the hand and cuticle. Other treatments are clear tincture of iodine mixed with equal parts of 70% isopropyl alcohol and applied under the cleft between the nail fold and plate, application of the combination of clotimazole and betamethasone, subsequent application of emollient lotions to lubricate the nascent cuticle as well as the hands, and, when the paronychia is slow to respond to conservative measures, intralesional corticosteroid administration. Bacterial infection of the paronychia is treated with antibiotics.

Trauma is the initiating event in essentially all cases of *ingrown nail*. The nail plate encroaches on or actually pierces the lateral nail fold with resulting edema, erythema, and infection.

Causes of ingrown nails include (1) pressure from tight-fitting shoes, (2) leaving spicules of nail that injure the nail fold after improper nail trimming, (3) overly curved or wider-than-normal nails, (4) onychomycosis, and (5) hyperhidrosis. Early stages of ingrown nails are best treated by removing the ingrown portion of nail with double-action nail clippers, treating infection with antibiotics, repeatedly inserting a hydrogen peroxide–saturated cotton-tipped applicator between the nail plate and nail fold during the period of nail regrowth to help prevent recurrence and keep the area free of debris. Properly fitting shoes must also be worn and onychomycosis treated by regular trimming or systemic antifungal therapy. In more advanced disease, lateral matricectomy must be performed to remove the offending nail and to permanently destroy that portion of the nail matrix and diminish the width of the nail plate.

BIOLOGY AND DISORDERS OF SWEAT GLANDS

(CM&S Chapter 137)

Sweat Gland Science

Eccrine sweating is unique to humans and apes and enables them to regulate rising body temperature due to heat or physical activity through the evaporative heat loss of eccrine sweating. Inability to regulate body temperature leads to hyperthermia and death. The eccrine sweat gland is a secretory as well as an excretory organ. Sweat is a dilute electrolyte solution containing mainly sodium, chloride, potassium, proteins, peptides, and inorganic compounds such as lactate, urea, and ammonia. Since profuse sweating causes an obligatory loss of water and electrolytes, the conservation of electrolytes by ductal reabsorption with the resultant secretion of hypotonic sweat is a vital function of the eccrine sweat gland (absent in patients with cystic fibrosis).

Anatomy of the Sweat Gland

There are three histologically and functionally distinguishable types of sweat glands: the eccrine, apocrine, and apoeccrine. Of these three types, it is the eccrine sweat gland that is primarily involved in thermoregulation. The eccrine sweat gland is innervated by the sympathetic nervous system. Its principal terminal neurotransmitter is acetylcholine. In humans, 2 to 3 million eccrine sweat glands are distributed over nearly all parts of the body. The eccrine sweat gland consists of two components: (1) the secretory coil, which secretes a nearly isotonic primary fluid, and (2) the duct, which reabsorbs sodium chloride in excess of water, releasing hypotonic sweat onto the skin surface. The size of the sweat gland, which varies as much as fivefold among different individuals, with gland size largely correlated with individual differences in the rate of sweating, may vary among regions of the body. When the maximal rate of sweating is measured, it ranges from 2 to 20 nL/min per gland.

Clinical Syndromes

Hyperhidrosis

Definition

In hyperhidrosis the eccrine glands produce excessive sweat in one or more anatomic locations. The axillae, palms, soles, and groin are commonly affected.

Clinical Description

Hyperhidrosis, or excessive sweating, is a source of great embarrassment to individuals afflicted with this condition. Hyperhidrotic patients are at particular risk for heat prostration when they are exposed to excessively high temperatures. Patients with axillary hyperhidrosis usually do not have bromhidrosis (abnormal sweat odor).

A number of systemic or local disorders can produce or accompany hyperhidrosis. Neurologic injury or disease affecting the autonomic system can overstimulate the eccrine sweat gland. Vascular disorders or injury can have the same effect. Metabolic disorders including diabetes mellitus, gout, hyperthyroidism, and porphyria, as well as hormonal disorders, fever, and shock, can also cause hyperhidrosis.

Pathogenesis

Although heat is usually responsible for an increase in sweating of the hairy surfaces, emotional stimuli control sweating of the palms and soles, and in some patients the axillae.

Differential Diagnosis

Systemic and local causes of hyperhidrosis should be considered (Table 8–2). In addition, there are variants of hyperhidrosis, such as night sweats, that are episodic or localized to specific regions.

Night sweats may be associated with systemic diseases such as tuberculosis, endocarditis, lymphoma, Hodgkin's disease, hyperthyroidism, diabetes mellitus, systemic vasculitis, pheochromocy-

---

TABLE 8–2. Differential Diagnosis of Hyperhidrosis

Neurologic injury or disease
  Spinal cord injury
    At or above T-6—automatic dysreflexia
    Cervical—orthostatic hypotension in quadriplegics with
      secondary hyperhidrosis
  Post-traumatic syringomyelia
  Peripheral neuropathies
    Familial dysautonomia
  Brain lesions
    Episodic hypothermia with hyperhidrosis
  Parkinson's disease
Vascular diseases
  Raynaud's disease
  Erythromelalgia
  Arteriovenous fistula
  Cold injury
Intrathoracic neoplasms of lesions
Systemic diseases
  Rheumatoid arthritis
  Diabetes mellitus
  Congestive heart failure
  Thyrotoxicosis
  Hyperpituitarism
  Pheochromocytoma
Drugs or poisoning
  Antidepressants
    Cyclobenzaprine (Flexeril)
    Fluoxetine
  Acrodynia (mercury)

---

toma, carcinoid syndrome, drug withdrawal, and dysautonomic states. The term *compensatory hyperhidrosis* is used to describe the occurrence of hyperhidrosis on the trunk and legs after a thoracic sympathectomy for the treatment of palmar hyperhidrosis, of facial hyperhidrosis in patients with generalized sweat retention syndrome, or of hyperhidrosis of the face and the upper trunk in patients with widespread diabetic neuropathy. Sweating, triggered by thermal stimuli or by physical exercise, presumably is due to an increased thermoregulatory need resulting from anhidrosis.

In unilateral circumscribed hyperhidrosis the hyperhidrotic area is usually sharply demarcated, measures no larger than 10×10 cm^2, and is present mainly on the face and upper extremities of otherwise healthy persons. The age at onset varies between 7 and 67 years. Patients typically notice a sudden onset of profuse sweating that lasts 15 to 120 minutes, precipitated by heat or physical exercise. Characteristically, there is no accompanying sensory or motor neuropathy. Sweating is not accompanied by flushing of the face, headaches, excessive salivation, lacrimation, vasodilation, or piloerection. The pathogenesis of circumscribed hyperhidrosis is unknown. Sweating may be partially controlled by local application of 25% aluminum salts, topical anticholinergic agents, or systemic clonidine, inhibiting central sympathetic outflow. Local tap water iontophoresis may also be tried. As a last resort, total excision of the affected area could be considered.

Physiologic gustatory sweating occurs in normal persons while eating certain hot, spicy foods. Although pathologic gustatory sweating is also precipitated by gustatory stimulation, it is usually unilateral, involving the preauricular or infra-auricular areas of the face. It can be mild or embarrassingly profuse. Pathologic gustatory sweating can be classified into several types according to its etiology.

Gustatory sweating due to hyperactivity of sympathetic function occurs in association with encephalitis, syringomyelia, or Pancoast's syndrome (invasion of the cervical sympathetic trunk by a tumor) and in three fourths of patients who have had an upper dorsal sympathectomy. Its pathogenesis is explained on the basis of preganglionic sympathetic regeneration or collateral sprouting resulting in aberrant synapses with postganglionic fibers in the superior cervical ganglion.

Gustatory sweating associated with peripheral autonomic and sensory neuropathy due to diabetic neuropathy is rare. Sweating is bilateral and widespread on the face, resembling exaggerated physiologic gustatory sweating.

Auriculotemporal (or Frey's) syndrome occurs in almost 100% of patients within 1 month to 5 years after having surgery of the parotid gland or preauricular area or after sustaining an injury to the preauricular region. The syndrome results from injury to the auriculotemporal nerve, which carries sensory fibers from the skin, parasympathetic fibers to the salivary glands, and sympathetic fibers to the sweat glands in the preauricular region. Gustatory sweating in Frey's syndrome is usually mild; only 10% of the patients may require treatment. Topical scopolamine cream (3% to 5%) and 20% aluminum chloride in ethanol have been used with variable success. Injecting alcohol around the auriculotemporal nerve has been reported to eliminate symptoms for several months. Tympanic neurectomy and interpositional fascia graft may offer permanent relief.

Treatment

Once systemic or local causes of hyperhidrosis are ruled out, choosing among treatment options depends on the severity, location of the problem, and the impact on activities of daily living.

On the soles excessive sweating is annoying. Simply changing socks more frequently and using absorptive powder may be sufficient. Likewise, continually drying the palms throughout the day is a simple, effective approach for many patients. Those with more difficult sweating problems can be treated with 0.1% formalin soaks several times a week, but there is a risk of producing contact dermatitis. Alternatively, 2% to 10% glutaraldehyde or 10% tannic acid in 70% alcohol can be painted on the involved areas daily. These topical approaches can also cause an irritant contact dermatitis. Perhaps the most practical approach is to employ powders containing tannic acid, salicylic acid, and talc frequently during the day to minimize the embarrassment of the ''wet handshake.''

Tap or deionized water iontophoresis can be used successfully in some patients for localized hyperhidrosis of the palms and soles. Cessation of sweating usually requires treatment of each palm or sole with 20 mA of current for 30 minutes daily. This approach may work by inducing plugging of the sweat gland pore.

Axillary hyperhidrosis sometimes responds to potent topical antiperspirants. Antiperspirants contain acidic salts of aluminum or zinc that function by temporarily occluding the sweat ducts. Deodorants contain various perfumes and antibacterial agents that are designed to mask the offending odors. Regular use of deodorant soaps helps to reduce the bacterial count and reduces the odor. For most people these simple hygienic approaches are sufficient. Aluminum chloride hexahydrate 20% in absolute alcohol is more effective than the commercial deodorants but may be irritating to axillary skin. This can be minimized by drying the axillae with a hair dryer before and immediately after application. Other antiperspirants must be avoided initially until the patient is accustomed to using the aluminum chloride. Baking soda can be substituted for other antiperspirants for its soothing and deodorant effects. After a few weeks of use at bedtime, this agent can be used in conjunction with commercial preparations. To minimize irritation the solution is applied once or twice a week, as infrequently as possible, to avoid dryness or irritation while still maintaining the anhidrotic effect. If simple application of aluminum chloride hexahydrate 20% is insufficient, then occlusion with plastic wrap nightly for two to three nights a week is performed.

In severe cases, systemic measures may be used initially in combination with or without topical agents. Anticholinergic drugs, such as propantheline bromide and glycopyrrolate, however, induce decreased salivation, loss of urinary bladder sphincter control, and reduction of gastrointestinal peristalsis. To minimize side effects, anticholinergics can be used periodically, before stressful situations.

For resistant localized axillary hyperhidrosis, direct excision of the sweat glands is an alternative. Simple surgical excision of the axillary vault can be employed to eliminate most sweating. It is not uncommon for eccrine sweat glands outside the original hyperhidrotic area to overcompensate gradually after surgery with increased sweating. It is important to first delineate the location of excess eccrine glands. The starch iodine technique can be used to identify the areas of most severe sweating. Starch is painted on a carefully dried axilla. When sweating resumes, a blue color appears on the areas of the greatest eccrine activity. This section of axillary skin can then be marked with a surgical pen and excised. Usually an area 7 to 10 cm long and 2 cm or more wide must be removed. These wounds are under tension, so extensive undermining must be performed, and a layered closure with subcutaneous absorbable sutures is preferred.

The newest surgical technique for treatment of hyperhidrosis of the axilla was developed from a modification of liposuction. A blunt cannula is used to suction out sweat glands residing in the subcutaneous tissue. Additionally, superficial liposuction just under the dermis causes lower dermal inflammation and subsequent fibrosis. This technique has the advantage of reducing the number of eccrine glands without the significance of scarring axillary resections. Only two 4-mm incisions are required and axillary hair is preserved.

As a last resort, patients with severe hyperhidrosis can also be treated by surgical ablation of the lumbar and supraclavicular sympathetic ganglia that control the specific sweating sites. Attendant side effects include postsympathetic neuralgia, phrenic nerve paralysis, Horner's syndrome, and compensatory hyperhidrosis in other areas.

Bromhidrosis

Definition

Bromhidrosis, also referred to as bromidosis or osmidrosis, is a condition of excess, abnormal, or offensive body odor whether either apocrine or eccrine secretion is implicated.

Apocrine bromhidrosis (exaggerated and offensive odor) is confined to the axilla and results from excessive apocrine sweat. Eccrine bromhidrosis usually affects the feet due to maceration from excessive sweating. Apocrine bromhidrosis appears after puberty with the enlargement of apocrine glands, while eccrine bromhidrosis may appear early in childhood.

Pathogenesis

Although freshly secreted eccrine and apocrine sweat is odorless, it provides a ready environment for the growth of bacteria, especially aerobic diphtheroids and micrococci. Odor results from bacterial, especially diphtheroids, degradation of short-chain fatty acids. The odor of plantar skin bromhidrosis results from decomposition of keratin by bacteria. The major odor-causing substance in axillary sweat is 5α-androstenone.

Differential Diagnosis

The two significant disorders that the clinician should consider are psychiatric disorders and olfactory lobe brain tumors. Some patients with psychiatric disorders believe that they have offensive body odor in the absence of bromhidrosis. They may resort to excessive bathing and deodorant use. Psychiatric help may be required to solve their emotional problems.

Treatment

The treatment approach for bromhidrosis is the same as for hyperhidrosis.

chapter 9

What Diseases Alter Mucous Membranes?

DISORDERS OF ORAL MUCOUS MEMBRANES

(CM&S Chapter 138)

Benign Neoplasms, Reactive Processes, and Systemic Disorders Affecting the Oral Cavity

Blue and Black Lesions

Pigmentation of the oral cavity may be due to a variety of causes: antimalarials, minocycline, adrenocorticotropic hormone, oral contraceptives, phenolphthalein, and zidovudine are medications that cause localized or diffuse hyperpigmentation of the oral mucosa; heavy metals may account for gingival and diffuse oral pigmentation; and systemic illnesses, including Addison's disease, neurofibromatosis, hemochromatosis, and Peutz-Jeghers disease, may be accompanied by various degrees of oral pigmentation. Diffuse patches of pigmentation on the buccal mucosa and gingiva are commonly present in dark-skinned persons.

Amalgam Tattoo. The most common cause of exogenous oral pigmentation is due to particles of amalgam fillings accidentally introduced into oral soft tissues. Clinically, macular lesions in shades of blue, gray, or black appear most commonly on the gingiva and alveolar mucosa.

Oral and Labial Melanotic Macules. Pigmented, usually solitary, well-circumscribed macules on the lips and in the oral cavity occur predominantly in 20- to 30-year-old women. These lesions are completely innocuous and have no malignant potential.

White and Yellow Lesions

Fordyce's Spots. Fordyce's spots, that represent heterotopic sebaceous glands, are small white or yellow papules usually appearing in clusters at various sites in the oral cavity. They are a normal finding in approximately 80% of patients and are most frequently seen on the buccal mucosa.

White Sponge Nevus. This autosomal dominant disorder is characterized by the development of asymptomatic oral white plaques in which the mucosa appears thickened and folded with a spongy texture. The buccal mucosa is the most frequently affected site, but severity and extent are variable. Extraoral lesions at other mucosal sites may be seen. The lesions are benign and do not undergo malignant transformation.

Keratosis Follicularis (Darier-White Disease). Oral lesions, present in 15% to 50% of patients, include white papules that appear most commonly on the palate and that may coalesce in a "cobblestoning" appearance, giving the palate a sandpaper surface.

Red and Pink Lesions

Pyogenic Granuloma. Pyogenic granuloma is a vascular proliferative lesion that is usually a response to trauma. It presents as an intensely red, sometimes ulcerated, pedunculated mass that bleeds easily on provocation. There is a predisposition for the maxillary anterior gingiva, and the growth is seen frequently in pregnant women. Treatment involves removal of the irritating stimulus and excision of the granuloma.

Papillary Hyperplasia. Papillary hyperplasia, a reactive process to ill-fitting dentures, is a benign condition of the palate in which diffuse red, papillary projections confined to the hard palate bleed easily on provocation. Treatment consists of prosthetic adjustment, removal of the denture at night, or surgical excision of fibrotic lesions.

Mucocele. The mucocele, a common oral lesion, is frequently the result of damage to the small duct of an accessory salivary gland, resulting in a pink, yellow, or slightly bluish, dome-shaped, fluctuant mass, usually on the lower lip. The mucous retention cyst, or ranula, occurs in the buccal mucosa and on the floor of the mouth. The treatment is surgical removal.

Fibroma. The fibroma is the most common oral mucosal lesion and represents a hyperplastic response to trauma. Fibromas are firm, exophytic, nodular or pedunculated lesions covered by normal pink mucosa, most commonly seen in areas subjected to trauma (e.g., lips and tongue). Treatment of fibromas consists of simple excision.

Mixed and Miscellaneous Lesions

Cowden's Disease. Papillomatosis, the classic feature of the disease, is histologically benign. Clinically, it is characterized by a cobblestoning appearance of white and pink coalescing papules, occurring on the lips, tongue, palate, gingiva, and buccal mucosa.

Melkersson-Rosenthal Syndrome and Cheilitis Granulomatosa. The Melkersson-Rosenthal syndrome consists of a triad of recurrent orofacial swelling, relapsing facial paralysis, and fissured tongue that occurs most frequently in the second and third decades of life in females. The complete triad is found in only 10% to 20% of patients. Cheilitis granulomatosa, consisting of swelling of one or both lips, is considered an oligosymptomatic form of the syndrome.

Labial swelling, which develops suddenly and is often unilateral and asymmetrical, is often the initial sign and the most consistent feature of these conditions. Recurrent, painless episodes are usual and increase in duration as the disease progresses. Intraoral involvement with swelling of the buccal mucosa, gingiva, and tongue are frequently observed and occasionally associated with erythema, erosions, and pain.

Facial paralysis, the initial symptom in 30% to 50% of patients, and facial swelling are usually unilateral and episodic. Fissured tongue, found in approximately 50% of patients, may be associated with burning and swelling. The onset of this condition occurs most commonly in the second and third decades of life and is more frequent among females.

Classical histologic findings are small noncaseating granulomas. The differential diagnosis includes Crohn's disease and sarcoid.

Systemic and intralesional corticosteroids produce adequate treatment results in the majority.

Geographic Tongue (Benign Migratory Glossitis). Geographic tongue occurs in up to 2% of the general population. It presents as irregular areas of denuded, atrophic mucosa outlined by white or yellow elevated margins on the dorsum and lateral borders of the tongue. In a cycle of healing and recurrence, the lesions migrate over the surface of the tongue, assuming constantly new configurations, thus leading to the term *migratory glossitis*. Some patients undergo spontaneous regression. Symptomatic patients may respond to topical steroids.

Hairy Tongue. A matted, asymptomatic layer appears on the dorsal surface of the tongue due to hypertrophy of the filiform papillae and a lack of normal desquamation. The papillae appearing as elongated hairs may be yellow, white, brown, and often black, depending on their staining by foods, tobacco, medication, and organisms.

Hairy tongue is seen in patients after radiation of head and neck malignancies and following the use of broad-spectrum antibiotics. Overgrowth of *Candida albicans* and chromogenic bacteria may occur and may be causative factors. The lesions generally disappear when the tongue is brushed with a toothbrush, causing desquamation of the papillae. Topical antifungal therapy and topical retinoids may hasten resolution.

Burning Mouth Syndrome. Burning mouth syndrome may be associated with infection, vitamin deficiency, and neurologic and metabolic disorders, but most cases are of unknown cause and occur in postmenopausal women. Although the entire mouth may be involved, patients complain predominantly of tongue burning.

Xerostomia. The causes of dry mouth are diverse. Xerostomia, prevalent in the elderly, may in part be due to reduced saliva production. Diabetes, diuretics, anticholinergic drugs, chemotherapy, local radiation therapy, immunosuppressive agents, as well as sarcoid and Sjögren's syndrome, all may produce salivary gland dysfunction.

Aside from a dry or burning sensation of the oral mucosa, patients with xerostomia may complain of difficulty eating, diminution of taste acuity, and discomfort when speaking. Additionally, there is an increased rate of mucosal infections, dental caries, and periodontal disease. Treatments include sugar-free, flavored chewing gum and pilocarpine, both which can stimulate salivation, and saliva substitutes.

Gingival Hyperplasia. Gingival hyperplasia may result from the chronic administration of phenytoin, cyclosporine, nifedipine, and diltiazem; from poor oral hygiene; from periodontal disease; from allergic contact stomatitis; and from leukemia.

Premalignant and Malignant Oral Disorders

Leukoplakia and Erythroplakia. *Leukoplakia* and *erythroplakia* are descriptive terms for white and red plaques, respectively, that cannot be scraped off. Common causes of leukoplakia include chronic irritation from smoking or chewing tobacco, sharp dental restorations, and cheek biting. Fewer than 10% of biopsy specimens of leukoplakia will reveal dysplasia or carcinoma. Leukoplakia that is verrucous and nodular, speckled with erythroplakia, or recurring in locations prone to the development of oral carcinoma (floor of mouth) is more likely to undergo malignant transformation. Most erythroplakic lesions, when examined histologically, reveal carcinoma in situ or frank carcinoma. All red plaques should be viewed with suspicion and subjected to biopsy.

Cheilitis Glandularis. Characterized by enlargement of the lower lip, which eventually results in eversion, cheilitis glandularis is caused by excessive mucus secretion of the lip's salivary glands, which appear red and swollen. With advanced disease, the lip becomes painful and permanently enlarged. The etiology of this condition is unknown and perhaps multifactorial; actinic damage, bacterial infections, use of tobacco products, and oral habits have all been implicated. Treatment of associated findings with or without the addition of intralesional steroids is suggested.

Squamous Cell and Verrucous Carcinoma. The tongue is the most common site for cancer of the oral cavity, followed by the lip and the floor of the mouth. Tobacco and alcohol, especially in combination, are major causes of oral carcinoma. Excessive exposure to ultraviolet light is another factor.

The classic appearance of a painless, nonhealing ulcer with elevated, rolled margins and induration is not always seen, especially in the early stages of the disease. Small areas of erythema, erosion, hyperkeratosis, or leukoplakia, if persistent, should be biopsied.

Oral verrucous carcinoma is a slow-growing malignancy characterized by a white, warty, friable lesion with little tendency to metastasize. It is frequently observed in patients who chew tobacco and is seen most commonly on the alveolar ridge and buccal mucosa.

Kaposi's Sarcoma. In contrast to the other forms of Kaposi's sarcoma, intraoral involvement is frequent in patients with acquired immunodeficiency syndrome (AIDS). Up to 50% of patients with AIDS may have oral involvement, and in 25% of cases the oral lesions represent the initial sign of HIV infection. Most lesions occur on the palate and gingiva. Multiple lesions are common. Treatments include radiation therapy, intralesional vinblastine, and systemic chemotherapy.

Ulcerative Disorders of the Oral Cavity

Oral ulcers result from a wide variety of causes. Traumatic ulcers such as those from sharp dental restorations, cheek biting, hot foods, or denture irritation are commonly observed and may be easily diagnosed by the history preceding their onset. Other frequent causes are allergic contact stomatitis to toothpaste, chewing gum, oral hygiene rinses, and cinnamates, and from systemic medications, most commonly antibiotics, chemotherapy, and cardiac drugs.

Ulcers that persist require a biopsy to exclude other causes, such as malignancies.

Recurrent Aphthous Stomatitis. Recurrent aphthous stomatitis (canker sores) is the most common cause of oral ulcerations, affecting approximately 25% of the general population. Aphthae are frequent in childhood and in young adulthood, but the severity decreases with age. Recurrent aphthous stomatitis has been divided into three types. Minor aphthous ulcerations, the most common form, account for 80% of cases. Episodes of single or multiple ulcerations, generally less than 1.0 cm, develop recurrently, with healing of lesions occurring in 7 to 14 days. Pain is minimal to moderate, and scarring does not usually occur. Major aphthous ulcerations (Sutton's disease), comprising 10% of cases, are characterized by larger and deeper ulcerations greater than 2.0 cm. The pain that results is usually severe, and healing, which takes 2 to 4 weeks, often leads to scarring. Herpetiform aphthae are similar to minor aphthae, with the exception of exhibiting large numbers (10–100) of 1- to 2-mm ulcerations.

Recurrent aphthous stomatitis occurs on the nonkeratinized mucosal surfaces; minor aphthae are most common on the labial and buccal mucosa, tongue, and floor of the mouth, while major aphthae frequently involve the soft palate and oropharynx.

The severity of aphthous ulcerations is variable. Some may experience only a few recurrent episodes, while others may develop continuous and debilitating ulcerations. The etiology is unknown, but factors that may induce recurrences include trauma and possibly stress, illnesses, and menses. Nicotine in cigarettes and smokeless tobacco may reduce the prevalence of recurrences.

Recurrent ulcerations may be a manifestation of nutritional deficiencies of iron, folate, and vitamin B_{12}. Patients with inflammatory bowel disease, AIDS, systemic lupus erythematosus, and viral infections may all exhibit ulcerations that are clinically indistinguishable from recurrent aphthous stomatitis. Patients with Behçet's disease or complex aphthosis (oral and genital ulcerations) demonstrate ulcers identical to recurrent aphthous stomatitis, and the three disease processes may actually represent a spectrum of one disease.

No treatment of recurrent aphthous stomatitis is uniformly effective or results in permanent remission. Topical benzocaine (Oragel), tannic acids (Zilactin), viscous lidocaine and tetracycline, or potent topical corticosteroids may alleviate the discomfort. In severe cases, systemic therapy with antibiotics, colchicine, dapsone, and prednisone may be beneficial. Major aphthae in patients with AIDS respond to thalidomide.

Oral Lichen Planus (see Chapter 2 in this text or Chapter 20 in CM&S). Only 10% to 20% of patients with oral lesions exhibit cutaneous evidence of lichen planus, whereas more than two thirds of patients with cutaneous disease have oral lesions.

There are three types of oral lesions: reticular (white lesions appearing linear, papular, or as plaques), atrophic (erythematous lesions), and erosive (ulcerative and bullous lesions). Lesions have a predilection for the buccal mucosa and tongue. Malignant transformation of oral lichen planus, which has been reported to occur with frequencies ranging up to 5%, is controversial.

All therapy for oral lichen planus is palliative. Most effective are potent topical corticosteroids applied to the oral mucosa supplemented with intralesional corticosteroids. In those patients whose disorder is refractory to this regimen, topical and systemic retinoids and cyclosporine may induce clinical remission.

Pemphigus (see Chapter 3 in this text or Chapter 74 in CM&S). Oral lesions are the initial manifestation of pemphigus in over 75% of cases. Oral lesions develop insidiously. Intact blisters are rarely observed, since they rupture rapidly and form large erosions with ragged borders. Pain, bleeding, swelling, and difficulty in mastication develop as the disease progresses. Any mucosal surface may be involved, but the soft palate is affected in most of cases.

Pemphigoid (see Chapter 3 in this text or Chapter 75 in CM&S). Oral lesions in bullous pemphigoid occur in 10% to 30% of cases. Small bullae and ulcerations are usually observed but, unlike pemphigus, are rarely the initial presenting features.

Oral manifestations of cicatricial pemphigoid are almost always encountered. The disease may be confined entirely to the oral mucosa. Desquamative gingivitis characterized by erythema, bleeding, swelling, and ulceration of the gums is the most common and characteristic presentation. Nongingival involvement is frequent and appears as bullae and ulcerations.

Epidermolysis Bullosa (see Chapter 3 in this text or Chapter 73 in CM&S). Oral involvement is common in all forms of inherited epidermolysis bullosa. Patients with recessive dystrophic epidermolysis bullosa have the highest frequency of oral disease (90%–100%) and the most severe involvement. In addition to widespread oral ulcerations, intraoral scarring often results in complete vestibular obliteration, ankyloglossia, and microstomia. Although 90% of patients with dominant dystrophic epidermolysis bullosa exhibit oral lesions, scarring does not occur.

Lupus Erythematosus (see Chapter 2 in this text or Chapter 24 in CM&S). Oral ulceration, one of the ARA criteria for the diagnosis of systemic lupus erythematosus, occurs in 25% of patients with systemic lupus erythematosus, most commonly on the hard palate, and is associated with active systemic disease. The lesions are usually asymptomatic. Nonspecific erythema accompanied by edema and petechial reddening of the hard palate is the most frequent oral finding in patients with systemic lupus erythematosus.

Erythema Multiforme (see Chapter 2 in this text or Chapter 22 in CM&S). Oral lesions are characterized by diffuse areas of erythema and bullae, which rapidly appear and rupture, forming ulcerations. A distinctive, whitish gray pseudomembrane of necrotic epithelium covers the ulcerations. Hemorrhagic crusting of the lips and severe oral pain causing inability to eat or swallow are features of erythema multiforme major.

Necrotizing Sialometaplasia. Necrotizing sialometaplasia is an uncommon, benign, inflammatory process of the salivary glands that is self-limited, lasting 5 to 6 weeks. Clinically, unilateral, painful, deep-seated ulcerations are observed in the majority of patients. Most cases occur on the hard and soft palate, although any mucosal site may be involved.

Crohn's Disease. Oral involvement in Crohn's disease occurs in approximately 15% of patients, with a greater prevalence in young, adolescent males. Diffuse swelling of one or both lips identical to granulomatous cheilitis is the most constant oral feature. Mucosal cobblestoning of the buccal mucosa and lips, linear or extensive ulcerations indistinguishable from recurrent aphthous stomatitis, and mucosal tags are additional findings.

Pyostomatitis Vegetans. Pyostomatitis vegetans is a marker highly specific for inflammatory bowel disease. In the majority of patients, bowel disease precedes the oral lesions and the severity of the oral disease parallels the activity of the gastrointestinal symptoms.

Multiple, yellow pustules on an erythematous base coalesce to form the pathognomonic "snail track" appearance. Lesions show a predilection for the gingiva, buccal mucosa, and palate. Oral vegetative nodules and hypertrophic gingiva may occur. Treatment of the underlying gastrointestinal disease will usually cause oral erosions to resolve.

Wegener's Granulomatosis. Oral ulceration may be seen in up to 60% of patients and may occasionally be the presenting sign of Wegener's granulomatosis. Painful and bleeding gingivitis starting in the interdental papillae early in the disease which progresses and results in exophytic, friable, and granular gingival tissue is pathognomonic of the disease.

Candidal Infection of the Oral Cavity

Candida is demonstrated in the oral cavity of more than 50% of healthy persons. Therefore, it is imperative to differentiate between commensalism and mucosal disease. Common factors that predispose to the development of oral candidiasis include immunosuppression, malnutrition and debilitation, malignancy, dental prosthetic devices, antibiotic therapy, infancy, old age and pregnancy, chronic oral diseases, xerostomia, and genetic and metabolic diseases. Oral candidiasis is an early and common manifestation of patients infected with HIV.

Candidiasis may appear in one of several forms. Thrush and pseudomembranous candidiasis are diagnosed by white, curd-like plaques, which can be partially removed. Atrophic candidiasis appears as mucosal erythema most frequently on the tongue and palate. Diffuse reddening of the hard palate in individuals who wear dentures continuously represents a form of atrophic candidiasis and has been termed *denture sore mouth*. Hyperplastic candidiasis may clinically present as leukoplakia and resemble squamous cell carcinoma, necessitating a biopsy. Median rhomboid glossitis, characterized by a smooth erythematous plaque on the posterior mid-dorsal surface of the tongue, is a form of localized, chronic candidiasis. Angular stomatitis is characterized by red, fissured crusts with or without ulceration at the labial commissures. The diagnosis of oral candidiasis is often made clinically and should be confirmed by cytology and culture and, if necessary, biopsy.

Antifungal treatment for oral candidiasis consists of nystatin suspension (400,000–600,000 units four times a day swish and swallow) or clotrimazole troches (10 mg dissolved in the mouth five times daily). Chlorhexidine 0.12% (3 teaspoonfuls as a rinse and expectorate) is useful as maintenance therapy rather than as a first-line antimycotic agent. Systemic therapy with ketoconazole, fluconazole, or itraconazole is often necessary in immunocompromised patients.

Acquired Immunodeficiency Syndrome. Oral lesions are common at all stages of HIV infection.

Oral Hairy Leukoplakia. In oral hairy leukoplakia, corrugated white patches and plaques that cannot be scraped off occur on the lateral margin of the tongue, frequently bilaterally. It occurs in up to 20% of HIV-infected patients, and it is most likely caused by repeated direct infection of superficial epithelial cells by Epstein-Barr virus from saliva.

Oral hairy leukoplakia should be differentiated from leukoplakia, candidiasis, lichen planus, geographic tongue, and white sponge nevus. Most patients require no therapy, since the lesions spontaneously remit. In those patients who are symptomatic, treatment with acyclovir, topical retinoic acid, and 25% podophyllum induces temporary remissions.

GENITAL DISORDERS

(CM&S Chapter 139)

Infections in the Genital Area

Bacterial Infections

Pyodermas

Staphylococcus aureus and group A hemolytic *Streptococcus* can cause the usual range of cutaneous pyodermas (i.e., impetigo, folliculitis, cellulitis, and abscesses). *S. aureus* frequently infects Bartholin's glands. An abscess of Bartholin's gland may require marsupialization in addition to systemic antibiotics.

Vulvovaginitis caused by group A hemolytic *Streptococcus* occurs in girls younger than 15 years of age. A vaginal discharge with erythema and labial swelling are presenting signs. Diagnosis is made by culturing vaginal swabs.

Erythrasma

Corynebacterium minutissimum, a gram-positive rod, causes erythrasma, which appears as a well-demarcated patch that may be seen in the inguinal and intergluteal folds. It is diagnosed by the demonstration of a coral-red fluorescence on examination under a Wood's light. A gram a day of erythromycin or tetracycline for 7 to 10 days is the usual therapy. Topical azoles and clindamycin in addition to measures aimed at keeping the involved areas clean and dry help to prevent recurrences.

Trichomycosis

Trichomycosis, a condition characterized by the presence of yellow or red nodules along the hair shafts that may stain clothing, is caused by two or three species of corynebacteria. Therapy consists of shaving the hair from the involved area. Washing with an antiseptic and keeping the involved area dry helps prevent recurrences.

Syphilis

The chancre, the primary lesion of syphilis, starts as a painless papule that enlarges and becomes an indurated ulcer. The bases of these ulcers teem with the etiologic spirochete, *Treponema pallidum,* which cannot be cultured but is easily seen on darkfield examination. Although typically single and painless, multiple chancres may occur and secondary pyogenic infection may render these chancres painful. These ulcers may be located anywhere on the genitalia and are frequently missed when they occur on the cervix or vagina. Nontender unilateral or bilateral inguinal adenopathy accompanies the chancre.

The secondary stage of syphilis is characterized by the appearance of a generalized eruption. On mucous membranes, grayish white, round, thin papules, known as mucous patches, are seen, while thicker, discrete to confluent, flat-surfaced white papules known as condylomata lata are also encountered in the moist genital and perianal areas in the second stage of syphilis. Like the chancre, these lesions teem with spirochetes and are very infectious (see Chapter 6 in this text or Chapter 108 in CM&S).

Nongonococcal Urethritis and Mucopurulent Cervicitis

In 50% of cases, nongonococcal urethritis and mucopurulent cervicitis are caused by *Chlamydia trachomatis* types D to K. These chlamydial infections are the most common sexually transmitted diseases. Although chlamydial infection of the lower genital tract in women may cause an irritating vaginal discharge, it is more often asymptomatic. Besides the cervix and urethra, the ducts of Bartholin's glands in women and the epididymis in men may also become infected. Ascending infection of the genital tract of women accounts for almost half the cases of pelvic inflammatory disease and 25% of subsequent cases of infertility. Diagnosis is made by culture or by a rapid direct immunofluorescent test.

Bacterial Vaginosis (Nonspecific Vaginitis)

Bacterial vaginosis is not a true infection but is a disturbance of the normal vaginal flora. About half of affected women are asymptomatic. The other half have a foul-smelling discharge that can cause vulvar irritation. For various reasons, such as chronic cervicitis or estrogen deficiency, the normal peroxide-producing *Lactobacillus*-dominated vaginal flora is replaced by anaerobic gram-positive streptococci and other anaerobes belonging to the *Gardnerella, Bacteroides, Mycoplasma,* and *Mobiluncus* species.

Three of the following four criteria are necessary for diagnosis: (1) a gray-white homogeneous discharge at the introitus; (2) a pH of greater than 4.5; (3) a "fishy," amine odor intensified by adding 10% potassium hydroxide; and (4) presence of "clue cells" on microscopic examination. "Clue cells" are desquamated vaginal epithelial cells whose surfaces are covered with bacteria so as to obscure their margins.

Bacterial vaginosis may remit spontaneously. The standard therapy is a week's course of metronidazole, 800 to 1200 mg in divided doses. An alternative to metronidazole is a week's course of clindamycin in a 2% cream or suppository.

Mycotic Infections

Dermatophyte Infection

Dermatophyte infection of the labia minora, penis, or scrotum almost never occurs.

Candidiasis

Candida infection in the genital area frequently manifests as an erythematous, macerated intertrigo with classic "satellite" pustules along the periphery. Most of these infections are caused by *C. albicans* strains.

The clinical hallmark of infection of the female genitalia with *Candida* is the presence of vulvitis, which may be erosive. Symptoms vary from pruritus to burning and dyspareunia. Candidiasis can present acutely as edema, erythema, white mucosal plaques, and a "cheesy" discharge at the vulva with "satellite" pustules on surrounding skin. As the condition becomes chronic, the surrounding skin becomes lichenified. Many patients with the recurrent, incapacitating form show only marked erythema, some edema, and minimal discharge.

Acute *Candida* infections tend to be more severe in the uncircumcised male and in women with undiagnosed, clinical diabetes. Other predisposing conditions are systemic antibiotic therapy, vulvar candidiasis in a sexual partner, or topical steroid therapy to the area. The genitalia become erythematous and swollen, with erosions and pustules. In the chronic form of penile candidiasis, the glans appears glazed and may progress to sclerosis and fissuring.

Approximately three fourths of adult women have vulvovaginal candidiasis at least once in their life. Approximately 20% of healthy asymptomatic women in the childbearing age have *Candida* in their genital tract. This vaginal carriage rate and the incidence of symptomatic vulvovaginal candidiasis are higher in pregnant women, in diabetics, in users of antibiotics and high-estrogen oral contraceptives, and in women frequenting clinics for treatment of sexually transmitted diseases. Several studies have failed to implicate subclinical diabetes, an intestinal reservoir, partner transmission, iron deficiency, and clothing and personal habits as predisposing factors in chronic or recurrent vulvovaginal candidiasis.

Diagnosis can be made in the office by microscopic examination of potassium hydroxide to treated vaginal discharge or skin scrapings. The presence of budding yeast and mycelia confirms the diagnosis. When candidiasis is suspected but the microscopic examination is negative, a culture is necessary.

Topical therapy is generally sufficient for *Candida* balanitis and vulvitis. In the presence of candidal vulvitis, the vagina also needs to be treated because the condition is vulvovaginitis. There are several effective topical preparations (tablets, suppositories, creams, and lotions) so that patient preference may guide the choice. Nystatin, a polyene antibiotic, and the numerous azole derivatives are beneficial. For the uncomplicated, episodic cases, azole derivatives in short courses or even single-dose regimens have been proven effective. Daily consumption of *Lactobacillus acidophilus*–containing yogurt has been found to decrease candidal colonization and infection. Systemic anticandidal therapy tends to be reserved for patients who have chronic recurrent vulvovaginal candidiasis or who are immunosuppressed.

Viral Infections

Molluscum Contagiosum

This infection is caused by a poxvirus, and classic lesions are dome-shaped, shiny or white papules with central umbilication.

This infection has joined the ranks of sexually transmitted diseases and can be quite extensive in persons with HIV infection. The differential diagnosis includes folliculitis and warts.

Herpes Simplex

Genital herpes simplex virus (HSV) infection, one of the most common sexually transmitted diseases, may be caused by HSV-1 or HSV-2. From 1976 to 1980, 16.4% of the U.S. population aged 17 to 74 years was found to be HSV-2 infected, while infection in prepubertal children is infrequent. As many as 50% of women whose sera are positive for HSV-2 antibodies are not aware of having genital lesions. Although HSV-1 infections occur in the genital area, thought to be caused by orogenital sex, most genital outbreaks are caused by HSV-2.

Genital herpes infection may be primary or recurrent. Primary infections occur in individuals with no history of previous outbreaks and absence of antibodies to HSV in their sera. They have an incubation period of 3 to 7 days. Paresthesias may precede the eruption by 2 to 3 days. The eruption consists of erythematous papules on a diffusely edematous and tender base. The papules develop into vesicles and pustules, coalescing and breaking down into ulcers that take as long as 2 to 4 weeks to heal. On average, virus may be cultured from these lesions for around 12 days. In severely immunocompromised patients, extensive, persistent, phagedenic, perianal herpetic ulcers are not uncommon. Primary genital HSV infections are more likely to be accompanied by systemic symptoms, cover a wider area (cervix, vagina, urethra, bladder, anus), and take longer to heal than recurrences. Systemic symptoms include low-grade fever, malaise, urinary retention, and regional lymphadenopathy. Primary HSV infections are likely to be accompanied by other sexually transmitted diseases. Within a year of recovering from primary genital HSV infection, 50% to 80% of patients develop a recurrence. Recurrent genital HSV infection is much milder than the primary infection. The lesions are fewer, smaller, and less painful and heal in 7 to 10 days. Viral shedding is reduced to 4 days, with a peak at 48 hours. Lesions consist of localized groups of vesicles, pustules, and shallow ulcers anywhere on the genital area. Systemic symptoms are less likely to occur.

The differential diagnosis of genital HSV includes all ulcerating sexually transmitted diseases, such as syphilis (primary and secondary), chancroid, lymphogranuloma venereum, and granuloma inguinale. Zosteriform primary HSV infection needs to be differentiated from herpes zoster. Recurrent genital ulcers may be a manifestation of recurrent genital aphthosis, inflammatory bowel disease, or Behçet's disease.

The gold standard for diagnosis is a positive culture that may yield results in 24 to 48 hours. For most clinical situations, a rapid, inexpensive, and fairly accurate test is a well-done Tzanck smear demonstrating multinucleated giant cells, intranuclear inclusions, or both. A comparison of Tzanck smears and viral isolation taken from vesicular lesions showed that Tzanck smears had a 90% predictive value when compared with positive cultures. Direct immunofluorescence, indirect immunoperoxidase, and viral isolation techniques yielded 71%, 76%, and 90% positive results, respectively, when specimens and smears were collected at the vesicular stage of the disease.

Treatment. The treatment of choice for primary genital HSV is systemic acyclovir. Except for severely immunocompromised persons or those who have systemic involvement, acyclovir is given orally, 200 mg five times a day for 10 days. When indicated, acyclovir may be given intravenously at a dose of 5 mg/kg every 8 hours for 7 days. Treatment of primary genital HSV infection does not prevent recurrences. Ancillary therapy during the acute stage of a primary infection includes bed rest as needed, baths or open-wet dressings, and pain management.

Treatment of recurrent genital HSV infection with acyclovir may be given continuously, 400 mg twice a day, or intermittently, starting in the prodromal phase, 200 mg to 400 mg three times a day. Signs and symptoms of recurrent disease are reduced, but viral shedding and, hence, possible transmission are not totally eliminated. Acyclovir-resistant strains are beginning to be seen in the immunocompromised group of patients.

The most important aspect of genital HSV infection is the prevention of neonatal herpes infection. Untreated neonatal HSV infection most often results in death or severe central nervous system disease.

Human Papillomavirus

Genital human papillomavirus (HPV) infection is most often a sexually transmitted disease with an incubation period of 2 to 3 months. The incidence of clinically evident HPV infection of the genital tract has increased remarkably in the past 2 decades, coincident with the increasing incidence of sexually transmitted diseases. The prevalence of subclinical HPV carriage has been demonstrated to be as high as 43% in women and 41% in men. There is strong epidemiologic and molecular biologic evidence of an association between genital HPV and carcinoma.

HPV infection of the genitalia may be viewed as *clinical, subclinical,* or *latent. Condylomata acuminata,* also known as genital warts, are the classic manifestation of HPV infection anywhere in the genital area and the urethral meatus. Single or multiple, discrete or coalescent, soft, cauliflower-like growths are most commonly seen on the moist, mucosal surfaces of the anogenital areas of both males and females. On nonmucosal areas, they become less papilliferous and more keratotic. Condylomata are most often associated with HPV types 6 and 11. Condylomata become more numerous and more resistant to therapy in immunosuppressed states such as pregnancy and acquired immunodeficiency syndrome, and during chemotherapy. The differential diagnosis includes condylomata lata of secondary syphilis, and verrucous carcinoma.

Flat papules and plaques may be solitary or multiple, discrete or confluent, skin colored, erythematous, or hyperpigmented with smooth, velvety, or verrucous surfaces. These lesions are analogous to flat warts on glabrous skin. The differential diagnosis includes vulvar intraepithelial neoplasia III (carcinoma in situ), lichen simplex chronicus, Paget's disease, psoriasis, and lichen planus.

Micropapillary forms are small, soft, smooth, pink papillations of the vulvar vestibule. As their relationship to HPV is controversial, it is probably best to adopt a position of watchful waiting when these lesions are encountered in asymptomatic women, unless examination of the rest of the genital tract reveals clinical evidence of HPV.

Subclinical or latent infection is present when the skin or mucosa appears normal by colposcopy, cytology, and histology. However, HPV DNA can be demonstrated by using molecular biologic techniques, particularly the extremely sensitive polymerase chain reaction (PCR) technique. Latent infection is thought to be responsible for recurrences at and around treatment sites, as demonstrated by the presence of HPV DNA in normal-appearing skin beyond the margins of treatment for anogenital condylomata and intraepithelial neoplasia.

The Papanicolaou smear is a very useful tool for screening the cervix and vagina for HPV infection. A positive result depends on the presence of "koilocytes," abnormally enlarged epithelial cells with abundant basophilic cytoplasm and hyperchromatic single or multiple nuclei that contain granular or densely staining chromatin, which are pathognomonic for HPV infection. These cells have a perinuclear halo that occupies a fourth to two thirds of the total cytoplasmic surface.

Treatment. Treatment of clinically evident genital HPV infection is destructive, nonspecific, and not reliably effective. For example, long-term cure rates after cryotherapy and salicylic acid are less than 50%. Before embarking on treatment, it is important to remember that spontaneous regression occurs about 30% of the time, that genital HPV infection is most often multifocal, involving contiguous structures, and that both local and systemic immunity play important roles. The indications for treatment are to (1) prevent spread; (2) alleviate symptoms such as itching and burning; (3) preserve normal function; (4) treat concomitant, dysplastic changes; and (5) alleviate disfigurement caused by the presence of clinical lesions.

Topical podophyllin, which arrests mitosis in metaphase, purified podophyllotoxin, the active ingredient in podophyllin, trichloroacetic acid, 5-fluorouracil, and liquid nitrogen cryotherapy are the most frequently used topical agents.

Electrosurgery. If the condylomata are large and extensive, a loop electrode may be used. Electrofulgination may be used for extensive, obstructive lesions.

Laser. The CO_2 laser is used for extensive lesions. The major disadvantage is the postoperative course, which is marked by severe discomfort, lasting for about 3 weeks after the procedure, and the relatively high recurrence rate.

Other Therapies. Recombinant interferon alfa is somewhat successful in the treatment of recalcitrant genital warts when injected intralesionally, and both alfa and interferon gamma are effective when given systemically.

Combination of several modalities of therapy such as laser-interferon or laser–5-fluorouracil is thought to decrease the recurrence rate after cessation of therapy.

There is general agreement that currently available therapies, no matter how aggressive, do not result in eradication of latent HPV infection. The use of proper barrier contraceptives is an important preventive measure. Once the presence of HPV infection is documented, regular surveillance such as by yearly or twice-yearly Papanicolaou smears and colposcopy is recommended.

Dermatoses

Aspects with particular relevance to their occurrence on the genital area are discussed in this chapter.

Intertrigo

Intertrigo usually appears as an erythematous, moist, macerated, and frequently malodorous dermatitis affecting flexural areas in the obese person during hot, humid weather. There is frequently superinfection with *Candida*. The differential diagnosis includes psoriasis, seborrheic dermatitis, erythrasma, and, in infants, Langerhans cell histiocytosis. It is responsive to a combination of open wet dressings or tub baths followed by a combination of 1% hydrocortisone mixed with 2% precipitated sulfur, miconazole, or iodoquinol in a light, greaseless base.

Psoriasis

Psoriasis may first appear or become a stubborn problem in the genital area. Lesions may vary from discrete scaly papules to erythematous, fissured plaques with macerated, white scales in the flexures. In the uncircumcised penis, lesions on the glans appear erosive. It is important to distinguish flexural psoriasis from diaper rash in infants and seborrheic dermatitis in adults because psoriasis takes longer to respond to therapy and is more likely to recur. Therapy is as for intertrigo, although a medium-strength topical corticosteroid may be used initially.

Contact Dermatitis

Irritant dermatitis may be caused by a chronic discharge, overcleansing, and therapeutic modalities such as trichloroacetic acid or 5-fluorouracil. Allergic contact dermatitis in the genitalia is frequently caused by preservatives (e.g., ethylenediamine, propylene glycol, formaldehyde releasers), medications (e.g., neomycin), fragrances, and latex (e.g., condoms). Therapy consists of discontinuing the offending agent followed by the use of topical steroids.

Lichen Simplex Chronicus

Lichen simplex chronicus refers to idiopathic chronic pruritus resulting in thickened skin from constant rubbing. It is otherwise known as pruritus vulvae when localized to the vulva. The skin becomes hyperkeratotic and hyperpigmented and resembles cobblestones, with broken-off hairs and prurigo nodules. The labia majora, mons, perineum, and scrotal sac are the areas most often involved. Histology is frequently necessary to differentiate this from other papulosquamous diseases mentioned in the previous section. The mainstay of therapy is topical steroids, and it is often necessary to start with a potent preparation for the first 3 to 4 weeks. Because itching is usually most intense as the patient is trying to fall asleep, sedating antihistamines taken before bedtime and the use of an icebag for immediate but temporary relief of pruritus are very helpful measures. Regular follow-up to monitor progress and provide encouragement is necessary for a good outcome.

Lichen Planus

Lichen planus can involve both the keratinized and mucosal surfaces of the genitalia. On keratinized skin, it looks like lichen planus elsewhere on the body. Annular lesions are frequently seen on the glans. On mucosal surfaces such as the uncircumcised glans, inner surface of the labia minora, vulva, and vagina there are prominent white, lacy patches bordering extensive erosions. Erosive lichen planus is one of the causes of desquamative vulvovaginitis. In the vulva and vagina, the erosive lesions of lichen planus can cause sclerosis, with eventual scarring. Pruritus may be present at the onset, but dyspareunia, burning pain, and spotting quickly supervene. Erosive lichen planus needs to be differentiated from lichen sclerosus, desquamative inflammatory vaginitis, and other erosive diseases that may affect the vulva (Table 9–1). The definitive diagnosis can be established on biopsy.

Therapy is difficult. Aggressive topical therapy with superpotent topical steroids, with or without intralesional steroids, is helpful. Systemic steroids, dapsone, antimalarial agents, retinoids, immunosuppressive agents, and topical steroids have at best been only temporarily palliative.

Lichen Sclerosus

Lichen sclerosus is the currently accepted terminology for a dermatosis that has been known as vulvar dystrophy, lichen sclerosus et

---

TABLE 9-1. Differential Diagnosis of Pruritus in the Genital Area

A. With minimal visible changes
   1. Associated with generalized pruritus from:
      Systemic disease—diabetes, chronic renal and
        hepatic diseases, Sjögren's syndrome, malignancy
      Paresthesias
      Psychogenic—delusions of parasitosis
   2. Localized to genital area
      Infestation—pediculosis pubis, early scabies
      Dermatitis—early irritant/allergic contact
B. With scaling/maceration/crusting or thickening of
  cutaneous/mucosal surfaces
   1. Infections—erythrasma, superficial dermatophyte,
      candidiasis, tinea versicolor, human papillomavirus
   2. Dermatitis—intertrigo, seborrheic dermatitis, allergic/
      irritant contact, lichen simplex chronicus
   3. Papulosquamous dermatoses—psoriasis, Reiter's, lichen
      planus, Darier's, lichen sclerosus/balanitis xerotica
      obliterans
   4. Neoplasias—VIN I to III; PIN I to III; squamous cell
      carcinoma, extramammary Paget's disease
C. With vaginal/urethral discharge
   1. Vulvovaginitis—from estrogen deprivation; candidiasis;
      from cervicitis caused by herpes simplex, gonorrhea,
      Trichomonas, and bacterial vaginosis
   2. Balanoposthitis—in uncircumcised males from
      accumulation of smegma; candidiasis, from urethral
      discharge caused by gonorrhea, *Trichomonas*, and
      nonspecific urethritis

atrophicus, kraurosis vulvae, and, in the male, balanitis xerotica obliterans. This dermatosis, which can affect any part of the body, occurs most often in the anogenital area of postmenopausal women, although it has been reported in all age groups of both sexes. Lichen sclerosus in prepubertal girls is rare, has a tendency to improve with increasing age, but may persist to adulthood. It is rare in males, and the glans and prepuce are often the only sites involved, with phimosis as the leading complication.

Lichen sclerosus in the genitalia appears as ivory-colored atrophic or white, hyperkeratotic papules that coalesce into shiny, sclerotic plaques leading to phimosis in males. In females, the plaques may become sclerotic, bullous, ulcerated, or hemorrhagic and the epidermis may be thin and shiny or thick and white. End-stage vulvar lichen sclerosus shows total loss of identifiable structures, and the introitus can be reduced to a slit-like opening. In women, the perianal area is frequently involved, giving rise to obstipation.

Early lichen sclerosus is generally very pruritic, but as it becomes chronic, symptoms secondary to erosions of stenotic orifices supervene. Depending on the stage of lichen sclerosus, the differential diagnosis may include lichen planus, lichen simplex chronicus, and the scarred end-stage of the different erosive conditions afflicting the genitalia. Multiple biopsy samples from noneroded lesions may be necessary to arrive at the correct diagnosis. Current therapy for lichen sclerosus relies on the use of superpotent topical steroids such as 0.05% clobetasol propionate. This results in rapid relief of symptoms with accompanying evidence of histologic improvement. Whether persistent use of these agents will eventually reverse the disease process is still not known.

Neoplasms

Benign Neoplasms

Benign neoplasms with special predilection for or importance in the genitalia are discussed here. Angiokeratomas are common lesions in the genitalia of older men and women. They are frequently multiple, dark red to purple papules, usually between 1 to 3 mm in diameter. When these lesions are numerous on the scrotum of a young male, the possibility of Fabry's disease (angiokeratoma corporis diffusum) might be considered. Angiokeratomas usually do not require therapy.

Bartholin's cyst is a cystic swelling in the posterolateral aspect of the vulvar vestibule caused by obstruction of Bartholin's duct. When sizable, it might cause pain. Because the obstruction tends to be recurrent, marsupialization is the treatment of choice.

Idiopathic calcinosis of the scrotum occurs as asymptomatic, grayish or yellowish white, firm nodules on scrotal skin. Draining lesions may be excised.

Pearly penile papules are small, smooth, dome-shaped or papillomatous papules occurring in the corona of the penis. They are a type of angiofibroma and are asymptomatic and require no therapy.

Nonvenereal sclerosing lymphangitis of the penis presents as asymptomatic purplish cords around the coronal sulcus of the penis. Despite its name, it is most likely a post-traumatic phlebitis of superficial penile veins. No therapy is needed.

Malignant Tumors

Intrapeithelial Neoplasia

Equivalent classification and terminology apply to vaginal, cervical, penile, and anogenital intraepithelial neoplasia. Squamous intraepithelial neoplasia of the external genitalia comprises carcinoma in situ, Bowen's disease, bowenoid papulosis, and erythroplasia of Queyrat. Multifocal lesions (bowenoid papulosis) are more common in young persons and are associated with HPV (most commonly, types 16, 18, 31, and 33). These lesions appear as multiple, white, skin-colored or hyperpigmented flat papules of varying sizes. Although some of these lesions may progress to invasive squamous carcinoma, most tend to follow a benign course, so that the currently accepted therapy is local destruction with careful longitudinal follow-up. Differential diagnosis of these multiple, discrete lesions includes flat warts, genital lentiginosis, and seborrheic keratoses. The solitary form of intraepithelial neoplasia, also known as Bowen's disease of the vulva or erythroplasia of Queyrat on the male genitalia, is more common in the older age group. This presents anywhere on the vulva of older women as a red or hyperpigmented, velvety to hyperkeratotic, pruritic plaque. In older men, it presents as a red, glazed patch, usually on the glans penis. These solitary lesions have a tendency to become invasive squamous cell carcinomas and are thus treated by excision, CO_2 laser vaporization, or 5-fluorouracil. Follow-up is important.

Extramammary Paget's disease appears in the anogenital areas of older men and women as well-dermarcated, pruritic, erythematous, scaly, or eczematous plaques. This condition should be considered if a red, scaly eruption on or near genital skin does not resolve with topical therapy. Extramammary Paget's disease encompasses three entities: a primary intraepidermal carcinoma with apocrine differentiation, carcinoma of apocrine glands that colonizes the adjacent epidermis, and intraepithelial spread from nearby internal carcinomas, such as those of the rectum or bladder. Because the area of involvement is generally larger than what is superficially visible, margin control is necessary during the excision process.

Squamous Cell Carcinoma

Verrucous carcinoma, also known as giant condyloma of Buschke and Lowenstein, can reach enormous sizes in both men and women. These are now considered a type of squamous cell carcinoma despite their bland histologic appearance because of their tendency to recur after, and despite, extensive surgery. Radiation therapy can cause the tumor to become more aggressive.

Squamous cell carcinoma of the scrotum is associated with contact with tar and mineral oils. Penile squamous cell carcinoma is almost never seen in circumcised males. It may present as red or white plaques, verrucous lesions, or ulcers. Treatment is generally surgical, with amputation and node dissection depending on the stage of the cancer.

Squamous cell carcinoma, although rare, is the most frequent malignancy found in the vulva. Most of the cases can likely be accounted for by progression of Bowen's disease, HPV infection, and lichen sclerosus. Squamous cell carcinoma may appear as verrucous lesions, red or white plaques, and ulcers. Therapy is mostly surgical with total vulvectomy and node dissection depending on the stage.

Vulvodynia

Vulvodynia is chronic vulvar discomfort characterized by the patient's complaint of burning, irritation, or rawness. Systematic investigation of the possible causes and therapies for vulvodynia is just now beginning. An algorithm for diagnosis is presented in Table 9–2.

Vulvar Vestibulitis Syndrome

Criteria for making a diagnosis of vulvar vestibulitis syndrome include (1) pain on penile entry (introital dyspareunia), (2) findings confined to focal erythema within the vulvar vestibule, and (3) exquisite tenderness on light palpation of erythematous areas. The typical patient complains of painful intercourse or inability to have intercourse. In those who are not sexually active, complaints range from pain on touching the vulvar vestibule to pain on tampon insertion, on prolonged sitting, on riding a bicycle, on crossing the legs, or on wearing tight jeans. Clinical findings are meager and confined to the vulvar vestibule, in which there is always erythema around the openings of Bartholin's ducts, at times accompanied by erythema around the openings of Skene's glands and around the ostia of minor vestibular glands at the base of the hymen. The cause remains unknown. Potential etiologies include trauma, HPV infection, and chronic candidiasis, but in most cases no cause is found.

Treatment includes discontinuing everything the patient has been using or taking and application of bland barrier preparations such as white petrolatum or zinc oxide supplemented with topical anesthet-

---

TABLE 9–2.   Differential Diagnosis of Vulvodynia

A. With visible lesions on mucocutaneous surfaces
 1. Vesiculopustules—recurrent herpes simplex, recurrent candidiasis, pustular psoriasis, Reiter's, chronic aphthosis, Behçet's disease, poststeroid vulvitis
 2. Ulcers—recurrent herpes simplex, chronic aphthosis, Behçet's disease, deep fungal infections, tuberculosis, pyoderma gangrenosum, Crohn's, malignant neoplasms
 3. Bullae—Hailey-Hailey disease, pemphigus vulgaris, cicatricial pemphigoid, benign bullous dermatosis of childhood, recurrent bullous drug eruptions
 4. Erosions—all of No. 3 above; lichen sclerosus, lupus erythematosus, desquamative lichen planus, desquamative vulvitis, atrophic vulvovaginitis
B. With tender, red spots in vestibule only
 1. Vulvar vestibulitis*
 2. Zoon's vulvitis
C. Without visible lesions
 1. Pudendal neuralgia—with demonstrable sensory alterations such as allodynia and hyperalgesia
 2. Other perineal pain syndromes—?sensory findings

---

*Except for vulvar vestibulitis syndrome, all of the above conditions may be seen in the male genitalia also.

ics such as lidocaine ointment or EMLA (eutectic mixture of prilocaine and lidocaine). For those with demonstrable *Candida* on potassium hydroxide or culture, systemic anticandidal therapy may be initiated and continued for 3 to 6 months after cultures have turned negative. Interferon alfa administered intradermally into the vestibule has provided temporary relief in women with idiopathic vulvar vestibulitis. For patients with long-standing (>2 years) entry dyspareunia of such severity as to almost totally prevent sexual intercourse, surgical excision of the vulvar vestibule with mobilization of the vaginal mucosa offers about a 65% rate of success. The long-term benefit from this procedure is unknown. In women presenting with vulvar vestibulitis after trauma from topical 5-fluorouracil or laser therapy, the symptoms most likely clear up spontaneously.

Pudendal Neuralgia

In pudendal neuralgia, the burning pain is unprovoked and extends outside the vulvar vestibule. It is often accompanied by a deep aching component with occasional paroxysms of severe lancinating pain. The similarity of these symptoms to those described for post–herpes zoster neuralgia and diabetic neuropathy suggested neuropathic pain in the area innervated by the pudendal nerve (S-2 to S-5).

Affected patients are usually in their mid 20s to mid 30s. Additional complaints include deep itching, formication, a painful burning sensation on light touch, discomfort or burning on movement of pubic hairs, entry to postcoital dyspareunia, and a sensation of labial swelling.

Visible changes are generally limited to mild erythema around the openings of the vestibular glands. Sensory testing of the area innervated by the pudendal nerve using a sharp-pointed stick and a cotton-tipped applicator reveals a variety of responses, including hypalgesia, hyperalgesia, and hyperpathia. Occasionally developing after a traumatic event, such as a bicycle accident, in the majority of cases the cause is idiopathic.

Drug therapy of the idiopathic cases relies on the use of tricyclic antidepressants (e.g., amitriptyline and imipramine) and topical anesthetics for milder cases and anticonvulsants for those with accompanying paroxysmal pain.

chapter 10

What Benign and Malignant Proliferations of Cells Affect the Skin, and How Are They Treated?

PHOTOCARCINOGENESIS

(CM&S Chapter 140)

Cells that proliferate in defiance of the normal restraints of the cell cycle give rise to tumors or neoplasms. Cells of benign growths remain clustered in a single group; once the cells invade surrounding tissues, the tumor is considered malignant. Cancers are categorized according to their origin, if it is known, or state of differentiation. Those arising from epithelial cells are termed carcinomas and in the skin they mainly consist of basal cell carcinomas (BCCs) and squamous cell carcinomas (SCCs). Melanomas arise from melanocytes.

Genetic changes that hyperactivate stimulatory genes (oncogenes) or inactivate inhibitory genes (tumor suppressor genes) are involved in the development of neoplasms. Such changes allow the abnormal cells to pass on their aberrant characteristics to their progeny (although epigenetic changes have been determined to play a part in some cases). The effect of activation of oncogenes is dominant, that is, only one of the two copies present in a cell need undergo the change. On the other hand, direct inactivation of tumor suppressor genes may have a recessive mode of action, that is, both copies of the gene have to be quiescent or absent in order to free the cell of their growth control properties. Aberrations in the cellular environment disrupt the delicate balance between the processes of growth, differentiation, and physiologic programmed cell death (apoptosis), and result in the formation of immortalized cells. Because cancers do not arise immediately after exposure to carcinogens, and because the chances for developing cancer increase with age, it is likely that multiple genetic alterations cooperate in the development of the neoplastic state.

Agents that cause genetic changes, or *mutagens* as they are termed, may present themselves to living organisms as chemicals, viruses, or as radiant energy. This chapter focuses on solar ultraviolet (UV) radiation, a naturally occurring environmental carcinogen associated with cancers of the skin. Lesions induced by UV radiation have unique characteristics that in effect, leave "signature" mutations on the affected genes. Thus far, mutations in the *ras* family of oncogenes and in the *p53* tumor suppressor gene have been characterized in skin carcinomas.

Photobiology of Solar Ultraviolet Radiation

Solar Ultraviolet in the Etiology of Skin Cancers

Basal and squamous cell carcinomas occur most frequently on sun-exposed regions of the body. The incidence of these neoplasms correlates with the amount of accumulated sun exposure and is inversely related to the protective action of skin pigments. It has been demonstrated, in studies using laboratory animals, that most of the deleterious effects arise from exposure to the UV component of sunlight. Recent advances using molecular techniques have confirmed the role of UV radiation in the etiology of epidermal neoplasms.

Solar Ultraviolet Spectrum

The UV region of the solar spectrum is divided into three parts; UVA (320 to 400 nm), UVB (280 to 320 nm), and UVC (200 to 280 nm). The shorter wavelengths of UV radiation reaching the earth's surface extend into the absorption spectra of nucleic acids and proteins, and energy in this region of overlap is absorbed into the skin, producing erythema, burns, and eventually keratoses. These biologic effects are brought about through damage at unsaturated chemical bonds, such as those in the bases of DNA and RNA, and in the aromatic amino acids of proteins. Epidemiologic and clinical studies indicate that UVB is responsible for the induction of most skin cancers in humans. For a long time UVA was believed to be noncarcinogenic, but recent studies have demonstrated both the carcinogenicity of UVA, as well as its ability to enhance the development of UVB-induced skin cancers.

Although UVC is a potent mutagen, it assumes a less significant role in the pathogenesis of human skin cancers because it does not pass through the stratospheric ozone layer. Additionally, transmission of solar radiation through the skin drops off sharply below 300 nm, thereby providing a natural barrier to the most harmful fraction of UV rays. Much public and scientific attention is now focused on measuring alterations in the ozone layer and the resultant shift in the intensity and wavelength spectrum of solar UV radiation reaching the earth's surface.

DNA Photoproducts Induced by Ultraviolet Radiation

DNA as Target in Photodamage

Several lines of evidence implicate DNA as the primary target involved in most of the biologic effects of UV irradiation:

1. The action spectra for mutagenesis, cellular transformation, and cell death closely follow the absorption spectrum for DNA.

2. Removal of photolesions from irradiated DNA by enzymatic photoreactivation reduces the incidence of UV-induced cellular transformation and tumor formation.

3. Introduction of protooncogenes damaged in vitro by UV radiation into normal cells leads to tumorigenic transformation.

4. Individuals suffering from DNA repair deficiency disorders such as xeroderma pigmentosum (XP) are sunlight sensitive and highly cancer prone.

Major Components of Photodamage

UV radiation damages DNA by direct interaction and also via the involvement of endogenous cellular photosensitizers. The predominant UV-induced DNA photoproducts are (1) the cis-syn diastereoisomers of cyclobutane-type pyrimidine dimers (Py $\diamond$ Py) and (2) the pyrimidine (6-4) pyrimidone lesions. These two major groups of UV photoproducts result from the covalent association of adjacent pyrimidines. The cyclobutane pyrimidine dimers are formed when the double bonds between the C5 and C6 carbon atoms of two adjacent pyrimidines become saturated, producing a four-membered ring structure. As a result of this dimerization, the angle between the bases is reduced and the DNA helix is distorted. The potential of photodimerization is enhanced by the presence of a 5' pyrimidine and lowered by a 5' purine, especially a guanine. Both photolesions appear to form preferentially in runs of tandemly located pyrimidine residues that are often "hot spots" of UV-induced mutations.

Minor Components of Photodamage

UV radiation also induces other types of DNA lesions, such as single-strand breaks, DNA-protein cross-links, and unstable pyrimidine photohydrates. The photohydrates are rare lesions (up to 100 times less frequent than pyrimidine dimers) formed by UVC and UVB in comparable amounts. In both instances cytosine photohydrates predominate over thymine photohydrates. UVA is also known to produce single-strand breaks and alkali-labile sites through the action of reactive oxygen species such as superoxide anion, singlet oxygen, and hydrogen peroxide. Occasional double-strand breaks have been observed in UV-irradiated DNA, but it is possible that they arise from lesions at closely opposed dipyrimidine sequences. Photoproducts involving purine bases in double-stranded DNA occur at a very low frequency.

Repair of DNA Photolesions

The DNA Repair Systems

Both cyclobutane dimers and (6-4) lesions, if left unrepaired, obstruct the progression of DNA and RNA synthesizing machineries and disrupt cellular processes. Thus, a number of repair pathways operate in human cells to overcome the harmful effects of DNA damaging agents. In the versatile repair pathway known as excision repair, a portion of the damaged strand is enzymatically excised and subsequently replaced using the intact opposite strand as template. The pathway consists of multiple steps, and genes involved at a number of stages have been identified. Proteins that bind preferentially to damaged DNA without any sequence specificity are thought to serve as markers that pinpoint the damage to the repair system. Such proteins may also function as "molecular matchmakers" that enhance the probability of interaction between other components of the repair complex and a damaged stretch of DNA in the absence of stabilizing effects arising from specific sequences. The enzyme photolyase is present in many species and mediates reactivation of cyclobutane dimers in the presence of long wavelengths of light.

Human Genetic Repair Deficiency Diseases

A number of genetic disorders arise from defects in the cellular system responsible for processing DNA damage. They are often associated with increased incidence of malignancies, mutagenesis, and chromosomal instability, with patients usually exhibiting radiation sensitivity from an early age. XP, Cockayne's syndrome, Bloom syndrome, and hereditary dysplastic nevus syndrome are examples of diseases in which the patients exhibit UV sensitivity.

Biologic Effects of Ultraviolet Radiation

Mutagenesis at DNA Photolesions

The genetic background of the individual is an important factor in determining the biologic consequences of UV radiation. For example, when exposed to UVB, persons with sun-sensitive (Type I) skin have a higher amount of pyrimidine dimer formation than do those with sun-insensitive (Type IV) skin. Both cyclobutane dimers and (6-4) lesions cause mutations in human cells. These mutations are predominantly $C \rightarrow T$ and $CC \rightarrow TT$ transitions at sequences containing adjacent pyrimidine nucleotides and have become the *signature* of UV-induced mutagenesis.

Photocarcinogenesis

Carcinogenesis is usually a multistep process involving initiation, promotion, and progression. For instance, a subthreshold dose of a DNA-damaging agent may initiate the process of carcinogenesis by inducing mutations at one or more sites in the DNA. These mutations may lie dormant for several years until subsequent exposure to tumor-promoting agents (which need not be carcinogenic in themselves) leads to the appearance of tumors. UV radiation is a potentially complete carcinogen because it does not require additional extraneous effectors as initiators or promoters. Rodent skin cancers induced by repeated exposure to UV radiation have provided researchers with excellent model systems for investigating the harmful effects of UV radiation because the etiology of these tumors is well defined and other known risk factors are carefully controlled. Either a single large dose, or the accumulation of several small doses of UV radiation, is sufficient to induce skin cancers in experimental animals. Skin cancer induction is usually associated with the appearance of precancerous lesions (actinic keratoses) at the site of UV exposure, indicating that the disease develops in multiple sequential stages that involve direct interaction between the carcinogen and the affected cells.

Photosuppression of Local and Systemic Immune Responses

Another rapidly emerging role of UV is at the level of interference with the immune mechanisms that protect against tumor development. The tumors induced in the above mentioned study, by chronic exposure to UV radiation, were highly antigenic and did not grow when transplanted to normal syngeneic recipients. All tumors grew readily in immunosuppressed mice, indicating that the rejection seen in normal mice was immunologically mediated. This suggested that the original tumor-bearing animals must have been immunocompromised in order for the tumors to have grown. Subsequent studies revealed that the UV-induced tumors from the agouti mice were immunogenic as well, bringing about a specific memory response during tumor regression, and that UV radiation suppresses specific immune responses, thereby allowing the growth of the tumors.

UV radiation exerts both local and systemic effects on the host's immune system. Local effects at the site of UVB exposure are mediated mainly via qualitative and quantitative changes in the Langerhans cells that reside in the epidermis. The number of these cells is decreased in irradiated murine skin; those remaining are morphologically altered and unable to present antigens to the Th2 subset of T helper cells. Moreover, under the influence of cytokines released from surrounding UV-induced keratinocytes, the Langerhans cells become converted to antigen-presenting cells that induce T cell tolerance. Yet another effect of exposure to UVB radiation is the recruitment of melanophages to the epidermis. The melanophages present antigens to suppressor cells, further down-regulating the local immune response.

Systemic immune suppression is associated with the release of immunomodulatory cytokines and immunosuppressive substances by UV-irradiated epidermal cells. The release of at least some of these factors seems to be wavelength dependent because UVB exposure suppresses delayed type hypersensitivity whereas UVA is responsible for decreasing contact hypersensitivity. Although cellular immune reactions such as delayed type hypersensitivity are suppressed, antibody production remains unaffected.

Molecular Mechanism of Ultraviolet-Induced Carcinogenesis

Molecular analysis of human skin cancers originating on sun-exposed body sites and mouse skin tumors induced by UV radiation has provided new information on the role of oncogenes and tumor suppressor genes in UV radiation carcinogenesis. In particular, mutations in *ras* and *p53* genes have been detected in both the human and murine skin cancers, suggesting that *ras* activation as well as *p53* inactivation plays a role in UV radiation carcinogenesis. Although the genes implicated in the pathogenesis of human and mouse skin cancers may be similar to those involved in other types of cancer, UV-induced skin cancers display unique UV-signature mutations ($C \rightarrow T$ and $CC \rightarrow TT$) at dipyrimidine sequences that are not commonly found in other types of human or mouse cancers.

MALIGNANT NEOPLASMS OF KERATINOCYTES

(CM&S Chapter 141)

Actinic (Solar) Keratosis

Definition

Actinic keratoses (AK), also referred to as solar keratoses, are keratoses induced by chronic ultraviolet radiation (UVA). Solar keratoses can be conceived of as evolving lesions of squamous cell carcinoma in situ, but because so few of them progress to invasive neoplasia, they are not usually considered malignancies. AKs typically begin to appear in the fourth and fifth decades, and increase in number with advancing years. Individuals who are fair-skinned, with blue eyes and red or blond hair, are particularly susceptible. Similarly, individuals whose occupation or recreation takes them out of doors are regularly affected.

Clinical Presentation

AKs are poorly circumscribed erythematous macules and papules, usually several millimeters to a centimeter in diameter, arising in a sun-exposed distribution. These lesions often have an adherent scale and are variably rough depending on the degree of hyperkeratosis. Lesions arising on the ears, the dorsal hands, and forearms tend to be much thicker and horn-like than those on the face. Some AKs are remarkably tender. Less commonly, AKs are hyperpigmented. Lesions arising on the lip (usually the lower lip) are referred to as actinic cheilitis, which typically is manifested by confluent scaliness, focal erosion, fissures, and lack of definition of the vermilion border.

The natural history of AKs is controversial. Malignant transformation rates of 0.24% have been cited; however, up to 20% of untreated AKs have reportedly transformed into squamous cell carcinomas (SCC).

Pathology

Common to all actinic keratoses is the presence of atypical keratinocytes along the basal cell layer (often budding off) and usually in the lower third of the epidermis, and disordered cornification marked by singly dyskeratotic keratinocytes, a diminished granular layer, and parakeratosis. A hallmark is alternating orthokeratosis and parakeratosis.

In some solar keratoses there is complete full-thickness atypia of the epidermis (called the bowenoid type). They may be indistinguishable from Bowen's type of SCC in situ.

Bowen's Disease

Definition

Bowen's disease refers to SCC in situ and may arise anywhere on the skin; however, when it occurs on the mucous membrane of the glans penis it is termed erythroplasia of Queyrat. It has a protracted course that over many years may progress to invasive SCC.

Clinical Presentation

Lesions are characterized by macules or plaques of scaly erythema up to several centimeters in diameter, and may simulate an inflammatory dermatosis. Some lesions are pigmented. The variable degree of hyperkeratosis and margination give rise to the following basic clinical patterns: (1) nodular crusted or ulcerated plaques; (2) less nodular lesions with a raised thread-like border; (3) scaly, keratotic plaques similar to large actinic keratosis; and (4) slightly elevated scaly flesh-colored plaques.

Bowen's disease most commonly arises on the head and neck but is noted to arise on sun-protected skin as well. It also can arise from the nail bed, palms and soles, and mucous membranes. Patients may have more than one lesion.

Pathology

Bowen's disease is SCC in situ in which atypical keratinocytes are arranged throughout the entire thickness of the epidermis. A loss of the granular layer with the production of parakeratosis is typical. Pagetoid spread may be seen, as well varying amounts of psoriasiform hyperplasia, hyperkeratosis, papillomatosis, and an extensive inflammatory cell infiltrate in the dermis. Some lesions can be atrophic and others heavily pigmented.

Pathogenesis

Chronic solar exposure as well as other forms of radiation, including ultraviolet light, psoralens and ultraviolet light, and inhalation of mustard gas are implicated in causing Bowen's disease. This neoplasm may occur as a late sequela of chronic arsenic toxicity or related to human papillomavirus infection.

Differential Diagnosis

Any persistent chronic scaling macule or plaque such as eczema, psoriasis, actinic keratosis, or superficial spreading basal cell carcinoma may suggest Bowen's disease.

Keratoacanthoma

Definition and Clinical Description

Keratoacanthoma (KA) has classically been considered a benign epithelial neoplasm. KA shares many clinical and histologic features with SCC, and some consider it to be a form of SCC that usually, but not invariably, involutes. They typically arise on sun-damaged, hair-bearing, light-colored skin in mid- to late life. Males are more commonly affected than females by a ratio of 2:1. The typical solitary KA is a distinctive, well-circumscribed, dome-shaped papule or nodule with a central keratin-filled crater. The lesion is rapidly progressive, reaching 1.0 to 2.5 cm over a 6- to 8-week period. After a stationary phase of 2 to 8 weeks, KAs typically spontaneously involute over a 2- to 8-week period, leaving an atrophic scar in their wake. Lesions morphologically consistent with KA may be SCC when examined histologically. Lesions recalcitrant to treatment and otherwise simulating SCC may represent typical KA histologically.

Waiting for a KA to involute can have disastrous consequences. The metastasis of an invasive SCC that morphologically simulated a KA is a paradigm of a clinical paradox: If a presumptive benign diagnosis can be proven incorrect by subsequent biologic activity, should not all such lesions be treated as malignant? It is for this reason that most authorities treat KA as a well-differentiated SCC.

Pathology

Keratoacanthoma has a distinctive symmetric exoendophytic proliferation of cornifying glassy eosinophillic squamous epithelium, having a central crater filled with orthokeratotic scale. At the edge of the lesion, well-differentiated squamous epithelium lip the opening to the crater, and the base of the lesion consists of irregular lobules that usually extend deep into the reticular dermis. There are varying amounts of cytologic atypical mitoses, as well as mixed inflammation with microabscesses and fibroplasias at the base of the lesion.

Squamous Cell Carcinoma

Definition

SCC is the second most common form of skin cancer, representing 20% of cutaneous malignancies. The incidence has been increasing at a rate of 4% to 8% since the 1960s. SCC most commonly affects individuals in mid- to late life, and most commonly arises in areas of chronic sun exposure. Cutaneous SCCs characteristically cause local tissue destruction. Cutaneous SCCs carry greater risk for metastases than does basal cell carcinoma (BCC), and in some instances have an explosive growth rate.

Clinical Presentation

The typical SCC is a hyperkeratotic, skin-colored to erythematous papule, nodule, or plaque arising on sun-damaged skin. Larger lesions may have subcutaneous extension.

The tendency for recurrence or metastasis is based on several parameters. The central zone of the face is an area at high risk for local recurrence. SCC arising on the temple, dorsal hands, lips, ear, scalp, and penis is at significant risk for metastases. Larger surgical margins are required to histologically clear SCC in these high-risk areas. SCC arising in areas of chronic ulceration, sinus tracts, and chronic osteomyelitis also has increased risk of metastases.

Size

The larger the tumor, the more likely the chance for local recurrence. Tumors less than 1 cm have a 99.5% cure rate by Mohs micrographic surgery, compared with 82.3% for tumors 2 to 3 cm, and 58.9% for tumors greater than 3 cm. A local recurrence rate of

7.4% for tumors under 2 cm in diameter, contrasted to 15.2% for tumors greater than 2 cm, has been reported. Margins of excision therefore are adjusted according to size, with a 4-mm margin recommended for tumors less than 2 cm, and 6 mm for tumors of 2 cm or greater.

Depth of Invasion

Lesions that penetrate through the dermis to the subcutaneous adipose tissue may occur up to 30% of the time. A local recurrence rate of 5.3% for tumors less than 4 mm in depth, compared with a rate of 17.2% for tumors 4 mm or greater, has been observed. Tumors greater than 1 cm in diameter, or of histologic grade 2 or higher, are more likely to extend to the subcutaneous tissue.

Degree of Histologic Differentiation

Less well differentiated SCC generally requires larger resections, and therefore has greater likelihood of local recurrence.

Metastases and Death Rates

Actinically derived SCC has an extremely low propensity for metastasis (0.3% to 3.7%). SCCs arising at specific high-risk sites such as the lip, ear, penis, scrotum, and anus carry much greater risk. Size greater than 2 cm, depth of invasion to at least 4 mm, and Broder's histologic classification of 2 or greater are various factors defining a tumor at higher risk for metastases. Additionally, underlying immunosuppression may significantly impact on propensity for metastasis. When SCC does metastasize, typically it is to regional lymph nodes. Five-year survival in patients with regional lymph node metastases is 26%, and 23% in patients with distant metastases.

Verrucous Carcinoma

Verrucous carcinoma is a clinicopathologic subtype of SCC. This low-grade, indolent neoplasm is usually exophytic with a wart-like appearance and may cause significant local tissue destruction, but carries a very low risk for metastasis. It characteristically arises on the foot (epithelioma cuniculatum), or on the glans penis (giant condyloma of Buschke and Lowenstein). When seen in the mouth (oral florid papillomatosis), hyperkeratosis is manifested by diffuse leukokeratosis.

Pathology

SCC most commonly consists of a proliferation of atypical squamous cells that originates in the epidermis and extends into the reticular dermis and below. Multiple, often atypical, mitoses are common. There are variable degrees of differentiation with individual cell keratinization or more organized cornification in the form of squamous eddies and horn pearl formations.

Histologic subtypes of SCC include spindle and acantholytic SCC. Verrucous carcinoma is a distinct clinicopathologic entity that is characterized by a large papillated exoendophytic proliferation that has hyperkeratosis and parakeratosis. It may be indistinguishable from a large condyloma because the bulbous rete in verrucous carcinoma contains very well differentiated squamous cells with little to no cytologic atypia.

Pathogenesis

Many etiologic factors exist in the development of SCC. The single most significant predisposing factor for the development of SCC is chronic ultraviolet light exposure. These include occupational chemical exposure (such as soot and other hydrocarbons, arsenic from medicinals, well water, and insecticides), x-irradiation, human papillomavirus infection, chronic thermal injury, chronic ulcers/sinus tracts/osteomyelitis, discoid lupus, and certain genetic disorders (e.g., xeroderma pigmentosum, epidermodysplasia verruciformis, recessive dystrophic epidermolysis bullosa, and oculocutaneous albinism).

Basal Cell Carcinoma

Definition

BCC is a malignant neoplasm of epithelial cells that resemble the germinative cells of hair follicles more than they do the cells of the basal layer of the epidermis. It is the most frequently encountered cancer in man.

Clinical Presentation

Basal cell carcinoma has multiple distinctive clinical forms, which can often be correlated with histologic subtypes. The various clinical forms of BCC include:

1. Nodular BCC. The most frequent form of BCC, this presents as a waxy, opalescent or translucent papule or nodule associated with overlying fine telangiectasias. Ulceration or erosion of the surface is a frequent finding. Histologically, these lesions may have an infiltrative or micronodular pattern. Subclinical extent may be significant, which frequently accounts for inadequate treatment. For this reason, such tumors are more likely to recur after therapy, and therefore are categorized as aggressive BCC. BCCs may occasionally be pigmented.

2. Morpheiform or sclerosing BCC. This subtype of BCC has a scar-like appearance. It presents as a dermal plaque with overlying epidermal atrophy in a sun-exposed distribution with a history of antecedent trauma. Subclinical extension is often great and treatment failures frequent.

3. Superficial BCC. This BCC subtype most commonly arises on the trunk and extremities. The tumors are characterized by an erythematous macule or patch with a fine scale or superficial erosion. This type of BCC is the type most frequently seen in chronic arsenism, and as a late sequela of radiation therapy. Individuals may have broad areas of superficial BCC that are multiple and disconnected. This true multicentricity is likely a field effect, with all affected tissue having similar local carcinogenic factors accounting for the tumor.

As with SCC, certain parameters define BCCs that pose greatest risk to affected individuals.

Location

The factors discussed for SCC are also wholly relevant for BCC.

Size

A cure rate for tumors less than 2 cm in diameter of 99.8%; 98.6% for tumors between 2 and 3 cm; and 90.5% for tumors greater than 3 cm has been reported with Mohs surgery.

Histology

Unlike SCC, BCC is not histologically graded according to degree of differentiation. However, several histologic subtypes are notoriously difficult to manage. In particular, micronodular, infiltrative, and morpheiform BCCs have a much higher incidence of positive surgical margins after surgical excision (18.6% to 33.3%) as compared with tumors with a nodular or superficial histologic pattern. BCC with marked squamous differentiation has been observed by some to be a more virulent tumor. As with SCC, the perineural space can serve as a conduit for significant subclinical tumor extension.

Pathology

Only the nodular, morpheiform, superficial, fibroepitheliomatous, and infundibulocystic types are well-established clinicopathologic entities. Keratotic, adenoid, infiltrating, micronodular, and pigmented BCCs are variations of these basic clinicopathologic entities. All basal cell carcinomas have in common the presence of basaloid cells arranged in varied aggregations with elongated nuclei palisading the periphery of some aggregations, neoplastic cells with hyperchromatic nuclei, and varying numbers of mitotic figures accompanied by karyorrhexis and pyknosis. Clefts between the neoplastic cells and the adjacent, often mucinous stroma are characteristic. The vast majority of the neoplasms show some attachment to the undersurface of the epidermis.

Nodular BCC is composed of large, rounded aggregations of basaloid cells. These lesions are often cystic as a consequence of central tumor necrosis or mucin deposition within the epithelial aggregations.

Superficial basal cell carcinoma is composed of multiple buds of basaloid cells that project from the basal layer of the epidermis into the papillary dermis, with varying amounts of fibroplasia, inflammatory cell infiltrate, and fibromyxoid change to the surrounding stroma. Morpheiform BCC is also known as sclerosing, fibrosing, and desmoplastic types of BCC. The neoplasm is composed of narrow cords and even strings of single cells that are branched and separated in a dense fibrotic and sclerotic stroma. Deep dermal invasion and subcutaneous involvement are not uncommon.

Squamous differentiation is common in BCC, especially in recurrent/persistent BCC, particularly near the dermoepidermal junction. Metatypical types of BCC are thought to be a variant with some squamous differentiation that has more nuclear anaplasia and an infiltrative pattern. Peripheral palisading is less obvious and the cells are large with more abundant pale-staining cytoplasm.

Pathogenesis

Like SCC, BCC is related to chronic UVR exposure. They are common on the head and neck of Caucasians between 40 and 79 years old. Risk factors include fair skin (that burns easily), Celtic or Scandinavian ancestry, and significant sun exposure; men are slightly more commonly affected.

Other significant risk factors for the development of BCC include prior injury such as trauma, burns, or vaccinations, x-irradiation, prior exposure to inorganic arsenic, immunosuppression, and certain genetic syndromes, such as xeroderma pigmentosum, nevoid BCC syndrome, and albinism. Nevus sebaceous and linear unilateral basal cell nevus are developmental hamartomas that may give rise to BCC.

Untreated or inadequately treated BCCs have an insidious growth pattern and may result in death. Metastasis from BCC is a rare event, with estimates of metastatic incidence ranging from 0.0028% to 0.1%.

Merkel Cell Carcinoma

Definition

Trabecular cell carcinoma or Merkel cell carcinoma is a primary neuroendocrine neoplasm of the skin that is commonly clinically diagnosed as a BCC. It may also mimic a BCC pathologically.

Clinical Presentation

It is slightly more prevalent in elderly females and occurs as a solitary lesion on the face, extremities, or buttocks. The clinical behavior of MCC is difficult to predict, but tends to be aggressive in nature. The 5-year survival rate for patients with regional disease is 30%.

This slow-growing asymptomatic papule or nodule rarely ulcerates. It presents as a pink to red or violet firm, dome-shaped, usually solitary, lesion. Lymph node involvement is present in greater than 50% of patients.

Pathology

Most Merkel cell carcinomas are dermally based masses of small round cells with scant cytoplasm and hyperchromatic nuclei and frequent mitoses and nuclear debris. Some lesions show the trabecular pattern that led to its original name of trabecular carcinoma of the skin.

The cells of Merkel cell carcinoma contain neurosecretory granules that can be seen by electron microscopy as membrane-bound dense-core structures. These granules and perinuclear whorls of intermediate filaments are ultrastructural hallmarks of Merkel cell tumors.

Differential Diagnosis

Clinically the firm, solid tumor of Merkel cell carcinoma must be distinguished from SCC, desmoplastic melanoma, amelanotic melanoma, metastatic carcinoma, BCC, and adnexal tumors. Biopsy is required to distinguish these.

Treatment

Management of this tumor begins with wide local excision with margins of 2.5 to 3 cm followed by careful and frequent follow-up examinations including palpation of lymph nodes, liver, and spleen. Periodic liver function tests and chest radiographs should be obtained and compared with baseline studies.

Prophylactic lymph node dissection or irradiation are advocated by some because of the high incidence of regional metastasis. Radiotherapy and adjuvant chemotherapy may be palliative in the early stages of the disease but are unproven in advanced disease.

TREATMENT

Treatment of Basal Cell and Squamous Cell Carcinoma, Bowen's Disease, and Solar Keratoses

Basal Cell Carcinoma

BCC can be treated with multiple modalities, providing 90% cure rates for primary disease in most instances. The preoperative biopsy helps determine the most appropriate treatment. Aggressive growth pattern tumors such as the morpheiform or sclerosing, micronodular, or infiltrative variants of BCC require excisional surgery with histologic margin control for adequate cure rates. Circumscribed growth pattern tumors, such as nodular and superficial BCC, do quite well with a variety of treatments, and in some circumstances, superficial or ablative surgery can result in less morbidity than full-thickness excisional surgery.

Cure rates for ablative surgery are less than the 90% figure quoted above for BCC exceeding 0.5 cm in diameter on the face and over 2.0 cm in diameter on the trunk and extremities. In these instances, excisional surgery is appropriate. BCC exceeding 0.5 mm in diameter of the central facial zone should be treated with Mohs micrographic surgery.

Squamous Cell Carcinoma

SCC can also be treated satisfactorily with different modalities. The therapeutic choice for SCC varies; however, histologic growth pattern is less important in SCC than clinical size and depth of invasion with the exception of rare histologic subtypes such as adenosquamous cell carcinoma. Poorly differentiated SCC may behave aggressively, but prognosis is often not affected by the degree of differentiation. SCC exceeding 1 cm in diameter and tumors that invade into the mid-dermis or deeper, particularly those involving cartilage and bone, are high-risk tumors. SCC of the lip, ear, temple, genitalia, and those associated with preexistent conditions such as radiation or burn scars are all higher risk tumors. In these instances, excisional surgery with careful margin control should be the treatment of choice. Postoperative radiation therapy may also be considered on a case-by-case basis.

Superficial or ablative procedures such as curettage and electrodesiccation, cryotherapy, and shave excision should be reserved for SCC in situ (Bowen's disease) or SCC that invades only the superficial dermis.

Solar Keratoses

Solar keratoses may require treatment to decrease pain, discomfort, pruritus, crusting, and progression to SCC. The rate of malignant conversion has been said to be less than 1%, but even this low rate of transformation translates into a significant 10% lifetime risk of developing invasive SCC.

Solar keratoses respond well to a variety of destructive modalities, especially liquid nitrogen, curettage, topical acids or caustics, 5-fluorouracil (5FU), and shave excision. A 3-week course of topical 5FU is useful for large areas of closely placed actinic keratosis with very diffuse borders or for actinic cheilitis, erythroplasia of Queyrat, and vulvar and intraoral leukoplakia. Temporary unsightly inflammatory changes and crusting of the precancerous skin usually occur about 5 to 15 days after starting twice-daily topical application of 1% to 5% 5FU.

Cryosurgery with liquid nitrogen for 10 to 15 seconds is highly effective. The most significant side effect is depigmentation. Bowen's disease of the skin requires two freeze-thaw cycles of 30 seconds each.

For hyperkeratotic lesions, shave biopsy, carried into the dermis, followed by curettage provides a more expedient and effective treatment modality than others.

Ablative Treatment Techniques

Curettage and Electrodesiccation

Curettage and electrodesiccation (C&E) has been used successfully with cure rates that approach 90% for nonaggressive growth pattern BCC and superficial SCC. Its limitations are based upon the experience of the surgeon, the carefulness and thoroughness of the curettage, and the depth and extent of the electrodesiccation as well as the number of cycles that are performed. C&E should be done initially with a large curette to debulk the tumor followed by a 2-mm curette to feel small extensions of superficial and nodular BCC and superficial well-differentiated SCC. The curette should be thoroughly used in every direction to eradicate all tumor extensions. Electrodesiccation should be performed by fulgurating a margin of clinically normal appearing skin around the curettage site, then carefully electrodesiccating the entire wound bed while maintaining a dry field to get a uniform depth of destruction. At least two, if not three, full cycles of curettage followed by electrodesiccation should be performed to obtain the documented 90% overall cure rate.

Cure rates for the treatment of BCC with C&E vary depending upon the site and clinical size of the BCC. BCCs of the trunk that approach 2 cm and above in diameter have much less satisfactory results with C&E than with other modalities. Because of the metastatic potential of SCC in immunocompromised patients, these SCCs should be removed by excision.

Disadvantages of C&E include prolonged wound healing (3 to 4 weeks before reepithelialization), especially on the lower extremity; the development of hypopigmented, slightly depressed or hypertrophic scars (the latter occurs over the dorsal hands, digits, shoulders, and chest); and tumor recurrence. Recurrent tumors can be deceptive and extensive with an infiltrative and perineural and poorly demarcated growth pattern beneath the scar. Because of a 40% to 50% recurrence rate after repeat C&E, non-melanoma skin cancer (NMSC) recurrent after C&E and sclerosing or aggressive growth pattern tumors should be treated with full-thickness excisional surgery with histologic margin control.

In summary, C&E offers an efficient and cost-effective means to eradicate primary nonaggressive growth pattern BCC and superficially invasive SCC. These wounds heal by second intention and can sometimes result in a better cosmetic outcome for large superficial tumors of the central trunk when compared with large elliptical excisions.

Cryosurgery

Cryosurgery for malignancies utilizes liquid nitrogen ($-195.8°$ C) delivered by cryogenic spray, cotton-tip applicators, and various cryoprobes. Freeze depth is most accurately determined by thermocouple, although many cryosurgeons feel comfortable estimating it. Cryosurgery is useful to eradicate superficial solar keratosis. Treatment of BCC requires two cycles of at least 60 seconds' thaw time for adequate clearance. The full thickness of the tumor must be frozen to $-40°$ C to $-70°$ C for complete necrosis. Ideally, as with C&E, preoperative biopsies to measure the extent of the tumor invasion are advised. Some cryosurgeons recommend curettage prior to freezing to help determine margins and to debulk the tumor.

Although cryosurgery is technically easy for the physician, it is not necessarily less invasive for the patient. Anesthesia is required because of the severe pain associated with the cold temperature and long freeze times, treatment results in an exudative, sometimes painful wound that heals over 3 to 4 weeks, and with atrophic hypopigmented scars.

Carbon Dioxide Laser Ablation

Carbon dioxide (CO_2) laser ablation is occasionally used to treat superficially invasive or in situ SCC (Bowen's disease) and superficial BCC with excellent results. The CO_2 laser offers some advantage over electrodesiccation because it can precisely de-epithelialize tissue when used in a defocused mode. Sophisticated superpulsed and ultrapulsed CO_2 lasers can limit the depth of penetration of heat. However, treatment with these expensive devices may be associated with high recurrence rates if thicker tumors or in situ tumors with follicular involvement are treated.

CO_2 ablative surgery is most useful for in situ SCC of the digits and the periungual regions. Here the CO_2 laser can remove the nail plate and allow easy access to involved nail bed.

In a similar fashion, SCC in situ of the penis and vulva, actinic cheilitis, and extensive solar damage of the vermilion can be adequately eradicated with CO_2 laser ablation with less risk of dysfunctional scarring than other modalities.

Excisional Techniques

Shave Excision

Superficial BCC, SCC in situ, and SCC invasive only to the superficial dermis can be extirpated with reasonable histologic margin control using tangential excision. Modalities vary and include simple scalpel shave excision, straight razor excision using the Gillette blue blade or single-edged razors, sharp scissors excision, and large planar blade excision. After debulking the tumor by curettage, a tangential excision is made around and under the curettage defect with a 2- to 5-mm margin of normal-appearing skin depending upon the preoperative size of the tumor. This disk or wafer of tissue should then be flattened and affixed to paper prior to placement in formalin to prevent excessive curling of the lateral edges.

Shave excisions or tangential excisions heal by second intention and thus should be performed in areas where the skin is thick, such as the central trunk. Atrophic hypopigmented or hypertrophic scars may result. Wound healing may be improved by avoiding or limiting the use of electrosurgery, Monsel's solution, or aluminum chloride for hemostasis. Occlusive biosynthetic dressings are most optimal.

Excision

Excisional surgery has been the standard of care for NMSC, and offers similar to slightly better cure rates (90%) than C&E or cryosurgery for primary tumors.

For recurrent disease, full-thickness excision is superior to nonexcisional modalities. Cure rates do not approach those of Mohs micrographic surgery (see below) because of significant differences in pathology processing and examination, which results in loss of margin control. The standard surgical margin for BCC up to 1 cm in diameter has been reported to be 4 mm to obtain 90% cure rates. For aggressive growth pattern BCC and for deeply invasive SCC, margins should be 6–9 mm. Curettage prior to excision for nonsclerosing growth pattern BCC can better estimate the horizontal and vertical extent of tumor infiltration.

Radiation

Radiation is an excellent choice for skin cancer of the central face, including the eyelids, nose, and lips. It is also often the ablative treatment of choice in skin cancer of the ears or large areas of the forehead and scalp. Radiation should be used cautiously in large lesions involving cartilage because of the risk of radionecrosis and chondritis. Radiation has the advantage of being able to treat all visible tumor plus subclinical disease without alteration of the anatomy. Cure rates with radiation vary depending on the tumor type, size, and location, and range, in general, from approximately 70% to

90%. Cosmetic results are often far superior to those achieved with surgery in certain anatomic sites.

The margin of normal appearing tissue included in the field of radiation is usually 5 mm in small tumors, and 10 mm in sclerosing or morpheiform BCCs. Well-differentiated SCCs are treated similarly to BCCs; however, poorly differentiated SCCs or those over 3 cm in size may spread to lymph nodes, and consideration should be given to the use of wider margins, or to even include regional lymph nodes in the radiation field.

Mohs Micrographic Surgery

Definition

Mohs micrographic surgery (MMS) first described by Dr. Frederic Mohs in 1941, utilizes microscopically controlled excision in the extirpation of cutaneous malignancies.

Technique

MMS is usually performed in the ambulatory setting. Under local anesthesia, the gross tumor is debulked with a curette, then is excised with a 1–3 mm margin using a scalpel blade angled at 30 to 45 degrees to the skin, slightly undercutting the tumor. The beveled edge allows simultaneous microscopic examination of the entire undersurface and epidermal edge of the excised layer of tissue. The patient waits on the premises (usually 30 to 60 minutes) while the tissue is being processed. An anatomic map is created corresponding to the exact orientation of the excised tissue with respect to the patient, and the frozen tissue sections are color coded. This allows the surgeon (who also serves as the pathologist) to determine the precise area of residual tumor (if any), thus minimizing unnecessary tissue removal. The procedure is repeated until a tumor-free plane is reached.

Indications

There are two major advantages of MMS in treating cutaneous malignancies (typically BCC and SCC). By examining 100% of the surgical margin there is no sampling error; thus a higher cure rate for all BCC and SCC (94–99%) results. It also removes the need for a safety margin, allowing the surgeon to spare as much tissue as possible while still obtaining the desired cure rate. Most primary skin cancers may be managed by less expensive surgical modalities. MMS is reserved for (1) situations in which the cutaneous malignancy is more likely to recur (e.g., subclinical tumor spread, perineural invasion, incompletely excised or recurrent tumors, aggressive histology, indistinct clinical margins, or tumors located on the nose, ears, eyelids, and perioral aeras); and (2) tumors that are in areas in which tissue conservation is important (e.g., lower nose, periorbital, periauricular, lips, digits, and genitalia).

Limitations of MMS

There are limitations of MMS. Only those tumors that may be easily identified with frozen sections may be treated with MMS.

Thus, tumors with discontiguous growth or those displaying satellitosis may not be optimal for MMS.

Patient-related limitations may be poor health, surgical phobia, or intolerance to local anesthesia. Technical limitations include mapping errors, poor sectioning, poor staining, and slide interpretation error. Advanced training in the technique is paramount.

Reconstruction with Flaps and Grafts Following Excision of Skin Cancer

Following skin cancer excision, the four general categories of management of the resulting defect are healing by second intention, side-to-side closure, skin grafting, and a variety of skin flaps. The decision to use a skin flap or graft to repair a wound should always be taken in the context of the local anatomy, tumor biology with likelihood of recurrence, and the desires and health of the patient. Healing by second intention or side-to-side closure is often the best option due to their relative simplicity. However, if these modalities are unable to close the particular defect, or if they will result in significant anatomic distortion or loss of function, flaps or grafts should be considered.

BENIGN NEOPLASMS OF THE EPIDERMIS

(CM&S Chapter 142)

Dermatosis Papulosa Nigra

Clinical Description

Dermatosis papulosa nigra occurs almost exclusively in the black population. It usually appears in early adulthood as multiple 1- to 5-mm asymptomatic, hyperpigmented papules on the face and neck, and it progresses with age. There have been no reports of malignant degeneration, and the lesions are not associated with any systemic diseases or syndromes. Dermatosis papulosa nigra may be a variant of seborrheic keratosis, epidermal nevus, or fibroepithelial papilloma (acrochordon).

Pathology

There is a slightly hyperkeratotic stratum corneum with an underlying acanthotic basaloid, slightly lobulated epidermis. There is fibrosis within the superficial papillary dermis.

Diagnosis and Differential Diagnosis

The clinical differential diagnosis includes multiple seborrheic keratoses, verrucae, fibroepithelial polyps, and, less likely, small, benign appendage tumors such as syringomas or trichoepitheliomas.

Treatment

Although often no treatment is needed, these small papules may be removed by curettage or scissors excision. Chemical peeling using alpha hydroxy acids will soften and flatten these lesions. Light electrodesiccation is successful but may result in hyperpigmentation or hypopigmentation.

Pale Cell Acanthoma

Clinical Description

Pale cell (or clear cell) acanthoma most commonly presents on the lower extremities, especially the thighs. It usually occurs in patients over 50 years of age but has been seen in children. Although most lesions are solitary, multiple lesions can occur simultaneously. These tumors present as nontender, erythematous papules or nodules ranging up to 1 cm in diameter. There can be a slight overlying scale and infrequent ulceration. These tumors are believed to be entirely benign.

Pathology

The histology is characteristic. The low-power appearance is similar to psoriasis, but the keratinocytes show an abrupt and marked cytoplasmic pallor. The cytoplasm is periodic acid–Schiff (PAS) positive and diastase labile, suggesting the presence of glycogen. At either edge of the lesion, the surrounding keratinocytes form a collarette, helping to demarcate the borders of the lesion.

Differential Diagnosis

The main clinical differential diagnoses include pyogenic granuloma, Kaposi's sarcoma and other vascular neoplasms, Spitz's nevi, and xanthogranulomas.

Treatment

The lesions are often solitary, and a shave or excisional biopsy with suture closure is effective therapy, as is cryotherapy.

Seborrheic Keratosis

Clinical Description

Seborrheic keratoses are macular or papular, velvety to verrucous lesions that vary in color from waxy yellow to dark brown. A greasy, hyperkeratotic scale is a helpful diagnostic clue. Seborrheic keratoses may occur in any site and vary in size from 1 mm to several centimeters. Stucco keratosis, a variant of seborrheic keratosis, occurs almost exclusively in acral locations.

Seborrheic keratoses are common in elderly Caucasian patients but are not limited to this population. They are unusual in childhood and increase in number and size with progressive age. They may be pruritic. These lesions are invariably benign, and there are no reports of malignant degeneration; however, basal cell carcinoma can coexist within a seborrheic keratosis.

Pathology

Seborrheic keratoses have several characteristic histologic appearances. Common to all forms is a proliferation of basaloid keratinocytes that have ovoid nuclei, without prominent nucleoli, small amounts of cytoplasm, and variable amounts of melanin. A characteristic feature is the ''horn pseudocyst'' (an invagination of loosely hyperkeratotic surface epithelium that on cross-sectioning appears cystic).

When seborrheic keratoses become irritated, there is a characteristic pattern of squamous eddies that form within the keratinocytic proliferation.

Differential Diagnosis

The clinical differential diagnosis of a seborrheic keratosis depends somewhat on the clinical appearance and includes verruca vulgaris, epidermal nevi, solar lentigines, and melanocytic neoplasms.

Treatment

A variety of treatments are effective, including electrodesiccation and curettage, cryotherapy, and shave excision.

CYSTS OF EPITHELIAL ADNEXAL ORIGIN

(CM&S Chapter 143)

Cysts are among the most common benign lesions encountered by dermatologists. To the clinician, ''cyst'' describes any round to dome-shaped mobile lesion that contains expressible material.

Cysts Lined by Squamous Epithelium

Cysts lined by squamous epithelium represent approximately 80% of all cysts. The appearance of cyst lining and contents of the cyst on histologic evaluation will determine the true origin of the cyst.

Infundibular Cysts

The majority of keratinizing cysts are infundibular, meaning they arise from the infundibular portion of the pilosebaceous unit. They are frequently termed *epidermal inclusion cyst*. These cysts occur primarily on the neck, chest, and face and have a predilection for periauricular areas, but also occur on the genitalia, where they frequently calcify. The distribution pattern closely mimics that of acne vulgaris. The male-to-female ratio is approximately 2:1. Infundibular cysts may be solitary or multiple and can range from 3 mm to several centimeters in diameter. Many contain a small punctum that marks the connection of the cyst to the overlying epidermis either by the pilar canal of a follicle or by a sinus tract. These cysts are lined by stratified squamous epithelium with a prominent granular layer and contain laminated keratin. Often these cysts rupture, resulting in suppuration, foreign body granulomatous reaction, and/or granulation tissue with chronic inflammation.

Eruptive Vellus Hair Cysts

Eruptive vellus hair cysts are multiple and clinically appear as a hyperpigmented papular eruption on the chest, abdomen, and flexural aspects of the extremities. The lesions are usually smooth but may be crusted, umbilicated, or keratotic. They tend to occur with greater frequency in children and adolescents. The condition is thought to represent a developmental anomaly of the vellus hair follicle. Microscopically, the cysts are lined by a thin layer of squamous epithelium and contain many cross-sections of vellus hair shafts.

Milia

Milia appear clinically as miniature epidermal inclusion cysts. They range from 0.5 to 2.0 mm. They are white to yellow and may be single or multiple. Milia occur primarily on the face with a predilection for the thin skin of the periorbital region. Primary and secondary forms have been described. Primary milia occur de novo in adults as well as in children. Patients give a history of using powder cosmetics or cleansing granules. Either of these products may be abrasive enough to invaginate portions of the vellus follicular ostia, leading to milia formation. Secondary milia occur as a consequence of healing of denuded areas of skin. They occasionally develop after trauma, such as dermabrasion or burns. Any disease that results in de-epithelialization may be predisposed to milia, especially the blistering conditions porphyria cutanea tarda and epidermolysis bullosa.

Milia are easily expressed after lancing the overlying skin with a No. 27 needle or a microsharp blade. It is helpful to express milia by compressing the lesion between two cotton-tipped swabs or with an extractor. Retinoic acid cream may be a useful adjuvant treatment to prevent further milia formation.

Trichilemmal (Pilar) Cysts

Trichilemmal cysts represent approximately 15% of excised lesions. They occur mainly on the scalp, where they present as smooth, firm, mobile nodules. Overlying hair growth is normal unless the cysts exceed several centimeters in size. A punctum is not typically seen, and inflammation is relatively uncommon. Trichilemmal cysts have thick walls and are more easily enucleated intact, compared with infundibular cysts, which tend to rupture easily. They can be solitary or multiple. When multiple, cysts are likely inherited as an autosomal dominant trait.

It is now thought that the term *trichilemmal cyst* most accurately describes this lesion. These cysts differ from infundibular cysts in having the squamous epithelial lining without the granular layer.

Proliferating Trichilemmal Cysts (Pilar Tumors of the Scalp)

Proliferating trichilemmal cysts are large, multilobulated nodules or exophytic lesions most commonly occurring on the scalp in women over 60 years of age. In many cases they cause overlying alopecia. These lesions are characterized by a well-circumscribed multicystic structure containing keratin with proliferating lobules of squamous epithelium with varying degrees of atypia that can be confused with squamous cell carcinoma. Like trichilemmal cysts, adequate treatment involves complete surgical excision.

Cysts Lined by Nonsquamous Epithelium

Steatocystoma Multiplex

Despite common misuse of the term *sebaceous cyst*, the steatocystoma is the only cyst that actually features sebaceous differentiation cells or lobules in its lining. The steatocystoma can occur singly (simplex) but most often occurs as a multiple lesion complex known as steatocystoma multiplex. It is inherited as an autosomal dominant condition.

Steatocystomas are usually small, ranging in size from 0.5 to 3.0 cm. They are first noted around the time of puberty. Approximately 25% of cases occur on the face; however, the chest, back, axilla, and groin areas can be affected.

These cysts are lined by few to several layers of squamous epithelial cells without a granular layer. A thick, wavy homogeneous eosinophilic cuticular lining is present, similar to that of the sebaceous duct. Frequently, sebaceous glands can be seen in the cyst wall.

Steatocystomas should be differentiated from eruptive vellus hair cysts. Steatocystomas discharge a yellowish oily material when gently lanced with a No. 11 blade, and this greatly aids in differentiating these two conditions.

Surgical excision of cysts is reasonable when they are few. Patients with a plethora of lesions should be approached more cautiously. Incision and drainage, cryosurgery, electrocautery, and CO_2 laser surgery have all been successful; however, the surgeon should weigh the consequences of having either the lesions or multiple small scars.

Hidrocystomas

Apocrine hidrocystomas are solitary cystic lesions that occur primarily on the face. They present as a translucent nodule with a bluish gray hue. Lancing these lesions gives rise to a gelatinous material. These cysts are characterized by one or many cystic spaces lined by columnar cells. The lining shows ''decapitation'' characteristic of apocrine secretion.

Eccrine hidrocystomas are often solitary. They range in size from 1 to 3 mm and are yellowish to slightly blue. They tend to be tense or firm to the touch. Differentiation of apocrine from eccrine hidrocystomas can be difficult clinically and, at times, histologically. A solitary cystic space usually lined by two layers of cuboidal epithelial cells characterizes the eccrine hidrocystoma.

Surgical Management of Keratinizing Cysts

The most frequently noted reasons for treating cysts includes painful inflammation, infection, desire for diagnosis, or cosmetic concerns. Inflamed and infected cysts should be identified since treatment differs from that of cysts that are quiescent.

Inflamed Cysts

Inflamed cysts present as erythematous, dome-shaped lesions that are tender to the touch. Inflammation occurs when a cyst ruptures and spills its contents into the dermis. Such cysts are commonly found in patients with acne who have squeezed or manipulated their lesions. Initial treatment should be conservative and include warm compresses along with an injection of triamcinolone acetonide (usually 2.5 to 5.0 mg/mL). These measures often hasten and encourage resolution. At the least, inflammation subsides and the cyst can then be treated as a quiescent cyst.

Infected Cysts

Infection tends to occur in large cysts that have been present for many years. Infected cysts are extremely tender, with erythema that extends well beyond the cyst margins. This is in contrast to inflamed cysts, in which the erythema localizes to the lesion site.

Complete excision of infected lesions should be postponed until infection is under control. This will avoid potential seeding of the infection. Proper management includes incision and drainage, systemic antibiotics, or a combination approach. Infected lesions should not be treated with intralesional steroids, since steroids may weaken the stromal collagen. This, in turn, leads to delayed healing and increases the incidence of wound dehiscence.

Some form of an anesthetic should be used. Once the area is anesthetized with either a topically applied refrigerant such as ethylchloride or anesthetic such as eutectic mixture of local anesthetics (EMLA), cream (prilocaine and lidocaine [Astra, Westborough, MA]) or local anesthesia, drainage of the cyst is initiated by using a large-gauge needle, such as a No. 14 or 16, or a No. 11 scalpel blade. The smallest drainage port possible should be attempted first. However, if drainage is not possible, the lesion should be incised.

When possible, incisions should be made along resting skin tension lines. Purulent drainage, which exits upon piercing the overlying skin and which may be increased with gentle lateral pressure, should be cultured. It is frequently followed by the typical cheesy foul-smelling keratinous debris characteristic of most cysts. An antibiotic such as erythromycin should be started empirically until culture results are final. Once the cyst is drained, saline lavage may further loosen and remove any remaining cyst wall fragments. If the cavity is large, iodoform-impregnated gauze or other packing material can be placed into the cavity to facilitate further drainage.

Infected wounds should not be sutured. It is customary to allow infected sites to heal by second intention.

Differential Diagnosis

If a punctum is visible, the diagnosis of keratinizing cyst is rarely questioned. Lesions of the cheek, such as cystic lesions of the parotid gland and swollen lymph nodes, should be distinguished. Lesions on the scalp that appear dome shaped may actually be nodules of obscure origin such as hemangiomas, cephaloceles, or dermoid tumors. Developmental anomalies may present as midline lesions. Thymic cysts, thyroglossal duct cysts, and bronchial cleft cysts present on the neck and cutaneous bronchogenic cysts occur in the lower part of the neck, the shoulders, and the chin as asymptomatic masses that can resemble benign subcutaneous cysts.

Treatment of Quiescent Cysts

Cysts that are neither inflamed nor infected are amenable to a wide variety of treatments, including excision, piezosurgery (pressure extraction), and electric current. Any approach should have as its goal complete removal or destruction of the cyst wall, without which recurrence is to be expected, leaving the lining behind to re-form the cyst.

The mobility of a cyst on palpation may indicate how bound down it may be to surrounding tissues. Freely mobile cysts usually indicate that the cyst wall is thin and not well connected to surrounding stroma. They also tend to have a visible punctum. These cysts are much more easily evacuated, giving an option for removal other than excision. Slightly movable cysts in areas of thicker dermis, such as the back, and firm to nonmobile cysts, which often have scar tissue tethering them into place, should not simply be evacuated. In such cases, the cyst as well as surrounding fibrotic tissue must be removed.

Steps to Removing Quiescent Cysts

Ballottement

Gently manipulate the cystic lesion before excision. The periphery of the cyst should be marked since the cyst generally feels larger than it is when removed. In most circumstances, the incision or excision should not extend beyond the palpable boundaries of the cyst. The anticipated incision line should be along skin tension lines.

Anesthesia

A solution of lidocaine with 1:100,000 epinephrine is adequate for most areas. It is best to infiltrate the area peripheral to the perceived outline of the cyst to avoid injecting directly into the cyst itself, which would place it under undue pressure and encourage it to rupture prematurely.

Removal

Cysts that appear superficial and are freely mobile or with a well-visualized punctum can be incised with a No. 15 blade or punched with a routine trephine device at the punctum site. By manually squeezing the incised area, the cystic contents will be extruded, followed by portions of or the entire cyst lining or sac. The sac is well recognized by its bluish gray shiny texture. To extract the remainder of the cyst sac, a fine forceps such as a mosquito forceps or a curette may be helpful. The cyst wall should be sent for pathologic evaluation because benign-appearing cysts have on occasion been found to be associated with squamous cell carcinomas or other neoplasms.

For slightly mobile and firmer cysts or those without a visible punctum, the approach is to excise the cyst in such a manner that the wall is completely removed. This can be done by dissecting the cyst from surrounding tissues and delivering it through a small incision or ellipse or by totally excising the cyst. The advantage of dissection is that a smaller wound site and therefore a smaller scar result. Dissection, however, requires greater skill since the risk of cystic rupture is higher. To dissect the cyst, a curved or elliptical incision is made within the palpable cyst boundaries. This should extend to just below the skin. The cyst wall should then become visible as a shiny layer. By using skin hooks and curved dissecting scissors, the cyst wall is separated from surrounding tissue by gentle undermining at a level between the cyst and the subcutaneous tissues surrounding it. The curve of the scissors tip should parallel the curve of the cyst wall. Complete separation of the cyst wall is possible if it is not bound down by fibrosis. In most cases, once the subcutaneous fat is reached, the cyst is easily freed up and can be gently "rolled" out of the excisional site. A cotton-tipped applicator or the blunt end of a scalpel handle may assist in this maneuver.

At times, it is impossible to avoid rupturing the cyst or spilling its foul-smelling debris into the surgical field. Debris should be completely removed, since it serves as a source of inflammation. The remainder of the sac and its contents may then be removed by further dissection without further spillage. The remaining dead space should be rinsed with normal saline to remove any residual debris before closure. Cauterization of the wound site usually suffices for hemostasis.

In closing the wound, it is essential to close any created dead space. Redundant skin edge tissue can be trimmed away and the fresh edges sutured together, being careful to avoid removing too much skin since this may put added tension on the wound. Redundant skin that is not trimmed will eventually settle into place.

At the close of the procedure, the patient should have assurance that the cyst has been completely removed. The decision to prescribe antibiotics should be left to the discretion of the surgeon.

NEOPLASMS OF THE PILOSEBACEOUS UNIT

(CM&S Chapter 144)

Introduction

Pilosebaceous neoplasms are best classified by their suspected cells of origin or differentiation. Pilosebaceous tumors can differentiate toward the hair bulb, inner and outer root sheath, sebaceous gland, and lining epithelium.

Pilar differentiation, in its most primitive form, is represented by small buds of basaloid epithelium that resemble embryonic hair germ. Advanced pilar differentiation is manifested by the formation of structures resembling those of the hair matrix, papilla, inner or outer root sheath, or hair shaft, alone or in combination. The overall architecture of the tumor also aids in defining it.

Basal cell carcinoma (see earlier in this chapter; see also Chapter 141 in CM&S) is a type of pilar carcinoma, with differentiation toward the germinative cells of the developing follicles. Other malignant follicular neoplasms are rare. The most common or most important tumors are reviewed herein.

Dilated Pore of Winer

Clinical Description

Dilated pore of Winer is a benign proliferation of epithelium, which forms a characteristic cone-shaped, giant follicular orifice. It appears at all ages on the trunk, head, and neck as small to large dermal nodules with a central, usually oxidized and black, keratin plug.

Differential Diagnosis

The differential diagnosis includes pilar sheath acanthoma, seborrheic keratosis, keratoacanthoma, giant comedo, and epidermal cyst.

Treatment

Excision (although not necessary) is curative.

Trichoepithelioma

Clinical Description and Epidemiology

Two forms of trichoepithelioma exist: the common, solitary (sporadic) form and the rare, multiple (autosomal dominant) form. These entities are distinct. There is an association between multiple trichoepitheliomas and multiple cylindromas.

Solitary lesions are pale or skin-colored papules that may reach 2 cm in diameter. The face of adults is the usual site. In the multiple form, many skin-colored to pink papules develop in childhood and are scattered on the face (especially nasolabial fold and preauricular cheek), neck, scalp, and upper trunk.

Pathology

Trichoepitheliomas share many features with basal cell carcinomas. They differ from basal cell carcinomas by lacking a connection to the overlying epidermis, being well circumscribed, and lacking the mucinous epithelial stromal clefts, myxoid stroma, and necrosis typical of basal cell carcinomas.

Differential Diagnosis

Trichoepithelioma can be confused with basal cell carcinoma, sebaceous hyperplasia, syringoma, hidrocystoma, and angiofibroma (adenoma sebaceum) of tuberous sclerosis. Biopsy is usually required to distinguish trichoepithelioma from basal cell carcinoma.

Treatment

The lesion is typically benign, and excision is curative. Rarely, malignant trichoepitheliomas (as well as basal cell carcinomas) may be seen in the multiple heredity cases.

Desmoplastic Trichoepithelioma

Clinical Description and Epidemiology

Desmoplastic trichoepithelioma is usually a small, sclerotic, depressed plaque found on the face of a young woman. These lesions are usually solitary (although a familial pattern of multiple desmoplastic trichoepitheliomas has been reported). The lesions appear to be unrelated clinically to trichoepithelioma.

Pathology

The lesion is similar to a morpheiform basal cell carcinoma, with scant strands of epithelium coursing between densely sclerotic stroma, but many other features of basal cell carcinoma are not seen in desmoplastic trichoepithelioma. The presence of a sharply circumscribed fibrotic stroma and the presence of thick rims of collagen immediately around strands of cytologically bland cells within it favor a desmoplastic trichoepithelioma.

Differential Diagnosis

Desmoplastic trichoepithelioma may be confused with morpheiform basal cell carcinoma, granuloma annulare, eccrine carcinoma, and syringoma.

Pilomatricoma

Clinical Description and Epidemiology

Pilomatricoma (calcifying epithelioma of Malherbe) presents as a deep, firm, nontender dermal or subcutaneous nodule ranging from 5 mm to 3 or 4 cm in diameter. The clinical presentation can range from an erythematous epidermal nodule, as seen in children, to a hard nodule that is flesh colored to blue-black in coloration. Children are frequently affected, and tumors often occur on the face or upper extremity.

Pathology

Pilomatricoma grows as a cystic structure that is usually present within the deep reticular dermis, which may show contiguity with follicular epithelium. There is a proliferation of small, basaloid cells, with dark nuclei, small nucleoli, and virtually no visible cytoplasm lining the cystic structure. Centrally, larger eosinophilic "shadow" cells with clear, nonstaining nuclei are apparent. These represent dying and dead keratinocytes derived from the lining wall.

Differential Diagnosis

The clinical differential diagnosis of pilomatricoma includes many deep dermal or subcutaneous benign tumors, cysts, and lipomas. The diagnosis is suspected if the nodule has a bluish hue.

Treatment

Complete excision is usually curative. Recurrence after supposed complete excision has been reported in up to 3% of cases.

Tricholemmoma and Cowden's Syndrome

Clinical Description and Epidemiology

Tricholemmomas are benign tumors that occur most often on the face in the solitary, nonhereditary form. Solitary tricholemmoma presents as a verrucous, hyperkeratotic, or smooth papule, which ranges from a few millimeters to over 1 cm in size.

The autosomal dominantly inherited form (Cowden's syndrome) is associated with internal malignancy. Cowden's syndrome consists of multiple tricholemmomas on the face that appear in the third or fourth decade. Patients also have benign keratoses of the distal extremities and fibromas and papillomas of the oral mucosa. These growths may appear as "cobblestones" on the lip. Multiple benign and malignant tumors often develop. The most prominent of these is carcinoma of the breast (up to 29% of women). The thyroid gland, gastrointestinal tract, ovaries, and uterus can also develop benign and malignant tumors.

Pathology

Histologically, there is an endophytic proliferation of large keratinocytes with abundant eosinophilic to clear cytoplasm. Hypergranulosis similar to viral changes may be seen on the surface. Surrounding the lesion, there is a markedly thickened, periodic acid–Schiff positive basement membrane, simulating the vitreous membrane of the outer root sheath of the hair follicle.

Differential Diagnosis

Both the solitary and multiple forms may look like verrucae.

Treatment

The solitary tumor is usually diagnosed and treated with the biopsy. Multiple lesions may be excised, electrodesiccated, or removed with the carbon dioxide laser. In addition, the patient should be evaluated, and followed closely, for the development of internal malignancies.

Sebaceous Hyperplasia

Clinical Description and Epidemiology

Sebaceous hyperplasia, the most common of all pilosebaceous tumors, is a disproportionate enlargement of sebaceous glands found on the forehead and cheeks of middle-aged or older individuals. These areas of hyperplasia consist of one or more 2- to 4-mm umbilicated papules that have a yellowish hue.

Pathology

Histologically, there is an increased number of mature sebocytes aggregated into large nodules that cluster around a central duct. The sebaceous lobules show proper maturation with only a single rim of basaloid cells at the periphery and mature sebocytes within the central portions of the lobules.

Diagnosis and Differential Diagnosis

Sebaceous hyperplasia must be distinguished from rhinophyma, basal cell carcinoma, nevus sebaceus, and dermal nevus. This can usually be determined clinically, based on the yellowish coloration and central dell that are usually present in sebaceous hyperplasia.

Treatment

Often, a tangential biopsy will provide diagnostic material as well as remove the lesion. Any destructive method, including curettage, cryotherapy, mild electrodesiccation, CO_2 laser surgery, or topical application of acids, is effective.

Sebaceous Adenoma and the Muir-Torre Syndrome

Clinical Description and Epidemiology

Sebaceous adenoma varies from a small nodule to an ill-defined plaque, usually yellow or tan-yellow in color, located on the face or scalp. They may arise within a nevus sebaceus. They usually arise on older patients, often in sun-damaged skin. Sebaceous adenoma (epithelioma or sebaceoma) is benign but may be a marker for an autosomal dominant, genetic syndrome: the Muir-Torre syndrome.

The Muir-Torre syndrome consists of multiple facial sebaceous adenomas, sebaceous epitheliomas, sebaceous carcinomas, keratoacanthomas, and gastrointestinal carcinomas, particularly adenocarcinoma of the colon. Carcinomas of the tracheobronchial tree, genitourinary tract, and endometrium have also been documented. Solitary sebaceous adenomas have been associated with the Muir-Torre syndrome. The skin lesions usually appear in childhood.

Pathology

Sebaceous adenomas have a lobular configuration, are located in the papillary and superficial reticular dermis, and have a connection to the epidermis. The relative amount of basaloid peripheral sebocytes is increased; however, there is a predominance of mature sebocytes over basaloid cells.

Differential Diagnosis

Clinical and histologic differential diagnosis includes sebaceous hyperplasia, basal cell carcinoma, and sebaceous epithelioma.

Treatment

Excision is curative. Family history should be sought and evaluation for Muir-Torre syndrome performed when indicated.

Sebaceous Carcinoma

Clinical Description and Epidemiology

Sebaceous carcinoma is quite rare and is usually found on the eyelids. It is an aggressive neoplasm, metastasizing first to regional nodes and later to the liver, lung, and brain. Approximately 33% of patients may develop metastases. The 5-year mortality rate is thought to be about 20%. Lesions appear as asymptomatic, firm, nonencapsulated nodules, usually on the upper eyelid.

Some lesions are associated with previous radiation treatment to the area for unrelated conditions. Sebaceous carcinoma is also seen in association with the Muir-Torre syndrome.

Pathology

Multiple lobules of basaloid, undifferentiated cells are present, mainly in the dermis. In the central portions of the lobules, more mature sebocytes are present.

In about half of cases, there is pagetoid spread of tumor cells with abundant, clear, foamy cytoplasm and nuclear atypia. In this situation, sebaceous carcinoma can be confused with Bowen's disease, extramammary Paget's disease, Merkel cell carcinoma, and amelanotic melanoma.

Differential Diagnosis

The clinical presentation of sebaceous carcinoma is subtle, and diagnosis can be difficult. The lesion can mimic ruptured cysts, blepharitis, conjunctivitis, chalazion, and later basal cell carcinoma, or other adnexal tumors. Diagnosis is usually a late one, and this contributes to the poor outcome of some patients.

Treatment

Treatment is surgical, with complete excision verified by negative margins. The Mohs technique has been used with some success for sebaceous carcinoma, although recurrences have been reported.

Metastatic disease to the lymph nodes of the neck occurs most commonly. Neck dissection, superficial parotidectomy, and radiation therapy are indicated in this circumstance.

NEOPLASMS WITH ECCRINE OR APOCRINE DIFFERENTIATION

(CM&S Chapter 145)

Tumors that differentiate toward the eccrine sweat coil or duct make up 1% of all cutaneous neoplasms. Most are benign and can often be controlled with simple excision. The traditional classification and nomenclature are based on differentiation and histopathologic pattern. The most common and clinically significant tumors are discussed in this chapter.

Eccrine Neoplasms

Syringoma

Clinical Description

Syringomas are benign, flesh colored to slightly yellow, soft, papules, usually found scattered on the lower eyelids. There is a female predilection, with slow onset at puberty, although rarely they may be eruptive.

Pathology

There is a well-circumscribed proliferation of small ductal structures embedded in a dense fibrous stroma in the papillary and superficial reticular dermis, without epidermal connections, that take on the appearance of a tadpole.

Diagnosis and Differential Diagnosis

Clinically, syringoma can be confused with sebaceous hyperplasia, eruptive xanthoma, and acne vulgaris.

Treatment

Reassurance is often the best therapy. If the patient desires treatment, syringomas can be unroofed with fine scissors and chemically cauterized, removed with a punch biopsy, or flattened to the contour of the surrounding skin by treating gently with electrodesiccation, or with the defocused beam of the carbon dioxide laser.

Apocrine Neoplasms

Extramammary Paget's Disease

Clinical Description

Extramammary Paget's disease is a rare adenocarcinoma usually restricted to the epidermis. It is an indolent disorder of the elderly that eventually can become invasive, metastasize, and cause death.

Extramammary Paget's disease presents as a well-circumscribed, reddish brown, itchy or painful plaque, usually in the anogenital region, although cases have been reported elsewhere. The plaque may be eroded, moist, or velvety.

In less than 10% of cases there is direct extension of an internal adenocarcinoma, especially those of the rectum, bladder, or prostate. Internal malignancy must be ruled out before planning therapy. Extramammary Paget's disease is histologically similar to mammary Paget's disease.

Diagnosis and Differential Diagnosis

It may take 5 to 10 years before a correct diagnosis is reached, because of confusion with other, more common, maladies such as tinea, contact dermatitis, psoriasis, and squamous cell carcinoma in situ (Bowen's disease).

Treatment

Extramammary Paget's disease eventually becomes invasive, and it is generally agreed that it should be excised if possible. The disorder always extends beyond the margin of obviously affected tissue and may be multifocal. The use of 5-fluorouracil cream to delineate more of the truly affected area has been reported to be helpful.

Extramammary Paget's disease should be excised with careful margin control, or recurrences are notoriously common. The cure rates obtained with Mohs micrographic surgery versus conventional excision are not significantly different if careful margin control is used in the conventional surgery. However, because Mohs micrographic surgery usually offers more accurate margin control and can be performed with the use of local anesthesia as an outpatient procedure, it is more often the chosen modality. The resected area is usually allowed to heal by secondary intention because of the high recurrence rate and possible multifocal nature of this tumor.

Mammary Paget's Disease

Clinical Description

Paget's disease of the breast appears as a solitary, unilateral, erythematous plaque that originates from the nipple. The lesion is sharply defined, and the vast majority of patients are women. The plaque is often crusted, oozing, or scaly and sometimes ulcerated.

This cutaneous lesion is almost always associated with an underlying carcinoma of the breast, from which it may be a direct extension. There is often metastatic disease to the axillary lymph nodes.

Pathology

Paget's disease is characterized by a proliferation of large cells with abundant pale-staining cytoplasm, interspersed between unremarkable keratinocytes, throughout the epidermis. These cells can be highlighted with a periodic acid–Schiff with diastase stain, and usually stain with antibodies to antibodies against epithelial membrane antigen and carcinoembryonic antigen.

Diagnosis and Differential Diagnosis

The differential diagnosis includes erosive adenomatosis of the nipple, nummular dermatitis, seborrheic dermatitis, psoriasis, and dermatophyte infection.

Treatment

The patient needs an evaluation for breast carcinoma and appropriate treatment.

VASCULAR MALFORMATIONS AND PROLIFERATIONS

(CM&S Chapter 146)

Vascular Birthmarks

Mulliken's classification simplifies vascular birthmarks based on the histology and natural history (Table 10–1). The vast majority of vascular birthmarks can be classified as either *hemangiomas* or *vascular malformations*. Hemangiomas are benign vascular neoplasms characterized by the rapid proliferation and slow involution of the endothelial lining of capillary walls.

In contrast, vascular malformations, the most common being the port-wine stain, are developmental anomalies of blood vessels that occur in utero. These lesions consist of ectatic vessels in which endothelial cell proliferation is normal. Vascular malformations may be composed of abnormal capillaries, veins, arteries, lymphatics, or combinations thereof.

Although this schema applies nicely to vascular birthmarks, it cannot be used for acquired vascular lesions, those beginning in older children or adults. In this setting, the term *hemangioma* or *angioma* is still used, both clinically and histopathologically, to describe many vascular neoplasms.

Hemangiomas of Infancy

Hemangiomas of infancy are benign neoplasms largely composed of capillaries and venules that are present or develop during the first few weeks of life and are characterized by a period of rapid growth followed by a period of slow involution leading to complete resolution in the majority of cases. They occur in about 1% to 2% of newborns and in 10% of 1-year-olds. Whites are more commonly affected, and premature infants have an increased incidence.

Hemangiomas are noted at birth in approximately 25% of cases and by 4 weeks in 88%. Deeper lesions are sometimes apparent until several months of age. Hemangiomas most commonly occur on the head and neck and less commonly on the trunk. Multiple lesions may occur.

Hemangioma precursors may appear as pale patches, thread-like telangiectasia with or without a pale halo, macular erythema, bluish discolorations, or small areas of skin ulceration and initially can be confused with nevus anemicus, a port-wine stain, or a bruise.

Dermal lesions are bright red, raised, and usually well-demarcated with a firm texture. Subcutaneous hemangiomas usually present as soft, enlarging masses with a bluish discoloration of the overlying skin. Lesions involving both the dermis and subcutis may share both appearances. Hemangiomas of infancy vary in size from a few millimeters to involvement of the entire face, the majority of a limb, or a significant portion of the torso.

Proliferation is most rapid between 3 and 6 months, but growth may continue until 12 months of age, and occasionally into the second year of life. After the proliferative phase, the lesion tends to plateau for months to several years, followed by a phase of slow involution. Lesions change in color from a bright crimson to a dull, faded red. Graying is first noted in the center and progresses centrifugally. The hemangioma gradually softens and becomes flabby. Complete resolution occurs in 50% to 60% of patients by 5 years of age, in 75% by age 7, and 90% by age 9. Hemangiomas involving the lip or nose may have poor outcomes after involution.

Complications

Approximately 40% of patients are left with some residual abnormality of the skin, including telangiectasia, atrophy, hypopigmentation, or scarring. Complications develop in about 20% of patients.

Ulceration usually occurs in large, rapidly growing, tense, superficial hemangiomas and results in scarring. Minor bleeding and superficial infections occur less frequently and are generally self-limited events.

Proliferating hemangiomas can lead to obstruction of critical anatomic structures. Patients with lesions involving the eyelids and orbit are at risk for developing permanent ophthalmologic sequelae. Amblyopia can occur even if the eye is closed for a few days.

Hemangiomas of infancy that obstruct the nasal passages, oropharynx, or subglottic area can cause respiratory failure. Those involving the maxillary and mandibular regions can cause dental malocclusion, and lesions in the parotid area can cause conductive hearing loss.

Infants with *diffuse neonatal hemangiomatosis* have multiple cutaneous hemangiomas in association with visceral hemangiomas, most often in the liver and gastrointestinal tract. Skin lesions, usually 1 to 10 mm in size, develop during the first few weeks of life, varying in number from a few to hundreds. Systemic complications include high-output cardiac failure, obstructive jaundice, gastrointestinal hemorrhage, respiratory failure, consumptive coagulopathy, and central nervous system bleeding resulting in a mortality rate of 80% in untreated patients. Multiple cutaneous hemangiomas without systemic involvement has been called *benign neonatal hemangiomatosis.* In general, spontaneous and uneventful involution of the hemangiomas occurs by 2 years of age. Infants with multiple cutaneous hemangiomas (especially with 10 or more) are best regarded as part of a continuum with variable degrees of cutaneous and visceral involvement.

The *Kasabach-Merritt syndrome* is a coagulopathy characterized by the platelet trapping within a hemangioma. It usually presents at birth or within the first few months of life. Typically, a large, rapidly enlarging hemangioma becomes tense, with taut overlying skin covered with petechiae and purpura. Other signs of low platelets may be seen. Most commonly, the subcutaneous lesions of the torso or extremities are affected. Death rates may still approach 20% to 30%, despite treatment.

Associated Syndromes

Hemangiomas of infancy may be associated with underlying structural malformations. Lumbosacral hemangiomas may be asso-

TABLE 10-1. Vascular Birthmarks

CONDITION	AGE OF ONSET	LOCATION	CLINICAL DESCRIPTION	SYSTEMIC MANIFESTATIONS	ASSOCIATED SYNDROMES	NATURAL HISTORY
Hemangioma of infancy	Birth to 6 wks	Variable	Raised, red, tense tumors; subcutaneous lesions with overlying bluish discoloration	Obstruction of vital structures; cardiac failure with extensive internal lesions	Kasabach-Merritt Sternal clefting Coarctation of aorta Dandy-Walker malformations	> 90% involute completely by age 9 years
Nevus simplex	Birth	Eyelids Forehead Nape of neck	Pink, irregular macules and patches	None	None	Facial lesions resolve by age 2 yrs; nuchal lesions persist
Capillary malformations (port-wine stain)	Birth	Anywhere; facial lesions may follow cutaneous innervation of trigeminal nerve	Red-violaceous patches, color deepens with age	Limb overgrowth	Sturge-Weber Cobb Phakomatosis-pigmento-vascularis Klippel-Trenaunay	Persist throughout life; may develop nodules within port-wine stain

Malformation	Onset	Location	Appearance	Hemorrhage	Associated syndromes/eponyms	Natural history
Venous malformation	Birth	Variable	Bluish-purple subcutaneous masses; can be solitary, localized, or diffuse	Hemorrhage of visceral lesions	Gorham's Maffucci's Blue rubber bleb nevus Cutis marmorata telangiectatica congenita	Lesions are persistent; may not be clinically evident until adulthood
Arteriovenous malformation	Birth	Variable	Pink to blue discoloration overlying a pulsatile mass	Potentially fatal hemorrhage, pain	See Combined malformations	Lesions are persistent; may not be clinically evident until adulthood
Lymphatic malformation	Birth	Anywhere	Single or multicystic lesions; subcutaneous lesions may resemble venous malformations or deep hemangiomas	None	See Combined malformations	Lesions are persistent; some cystic lesions may spontaneously collapse
Combined malformations	Birth	Variable	Variable	Variable	Klippel-Trenaunay Parkes-Weber Wyburn-Mason Riley-Smith Bannayan-Zonana Proteus	Persistent

567

ciated with spinal and genitourinary anomalies, and large facial hemangiomas can occur with the Dandy-Walker malformation and other posterior fossa abnormalities.

Pathology

Early hemangiomas of infancy demonstrate solid masses and strands of cells with few if any discernible lumina. Small vascular channels lined by plump endothelial cells gradually increase in number.

Diagnosis and Differential Diagnosis

The diagnosis of superficial hemangiomas rarely requires more than a complete history and physical examination. Occasionally, deep hemangiomas may be slow to involute and may be confused with a static vascular malformation. Hemangiomas presenting as a high-flow mass at birth may be mistaken for an arteriovenous malformation (AVM). Magnetic resonance imaging is the most reliable noninvasive technique for distinguishing deep or visceral hemangiomas from vascular malformations, meningoceles, dermoid cysts, and other neoplastic processes.

Treatment of Hemangiomas

The vast majority of hemangiomas eventually involute without complications and require no treatment. The lesions(s) should be monitored on a regular basis during the proliferative phase. Early treatment with the pulsed dye laser may prevent ensuing proliferation, irreversible cutaneous changes, and disfigurement. Growth of a deeper component may not be inhibited by this method, and hemangiomas with a significant deep component are not likely to benefit from pulsed dye laser therapy alone.

Medical therapies such as corticosteroids and interferon-alfa are usually necessary if functional impairment, involvement of vital structures (such as the airway, liver, or gastrointestinal tract), coagulopathy, or irreversible cutaneous changes ensue. Prednisone or prednisolone, 2 to 4 mg/kg per day, is usually given orally and, depending on the age of the patient, generally must be continued for one to several months before gradual tapering. A response is usually evident within a few days to weeks. Approximately one third of hemangiomas shrink dramatically, one third stop growing but do not shrink significantly, and one third do not respond.

Interferon-alfa 2α and 2β, 3 million units/m^2 per day injected subcutaneously, usually accelerates regression of lesions; however, 6 to 12 months of continuous therapy may be required.

Port-Wine Stains

Definition

Port-wine stains (nevus flammeus) are superficial vascular malformations. They always occur at birth and, unlike hemangiomas, do not resolve. Lesions are usually isolated but may be associated with other vascular malformations or occur as a component of a variety of congenital syndromes.

Clinical Description

Port-wine stains occur in approximately 0.3% of neonates. The size of the lesions varies from several millimeters in diameter to more than 50% of the body surface area. Although the face and neck are most commonly involved, any site may be affected. About one half of facial port-wine stains are restricted to one of the three trigeminal sensory areas. The mucous membranes are often involved contiguously with the dermal capillary malformation. Extensive facial port-wine stains are more likely than small isolated lesions to be associated with truncal and extremity lesions as well as with neurologic, ophthalmologic, and other congenital abnormalities.

The generalized erythema commonly seen in newborns may prevent accurate diagnosis for several weeks. The size of the lesion increases proportionately with the growth of the child, and the color generally deepens from light pink to red to dark purple with age. Progressive darkening and cutaneous hypertrophy of initially macular lesions occur in approximately two thirds of patients by age 45. Lesions may develop a ''cobblestone'' texture and can become studded with angiomatous nodules, including pyogenic granulomas.

Pathology

Port-wine stains are characterized by ectasia of capillaries located in the papillary and superficial reticular dermis. Early lightly colored lesions may be virtually identical histologically to normal skin. As the patient ages, the vessels in the port-wine stain progressively dilate and there is stasis of erythrocytes.

Diagnosis and Differential Diagnosis

A complete history and physical examination are usually sufficient to correctly diagnose a port-wine stain. Occasionally, a nevus simplex (salmon patch) or hemangioma precursor may be mistaken for a port-wine stain. Early proliferation of hemangiomas helps distinguish them from port-wine stains.

Management of Capillary Malformations

Patients with port-wine stains corresponding to the first branch of the trigeminal nerve (V1) are at risk for Sturge-Weber syndrome. Similarly, those with involvement of the upper or lower eyelid (or both) may have associated glaucoma and should be evaluated regularly by an ophthalmologist. Those with port-wine stains of the lower extremity need periodic leg-length measurements during early childhood to evaluate for limb hypertrophy. The pulsed-dye laser can dramatically improve port-wine stains.

In addition to efficacy and safety, a major advantage of pulsed-dye laser treatment has been a decreased need for anesthesia. Many adults can tolerate the procedure without local anesthesia. Most younger children, however, require sedation as well as the use of local, topical, regional, or general anesthesia in the treatment of medium to large lesions. Multiple treatments are required to obtain the maximum benefit. It is rare to see complete clearing in one or two sessions, as may be noted with a continuous-wave laser source. Although one study reported complete clearing of all patients after six treatment sessions, other studies have noted significant but incomplete clearing after multiple treatments. The degree of clearing is, in large part, related to the anatomic location of a port-wine stain. Facial port-wine stains usually respond most quickly, except those over the central portion of the face, in particular, the second branch of the trigeminal nerve, which respond more slowly

Continuous-wave lasers, such as the argon and continuous-wave tunable dye lasers, may be used to treat the hypertrophic component of port-wine stains.

Nevus Simplex (Salmon Patch)

Nevus simplex (stork bite) is a vascular birthmark seen in 25% to 40% of all newborns. The lesions are composed of ectatic dermal capillaries that are presumed to be the result of persistent fetal circulation. Sites of predilection include the glabella, eyelids, and most commonly, the nape of the neck. The lesions are light pink to scarlet, flat, and easily blanched and usually deepen in color with vigorous activity, fever, crying, or increases in ambient temperature. These lesions fade over time with complete resolution occurring by age 3 in the vast majority of cases. Nevus simplex of the nape of the neck and some glabellar lesions may persist into adulthood. Lesions usually respond to pulsed-dye laser within two or three treatments, but therapy is not usually indicated unless the lesions persist beyond 3 years of age.

Other Malformations (Venous, Arteriovenous, Lymphatic, and Combined)

Definition

Like port-wine stains, vascular malformations of veins, arteries, and lymphatic vessels are anomalies that occur during embryogenesis. Although they are almost always present at birth, the correct diagnosis may not be apparent until later in life. Vascular malformations may occur singly or as combined lesions and may affect cutaneous, subcutaneous, and visceral structures.

Venous Malformations

These low-flow vascular lesions usually present as a faint-blue patch or soft-blue mass, often with ill-defined borders. Lesions are usually present at birth but may occasionally become evident later. Venous malformations (VMs) are generally soft and compressible and have no increased skin temperature, thrill, or bruit. Over time, they may slowly enlarge, owing to increasing ectasia. Firm areas may become evident as the result of phleboliths, thrombosis, or hemorrhage. Swelling and/or pain may be episodic, owing to thrombosis or hemorrhage. A chronic consumption coagulopathy may occur in large VMs.

Craniofacial and limb VMs may require treatment because of involvement and compression of adjacent structures or distortion of facial features. MRI can be used to delineate the extent of the lesions, and Doppler flow studies can rule out an arteriovenous malformation.

Percutaneous sclerotherapy may decrease extensive VMs where

surgical removal is not possible. Custom-made elastic stockings are an important part of the management of VMs, usually necessary on a life-long basis.

Cutis marmorata telangiectatica congenita (congenital phlebectasia) is characterized by reticulated mottling of the superficial vasculature with areas of decreased perfusion and other areas with dilated venules and capillaries. When the distribution is localized, it tends to be sharply demarcated with strict observation of the midline. The condition is present at birth and tends to improve with age, although some lesions remain relatively fixed. Associated cutaneous findings include port-wine stain, atrophy of the skin overlying the dilated vessels, and superficial ulceration with scarring. Other associated anomalies include hyperplasia or hypoplasia of an affected limb, skeletal abnormalities, mental retardation, and glaucoma in cases with periorbital involvement.

Arteriovenous Malformations

Arteriovenous malformations (AVMs) are high-flow vascular malformations that can involve any structure, including the skin, subcutaneous tissues, musculoskeletal system, and the viscera. In contrast to other malformations, AVMs often go undiagnosed until adulthood, where they can be precipitated by puberty, pregnancy, trauma, or surgery. They present as faint-pink or bluish macules or a pulsating mass. Symptoms include a sensation of dependent heaviness, throbbing or stabbing pain, pulsation or thrill, hyperhidrosis or hypertrichosis overlying the lesion, and hyperthermia.

Lesions are usually solitary but may involve much larger areas of vasculature than are evident at the outset. Lesions often recruit new vessels, particularly after trauma or surgery. Auscultation for bruits may help differentiate AVMs from hemangiomas and other vascular malformations. Duplex Doppler studies and magnetic resonance imaging can help assess the lesions, but angiography is always required before therapy.

If AVMs remain quiescent during childhood, no treatment may be necessary until after puberty. If complications develop, superselective arterial embolization may be palliative, or embolization followed by complete surgical excision may be performed. Partial embolization or resection can result in severe and uncontrollable recurrences.

Lymphatic Malformations

Lymphatic malformations are localized or diffuse malformations of the lymphatic vessels. Solitary lymphatic cysts, so-called cystic hygromas, are most common on the neck and frequently communicate with adjacent lymphatic structures. Localized multicystic lymphatic malformations of the skin and mucosa, so-called lymphangioma circumscriptum, present as clusters of clear, fluid-filled vesicles that often become discolored by bleeding from surrounding capillaries. These lesions often have deeper components that are not initially evident, but become apparent if the lesion recurs after a "complete excision." Extensive lymphatic malformations usually present with lymphedema of an extremity, often in association with more superficial vesicular skin lesions. Deeper connective tissues and viscera may be affected. Recurrent leakage of lymph, recurrent cellulitis, and cosmetic disfigurement can occur.

Histologically, throughout the superficial and deep dermis and subcutis, there are dilated, thin-walled vessels whose lumina contain frothy-appearing proteinaceous material and are devoid of erythrocytes unless the lesion has been traumatized. In lymphangioma circumscriptum, round, dilated lymphatic vessels are present just beneath a hyperplastic and hyperkeratotic epidermis.

Some superficial lymphangiomas may benefit from carbon dioxide laser therapy. The deeper components may recur after any surgical technique, including laser ablation, electrosurgery, cryotherapy, and superficial excision. Many of these techniques may lead to scarring, which may be hypertrophic. Continuous wave visible light lasers may be of benefit, if there is a venous or capillary component. For diffuse lymphatic malformations, support garments may decrease progressive lymphangiectasia.

Complex and Combined Vascular Malformations

Virtually any vessel type may combine with another to cause combined malformations. *Klippel-Trenaunay syndrome* is characterized by soft tissue hypertrophy and bony overgrowth of an extremity (usually a lower extremity) in association with an overlying port-wine stain. The port-wine stain is present at birth, but the other abnormalities may not be evident in infancy. The capillary malformation almost always has an associated venous or lymphatic malformation. The enlargement of the limb is due to increased soft tissue and bone and is often disproportionate, with hypertrophy of the toes and feet being more prominent. Deep venous aplasia or hypoplasia may also be present and may lead to disastrous consequences if sclerotherapy or vein stripping is undertaken.

In the *Parkes-Weber syndrome,* limb hypertrophy is seen in association with multiple arteriovenous fistulas and an overlying port-wine stain. Venous anomalies are not usually present, and extremity overgrowth is proportionate without accentuation of the feet or toes. Congestive heart failure, due to a high-flow state, results in a poor prognosis.

Syndromes Associated with Cutaneous Vascular Malformations

The *Sturge-Weber syndrome* (SWS) is characterized by a facial port-wine stain and leptomeningeal and choroidal angiomatosis, but partial SWS can occur with only skin and central nervous sytem or eye involvement as well. The location and extent of the port-wine stain determine the risk for the development of SWS. Only patients with V1 port-wine stains can develop SWS, but because of overlap in the distribution of V1 and V2 enervation, patients with infraorbital port-wine stains may be affected. Those with V1, V2, and V3 or bilateral port-wine stains are at highest risk (approximately 25%) for developing the syndrome.

The most common neurologic findings are seizures, usually beginning in the first year of life, and mental retardation. A variety of other neurologic findings may occur.

The most common ophthalmologic finding is ipsilateral choroidal angiomatosis, which may lead to retinal dysfunction, anterior displacement of the retina with resultant amblyopia, retinal detachment, ectopic bone formation, and retinal degeneration. Glaucoma occurs in up to three fourths of patients. It is most often associated with ipsilateral port-wine stains of both the upper and lower eyelids.

Skull roentgenograms (after age 1 year), computed tomography, or magnetic resonance imaging may demonstrate characteristic railroad track–like calcifications of the brain parenchyma.

The *blue rubber bleb nevus syndrome* is characterized by multiple cutaneous venous malformations of the skin (usually trunk and upper extremities) and gastrointestinal tract (especially the small bowel). The skin lesions may be present at birth or during childhood and increase in size and number over time. They range from a few millimeters to several centimeters in diameter, may be spontaneously painful, or may be associated with hyperhidrosis. Recurrence after surgical excision is common. Besides the gastrointestinal tract, the respiratory tract, central nervous system, eye, liver, spleen, and genitourinary tract may be involved. Bleeding requiring transfusion or surgery frequently occurs, and acute massive gastrointestinal hemorrhage is the most common cause of death.

Maffucci's syndrome, a congenital, nonhereditary disorder of mesodermal dysplasia, is characterized by the presence of dyschondroplasia and multiple subcutaneous venous malformations. Onset is usually during childhood. The skeletal changes result from a defect in endochondral ossification that leads to irregular growth (dyschondroplasia), cartilage proliferation, and the eventual formation of endochondromas. The lesions most commonly involve the distal extremities, although they may involve the spine, thorax, pelvis, and skull.

Malignant transformation of endochondromas to chondrosarcomas has been noted in up to 20% of patients. Vascular lesions are also at risk for sarcomatous degeneration.

Acquired Vascular Proliferations

A variety of acquired vascular proliferations exist, such as Kaposi's sarcoma, cherry (senile) angiomas. Some are clearly hamartomatous, hyperplastic, or neoplastic, whereas others are difficult to classify. Only one neoplasm, angiosarcoma, is universally accepted as malignant.

Hyperplasias of Blood Vessels

The most common form of vessel hyperplasia is due to venous stasis (see Chapter 2 in this text or Chapter 65 in CM&S).

Acroangiodermatitis

Definition. Acroangiodermatitis (pseudo-Kaposi's sarcoma), an exaggerated form of venous stasis, is a superficial localized form of vascular hyperplasia due to abnormal blood flow. Cases due to venous hypertension alone have been termed acroangiodermatitis of Mali, whereas those associated with an arteriovenous shunt have been termed the *Bluefarb-Stewart syndrome*.

Clinical Description. Acroangiodermatitis usually presents on the legs or feet as circumscribed coalescent red to purple papules. Associated underlying cutaneous findings include chronic venous insufficiency, paralysis of the affected limb, an arteriovenous shunt, or damage to vessels from amputation or intravenous drug abuse.

Pathology. Biopsies of acroangiodermatitis show exaggerated venous stasis.

Diagnosis and Differential Diagnosis. The diagnosis of acroangiodermatitis should be considered if purplish papules or nodules arise on the skin of the toes or on an amputation stump. A triangular distribution over the dorsal first and second toes is characteristic. The differential diagnosis includes Kaposi's sarcoma and angiosarcoma.

Treatment. Correction of arteriovenous shunting or other underlying condition or the use of pressure garments may improve the condition or help prevent its progression.

Reactive Angioendotheliomatosis

Definition. Reactive angioendotheliomatosis is a rare condition in which endothelial cells and pericytes proliferate as the result of several different stimuli that have in common the occlusion of vascular lumina. Reactive angioendotheliomatosis is a self-limiting condition that occurs in patients with systemic diseases, including endocarditis, vasculitis, disseminated intravascular coagulation, and cryoglobulinemia. Its lesions are erythematous, purple or blue papules that are usually on the limbs, face, or trunk, and, in cases due to cryoglobulinemia, on the acra. It appears to be mediated by the blockage of the lumina of small vessels.

Pathology. Histologic features include small clusters or tufts of vessels with rounded shapes that are invested by pericytes and sometimes by myxoid connective tissue.

Treatment. The treatment of reactive angioendotheliomatosis is to treat the underlying systemic condition. Once the vaso-occlusive stimulus is removed, cutaneous lesions slowly involute.

Telangiectases

Telangiectases are due to ectasia of preexisting blood vessels with minimal proliferation of endothelial cells, pericytes, or smooth muscle, unlike in vascular neoplasms. In *angioma serpiginosum,* small pinhead-sized erythematous puncta are arranged in circinate or serpentine patterns. Any site can be affected. Dilated capillaries are present in enlarged dermal papillae. *Spider angioma* (nevus araneus) occurs on the upper trunk and face as a central punctum from which fine vessels radiate. They are sensitive to estrogen and appear/enlarge during pregnancy and in patients with cirrhosis. *Venous lakes* are blue papules that occur on the face of older patients, favoring the lips and ears. Elastosis of the walls of vessels due to actinic damage weakens the vessel wall, allowing dilatation. Lesions whose lumina house thrombi have been termed *thrombosed capillary aneurysms.* In *generalized essential telangiectasia,* there are small lesions that resemble spider angiomas over much of the cutaneous surface. The condition is an autosomal dominant, has its onset in the fourth decade, and mostly affects women. In *unilateral nevoid telangiectasia,* the dermatomes innervated by either the trigeminal or third or fourth cervical nerves are the sites of telangiectases, which can either present at birth or in later life, when they may increase with estrogens. Secondary telangiectases can be due to collagen vascular diseases, actinic damage, and other causes.

Treatment of Telangiectasia. Treatment depends on the location and extent of lesions. Small well-localized lesions may be treated with electrocautery using an epilating needle or continuous wave or pulsed-dye laser using a yellow light source. Larger areas on the upper body are best treated with laser; those on the legs are usually treated with sclerotherapy. Venous lakes are best treated with laser or in some cases, injected with a sclerosing agent.

Benign Vascular Lesions

Benign vascular neoplasms of the skin include proliferations with capillary, venular, smooth muscle, arteriolar, and venous composition and varying components of endothelial cells, pericytes, smooth muscle, and glomus cells.

Pyogenic Granuloma (Lobular Capillary Hemangioma)

Definition. Pyogenic granulomas (PGs) are neither pyogenic nor granulomatous. Instead, they are lobular proliferations of capillaries and venules that present as exophytic lesions and are often related to minor trauma.

Clinical Features. PGs are typically glistening red or pink excrescences that rapidly evolve into pedunculated papules or nodules with eroded surfaces that eventually reepithelialize. Common sites are the lips, periungual skin, and face. They frequently arise on the gums and lips in pregnant women. They often bleed, at times profusely. PGs can arise within preexistent vascular malformations such as nevus flammeus or spider angiomas.

Pathology. Early PGs appear as volcanic protrusions of ulcerated granulation tissue. Mature lesions are characterized by lobules of small round vessels intermingled with ectatic vascular spaces and spindled pericytes. These lobules are divided by myxoid to fibrous connective tissue bands.

Pathogenesis and Etiology. PGs are most likely hyperplasias rather than neoplasms, as they are often induced by trauma, hormones, or drugs, such as retinoids and oral contraceptives.

Diagnosis and Differential Diagnosis. The diagnosis of PG is often made clinically. The differential diagnosis includes Kaposi's sarcoma, bacillary angiomatosis, and nodular amelanotic melanoma.

Treatment. Treatment depends on the size and location of the lesion. Often curettage and electrodesiccation is sufficient. Other options include pulsed-dye, continuous wave visible light, or carbon dioxide laser, cryotherapy, and surgical exision. Recurrences and the development of multiple satellite lesions after therapy are relatively frequent.

Angiolymphoid Hyperplasia with Eosinophilia

Definition. Angiolymphoid hyperplasia with eosinophilia (ALHE) is a benign proliferation of large, protuberant cells that is often accompanied by dense lymphoid infiltrates and frequently by peripheral or lesional eosinophilia. It is unknown whether the condition is hyperplastic or neoplastic.

Clinical Description. Lesions of ALHE are smooth-surfaced, tan, pink, red, or brown papules or nodules often found on the skin of the head, with a predilection for the area around the ears. Although usually asymptomatic, they can be painful, and because some of them are associated with an underlying AVM, they may be pulsatile. Multiple lesions are common, and eruptive presentation is occasional.

Pathology. ALHE is generally a well-circumscribed dermal proliferation of discrete thick-walled vessels lined with epithelioid endothelial cells that bulge into the lumen. Lymphocytic and eosinophilic infiltration varies from scant to dense.

Diagnosis and Differential Diagnosis. The differential diagnosis includes eosinophilic folliculitis. The diagnosis of ALHE is made on biopsy.

Treatment. Individual lesions of ALHE can be removed surgically. Care should be taken to adequately excise the arteriolar and venous segments at their bases. Intralesional corticosteroid therapy is sometimes successful.

Glomus Tumors

Definition. Glomus tumors are benign neoplasms characterized by vascular spaces surrounded by a proliferation of modified smooth muscle cells resembling the arrangement seen in the arteriovenous glomus—a cuff that surrounds the shunt between arterioles and veins on the skin of the digits and elsewhere. Glomus tumors are relatively solid, whereas glomangiomas have fewer glomus cells arranged around ectatic vessels.

Clinical Description. Glomus tumors are solitary red or purple nodules found on the skin of the fingers or toes, sites rich in normal glomus apparatus. Subungual papules can erode underlying bone and cause nail dystrophy. Glomus tumors generally occur in adults and are included in the spectrum of painful cutaneous tumors along with angioleiomyoma, neurilemoma, eccrine spiradenoma, and leiomyoma. Lancinating pain can follow a gentle touch or exposure to cold.

Multiple lesions (glomangiomas) affecting other sites can have a similar appearance but are less often painful.

Diagnosis and Differential Diagnosis. A solitary painful red acral papule is likely to be a glomus tumor. The diagnosis is almost always confirmed histologically.

Treatment. Excisional biopsy is usually curative.

Angiokeratoma

Definition. The angiokeratomas are a group of benign vascular neoplasms in which marked dilated, thin-walled vessels are situated beneath a hyperplastic and hyperkeratotic epidermis.

Clinical Presentation. Each type of angiokeratoma has a characteristic clinical setting. In solitary angiokeratoma, there is a well-circumscribed dark-red, scaly papule of at least 0.5 mm in diameter, which is often found on the leg. Multiple lesions sometimes occur. Thrombosis may cause the lesion to appear black, simulating melanoma. Angiokeratoma of Mibelli occurs largely as small multiple lesions on the skin of the dorsal toes (and sometimes fingers) in patients with cold intolerance and, sometimes, perniosis. Angiokeratomas of Fordyce are multiple lesions on the scrotal or vulvar skin and sometimes that of the adjacent abdomen or thigh. Angiokeratoma corporis diffusum is a component of several metabolic diseases, including Fabry's disease (X-linked recessive α-galactosidase A deficiency disease that results in ceramide trihexidose accumulation in several organs). In angiokeratoma corporis diffusum, many small papular angiokeratomas occur around the waist and at other sites. Angiokeratoma circumscriptum is a rare condition in which a solitary plaque composed of contiguous papular angiokeratomas occupies a large area of skin.

Differential Diagnosis. The differential includes cherry hemangioma, nevi, and cryoglobulinemia. Angiokeratoma of Mibelli can sometimes be difficult to distinguish from cryoglobulinemia or perniosis, but its lesions are more sharply circumscribed.

Treatment. Solitary angiokeratomas are cured by simple excision. Multiple angiokeratomas can be excised, frozen, electrodesiccated, or treated with lasers.

Cherry Hemangioma

Definition and Clinical Presentation. Cherry hemangiomas (senile hemangiomas) are small, bright-red papules composed of ectatic vessels. They arise in middle age, usually on the abdomen.

Pathology. A gently domed proliferation of dilated, thin-walled vessels is present in the papillary dermis.

Differential Diagnosis. The differential diagnosis includes petechiae and other benign vascular lesions. Minute lesions can be confused with petechiae.

Treatment. Lesions can be treated with shave excision, light electrocautery, cryotherapy, or laser therapy.

Angiosarcoma and Its Variants

Definition. Angiosarcoma is a highly malignant neoplasm whose cells differentiate toward blood, vascular, or lymphatic endothelium.

Clinical Presentation. Classic angiosarcoma of the skin occurs in only a few settings, such as the scalp and face of elderly patients, lymphedematous limbs, and skin that has been irradiated. Angiosarcoma of the head of elderly patients presents as an ill-defined bruise-like patch, usually involving the central or upper face, the scalp, or both. Over time, plaques develop, and blue or purplish nodules emerge. The best known presentation of angiosarcoma due to lymphedema is the Stewart-Treves syndrome, in which the disease develops in the arm of a patient who has undergone a mastectomy and axillary lymph node dissection for breast carcinoma. Postradiation angiosarcoma is rare and generally follows irradiation by a decade or more. The lower abdomen has been a common site.

The classic forms of angiosarcoma grow relentlessly and almost always recur following resection. They metastasize to lymph nodes and to the lungs.

Pathology. In patches of angiosarcoma, jagged vessels lined by endothelial cells with large and often protuberant hyperchromatic nuclei infiltrate between reticular dermal collagen bundles. Nodular lymphocytic infiltrates are often present. Nodules or plaques of angiosarcoma have a more solid growth pattern with either spindled or epithelioid cells predominating. Erythrocytes are usually present in the slit-like interstices between these cells.

Diagnosis and Differential Diagnosis. The diagnosis of angiosarcoma is often made clinically if the presentation is of one of its classic forms, and it is confirmed by biopsy. The clinical differential diagnosis of a flat red patch on the face or scalp of an adult is broad, but if the lesion is of recent onset, angiosarcoma becomes more likely. Histologic findings in patches of angiosarcoma can be difficult to distinguish from those of Kaposi's sarcoma.

Treatment. Early diagnosis and complete excision with wide and deep margins is the best approach to classic angiosarcoma. Locally recurrent disease has a grim prognosis. Radiation therapy can be useful for extensive lesions.

NEOPLASMS OF MUSCLE AND FAT; LIPOSUCTION SURGERY OF FAT HYPERTROPHY

(CM&S Chapter 147)

Tumors of Muscle

Leiomyoma

Clinical Description. Cutaneous leiomyoma may present as a group of superficial pinhead to pea-sized firm nodules on the skin of the back, face, or extensor surfaces of the extremities. The lesions may aggregate in linear or arciform patterns or plaques. Solitary subcutaneous leiomyomas vary from pea sized to walnut sized and are prevalent on the extensor surfaces of the lower extremities, scrotum, labia majora, and nipples. Pain may be prominent.

Pathology. Pilar leiomyomas present within the reticular dermis as an unencapsulated tumor that consists of spindle cells, often with blunt-ended (''cigar-shaped'') nuclei, that have perinuclear vacuoles. Genital leiomyomas are similar but more cellular.

Angioleiomyomas are sharply delineated from the surrounding tissue by a true capsule and are deeper, usually in the deep reticular dermis or subcutaneous tissue. Several slit-like or stellate endothelial-lined vascular spaces surrounded by concentric smooth muscle coats arranged in fascicles are a characteristic feature. Focal hemorrhage, vascular thrombosis, myxoid stroma, or fat cells may be seen.

Pathogenesis. It appears that cutaneous leiomyomas arise from any type of normal smooth muscle. The superficial tumors arise from the pilar arrector muscles, dartos muscle, or mamillary muscle. Angioleiomyomas arise from the muscular wall of blood vessels (usually veins). Multiple leiomyomas are often familial.

Differential Diagnosis. Clinically, pilar leiomyomas may be difficult to differentiate from other tumors such as dermatofibromas and other spindle cell neoplasms, although the presence of pain particularly on cold stimulation is highly suggestive.

Treatment. The degree of symptoms and extent of involvement determine the therapy. Solitary lesions and smaller plaques can be excised with a layered closure.

If there is a family history, genetic counseling should be considered. In women affected with multiple cutaneous leiomyomatosis, the uterus should be examined for involvement.

Leiomyosarcoma

Clinical Description. This solitary malignant tumor of smooth muscle is rare in either the cutaneous or subcutaneous tissue forms. The cutaneous variant arises from the arrectores pilorum or genital smooth muscle, while subcutaneous leiomyosarcomas arise from vascular smooth muscle. This is an important distinction, since the prognosis of these two tumors is vastly different. The dermal tumors only rarely metastasize, but the subcutaneous ones do so in 30% to 40% of cases. The most common site of metastasis is the lung.

These poorly circumscribed tumors do not have a distinctive clinical appearance and usually become suspicious because of rapid enlargement or ulceration. While seen in any location, they are frequently present on the extremities.

Pathology. The cutaneous leiomyosarcomas are composed of interlacing fascicles of atypical spindle-shaped cells. The spindle cells vary within and between tumors from benign-appearing smooth muscle cells to highly anaplastic multinucleated giant cells. In general, the cells are larger, plumper, and more hyperchromatic than their benign counterparts. Mitoses vary from rare to more than one per high-power field.

Differential Diagnosis. Histologically, leiomyosarcomas must be differentiated from other spindle cell neoplasms. Rare cases may also require electron microscopy.

Treatment. Survival improves with early detection and adequate excision. Although the tumor is easily enucleated, re-excision of the area is necessary. Wide local excision offers as good a chance at survival as an amputation. Postoperative radiation (but not chemotherapy) may provide effective adjuvant therapy.

Rhabdomyoma

This benign nodule of striated muscle may represent a hamartoma and is usually a well-circumscribed cutaneous mass. Rhabdomyomas can be seen in adults or fetuses. Fetal rhabdomyomas usually appear in young boys as subcutaneous tumors near the ear. In women, rhabdomyomas may appear as genital polyps in the vaginal or vulvar areas. In adult men, these tumors localize in the muscles of the head and neck region.

Pathology. Rhabdomyomas are well-defined tumors that are surrounded by compressed connective tissue. The tumor is composed of large, round to polygonal cells with eosinophilic cytoplasm and eccentric nuclei that are separated from each other by a thin layer of fibrovascular tissue. Cross-striations are classic but not seen in all cells. A distinctive feature is the presence of rod-like crystalline structures of the cytoplasm that are thought to represent Z-band material.

Differential Diagnosis. Rhabdomyomas can be histologically confused with granular cell tumors and hibernomas.

Treatment. Local excision is curative.

Rhabdomyosarcoma

Rhabdomyosarcomas are seen primarily in children as soft tissue masses alone or within congenital nevi. They may present as surface nodules singly or as multiple small lesions.

Pathology. Cutaneous rhabdomyosarcomas that are likely to be encountered by dermatologists include embryonal rhabdomyosarcoma and alveolar rhabdomyosarcoma. The least differentiated embryonal rhabdomyosarcomas are composed of cells that are small, round to oval basophilic nuclei without discernible cytoplasm or other distinctive features. A high mitotic rate is frequently present. More differentiated cells demonstrate larger vesicular nuclei and intensely eosinophilic cytoplasm. Highly differentiated embryonal rhabdomyosarcomas are composed of spindle-shaped or strap-shaped cells with some cells demonstrating abundant eosinophilic cytoplasm and cross-striations.

Diagnosis and Differential Diagnosis. The diagnosis is made histologically with immunoperoxidase, demonstrating myoglobin, or with electron microscopy, showing myofilaments. The histologic differential diagnosis includes other round cell neoplasms, such as Ewing's sarcoma, lymphomas, Merkel cell carcinoma, neuroendocrine tumors, and oat cell carcinoma.

Treatment. Treatment is by complete surgical excision followed by chemotherapy or radiation therapy.

Tumors of Fat

Nevus Lipomatosus Superficialis

Clinical Description. Nevus lipomatosus superficialis is a rare lesion that is usually asymptomatic. It appears as a circumscribed group of skin-colored to pale yellow soft nodules that often have a folded surface. They appear chiefly in the pelvic or gluteal areas and are usually present at birth.

Pathology. Nevus lipomatosus superficialis is a benign malformation that is both exophytic and endophytic. Microscopically, it demonstrates a normal or slightly attenuated epidermis associated with a dermal proliferation of mature lipocytes in the reticular dermis that may extend to the papillary dermis. The lipocytes are usually aggregated around blood vessels but may be solitary between collagen bundles.

Differential Diagnosis. Nevus lipomatosus superficialis is clinically difficult to differentiate from other tumors that are soft and polypoid such as soft fibromas and neurofibromas. Clinical information that favors a diagnosis of nevus lipomatosus superficialis includes presence at birth, large tumor or plaque, and presence of linear lesions. A pedunculated architecture favors a soft fibroma.

Lipoma

Clinical Description. Lipomas are common lesions seen primarily on the trunk (but may appear anywhere). They are usually solitary, but may be multiple, and range in size from a few millimeters to 20 or more centimeters. Most lipomas are painful when compressed.

A familial form, *multiple familial lipomatosis,* is autosomal dominant. Hundreds of lesions may be seen over the entire body. *Madelung's disease,* or benign symmetrical lipomatosis, is a form of multiple lipomatosis in which the lesions are poorly circumscribed and congregate especially around the neck and occiput, giving a "horse collar" appearance.

Pathology. Lipomas resemble normal adipose tissue both grossly and microscopically. They are typically well defined by a fibrous pseudocapsule, but they may demonstrate an infiltrative growth pattern into surrounding normal tissue such as muscle. The fat cells of lipomas are indistinguishable from normal fat cells, although they are generally more variable in size and may be larger. The lipomas of adiposis dolorosa (Dercum's disease), benign symmetrical lipomatosis (Madelung's disease), and familial multiple lipomatosis, which is autosomal dominant, are indistinguishable from ordinary lipomas.

Differential Diagnosis. Clinically, lipomas may be confused with epidermoid cysts, other benign fatty tumors, and liposarcomas. The histologic differential diagnosis of classic lipomas would include normal adipose tissue and well-differentiated liposarcoma. Well-differentiated liposarcomas can be difficult to distinguish from lipomas but can usually be differentiated clinicopathologically. Liposarcomas are larger, demonstrate insidious growth, and are more likely to infiltrate normal structures. Microscopically, hyperchromatic nuclei and multivacuolar lipoblasts support the diagnosis.

Treatment. Excision or liposuction surgery is employed for lipomas.

Angiolipoma

Clinical Description. These lesions are similar to but smaller and more mobile than lipomas. Angiolipomas are primarily located on the arms and the trunk, and may be painful.

Pathology. Microscopically, the tumor is delineated from the surrounding normal tissue by a thin fibrous pseudocapsule (although they may be infiltrative). The tumor is composed of mature lipocytes interspersed with variable numbers of thin, branching vascular spaces. Microthrombi within the vessels are characteristic. Fibrosis between the fat cells and vasculature may be seen.

Differential Diagnosis. Clinically, angiolipomas resemble lipomas and other fatty tumors; however, the presence of pain favors the former. The histologic differential diagnosis includes routine lipoma, capillary hemangioma, Kaposi's sarcoma, and angiomyolipoma.

Treatment. Surgical excision is required.

Spindle Cell Lipoma

Clinical Description. Clinically, these usually appear as painless, small, solitary, firm subcutaneous masses. They are seen primarily on the upper back and neck, and are slow growing.

Pathology. Microscopically, it is a lobular tumor with sharply delineated borders composed of an admixture of mature lipocytes and uniform-appearing spindle cells. In some areas the lipocytes predominate, elsewhere complete replacement of the fat by the spindle cells may be seen. The stroma varies from myxoid to collagenous.

Differential Diagnosis. Clinically, spindle cell lipomas are impossible to differentiate from other benign and malignant fatty tumors, and the diagnosis is established histologically. The histologic differential diagnosis of spindle cell lipoma includes liposarcoma and fibrosarcoma.

Hibernoma

Hibernomas are well-circumscribed rare benign tumors that clinically resemble lipomas. They are usually solitary, mobile and symptomatic, and are found on the back, neck, or axilla. They have a lobular architecture and a distinct tan to brownish color—hence the name "brown fat." The lobules are separated by vascular interlobular septa and are composed of distinctive lipocytes that may entirely fill the lobules or be intermixed with white fat cells. The distinctive hibernoma or "mulberry" cell demonstrates a centrally placed nucleus with eosinophilic, granular, or multivacuolated cytoplasm.

Hibernomas are the only known benign tumors of brown fat. In humans, brown fat is seldom found past infancy.

Differential Diagnosis. Hibernomas demonstrate such a distinctive histologic appearance that confusion with other tumors is unlikely. Hibernomas with prominent eosinophilic granular cytoplasm may be confused with granular cell tumors; the multivacuolated cytoplasm in at least some of the cells will exclude these possibilities. Liposarcomas can be excluded on the basis of increased cellularity and cytologic atypia.

Treatment. Surgical excision is curative.

Lipoblastoma

Lipoblastoma is a rare benign tumor of immature white fat that occurs in young children. It may be well-circumscribed lobular or diffuse in its growth pattern. Lipoblastomas are distinctly less yellow-orange than normal fat or routine lipomas and may be gelatinous.

Pathology. Microscopically, lipoblastomas resemble fetal fat, with lobules separated by highly vascularized septa and a variably myxoid stroma. The immature fat cells may vary from spindle- or stellate-shaped cells to lipoblasts. Lipoblasts are smaller than mature lipocytes and contain cytoplasmic lipid droplets, at times with a "signet ring" appearance.

Differential Diagnosis. Clinically, lipoblastomas cannot be differentiated from other fatty tumors, although the young age at the time of presentation is suggestive. Histologically, lipoblastomas may simulate liposarcoma; however, the lobular architure is lacking in the latter.

Treatment. Treatment is by surgical excision.

Liposarcoma

Clinical Description. Liposarcoma occurs most frequently on the lower legs of adults 40 to 60 years old and is rare in children. The tumors are often greater than 10 cm in diameter with poorly defined margins, hemorrhage, and necrosis. The tumor enlarges rapidly and is painful and nonmobile.

Pathology. There are four main subtypes; however, mixed patterns may occur. *Myxoid liposarcomas* are the most common subtype and are characterized by an admixture of lipoblasts, signet ring cells, and mature lipocytes associated with a myxoid stroma and prominent vascularity. *Round cell liposarcomas* are closely related to myxoid liposarcomas but have a higher mitotic rate and more cellularity and cytologically atypical, often signet ring, round cells. *Well-differentiated liposarcomas* are composed primarily of seemingly mature lipocytes that demonstrate an infiltrative growth pattern and more variation in size versus normal fat or lipomas. Scattered pleomorphic multinucleated cells are seen. Mitoses are rare. *Pleomorphic liposarcomas* demonstrate large hyperchromatic nuclei with irregular nuclear contours due to lipid vacuoles. Multinucleated giant cells and atypical mitotic figures are commonly present.

Differential Diagnosis. Liposarcomas may be difficult to differentiate from other benign fatty tumors and sarcomas. Liposarcomas are more painful, arise deeper, and are more infiltrative than benign fatty tumors. Cytologic atypia and lipoblasts or signet ring cells favor lipoblastoma. Diagnostic features may be focal.

Treatment. Treatment is with excision. Metastasis to lungs can occur.

Liposuction Surgery of Fat Hypertrophy

Many individuals develop localized adiposities (''love handles'') that apparently respond to weight gain or loss differently than fat stores elsewhere in the body. Because these areas often do not respond to weight loss or excercise, liposuction may be helpful.

In recent years, liposuction surgery has been adapted for the treatment of lipomas. Liposuction removes fat by using a cannula attached to a source of negative pressure. The fat is suctioned out in a tunneling fashion rather then en bloc to prevent large dead spaces, seromas, and hematomas. Instead of sharply removing the entire lipoma, the tumor is extensively suctioned, leaving multiple tunnels throughout the lesion. Healing and contraction of these tunnels shrink the size of the tumor. Liposuction and curettage of a lipoma are both time-consuming procedures that may take twice as long as excision. However, the advantage of liposuction over standard surgical excision is the small incision (3 to 4 mm). It also allows better recontouring of the area. Alternatively, a small surface incision (1 to 2 cm) is made, and with blunt dissection or curettage the lipoma is removed in fragments.

The chief areas where liposuction is performed are the upper thighs, abdomen, and flanks. Other conditions that may benefit include male pseudogynecomastia and as an adjunct to surgical reduction mammoplasty.

Complications of liposuction include infection (especially after multiple procedures), necrotizing fasciitis, blood loss (potentially massive), inadvertent puncture of adjacent ulcers, and death from anesthesia or, rarely, the above complications. In general, liposuction is a relatively safe procedure, if done correctly. Tumescent local anesthesia, which involves infiltration of large volumes of dilute lidocaine and epinephrine, significantly decreases the amount of blood loss.

Undesirable sequelae post-liposuction include contour abnormalities (more likely with larger cannulas in superficial areas), hematomas/seromas, cutaneous loss of sensation (usually temporary), and edema. Patients should be aware that changes may not be obvious until 3 or more months after the procedure.

NEURAL TUMORS (OTHER THAN TUBEROUS SCLEROSIS AND NEUROFIBROMATOSIS)

(CM&S Chapter 148)

Cutaneous neural tumors can be classified into two major groups: those derived from peripheral nerves and those from ectopic or heterotopic neural tissue (Tables 10–2). The features of clinically important benign neural tumors are covered in Table 10–3.

TABLE 10-2. Classification of Cutaneous Neural Neoplasms

TUMORS OF THE PERIPHERAL NERVES	TUMORS OF ECTOPIC OR HETEROTOPIC NEURAL TISSUE

True neuromas
  Traumatic type
  Palisaded, encapsulated
    type
True nerve sheath tumors
  Schwannoma
  Neurofibroma
  Nerve sheath myxoma
  Granular cell tumor
  Malignant nerve sheath
    neoplasms
	Nasal glioma
	Extracranial meningioma
	Neuroectodermal tumors
	  Peripheral
	    neuroepithelioma
	    (neuroblastoma)

TABLE 10-3. Clinical Features of Clinically Important Benign Neural Neoplasms*

	TRUE NEUROMAS†		NERVE SHEATH NEOPLASMS‡		
	Traumatic Neuroma	**Palisaded Encapsulated Neuroma**	**Neurofibroma (Common, Solitary Type)**	**Schwannoma (Neurilemmoma)**	**GRANULAR CELL TUMOR**
Incidence Age	Uncommon Any	Rare Adults (mean age, 45.5 years)	Very common Adults (20–60 years)	Uncommon Adults (20–50 years)	Rare Adults (30–50 years)
Gender		1:1 = M:F	1:1 = M:F	F > M	1:3 = M:F
Number	Usually solitary	Usually solitary	Usually solitary	Usually solitary	Usually solitary
Location	At sites of trauma, surgical scars, amputations	90% face, 10% elsewhere	Trunk, head	Flexor aspects of extremities, head	30% tongue, 70% elsewhere, mainly head and neck
Size	0.5–2 cm	0.2–0.6 cm	0.2–2.0 cm	0.3–3.0 cm	0.5–3.0 cm
Clinical appearance	Skin-colored, firm papules or nodules	Skin-colored or pink, rubbery, firm papules or nodules	Skin-colored, soft or rubbery papules or nodules, sometimes pedunculated	Soft, pink, yellow smooth-surfaced nodules or tumors	Skin-colored, brownish red raised, firm nodules; may have ulceration and verrucous surface
Symptoms	Variable, tingling, itching, lancinating pain	Asymptomatic	Asymptomatic; "buttonhole" sign may be present	Asymptomatic; rarely painful, tender or paresthesia; occasionally freely movable	Asymptomatic or occasionally tender or pruritic

Continued

TABLE 10-3. Clinical Features of Clinically Important Benign Neural Neoplasms* *(Continued)*

| | TRUE NEUROMAS† | | NERVE SHEATH NEOPLASMS‡ | | |
	Traumatic Neuroma	Palisaded Encapsulated Neuroma	Neurofibroma (Common, Solitary Type)	Schwannoma (Neurilemmoma)	GRANULAR CELL TUMOR
Association	Nerve regeneration secondary to trauma	A variant is part of multiple mucosal neuromata syndrome, marfanoid habitus, neuroendocrine neoplasms	If multiple, may be part of von Recklinghausen's disease (10%)	Rarely with von Recklinghausen's disease or central nervous system tumors	10% multiple; predilection for blacks; rare in children
Histology	Poorly organized tangle of fasicles encapsulated by a fibrous sheath	Well circumscribed, encapsulated, composed of uniformly arranged fascicles of spindle cells	Unencapsulated, variably circumscribed, composed of disorganized slender spindle cells with a variable stroma	Well circumscribed, encapsulated, hypercellular areas with palisading of nuclei, and hypocellular areas with degeneration	Poorly circumscribed collection of cells with granular, abundant cytoplasms, S-100 positive

Clinical differential diagnosis	Hypertrophic scar, dermatofibroma, granuloma	Dermal nevi, basal cell carcinoma, neurofibroma	Dermal nevi, dermatofibroma, neuroma, soft fibroma	Lipoma, angiolipoma, adnexal tumors, dermoid or pilar cysts, leiomyoma, ganglion	Dermatofibroma, neurofibroma, adnexal tumor, dermal nevi
Other	"Rudimentary supernumerary digit" is considered as variant	May be induced by minor trauma	Plexiform variant is pathognomonic for von Recklinghausen's disease	May be multiple; syndrome of "schwannomatosis"	Visceral forms occur; malignant transformation may occur (3%)

*Treatment for all five tumors is simple, complete excision.
†Proliferations of neural tissue in which Schwann cells and axons are present in roughly equal numbers.
‡Proliferations of the endoneural or perineurial nerve sheath elements of cutaneous nerves.

FIBROUS NEOPLASMS

(CM&S Chapter 149)

Dermatofibroma

Clinical Description

Dermatofibroma is a common fibrohistiocytic tumor that has been called by a number of names, including fibrohistiocytoma and sclerosing hemangioma. Dermatofibromas occur as asymptomatic papules or nodules on the extremities in approximately 80% of cases. The legs of women are a common location, possibly as a result of shaving or other minor trauma. Dermatofibromas most frequently affect individuals in early to middle adult life. Although usually solitary, in about 20% of patients multiple lesions will be found, and there are reports of generalized dermatofibromas, especially in immunosuppressed patients and in patients with systemic lupus erythematosus.

The typical dermatofibroma presents as a slow-growing, round to oval, firm nodule with a dermal component that is attached to the overlying skin. It ranges in size from a few millimeters to several centimeters. Some lesions are dome shaped, while others appear depressed. The color can range from red-brown to dusky brown. The surface of the lesions may be smooth or rough. The clinical differential diagnosis includes scar, atypical nevus, and melanoma. A simple maneuver to help confirm the diagnosis can be done by applying lateral compression, which causes the central portion of the dermatofibroma to "dimple."

Pathology

Dermatofibromas are usually well-circumscribed nodules confined to the dermis that are composed of plump fibroblasts arranged as intersecting fascicles. Although most dermatofibromas are easy to diagnose clinically and histologically, occasionally several variants pose a dilemma in the differential diagnosis with malignant lesions.

The presence of cytologic atypia in some dermatofibromas could be a problem in distinguishing them from atypical fibroxanthoma. Dermatofibromas with atypical cells have mononucleated and multinucleated cells with large pleomorphic and hyperchromatic nuclei, some of which have prominent nucleoli. Despite the striking nuclear atypia, these lesions are characterized by rare mitotic figures. If mitoses are present, they are not atypical. This latter feature distinguishes dermatofibroma with atypical cells from atypical fibroxanthoma, in which typical and atypical mitotic figures are common.

Dermatofibromas are usually confined to the dermis. However, when they are composed predominantly of fibroblasts and extend to the subcutaneous tissue, it can be difficult to distinguish them from an early lesion of dermatofibrosarcoma protuberans.

Treatment

Dermatofibromas are most frequently found on the leg in women. They are frequently left untreated because the result is often no better in appearance than the lesion itself. If the decision to treat is made, there are several approaches. For smaller lesions that protrude above the skin surface, tangential shave excision is often an excellent treatment. Cryosurgery may eliminate the discoloration as well as flatten out the raised portion of the nodule. In larger symptomatic lesions, simple excision is the treatment of choice.

Dermatofibrosarcoma Protuberans

Clinical Description

Dermatofibrosarcoma protuberans is a soft tissue low-grade sarcoma of the skin of intermediate malignancy that should be separated from both benign and malignant fibrohistiocytoma. Dermatofibrosarcoma protuberans has a pronounced tendency to recur but is of low metastatic potential.

The tumor typically presents from ages 20 to 50 years. The most common site of occurrence is the trunk and proximal extremities, followed by the head and neck area and distal extremities. Dermatofibrosarcoma may arise after skin trauma or in scars.

Dermatofibrosarcoma protuberans appears initially as a dusky, indurated plaque that often escapes recognition for an extended period of time. The color can range from brown to bluish red, and there often is a bluish or reddish discoloration of the surrounding skin. Initial lesions are usually flat, or in some cases even depressed. Over time, the plaque areas steadily become larger and gradually nodules develop within the sclerotic area, but they usually remain asympatomatic.

Advanced lesions are usually recognizable, but early dermatofibrosarcoma protuberans may resemble scar tissue or morphea. Once nodules begin to develop, intermediate lesions can be confused with larger dermatofibromas.

Pathology

Plaque lesions of dermatofibrosarcoma protuberans are characterized by a flat surface, lower cellularity, lack of a storiform pattern, and slender spindle-shaped neoplastic cells with uniform nuclei arranged in long horizontal fascicles parallel to the skin surface. The nodular stage of dermatofibrosarcoma protuberans is characterized by higher cellularity and slender to oval cells arranged as short intersecting fascicles in the typical "storiform" pattern. The cells have slender to oval nuclei with a variable degree of hyperchromatism. Mitoses are frequent, unlike the plaque stage, and range from 3 to 5 per 10 high-power fields. Because plaques extend beyond the nodules and infiltrate the surrounding tissues as thin layers of slender, spindle-shaped cells that blend with the normal connective tissue cells, the surgical margins of excision may be very difficult to evaluate.

Treatment

Dermatofibrosarcoma protuberans grows by direct extension spreading outward and downward with irregular tracts of tumor following along paths of least resistance. The tumor can invade to involve deeper structures, including muscle and even bone. Recurrences are common because the infiltrating growth pattern extends well beyond the clinical margins, but metastases are infrequent. Cases that metastasize are almost always recurrent tumors with a considerable time interval between diagnosis and metastasis. When metastases do occur, the lung is the most common target organ, followed by the regional lymph nodes.

Dermatofibrosarcoma protuberans has a strong propensity to recur even after wide excision. Recurrence rates range from over 40% with 2-cm margins of excision to 11% with 3-cm margins taken beyond clinically involved skin and extending down to and including fascia. Recurrences of dermatofibrosarcoma protuberans typically occur within 3 years and are mainly due to incomplete excision. Because this tumor grows with very irregular projections that extend far beyond the clinical borders, it is difficult to determine adequate surgical margins.

Current recommendations for the surgical treatment of dermatofibrosarcoma protuberans call for wide excision with a 3-cm or greater margin down to and including fascia. There is no evidence to indicate that prophylactic lymph node dissection is warranted. Mohs' micrographic surgery has shown great promise in treating this tumor in an effort to preserve tissue, especially in the head and neck region. In 21 cases so far reported with this technique, there have been no recurrences at 5-year follow-up.

Atypical Fibroxanthoma

Clinical Description

Atypical fibroxanthoma most commonly presents on the nose, cheek, and ear regions of elderly patients. It usually appears as an asymptomatic solitary nodule or nodular ulcer. Typically, the tumor is less than 2 cm, and as it enlarges it may erode and ulcerate. However, lesions on the extremities are often larger, less well demarcated, and extend deeper.

The clinical differential diagnosis includes squamous cell carcinoma, basal cell carcinoma, epidermoid cyst, and ulcerated pyogenic granuloma. Atypical fibroxanthoma is best thought of as a superficial form of malignant fibrous histiocytoma. It usually pursues a relatively benign course, but rarely has the tumor metastasized to regional lymph nodes.

Pathology

Atypical fibroxanthoma is characterized histopathologically by a predominantly dermal expansile nodular growth on chronically sundamaged skin of elderly patients that abuts the overlying thinned epidermis and may extend into the upper portion of the subcutaneous fat. The neoplasm is composed of atypical cells with fibroblastic and histiocytic differentiation. The fibroblastic cells are spindle shaped and arranged as long fascicles and admixed with larger cells with histiocytic differentiation that have abundant foamy cytoplasm. In both types of cells, the nuclei are large, pleomorphic, and hyperchromatic; the cells are frequently multinucleated. There are many typical and atypical mitotic figures.

Treatment

Surgical excision is the recommended treatment. Because these tumors can extend into the superficial subcutaneous tissue, excision with margin control is recommended. A 1-cm margin is considered acceptable.

MELANOCYTIC NEVI

(CM&S Chapter 150)

Benign Melanocytic Neoplasms: Congenital and Acquired Nevi

Definition

A melanocytic neoplasm refers to a ''new growth'' composed of cells with differentiation toward melanocytes. These may be benign (i.e., melanocytic nevi) or malignant (i.e., melanoma). Melanocytes are cells derived from the neural crest and are demonstrable in the epidermis by the eighth week of gestation. They may assume a number of different shapes and forms. Some of the morphologic variants of melanocytes include cells that are small and round, large and round, pagetoid, balloon, oval, spindle, cuboidal, epithelioid, multinucleated, and dendritic. Any of these cell types may be present in greatest number in a given melanocytic nevus, which explains the large number of variants that have been described.

Clinical Description and Pathology

Intraepidermal Melanocytic Proliferations

Intraepidermal melanocytic proliferation refers to an increase in the number of melanocytes confined to the epidermis usually associated with epidermal hyperpigmentation. *Ephelides,* also known as freckles, are small, tan, uniformly pigmented macules that are usually 1 to 3 mm in diameter. They are induced by ultraviolet irradiation and are seen most commonly in persons with Fitzpatrick skin type I or II. They darken with exposure to ultraviolet irradiation and fade when light exposure diminishes. Histologically, there is a slight increase in the amount of melanin in the basal cell layer with a normal number of melanocytes.

Lentigo is a Latin word that means ''lentil shaped'' and has come to mean any lentil-shaped spot on the skin like a freckle. For this reason, lentigo should not be used in an unmodified fashion. The simple lentigo (*lentigo simplex*), a very common lesion, is a macular or slightly raised area of brown or brownish black pigmentation that is usually round or oval and less than 5 mm in diameter. There may be slight scaling on the surface, but skin surface markings are unaltered. Pigmentation is usually uniform. These lesions usually arise in childhood and are generally few in number, although they may be present in great numbers in patients with certain syndromic disorders such as the Peutz-Jeghers syndrome. In many cases, lentigines develop into junctional and compound nevi, although others may remain stable throughout life. Histopathologically, there is an increase in the number of small typical-appearing melanocytes at the dermoepidermal junction with an increase in the amount of melanin in the epidermis and cornified layer.

A number of intraepidermal melanocytic proliferations may arise as a consequence of ultraviolet irradiation. The *PUVA lentigo* is a macular pigmented lesion that develops on the skin of patients receiving photochemotherapy and that is characterized histologically by the presence of an increased number of large, somewhat atypical melanocytes confined primarily to the basal cell layer and associated with hyperpigmentation.

Solar lentigines are macular tan-brown pigmented areas in the skin that vary from 0.1 to 1 cm or greater in diameter and usually develop as a consequence of long-standing sun exposure. Histologically, there are epithelial changes characterized by rounded buds of keratinocytes at the tips of epidermal retia, distinct from the thinner, more delicate elongated epidermal retia seen in simple lentigines. Solar lentigines may remain stable or can evolve into reticulated seborrheic keratoses. When dense infiltrates of lymphocytes arise within these lesions, the term *benign lichenoid keratosis* or *lichen planus–like keratosis* is applied.

Mucosal lentigines develop on the oral or genital mucosa and are characterized by diffuse tannish to dark brown macular pigmentation that may range from less than 0.5 cm to several centimeters in diameter. Histologically, there is an increase in melanin in the basal keratinocytes with an increase in the number of dendritic melanocytes in the epithelium without cytologic atypia.

Café-au-lait macules are well circumscribed tan macules that range from 1 to 20 cm in diameter. These lesions are characterized by an increase in the numbers of melanocytes at the basal cell layer of the epidermis as well as an increase in the amount of melanin.

Melanocytic Nevi

The word ''nevus'' refers to an abnormal or faulty growth in the skin that is generally synonymous with the term *hamartoma*. *Melanocytic nevus* refers to an abnormal but benign proliferation of melanocytes in the skin that is generally associated with the formation of nests of cells. Although there may be many different varieties of nevi, the most common are those in which melanocytes are situated mostly at the dermoepidermal junction, known as *junctional melanocytic nevi*, *compound melanocytic nevi* in which there are nests of melanocytes at the dermoepidermal junction as well as in the dermis, and *intradermal melanocytic nevi* in which melanocytes are situated predominantly within the papillary and reticular dermis. Nevi may be present at the time of birth or may be acquired. They are relatively rare in infancy, increase in frequency during childhood and adolescence, reach a plateau in middle age, and undergo slow resolution with advancing age. It has been estimated that the average number of nevi in whites is 20 by the time the individual has reached 20 years of age.

Simple lentigines, junctional nevi, compound nevi, and *intradermal nevi* lie on a continuum of evolution. In childhood, most acquired melanocytic nevi are composed of melanocytes that proliferate at the dermoepidermal junction forming *junctional nevi.* Over time, nests of melanocytes migrate into the upper papillary dermis to form *compound melanocytic nevi.* Eventually, the junctional component diminishes and virtually all the melanocytes are situated in the papillary and reticular dermis. Clinically, junctional nevi are usually small, round, flat, or slightly raised, light brown to dark brown or black macules on the skin that range from 1 mm to 1 cm in greatest diameter. Compound nevi are raised, often papillomatous lesions that are usually circular. They may assume colors that range from skin colored and light tan to brownish black. Intradermal nevi are usually brownish to skin-colored papules characterized by a smooth or papillary surface and a soft rubbery texture.

Differential Diagnosis

Junctional nevi, especially those on the volar skin of acral surfaces, may be confused with hemorrhage into the cornified layer that develops after trauma, traumatic tattoos, thrombosed hemangiomas, as well as evolving melanoma. Melanomas are generally broader, asymmetrical, and have a poorly circumscribed border in contrast to junctional nevi, which are small, symmetrical, and well circumscribed. Compound nevi may be confused clinically with basal cell carcinoma, molluscum contagiosum, verrucae, and sebaceous gland hyperplasia, while intradermal nevi may be confused with skin tags and other benign epithelial lesions.

Variants of Melanocytic Nevi

Spitz nevi generally have features of compound or intradermal nevi clinically but often have a somewhat yellowish or orange color. They most often occur in children but may be seen in any age group and are quite common in young adults. They occur on any part of the body but are usually present on the face, trunk, or extremity. Although they are usually solitary, they may be numerous and widespread or grouped. Histologically there may be features similar to melanoma, because the cells that make up the lesions are large with abundant eosinophilic-staining cytoplasm. Clinically, Spitz nevi are usually thought to be benign but they are often confused with other nonmelanocytic lesions, such as pyogenic granuloma, dermatofibroma, or juvenile xanthogranuloma.

Halo nevus refers to a melanocytic nevus surrounded by a depigmented halo of otherwise normal skin. It is seen most commonly in older children and young teenagers. Patients can develop depigmented halos around several nevi simultaneously. Histologically, there is a striking lymphocytic infiltrate admixed with nevus cells in the dermis and at the dermoepidermal junction with a loss of epidermal melanocytes in the depigmented halo area.

Nevus spilus, also known as a speckled and lentiginous nevus, is clinically characterized by a flat, macular area that is usually darker than the surrounding skin, resembling a café-au-lait macule, and speckled dark central lentigo-like lesions, which are nevi.

Many benign melanocytic nevi are characterized by proliferations of melanocytes that are situated wholly in the dermis. These are thought to arise from dermal melanocytes that became arrested in the dermis before birth and never reached the basal cell layer, the normal location of melanocytes in the skin. *Mongolian spot, nevus of Ota,* and the *nevus of Ito* all are characterized by proliferations of dendritic melanocytes in the dermis. Mongolian spot clinically appears most commonly as a macular blue-gray pigmentation at birth on the sacral area. The lesion is quite common in dark-skinned persons, being present in over 90% of Asian infants, although it is less common in whites, being seen in only 1% of infants. The nevus of Ota and the nevus of Ito, are characterized by diffuse grayish blue patches involving the face and sclera and the acromioclavicular region, respectively.

The *blue nevus* is an area of bluish gray or blue-black dermal pigmentation produced by heavily pigmented melanocytes in the deep papillary and reticular dermis. The "blue" color is a result of the transmission of black from melanin in the dermis through the dermis in association with the surrounding contrast of the normal skin color. There are classically two forms, the cellular blue nevus and the common blue nevus. In the "common" type, dendritic melanocytes are found singly or in small aggregations, usually in the reticular dermis and often centered around appendages, vessels, and nerves. Cellular blue nevi possess both spindle and dendritic melanocytes, although larger cells with neural differentiation may also be present. Features of blue nevi may be observed in combination with other types of benign melanocytes. In such cases, the term *combined nevus* is appended to these lesions. Blue nevi must be distinguished from heavily pigmented nodular melanoma.

Congenital Melanocytic Nevi

A congenital melanocytic nevus refers to a melanocytic nevus that is present at the time of birth. These lesions are present in 1% of all newborns and have been divided into three sizes: small lesions less than 1.5 cm in diameter, intermediate-sized lesions 1.5 to 20 cm in greatest diameter, and giant lesions with a diameter of greater than 20 cm. At birth, these may be pale macules that over the course of time become darker and may develop outgrowths of terminal hair. Both pigment and hair growth increase at puberty. Histologically, there may be junctional, compound, and intradermal variants. Generally, there is an increase in the number of melanocytes at the epidermal basal cell layer with minimal cells in the papillary dermis and numerous melanocytes involving the upper reticular dermis, sometimes in a band-like configuration. Nevus cells are also present between the collagen bundles in the reticular dermis and may be present prominently around blood vessels and adnexal structures.

The likelihood for the development of melanoma in association with these lesions appears to be proportionate to the size of the lesion. There is a well-documented risk for malignant degeneration in giant congenital nevi, but for small and intermediate-sized congenital nevi, it is extremely low.

Differentiation Between Benign and Malignant Melanocytic Lesions

"Suspicious" pigmented lesions are those in which there is clinical concern about the possible diagnosis of melanoma and are defined as those with the clinical features of asymmetry, irregular borders, jet-black or variegated colors (especially with shades of red, grayish-white, and blue-gray), or diameter greater than 6 mm. Additionally, any pigmented lesion with a history of recent growth, color change, tenderness, pruritus, or bleeding is suspicious. A family or personal history of melanoma or atypical nevi is also important. A biopsy to rule out melanoma is indicated for suspicious pigmented lesions.

Biopsy Techniques

Excisional Biopsy

Complete excision of a pigmented lesion suspicious for melanoma is desired. This is the first stage of a two-stage procedure if the lesion is, in fact, a melanoma. The second stage consists of a wide local excision to the fascia with margins ranging from 0.5 to 3 cm, dependent on the Breslow depth of invasion. The excision is designed with the long axis corresponding to the relaxed skin tension lines. The length-to-width ratio may range from 2 : 1 to 4 : 1, depending on anatomic location and skin elasticity. The optimal angle at the tip of the ellipse is 20 degrees. After perpendicular incision of the skin, the tissue is removed with scissors or scalpel at a uniform depth and placed in 10% formalin solution. If necessary, undermining may be achieved to provide greater skin mobility. After meticulous hemostasis with spot electrocoagulation, the wound is closed in a standard two-layer closure with absorbable and nonabsorbable sutures or with a simple cutaneous closure with nonabsorbable sutures.

The excisional saucerization represents a modification of the excision technique. No sutures are used, and the wound heals by second intention (granulation). The scalpel is placed on the skin at a 45- to 60-degree angle. The skin is cut with the scalpel or scissors through the dermis to the underlying adipose tissue and removed. Meticulous hemostasis is achieved with spot electrocoagulation, chemical cautery (aluminum chloride, Monsel's solution), or fibrin foam. Second intention healing usually occurs over 3 to 6 weeks, depending on the size of the wound. A shave biopsy through the dermis is never recommended for any suspicious pigmented lesion, owing to the risk of transection of the lesion.

Incisional Biopsy

Three types of incisional biopsies — punch biopsy, elliptical incisional biopsy, and saucerization are acceptable for a biopsy of a suspicious lesion and are useful for relatively large lesions when complete excision is difficult. Removal of the most elevated and/or clinically suspicious area of the lesion to the adipose tissue is indicated during any incisional biopsy. Incisional biopsy does not increase the risk of metastasis of a melanoma.

Due to the risk of progression to melanoma in large congenital nevi, excision is often recommended. This can be accomplished by the use of serial excisions or tissue expansion. Tissue expansion is performed by gradual inflation of a balloon-type device placed beneath the skin. Once the desired degree of tissue expansion has been achieved after a period of about 6 weeks, the tissue expansion device is removed. The adjacent lesion is then excised, and the expanded tissue is used to reconstruct the surgical defect.

Advantages of tissue expansion over conventional reconstructive techniques include the ability to biologically greatly increase the amount of skin available for soft tissue reconstruction, providing excess adjacent donor tissue with good to excellent tissue match in terms of color, texture, and hair-bearing properties of particular importance for maximal cosmesis on the face and scalp, and the fact that it can usually be performed in children younger than 1 year of age. Disadvantages include the need for two operations, multiple infusions of saline into the expander during the expansion process over a period of several weeks, and disfigurement, which usually occurs as the expansion process proceeds. Complications include infection, hematoma, seroma, pain, mechanical device failure, exposure or extrusion of the expander, tissue necrosis, and bone resorption.

Atypical Melanocytic Nevi

Definition

Atypical melanocytic nevus, formerly termed "dysplastic nevus," refers to a benign melanocytic neoplasm that displays a characteristic constellation of clinical and histologic findings that in some forms has been associated with the development of malignant melanoma. The term *dysplastic nevus* is controversial. The term *nevus with architectural disorder* or Clark's nevus has been suggested to be substituted for the pathologic description. Because the phrase "dysplastic nevus" is firmly entrenched in clinical practice and in the literature, it is likely to be used for some time to come. Although *atypical nevus* is used synonymously with *dysplastic nevus* in this chapter, the terms are in transition. For a diagnosis of atypical nevus to be rendered with certainty, clinicopathologic correlation is recommended.

Clinical Description

Clinical criteria that are characteristic of atypical nevi include melanocytic lesions with variegated colors of tan, brown, and, frequently, areas of dyspigmentation; irregular angulated outlines; and size 5 to 10 mm or larger with location predominantly on the back, chest, abdomen, and arms. They may be solitary or present in multiplicity. Individual lesions may have a central papular component surrounded by a "halo" of brown, or they may appear as mamillated plaques.

Pathology

The histologic features of atypical nevi, while not entirely specific, consist of nests of melanocytes at the dermoepidermal junction at the bases and sides of epidermal retia, elongation of epidermal retia, slight coalescence of nests of junctional melanocytes, fibrosis surrounding epidermal retia, and a sparse infiltrate of lymphocytes in the papillary dermis. Four histologic features that are generally found include "basilar melanocytic hyperplasia," "random" cytologic atypia, a sparse lymphocytic infiltrate in the dermis, and lamellar fibrosis.

Diagnosis and Differential Diagnosis

The most important feature of atypical nevi is that their presence has been correlated with melanoma risk. The familial melanoma syndrome associated with multiple unusual-appearing nevi is well accepted; however, significant controversy still exists with regard to precisely what is required to establish that diagnosis.

A number of different clinical subsets have been created depending on the presence or absence of atypical nevi and melanoma in family members. The sporadic subtypes are only weakly correlated with melanoma risk if at all. On the other hand, persons with multiple atypical nevi and a strong family history of melanoma in first-degree relatives are at risk for the development of melanoma that may reach 100% over the course of a lifetime. Approximately 32,000 persons in the United States have the familial atypical nevus syndrome. The prevalence of sporadic atypical nevi has been estimated to range from 5% to 53% of populations in different studies. Melanoma risk correlates more with the total nevus density or nevus number than morphologic features of individual lesions. The most reasonable conclusion is that patients with atypical nevi and a personal or family history of melanoma are those afflicted with the familial form of the disorder and are at greatest risk for the development of melanoma. Those with many nevi, regardless of clinical or histologic features, are also at increased risk for the development of melanoma, albeit less than patients with the familial atypical nevus syndrome.

It remains controversial as to whether atypical nevi are truly precursors of melanoma or whether they serve primarily as markers for an increased risk of melanoma development. Most patients with familial atypical nevus syndrome who develop melanoma most commonly develop them on normal skin where there is no preexisting melanocytic nevus. Nevertheless, the existence of atypical nevi seen histologically in association with melanoma has been estimated to range from less than 1% to 83%, likely a consequence of overinterpretation of melanocytic proliferation at the edge of melanoma as representing residual atypical nevus

A rational approach to managing patients with the atypical nevus syndrome is essential. The most important aspect of the diagnosis lies in distinguishing atypical nevi from melanoma. Atypical nevi are "stable" lesions and do not tend to increase rapidly in size or change appreciably in color. Careful observation should enable clinicians to distinguish between these because evolving melanoma tends to become darker and change in size and shape over time. Careful observation over time should help distinguish the two.

Treatment

In that many patients with atypical nevi have numerous lesions, wholesale biopsy, excision, and removal is not feasible. One alternative that has been proposed is that a series of regional photographs be taken for baseline documentation of the clinical morphology of lesions followed by periodic observation and comparison. In patients with only a few lesions, follow-up at 12-month intervals is generally considered sufficient. In patients with a personal or family history of melanoma, careful observation at up to 4-month intervals is necessary. Any lesions documented to have changed should be subjected to biopsy. Furthermore, family members of index cases should be examined. All affected patients should be advised to avoid potential carcinogens such as ultraviolet irradiation that could lead to a synergistic effect with regard to the development of melanoma.

MELANOMA

(CM&S Chapter 151)

Definition

Cutaneous melanoma arises from malignant melanocytes located in the skin. Noncutaneous primary sites of melanocytes also include mucosal epithelia, retina, and leptomeninges.

Clinical Description

Epidemiology

In the United States, the incidence of melanoma has almost tripled in the past four decades, faster than that of any other cancer. This rise is not explained by any temporal change in diagnostic criteria, although early detection efforts may be contributing to some degree. Approximately 32,000 Americans will be found to have melanoma in 1994, and 6900 will die from the disease. Projections suggest that by the year 2000, 1 in 90 Americans will develop melanoma. Melanoma affects all adult age groups, with the median age at diagnosis being 53.

While the current 5-year survival rate of 83% represents a vast improvement over the 49% rate in 1950, the mortality rate has increased almost 150% in the United States in the past 40 years.

The precise etiology of melanoma is unknown. Of the major risk factors for melanoma (Table 10–4), the importance of genetic factors is reflected in the fact that about 6% of persons with melanoma

TABLE 10-4. Summary of Risk Factors for the Development of Cutaneous Melanoma

RISK FACTOR	RELATIVE RISK*
Adulthood (≥ 15 yr)	88
Pigmented lesions:	148
Dysplastic mole(s) (and familial melanoma)	
Dysplastic mole(s) (but no familial melanoma)	7–64
Lentigo maligna	10
Higher than average number of benign nevi	2–64
Congenital mole	17–21
White race (vs. black)	12
Previous cutaneous melanoma	5–9
Cutaneous melanoma in parents, children, or siblings	2–8
Immunosuppression	2–8
Excessive sun exposure	3–5
Sun sensitivity	2–3

*Degree of increased risk for persons with the risk factor compared with persons without the risk factor. Relative risk of 1.0 implies no increased risk.
Modified with permission from the New Engl J Med 1991;325:171–182.

have a family history of this cancer; also, those with a family history of melanoma in parents or offspring have an estimated eightfold increased risk of developing the disease themselves.

Epidemiologic and case control studies suggest a role for sunlight in the pathogenesis of melanoma. Although radiation in the ultraviolet B (UVB) range (290–320 nm) may be causative, the precise action spectrum for human melanoma remains unknown. The risk of melanoma appears to depend more on intermittent recreational sun exposure, especially early in life, than on simple cumulative sun exposure. Worldwide, the incidence of melanoma generally correlates inversely with latitude, with rates higher in locations closest to the equator and progressively lower in areas closer to the poles. Whites, especially those of type 1 or 2 skin, have much higher rates of melanoma than nonwhites. Blistering sunburns in childhood or adolescence are linked with increased rates of melanoma later in life. Migration studies suggest that childhood or adolescence represents a "critical period" for UV burn. Furthermore, in xeroderma pigmentosum, a rare autosomal recessive disorder characterized by deficient repair of UVB-damaged DNA, there is a 1000-fold increased rate of skin cancer, including melanoma.

However, not all evidence readily links UV light with melanoma. Melanoma rates are relatively low in persons with outdoor occupations. Except for the lentigo maligna melanoma subtype, melanoma does not regularly occur on maximally sun-exposed skin, such as the face. Only one study has documented UV-induced melanoma in animals.

Many speculate that increased recreational sun exposure has contributed to the rising incidence of melanoma through changes in personal habits, ozone depletion, and perhaps use of sun beds and tanning parlors.

Clinical Presentation

Because cutaneous melanoma is a uniquely visible tumor, the early detection and recognition of melanoma is the key to possible cure. An ABCD guideline helps the observer to suspect the diagnosis of melanoma in any pigmented lesion: A—asymmetry, B—border irregularity, C—color variegation or dark color, and D—diameter of more than 0.6 cm (the size of a pencil eraser). The possibility of melanoma should be considered when a patient reports a new pigmented lesion or a change in a preexisting mole, such as a change in the color, size, shape, or surface. Melanoma is typically asymptomatic. Hence, the visual examination remains the most reliable means of identification.

Melanoma can occur anywhere on the skin surface but not infrequently occurs on the back and other areas that are difficult for persons to inspect themselves. Because patients with melanoma on such areas may be unaware of the existence of these lesions, early detection by physicians, nurses, spouses, family members, and others can be exceedingly important.

The four classic histogenetic types of melanoma are defined by their clinical and histologic characteristics and by the history of progression of the lesion. Regardless of type, nearly all cutaneous melanomas begin as proliferations of neoplastic melanocytes within the epidermis and sometimes its epithelial adnexal structures—eccrine ducts and hair follicles, a stage termed *melanoma in situ*.

Lentigo maligna is most commonly seen in atrophic sun-damaged skin of the head and neck in patients in the fifth decade or older. It begins as an irregularly bordered tan or brown macule and typically enlarges over many years to become an irregularly shaped patch. In time, one or more papules or nodules can develop within the patch. The raised areas can be the same color as the patch, or any shade of pink, red, and brown. Palpable areas within a lentigo maligna herald the presence of invasion, and the lesion is then termed *lentigo maligna* melanoma (LMM). The actual size of a lentigo maligna or LMM is often underestimated clinically.

Superficial spreading melanoma can occur anywhere on the skin. It rarely arises before the fourth decade of life and appears to evolve more rapidly than LMM. By the time that most lesions are recognized, they are more than 2.5 cm in diameter and may be palpable. They often have angulated or notched borders. There is great variability in the color of these lesions, and shades of pink, red, tan, brown, and black are often haphazardly arranged. Papular or nodular areas signify invasion of the dermis and can be ulcerated.

Nodular melanoma appears clinically as a papule or nodule of melanoma. Nodular melanoma is most common on the trunk in men and on the legs of women. It evolves rapidly, seemingly within months, and is elevated when first encountered. Most nodular melanomas are 1 to 2 cm at the time that they are diagnosed, which is most often in the fifth decade of life. Their color ranges from pink in amelanotic lesions to black or "thundercloud gray."

Acral lentiginous melanoma is found on the palms, soles, and nail beds. Not all melanomas on these sites are of this type. Acral lentiginous melanoma is defined in part by its histologic appearance, and some acral melanomas are of the superficial spreading or nodular varieties. Acral lentiginous melanoma appears to be equally common in all races and is the only form of melanoma consistently found in dark-skinned individuals. Its peak incidence is in persons of 65 years of age or older. It presents as a dark-brown patch with irregular borders, within which papules, nodules, or plaques can supervene. Subungual melanoma may extend onto the skin of the proximal nail fold, a finding known as Hutchinson's sign.

In addition to the classic forms of melanoma, some unusual ones can be suspected clinically. Melanoma arising in a congenital nevus presents as an area of change within the lesion. Mucosal melanoma can present to the dermatologist as a dark patch that spills over onto the cutaneous surface of the lip, genitalia, or anus. Mucosal melanomas are histogenetically similar to acral lentiginous melanomas.

Regression of melanoma is a cell-mediated immune process whereby lymphocytes destroy the cells of a melanoma, in whole or in part. Regression of a flat area of melanoma results in a white or gray area within it. Complete regression of melanoma can account for the inability to find a primary lesion on examination of a patient with metastatic melanoma. Halo reactions or even patches of vitiligo can also occur around melanomas and around benign nevi.

Invasive melanomas in which spindled cells predominate can induce desmoplasia. Desmoplastic melanoma presents as a firm plaque that is often amelanotic. Areas of desmoplastic melanoma occur more frequently in the lentigo maligna and acral lentiginous variants. Desmoplastic melanoma can also be found without any evident flat area of melanoma, and if amelanotic, this form is particularly difficult to diagnose.

Pathology

Most cutaneous melanomas begin as an intraepidermal proliferation of melanocytes, designated melanoma in situ when they meet the following criteria: (1) increased frequency of predominantly basilar melanocytes, or melanocytes dispersed at all levels of the epidermis (pagetoid spread); (2) a relatively monomorphous population of markedly atypical melanocytes; and (3) both of the above present for a minimum breadth, such as one high-power field, or 0.5 to 1 mm.

One theory proposes that tumor progression in melanoma can be divided into so-called radial and vertical growth phases, linked to the biologic properties of the neoplastic cells. In radial growth phase, neoplastic melanocytes spread centrifugally within the epidermis, and sometimes appear to infiltrate the papillary dermis as small nests or single cells. In the vertical growth phase, neoplastic melanocytes acquire the ability to form larger nodules. The radial growth phase appears to lack metastatic potential. The vertical growth phase signifies a focal qualitative change resulting in a population or clone of cells that have a growth advantage over the surrounding population.

Superficial Spreading Melanoma

Superficial spreading melanoma, the most common type of melanoma (about 70% of all melanomas), histologically presents with a prominent intraepidermal proliferation of malignant melanocytes that are at least focally scattered in single-cell array throughout the epidermis. Because the distribution of these cells resembles that of the cells of Paget's disease, the pattern is often called pagetoid. The pagetoid cells may spread up to and include the granular cell layer or may be confined to the lower portions of the epidermis. The cells have abundant cytoplasm, are epithelioid, and contain round large nuclei. The epidermis itself is frequently hyperplastic but may be of normal thickness or even atrophic.

The radial growth phase of superficial spreading melanoma may be entirely intraepidermal (melanoma in situ or Clark level I [see Prognostic Factors and Staging]). More often, however, single cells or small clusters of cells similar in character to those in the intraepidermal component fill the dermis (Clark level II).

The fully evolved vertical growth phase may be defined by expansile nodule formation in the papillary dermis, but some vertical growth phases do not form expansile nodules, instead extending directly into the deep portions of the skin.

Expansile-nodule formation (Clark level III disease) represents the fully evolved vertical growth phase, which may extend into the reticular dermis (Clark level IV) and infiltrate the subcutaneous fat (Clark level V).

Lentigo Maligna Melanoma

LMM comprises about 5% of all melanomas and occurs most commonly on the maximally sun-exposed skin of the head and neck. The radial growth phase, lentigo maligna, is characterized by a mainly basilar or lentiginous proliferation of atypical melanocytes that is associated with an atrophic epidermis, extension of this cellular proliferation along the dermoepidermal junction of appendages (in many instances), and prominent solar elastosis of the dermis. With progression, cells are often spindle shaped and form dyscohesive nests along the dermoepidermal junction; they frequently involve the skin appendages. With further progression, the cells often take on an epithelioid cell appearance, resembling the cells of superficial spreading melanoma.

The invasive component of LMM, which early on can be difficult to recognize, is most commonly composed of spindle cells, with epithelioid cells and small round melanoma cells occasionally observed.

Acral Lentiginous Melanoma

Acral lentiginous melanoma, accounting for about 2% to 10% of all melanoma, is a pattern of melanoma involving the palms, soles, and nail apparatus. The histologic changes that occur in the radial growth phase of acral lentiginous melanoma involve a predominant proliferation of large, highly atypical cells frequently associated with prominent melanin production along the dermoepidermal junction in a hyperplastic epidermis.

Nodular Melanoma

Nodular melanoma (NM), accounting for about 15% to 30% of all melanoma, conceptually represents direct tumor progression to the vertical growth phase. If this tumor arises from a de novo proliferation of basilar melanocytes or a radial growth component, the vertical growth phase rapidly follows. In most instances, little or no intraepidermal remnant is adjacent to the expansile nodule that forms in the papillary dermis. Most cases of NM are at least Clark level III lesions when first recognized.

Diagnosis and Differential Diagnosis

A number of melanocytic and nonmelanocytic lesions mimic melanoma. Ordinary melanocytic nevi enlarge, darken, or increase in number at certain times in life, such as during puberty or pregnancy. However, as a rule, most melanocytic nevi change together, whereas the changes of melanoma may stand out in a distinctive way. Melanocytic nevi arise in childhood, adolescence, or young adulthood and are characterized by regular borders and even pigmentation (sometimes with a regular stippled pattern). The common type of blue nevus, a smooth nodule that is ''gun metal'' or blue-black in color, is generally less than 1 cm in diameter; has a well-defined, regular border; and usually occurs on the buttocks, presacral area, or dorsa of the hands or feet. Lentigo simplex is usually less than 5 mm in diameter and is a sharply defined, oval, uniformly pigmented (or regularly stippled) tan-brown or black macule; it may have a reticulated (net-like) pigmentation pattern. Solar lentigines, commonly called ''freckles'' or ''liver spots,'' appear as lightly pigmented, tan macules or patches in sun-exposed areas.

Nonmelanocytic pigmented lesions that may resemble melanoma include seborrheic keratosis, pigmented basal cell carcinoma, appendage tumors, and vascular lesions. Vascular lesions that may look like melanoma include ulcerated pyogenic granulomas, which can resemble amelanotic melanoma; hemangiomas; angiokeratomas; Kaposi's sarcoma; and hemorrhage beneath a nail plate, which can simulate subungual melanoma.

The major class of precursor lesions, dysplastic nevi (atypical moles), are larger than common melanocytic nevi and have clinical features (such as haphazard pigmentation and irregular borders) that are qualitatively similar to but quantitatively not as extreme as those seen in melanoma. Histologically, they differ from common melanocytic nevi in their atypical architectural, cytologic, and stromal features (see Chapter 9 in this text or Chapter 150 in CM&S).

Other melanoma precursor lesions include the rare giant congenital melanocytic nevi, which carry at least a 6% to 7% lifetime risk of malignant transformation. Small to medium-sized congenital melanocytic nevi appear also to be precursor lesions, although the lack of definitive histologic criteria distinguishing these lesions from acquired nevi of similar size complicates proper analysis of this issue.

Histologic Differential Diagnosis of Melanoma

Spitz nevus, pigmented spindle-cell nevus, dysplastic nevus, halo nevus, combined nevus, recurrent nevus, and cellular blue nevus are commonly mistaken for melanoma.

Treatment

The treatment of melanoma includes surgery of the primary lesion, prognostic factors and staging, consideration of adjuvant therapy, and treatment of metastatic disease.

Biopsy Technique for Suspected Melanoma

Histologic interpretation of the biopsy specimen can confirm the diagnosis of melanoma and, by enabling measurement of the thickness of the neoplasm, help determine the patient's prognosis, appropriate surgical management, and potential need for other therapy.

Before performing the diagnostic biopsy, the physician should palpate the regional draining lymph nodes and record the presence or absence of adenopathy. The diagnostic procedure of choice is a biopsy that conservatively excises the entire lesion. Removal in toto permits the pathologist to evaluate the full breadth and depth of the lesion and also prevents sampling error. Exceptions to the rule of biopsy in toto fall into three categories: (1) lesions so large that complete conservative excision would require significant surgery such as a skin flap or graft; (2) lesions located in anatomic sites where complete removal would cause an unacceptable cosmetic deformity (should the diagnosis prove to be benign); and (3) fragile patient health status.

The margin of the excision need be no more than 1 mm outside the visible edge of the lesion. The orientation of the ellipse should be located parallel to the lymphatic drainage (rather than along the relaxed skin tension lines) to facilitate future definitive surgery, should the biopsy reveal the lesion to be melanoma. The depth of the incision should extend into the subcutaneous fat but need not be carried down to the underlying muscular fascia. The remainder of the procedure follows conventional excisional skin surgery.

An incisional biopsy does not compromise survival of the patient, and there is no evidence that ''seeding'' of tumor occurs with biopsy in parte.

Prognostic Factors and Staging

The 5-year survival rates for melanoma decline steadily with increasing clinical stage (Table 10–5). Traditionally, melanoma was staged according to whether disease was confined to skin (stage I) or to nodes (stage II) or was metastatic (stage III). The American Joint Commission on Cancer (AJC) has proposed a revised four-stage system, dividing traditional stage I lesions into two categories at the 1.50-mm mark. In addition, the prognosis depends on a number of other factors. The two classification systems for melanoma confined

TABLE 10–5. Staging Systems for Melanoma

TRADITIONAL THREE-STAGE SYSTEM

Stage	Criteria	5-Year Survival Rate
I (thickness categories)	Skin	80%
≤0.75 mm		96%
0.76–1.49 mm		87%
1.50–2.49 mm		75%
2.50–3.99 mm		66%
≥4.00 mm		47%
II	Nodal involvement	36%
III	Distant metastases	5%

AMERICAN JOINT COMMITTEE ON CANCER STAGING SYSTEM*

Stage	Criteria
IA	Localized melanoma, ≤0.75 mm, or Clark level II (T1, N0, M0)
IB	Localized melanoma, 0.76–1.5 mm, or Clark level III (T2, N0, M0)
IIA	Localized melanoma, 1.5–4 mm, or Clark level IV (T3, N0, M0)
IIB	Localized melanoma, >4 mm, Clark level V (T4, N0, M0)
III	Limited nodal metastases involving only one regional lymph node basin, or <5 in-transit metastases but without nodal metastases (any T,N1, M0)
IV	Advanced regional metastases (any T,N2,M0) or any distant metastases (any T,any N,M1 or M2)

*When the thickness and level of invasion criteria do not coincide within a T classification, thickness should take precedence.
Reprinted with permission from the New Engl J Med 1991;325:171–182.

to the skin, are the five Clark levels of invasion and Breslow's vertical tumor thickness (as measured by an ocular micrometer from the top of the granular cell layer to the deepest point of tumor penetration). Vertical tumor thickness (in millimeters) has been confirmed as the best prognostic indicator for melanoma confined to the skin. For localized melanoma, discrete thickness categories mark where survival rates decline most rapidly. For example, most patients with thin stage I lesions (lesions ≤ 0.75 mm thick) can expect prolonged disease-free survival and even cure after treatment, whereas those with thicker lesions (> 4.0 mm) have much higher likelihood of dying of metastatic disease. The limited data available suggest that melanoma in situ is associated with relative 5-year survival rates approaching 100%.

In addition to tumor thickness, a number of other clinical and histologic factors affect prognosis for localized melanoma. Anatomic site of the melanoma is one important factor; with equivalent thickness, lesions on the scalp, hands, and feet appear to carry a poorer prognosis. Older patients and men have a poorer prognosis than younger patients and women, but these differences largely reflect variations in thickness and site.

Histologic features associated with an unfavorable prognosis include high mitotic activity, the presence of microscopic satellites of tumor (defined as discrete nests of tumor cells more than 0.05 mm in diameter located in reticular dermis or subcutaneous fat and separated from the bulk of the tumor by normal tissue), the presence of a vertical growth phase, ulceration, and increased tumor volume. DNA aneuploidy measurements by flow-cytometry techniques may also have prognostic value. The histopathologic subtype does not appear to be of major prognostic significance. The difference in 5-year survival for the different subtypes tends to reflect varying tumor thickness at the time of presentation.

The overall 5-year survival in stage II (AJC stage III) disease is about 30% to 35% but varies according to the clinical status of the nodes (macroscopic versus occult metastases) and the number of nodes involved with the tumor. Stage III (AJC stage IV) disease is generally incurable and has a median survival of 6 months. Common sites for the dissemination of melanoma include the skin, lymph nodes, bone, lungs, liver, spleen, and especially the central nervous system. Like lung cancer and breast cancer, melanoma commonly metastasizes to the brain.

In evaluating the newly diagnosed melanoma patient, the clinician should perform a thorough history and physical examination. In the absence of signs or symptoms of metastasis, laboratory or radiologic tests, aside from baseline chest radiography and possibly serum transaminase and alkaline phosphatase, are not routinely necessary for staging purposes.

Surgical Excision of Stage I Melanoma

Although wide surgical excision has been the accepted treatment for stage I (AJC stages I and II) melanoma, newer data suggest that narrower margins may suffice.

Based on several studies comparing narrow and wide excesions that demonstrate increased local recurrences but no reduction in long-term survival in those randomized to narrow excision, recommendation for definitive therapeutic melanoma surgery for lesions up to 1 mm in thickness is a 1-cm margin of normal skin surrounding the tumor or biopsy area. In situ lesions can safely be removed with 0.5-cm margins. The recommendation for lesions greater than 1 mm in thickness continues to be a 2-cm (or 3-cm) margin of healthy surrounding skin.

If a lymph node dissection is planned, the long axis of the excision should be oriented toward the regional draining lymph node group. This tenet of surgical oncology takes precedence over orientation parallel to relaxed skin tension lines. The depth of the excision should extend to but not include the underlying muscular fascia.

Lymph Node Dissection

Patients with melanoma and palpable lymph nodes require therapeutic lymph node dissection for diagnostic and therapeutic purposes. However, there is no clear consensus regarding the efficacy of elective lymph node dissection. Although nonrandomized studies do suggest a benefit for patients with intermediate-thickness primary lesions (1.00- to 4.00-nm thickness), neither of the two prospective randomized node dissection studies performed to date demonstrated improved survival for patients treated with immediate prophylactic (versus delayed therapeutic) node dissection.

Adjuvant Therapy

After surgery, patients require regular follow-up because of the risk of metastasis and increased risk of a second primary cutaneous melanoma. Patients with nodal disease or thick primary lesions who are at high risk for recurrence of distant metastasis need effective adjuvant therapy to prolong the disease-free survival. Many adjuvant strategies have been employed, including chemotherapy, nonspecific immunotherapy (e.g., bacillus Calmette-Guérin, *Corynebacterium parvum*, levamisole, and transfer factor), active specific immunotherapy, chemoimmunotherapy, adjuvant isolated regional perfusion for extremity melanoma, and radiation therapy. However, none of these strategies have definitively improved survival.

Treatment of Metastatic Disease

Because widespread metastatic melanoma is generally incurable, the goal of treatment should be palliation. In deciding from among the treatment options, the clinician must consider the site and extent of metastases, the tempo of the clinical course, and the overall performance status of the patient. Traditionally, chemotherapy, radiation, and surgery have been the first approaches. Of the chemotherapeutic agents, the most commonly used single agent is dacarbazine, which has an aggregate response rate of approximately 15% to 25%. These responses are usually partial, of short duration (3 to 6 months), and more likely to occur in skin, soft tissue, node, and lung metastases than other sites. Compared with single agents, combination chemotherapy has not appreciably improved remission and survival rates. Isolated limb perfusion, used principally with melphalan and hyperthermia, clearly palliates locally advanced melanoma of the extremity, but its impact on overall survival is still a matter of debate.

At one time considered a radioresistant tumor, metastatic melanoma can respond to radiation therapy. The complete response rate is roughly 25%, and the partial response rate of treating metastatic nodules is approximately 35%.

Complete surgical excision of accessible, limited metastases may be associated with prolonged survival; more often, however, widespread metastases will preclude the possibility of surgery.

Early Detection and Prevention

The contrast between near-certain death from metastatic disease and possible cure of thin melanoma underscores the potential of prevention and early detection. The theoretical appeal of the early detection of melanoma and other skin cancer lies in the fact that these conditions are increasingly common, early disease has a high survival rate, and the screening examination (a visual examination by a qualified observer) is noninvasive, takes several minutes, and is regarded as reliable in diagnostic settings. However, formal screening for melanoma is in its infancy, and few data are available on its yield and efficacy.

At the present time, recommendations are for high-risk persons to minimize sun exposure, use sunscreens when possible, and, until more data emerge, be encouraged to perform regular self-examination of the skin. The management of patients with small to medium-sized congenital nevi is controversial; for now, patients should consider excision of the lesion at puberty, when surgery under local (not general) anesthesia is feasible.

Proper monitoring of patients with atypical moles should help prevent melanoma-related deaths. Recommendations are at least once- or twice-yearly skin examinations (with selective excision of the most atypical or changing pigmented lesions) for persons with atypical nevi.

MASTOCYTOSIS

(CM&S Chapter 152)

Definition

Mastocytosis is a heterogeneous group of disorders characterized by increased numbers of mast cells in a variety of tissues, most often the skin.

Clinical Description

Mast cell disease occurs in all races and affects both sexes equally. The peak incidence of mastocytosis is in children, especially before the age of 6 months. There is a second peak in young adults. Mastocytosis tends to be transient in children and chronic in adults.

Mastocytosis may be limited to one organ or may be classified as systemic if more than one organ system is involved. The disease may be further classified prognostically as indolent, aggressive, or associated with mast cell leukemia or other hematologic abnormalities.

General Features of Cutaneous Mastocytosis

Although there is overlap, patients with cutaneous mastocytosis are classified into those with solitary mastocytoma, urticaria pigmentosa, diffuse or erythrodermic mastocytosis, or telangiectasia macularis eruptiva perstans. The number of dermal mast cells in cutaneous mastocytosis varies from a relatively small number that is clinically undetectable to larger aggregations forming papules, nodules, or diffuse thickening of the skin. Papular or nodular lesions may have a yellowish hue. Darier's sign is the development of urtication and a delayed, axonally mediated erythematous flare elicited by rubbing or other minor trauma to a lesion. Such physical stimulus causes mast cell degranulation with the release of mast cell mediators and local tissue effects of vasodilatation, increased vascular permeability, and edema. In addition, cutaneous mastocytosis may be hyperpigmented due to increased epidermal melanin pigment. Patients may have prolonged dermographism or flushing, or pruritus, occasionally without visible skin lesions. Lesions in infants occasionally form tense blisters that usually heal without scarring unless secondary infection occurs. Unusual severe complications in infancy include hypotension and shock, severe diarrhea and dehydration, and a bleeding diathesis.

Mastocytoma

The term *mastocytoma* refers to nodular infiltrates of mast cells that may be isolated or generalized. Solitary mastocytomas occur almost exclusively in the first 2 years of life and are often present at birth. They occur on the trunk and extremities and range in size from 5 to 60 mm in diameter. Darier's sign, epidermal pigmentation, the formation of vesicles or bullae, and localized flushing are common. These lesions may occasionally be followed by extensive involvement within 1 or 2 months. Lesions that are truly solitary usually regress completely or become asymptomatic and rarely persist into adulthood.

Urticaria Pigmentosa

Patients with *urticaria pigmentosa*, the most common form of cutaneous mastocytosis, present with up to several thousand individual round-to-oval red-brown macules and papules that urticate. These occur over the trunk and extremities and may coalesce at times, giving a cobblestone appearance with exaggeration of the normal skin markings. Pruritus, dermographism, flushing, telangiectasia, and petechiae or ecchymoses can occur in lesions or in clinically normal skin. Most patients, particularly children, have an extremely good prognosis. Over half will clear by adolescence, and most of the remainder have only residual, lightly pigmented asymptomatic macules. Later-onset lesions are more likely to persist or progress slowly and remain symptomatic. Perhaps 25% of patients with adult-onset urticaria pigmentosa develop systemic mastocytosis.

Diffuse and Erythrodermic Mastocytosis

Diffuse infiltration of the skin is rare and occurs almost exclusively in infants, although it may persist into adult life. Blisters in the neonatal period may be the first indication of diffuse involvement, with later development of a "doughy" thickening of the skin. Involvement may be limited to large plaques or may include the entire skin surface. The skin may have a normal, hyperpigmented, or red color, and the surface may be smooth or covered with minute papules, causing a resemblance to grain leather. Scattered nodules and larger papules as well as urticaria pigmentosa type lesions may be seen. When the dermal mast cell infiltrate is dense, the skin may look similar to pseudoxanthoma elasticum. Although diffuse cutaneous mastocytosis often resolves spontaneously, these patients are at higher risk of systemic involvement, severe complications, and persistence of mastocytosis into adulthood.

Telangiectasia Macularis Eruptiva Perstans

Telangiectasia macularis eruptiva perstans is rare and occurs almost exclusively in adults. The lesions tend to be widespread and may involve the face. The lesions consist of telangiectases on an erythematous or hyperpigmented macular background. Darier's sign may be evident.

Systemic Mastocytosis

The vast majority of patients with cutaneous mastocytosis do not have systemic involvement, although bone involvement may be detected in 10% of patients with urticaria pigmentosa. Many patients with systemic mastocytosis have indolent disease that can be controlled pharmacologically. The skeletal and hematopoietic systems are common extracutaneous sites. The reticuloendothelial system, liver, gastrointestinal system, and cardiovascular and central nervous systems may also be involved. Systemic complaints include nausea, vomiting, diarrhea, episodic abdominal pain, weight loss, headache, fatigue, episodic flushing, chest pain, tachycardia, hypotension, syncope, or dizziness. These symptoms may be caused by chemical mediators released systemically or locally from mast cells. Malabsorption, gastritis, and peptic ulcer disease with hemorrhage or perforation are associated with hyperchlorhydria caused by high levels of histamine. Steatorrhea, hepatosplenomegaly, anemia, myelodysplastic and myeloproliferative syndromes, lymphoma, and leukemia may occur. In cases of mastocytosis associated with serious hematologic abnormality or malignancy, the overall prognosis is determined by the response of these associated conditions to therapy. True mast cell leukemia is very rare and has a dismal prognosis.

Pathology

Generally, there is an accentuation of normal mast cell distribution (perivascular, perineural, near-epithelial surfaces). The degree of infiltration varies widely from the subtle superficial perivascular mast cell infiltrates of telangiectasia macularis eruptiva perstans to the massive infiltrates that may extend into the subcutaneous fat seen in mastocytomas and nodular lesions.

Mast cells are monotonous with round-to-oval nuclei and a finely granular cytoplasm that shows metachromasia in Giemsa- or toluidine blue–stained sections.

Pathogenesis and Etiology

Most of the symptoms of mast cell disease are caused by mast cell mediators that can be released by a number of factors. Nonspecific complement and nonimmunologic stimuli include physical trauma and changes in temperature, venoms from snakes and insects, polypeptides found in shellfish, and a number of drugs such as aspirin, alcohol, narcotics, radiographic contrast dyes, and various drugs associated with anesthesia. The mediators released from stimulated mast cells include histamine, arachidonic acid and its metabolites (e.g., prostaglandins and leukotrienes), cytokines, and neutral proteases. Locally, they induce urtication, vasodilatation, and pruritus; systemically, they contribute to anaphylaxis or gastrointestinal and central nervous system disturbances.

Diagnosis and Differential Diagnosis

The diagnosis of cutaneous mastocytosis can be established when lesions of classic morphology with a positive Darier's sign are identified. No further diagnostic investigation is needed in young children with limited disease. Skin biopsy is the most common and most effective confirmatory test. Anesthetic without epinephrine infiltrated adjacent to the lesion rather than directly into it is recommended to avoid mast cell degranulation.

In patients with extensive, persistent, or progressive cutaneous disease, a baseline radiologic survey may be considered. A radiologic survey and bone scan are indicated in any patients with symptoms referable to the skeletal system. Bone marrow biopsy is indicated in individuals with hematologic abnormalities.

The differential diagnosis of cutaneous mastocytosis includes pigmented, telangiectatic, and nodular lesions as well as pruritus, dermographism, and flushing. The presence of Darier's sign allows easy differentiation of individual lesions in most cases, but in older patients, Darier's sign may be absent. Papular lesions of mastocytosis may resemble eruptive xanthomas, and lesions in infants may resemble impetigo or Langerhans cell histiocytosis. Both the carcinoid syndrome and mastocytosis may present as episodic flushing and nonspecific gastrointestinal and cardiovascular symptoms; flushing associated with carcinoid syndrome is evanescent, typically lasting 10 minutes or less whereas that of mastocytosis typically lasts 30 minutes or longer. Urine 5-hydroxyindoleacetic acid is usually elevated in the carcinoid syndrome. Occasionally, patients may present with few or no skin lesions and pruritus or a constellation of vague complaints (inability to concentrate, headache, fatigue, dizziness, syncope, nausea, vomiting, diarrhea, abdominal pain, weight loss, episodic flushing, tachycardia, or chest pain). A therapeutic trial of antihistamines or sodium cromoglycate may confirm the diagnosis.

Treatment

Reassurance of the usual benign course of this disease and avoidance of specific factors known to trigger mast cell degranulation may be sufficient. Therapeutic intervention is generally directed at amelioration of symptoms; however, in certain situations, therapy may be directed against specific cutaneous lesions. Acceptable temporary cosmetic results may be obtained by treatment with potent topical corticosteroids. Excision of symptomatic solitary mastocytomas may rarely be indicated if, for example, severe cardiovascular or respiratory symptoms are being produced.

Patients with extensive involvement or prominent cardiovascular symptoms should be taught to recognize and manage anaphylaxis and should be cautioned that they may be at increased risk for adverse reactions when undergoing general anesthesia.

Histamine receptor antagonists are the primary therapy for control of symptoms. Therapy may be begun with a single type 1 histamine (H_1) receptor antagonist. After maximum tolerated levels are achieved, another may be added. H_2-receptor blockers may help control the gastrointestinal effects associated with hyperchlorhydria. Oral disodium cromoglycate may prevent release of mediators and thus control diarrhea. Dosages are 20 to 40 mg/kg in four divided doses in patients younger than 2 years, 100 mg four times a day for ages 2–12, and 200 mg four times a day for adults. Two or 3 weeks of treatment may be required for a maximum clinical response.

Photochemotherapy with psoralens and ultraviolet A radiation (PUVA) may decrease itching and provide cosmetic benefits. The benefits, however, are temporary. Systemic corticosteroids and interferon alfa may be beneficial in patients with severe mastocytosis. In patients with aggressive systemic disease or with hematologic malignancies, death usually results from bleeding from thrombocytopenia. Splenectomy is controversial but may be recommended in a selected group of patients.

LANGERHANS CELL HISTIOCYTOSIS

(CM&S Chapter 153)

Definition

Langerhans cell histiocytosis (the term preferred to histiocytosis) comprises a broad spectrum of clinical diseases having proliferation of Langerhans cells in common. The most limited form includes skin lesions of congenital self-healing reticulohistiocytosis and solitary, indolent lesions (eosinophilic granulomas) of bone or other organs. Multifocal Langerhans cell histiocytosis lesions of the head classically produce diabetes insipidus, proptosis, and lytic bone lesions (Hand-Schüller-Christian disease) or, more commonly, an incomplete form of this triad. Disseminated, often fatal involvement of viscera and skin (Letterer-Siwe disease) constitutes the acute, fulminant end of the Langerhans cell histiocytosis spectrum. Whether Langerhans cell histiocytosis is a proliferative or reactive group of disorders remains controversial.

Clinical Description

Langerhans cell histiocytosis can occur at any age but onset is most common between 1 and 15 years of age. In general the Letterer-Siwe form occurs in infants, Hand-Schüller-Christian disease in older children, and solitary eosinophilic granuloma in young adults.

Skin lesions may be the sole manifestation of Langerhans cell histiocytosis; they occur in almost all patients with Letterer-Siwe disease and up to half of patients with Hand-Schüller-Christian disease. Lesions include erythematous, brown, or yellow papules, plaques, nodules, vesicles, pustules, ulcers, and purpura. The typical distribution is in flexural and seborrheic regions such as the scalp, hairline, retroauricular areas, axillae, groin, and perineum. Skin lesions are often hemorrhagic in patients with Letterer-Siwe disease.

Congenital self-healing reticulohistiocytosis is a limited form of Langerhans cell histiocytosis. It is present at birth or shortly thereafter and involutes spontaneously within the first year of life. Affected infants have multiple or, rarely, solitary red-brown or purple-blue nodules on the torso and extremities. The nodules ulcerate and heal with hyperpigmentation and atrophic scarring. Systemic involvement is absent, except for occasional hepatomegaly or hematologic abnormalities.

Eosinophilic granulomas are the most common manifestation of Langerhans cell histiocytosis. They may occur in any organ, including skin and lung, but have a predilection for flat bones, particularly of the calvaria. Lesions are asymptomatic or painful; infiltration of vertebral bodies can lead to collapse and spinal cord compression. Radiographs show well-demarcated radiolucencies.

Neurologic signs and symptoms in Langerhans cell histiocytosis, which result from widespread dissemination or direct extension of calvarial lesions, range from headaches to seizures. Otolaryngologic and oral manifestations are common and can be the presenting complaint. They include otitis, aural discharge, hearing loss, gingival bleeding, loosening of teeth, and buccal ulceration. Pulmonary, hepatic, and hematologic manifestations are associated with disseminated disease.

Hematologic manifestations include pancytopenia and bleeding diathesis due to hypersplenism or bone marrow infiltration; hemolytic anemia and peripheral eosinophilia may also occur.

In addition to a complete history and physical examination, recommended laboratory evaluation includes assessment of the complete and differential blood cell count, reticulocyte count, erythrocyte sedimentation rate, direct and indirect Coombs test, liver function tests, serum amylase level, prothrombin and partial thromboplastin times, serum protein electrophoresis, urinalysis, urinary specific gravity after water deprivation, chest films, and skeletal survey. Additional studies, such as pulmonary function testing, arterial blood gases, and bone marrow biopsy, should be based on clinical suspicion or abnormal findings from screening tests. Tests of immunologic function are indicated in disseminated cases.

Pathology

The dermis has a diffuse, nodular, or occasionally perivascular infiltrate of mononuclear Langerhans cells, each 15 to 25 μm in diameter, having a moderate amount of homogeneous, eosinophilic or pale cytoplasm, a lobular nucleus with a central, longitudinal groove (''coffee bean'' appearance) or hilar indentation (''kidney'' appearance), and a small nucleolus. There is not significant nuclear cytologic atypia. Epidermotropism of the Langerhans cells is common, and ulceration may occur. The infiltrate may be composed almost entirely of Langerhans cells, particularly in cases of Letterer-Siwe disease, or may be admixed with eosinophils, lymphocytes, and phagocytic macrophages.

Identifying the pathognomonic Langerhans cells in the infiltrate by immunohistochemistry using S-100, and HLA DR confirms the diagnosis, but electron microscopy remains the diagnostic standard.

Differential Diagnosis

The clinical differential diagnosis of cutaneous lesions of Langerhans cell histiocytosis includes seborrheic dermatitis, Wiscott-Aldrich syndrome, acrodermatitis enteropathica, cutaneous lymphoma, and other histiocytic syndromes, such as xanthoma disseminatum.

Treatment

Therapeutic decisions depend on symptoms and extent of disease. For limited disease, such as solitary eosinophilic granuloma, simple excision may be curative. Spontaneous regression is also possible. Intralesional corticosteroid injection (50 to 150 mg methylprednisolone for bone lesions) or local radiation therapy (6 to 10 Gy) is often effective for local disease. Patients with extensive cutaneous disease may respond to psoralen photochemotherapy (PUVA) (two to four times per week for several months) or topical nitrogen mustard (10 mg in 50 mL normal saline applied daily). Patients with disseminated disease may require prednisone, alone or in combination with cytotoxic agents such as vinblastine, methotrexate, and 6-mercaptopurine; at present, etoposide (150 mg per day for 3 days intravenously repeated in three to six cycles) seems to be the most active chemotherapeutic agent.

MULTICENTRIC RETICULOHISTIOCYTOSIS

(CM&S Chapter 154)

Definition

Multicentric reticulohistiocytosis is a rare, systemic, histiocytic disorder that involves primarily the skin, mucosa, and joints. Skin lesions may precede, accompany, or follow development of polyarthritis, and nearly half of the patients develop life-long disabling arthritis.

Clinical Description

The age at onset of multicentric reticulohistiocytosis is most frequently in the fourth decade, but the disorder can occur at any age. White females are typically affected. Cutaneous eruptions of papules and nodules have a cephalocaudal distribution, with the face, scalp, neck, hands, and forearms most often involved. Classically, papular lesions occur on the hands in a periungual distribution, resembling beads. Oral involvement occurs in half of the cases, with lips, buccal mucosa, tongue, and nasal septum being the most common sites. Lesions may be pruritic and may wax and wane. Patients often present with pain and swelling of the joints, and typically the arthritis and joint damage is very rapid. Destruction of the distal and proximal interphalangeal joints often results in an opera-glass–shaped deformity of the hands. The shoulders, knees, wrists, hips, feet, ankles, elbows, and spine can also be involved. Arthritic symptoms may also wax and wane; as a general rule, multicentric reticulohistiocytosis will spontaneously disappear in about 8 years.

Pathology

Microscopically, a circumscribed but unencapsulated proliferation of histiocytes in the dermis is seen. The majority of the infiltrate is composed of multinucleated giant cells with abundant eosinophilic, finely granular, ground-glass cytoplasm.

Diagnosis and Differential Diagnosis

The diagnosis is straightforward given the clinical and histopathological findings. Rheumatoid arthritis can show similar findings.

Treatment

Treatment is generally unrewarding. Anti-inflammatory agents may provide some relief to arthritic symptoms, but they do not alter the course of the disease. Chemotherapeutic agents such as azathioprine, cyclophosphamide, and methotrexate have been tried with some success.

OTHER HISTIOCYTOSES OF CHILDHOOD

(CM&S Chapter 155)

The histiocytoses of childhood are a group of diseases with localized or generalized proliferations of cells of the monocyte-macrophage and/or dendritic cell systems (Table 10–6). The cells of both systems are derived from monocytes, which in turn originate from a bone marrow stem cell.

Juvenile Xanthogranuloma

Clinical Description

Juvenile xanthogranuloma is a benign histiocytic tumor that occurs most commonly in infancy and early childhood and tends to be self-healing. Identical lesions can occur in adults. The pathogenesis of this tumor is unclear.

TABLE 10-6. The Histiocytoses of Childhood

CLASS I: DENDRITIC CELL HISTIOCYTOSES

Langerhans cell histiocytosis
Indeterminant cell histiocytoma

CLASS II: HISTIOCYTOSES OF MONONUCLEAR PHAGOCYTES OTHER THAN LANGERHANS CELLS

Juvenile xanthogranuloma
Benign cephalic histiocytosis
Generalized eruptive histocytoma
Xanthoma disseminatum
Sinus histiocytosis with massive lymphadenopathy
Multicentric reticulohistiocytosis

CLASS III: MALIGNANT HISTOCYTIC DISORDERS

Monocytic leukemia
Malignant histiocytosis
True histiocytic lymphoma
Malignant Langerhans cell histiocytosis

The lesions of juvenile xanthogranuloma generally erupt as one or several small erythematous papules that develop into 2- to 20-mm yellowish-red nodules that frequently have telangiectases or may appear somewhat hyperpigmented in dark-skinned individuals. Lesions tend to slowly flatten as they resolve and frequently heal with small atrophic scars.

Lesions of juvenile xanthogranuloma occur most commonly on the upper part of the body. Ocular involvement is the most common extracutaneous manifestation, and lesions affecting the iris can lead to anterior chamber hemorrhage and glaucoma. Mucous membranes are occasionally involved, and lesions have been reported in skeletal muscle, lungs, liver, spleen, testes, ovaries, colon, kidneys, heart, and bones.

Pathology

Early lesions show a diffuse infiltration of spindle-shaped fibro-histiocytic cells. As the lesion matures, a mixed cellular infiltrate with histiocytes, lymphocytes, eosinophils, and occasional neutrophils and plasma cells is seen. Touton giant cells, characterized by the wreath-like arrangement of multiple nuclei, are typically present.

Differential Diagnosis

The differential diagnosis of juvenile xanthogranuloma includes mastocytoma, benign cephalic histiocytosis, eruptive histiocytomas, xanthoma disseminatum, and Langerhans cell histiocytosis.

Treatment

Surgical excision is usually curative, but treatment is generally unnecessary in children unless the lesions are symptomatic, since cutaneous lesions tend to resolve spontaneously. Adults may desire removal of lesions because juvenile xanthogranuloma arising in adulthood is frequently persistent. An ophthalmologic examination is recommended for children with skin lesions of juvenile xanthogranuloma to rule out ocular involvement. Surgery or radiation therapy may be indicated for ocular lesions.

Xanthoma Disseminatum

Xanthoma disseminatum is a rare sporadic histiocytic disease that occurs in both children and adults. Skin lesions are typically red-brown to yellow and tend to be most prominent on flexural surfaces, where they develop in clusters and may become confluent. The eyelids and conjunctiva may be involved, and the lips, pharynx, and larynx characteristically become infiltrated, occasionally resulting in respiratory difficulty. Diabetes insipidus is the only characteristic sign of systemic disease.

Histopathologically, lesions are similar to those of juvenile xanthogranuloma, showing the presence of foamy histiocytes, inflammatory cells, and Touton giant cells.

The skin lesions tend to be self-healing, with spontaneous resolution occurring over a 2- to 40-year period. Diabetes insipidus, when present, tends to be mild and may also resolve spontaneously. Troublesome cutaneous, mucosal, and ocular lesions have been managed successfully with conservative surgical excision and electrocauterization. Xanthoma disseminatum responds poorly to chemotherapy and radiation.

Malignant Histiocytoses

Acute monocytic leukemia, malignant histiocytosis, and histiocytic lymphoma are malignancies of the monocyte–macrophage system of cells. Although they have been separated on clinical grounds, they form a spectrum of related entities and it is not always possible to differentiate them.

Monocytic leukemia is a malignancy that primarily affects the bone marrow and blood of infants. Extramedullary single or multiple skin involvement is common and may present as nodules. Histologically, the skin biopsy specimens show a dermal and subcutaneous infiltrate of closely packed, uniform, round cells with oval or slightly indented nuclei and moderate nongranular cytoplasm. Frequent mitoses are seen, but hemophagocytosis is not observed. Chemotherapy is the treatment of choice.

Malignant histiocytosis and true histiocytic lymphoma originate theoretically from tissue macrophages. Malignant histiocytosis predominantly involves the sinuses of lymph nodes, while true histiocytic lymphoma effaces the lymph node architecture, similar to other non–Hodgkin's lymphomas. Both are rare entities.

Malignant Langerhans Cell Histiocytosis

Malignant Langerhans cell histiocytosis or malignant histiocytosis X has been reported to be a distinct clinicopathologic entity that occurs predominantly in men. Multisystem organ involvement is typically present, while skin lesions consisting of widespread papules and nodules occur less frequently. These lesions frequently developed central necrosis and ulceration as the disease progressed.

Infiltrating cells in this disease are cytologically atypical with nuclear pleomorphism and enlarged nucleoli, and cells tend to occur singly rather than in syncytium-like sheets. All reported cases of malignant Langerhans cell histiocytosis have been rapidly fatal despite aggressive therapy with surgery, chemotherapy, and radiation therapy.

CUTANEOUS LYMPHOID HYPERPLASIA

(CM&S Chapter 156)

Definition

Cutaneous lymphoid hyperplasia is a clinically benign, usually localized dermatosis characterized by dense lymphoid infiltration of the skin that may be idiopathic or secondary to a recognized foreign antigen such as bites, stings, infestations, infection of foreign substances, drugs, and infection with *Borrelia burgdorferi*. Lymphocytoma cutis, pseudolymphoma, Spiegler-Fendt sarcoid, and lymphadenosis benigna cutis are synonyms for cutaneous lymphoid hyperplasia. In addition to being a principal lesion, cutaneous lymphoid hyperplasia may occur as part of a distinct disease such as Kimura's disease, angiolymphoid hyperplasia with eosinophilia, or systemic drug-induced lymphoid hyperplasia (e.g., secondary to phenytoin).

Clinical Description

Cutaneous lymphoid hyperplasia can involve any area of the skin but is most common on the face. The majority of cases present as a solitary or localized cluster of asymptomatic, erythematous to violaceous, papules or nodules that can coalesce into a plaque. Uncommonly, the lesions may be widespread over a body region or even generalized in their cutaneous distribution. In cutaneous lymphoid hyperplasia that is not part of some other systemic lymphoid hyperplasia syndrome, constitutional symptoms are absent. There are no associated extracutaneous physical findings or laboratory abnormalities.

Pathology

Histologically, cutaneous lymphoid hyperplasia exhibits a patchy or confluent dense lymphoid infiltrate throughout the dermis that spares the epidermis and is separated from it by a narrow, so-called grenz zone. There is generally a heterogeneous mixture of large and small lymphoid cells and histiocytes (macrophages, Langerhans cells, other dendritic cells).

Immunophenotypic studies have shown that most cases of cutaneous lymphoid hyperplasia consist of a mixture of reactive polytypic B cells, T cells, macrophages, and dendritic cells. The B cells are often organized into primary and secondary lymphoid follicles analogous to those occurring in reactive lymphoid tissues. Occasionally, B cells are rare or absent and the infiltrate is composed predominantly of T cells.

Differential Diagnosis

Diseases that produce localized red or purple cutaneous papules, nodules, or plaques are the main disorders that should be considered in the clinical differential diagnosis of cutaneous lymphoid hyperplasia (Table 10–7). Various forms of lymphoma and leukemia are the major diseases involved in the histopathologic differential diagnosis.

Treatment

Lesions of cutaneous lymphoid hyperplasia that are not cosmetically or functionally problematic for the patient can be followed without specific therapy. Some lesions may eventually undergo regression, either spontaneously or in response to biopsy. Given the relatively high prevalence of monoclonality among cases of cutaneous lymphoid hyperplasia and reports of progression to overt lymphoma in some cases, long-term follow-up of patients is warranted regardless of therapy.

Localized lesions are often amenable to surgical resection, and smaller lesions are often diagnosed and treated simultaneously by excisional biopsy. Cryotherapy has also been reported to be an effective surgical modality. Lesions generally improve with intralesional corticosteroid therapy. Topical and systemic corticosteroids have also been used with success. Antimalarial agents have been used to treat the generalized variant of cutaneous lymphoid hyperplasia. Recalcitrant cases can be treated with various forms of radiation therapy and usually exhibit rapid resolution. Relapse within the original or new sites may sometimes occur with any of these treatments.

TABLE 10–7. Differential Diagnosis of Cutaneous Lymphoid Hyperplasia

CLINICAL
Granulomatous
Adnexal tumor
Granuloma faciale
Leukemia
Lupus erythematosus
Lymphoma
Metastatic neoplasm
Nodular granulomatous lesion (e.g., deep fungal)
Nodular infiltrative lesion (e.g., nodular amyloidosis)
Soft tissue tumor

LYMPHOMATOID PAPULOSIS

(CM&S Chapter 157)

Definition

Lymphomatoid papulosis is a self-healing eruption whose lesions are clinically benign but histologically contain malignant-appearing cells. Despite the alarming histologic resemblance to lymphoma, individual lesions usually regress spontaneously within a few weeks.

Clinical Description

Lesions first appear as red, painless, nonpruritic papules that undergo central necrosis, sometimes with scale, and heal with scarring, often leaving a depigmented or hyperpigmented area. There may be few to more than 100 lesions, which are usually smaller than 1 cm (up to 2 cm). Individual lesions regress spontaneously in 4 to 6 weeks. Some lesions develop while others regress. Lesions may be random, symmetrical, clustered, or disseminated. The buttocks, trunk, legs, and arms are most often involved. Palms, soles, digits, face, scalp, and genitalia can be affected. Mucous membranes are spared. Papules sometimes coalesce to form nodules, plaques, or ulcers.

Incidence and Prevalence

The range of onset is from infancy to the eighth decade (median age is in the fourth or fifth decade), with an equal distribution between males and females. The overall prevalence of lymphomatoid papulosis is difficult to estimate but appears to be rare.

Association with Lymphoma

Lymphomatoid papulosis is preceded by, coexistent with, or followed by a malignant lymphoma in an estimated 10% to 20% of cases, usually mycosis fungoides, Hodgkin's disease, or CD30-positive large cell lymphoma. The time to develop lymphoma is highly variable, but a median of 13 years has been observed. Although the risk to develop lymphoma appears low, one recent report indicates that the risk may be higher, approaching 80%, when patients are followed for 15 years or longer.

The prognosis for these lymphomas appears to be better than for the same lymphomas arising de novo. The risk of developing lymphoma appears much higher for males than for female patients with lymphomatoid papulosis and appears to be lowest for patients who have lymphomatoid papulosis lesions of type B histology and highest for patients with diffuse large cell type lesions.

Pathology

The histology of lymphomatoid papulosis is characterized by an atypical lymphoid infiltrate of varied density (depending on stage of the lesion at biopsy). The atypical cells may be large with multilobed nuclei and prominent eosinophilic nucleoli (type A) or may be small with cerebriform nuclei and epidermotropism (type B). Mitoses are common, scattered mixed inflammatory cells are often present.

Pathogenesis and Etiology

Lymphomatoid papulosis is a clonal proliferation of T lymphocytes in most cases. A clonal relationship between lymphomatoid papulosis and malignant CD30-positive anaplastic large cell lymphoma or Hodgkin's disease has been demonstrated in several cases. Lesions of lymphomatoid papulosis (especially type A) often contain aneuploid cells. More abnormal chromosomes have been documented in anaplastic lymphomas that arose from lymphomatoid papulosis, suggesting a progression to a more malignant phenotype.

The etiology of lymphomatoid papulosis is an enigma. A relationship among prior or coexisting lymphoproliferative disorders, radiation therapy, and mosquito bite hypersensitivity reactions has been noted.

Diagnosis and Differential Diagnosis

Lymphomatoid papulosis is a combined clinical and pathologic diagnosis requiring spontaneously regressing papulonodular lesions that appear in crops without a history of exposure to drug, toxin, or allergen together with histology showing large atypical Reed-Sternberg–like cells surrounded by inflammatory cells. The distinctive immunopathology reveals Ki-1 (CD30)-positive cells with aberrant expression (deletion) of T-cell antigens. Histologically, lymphomatoid papulosis can be difficult to differentiate from some anthropod bite reactions, pityriasis lichenoides et varioliformis acuta, and mycosis fungoides.

Lymphomatoid papulosis comprises the benign end of a spectrum of lesions that ends in Ki-1 (CD30)-positive malignant lymphoma. However, individual lesions of Ki-1–positive lymphomas are larger than 2 cm and show delayed, incomplete, or no clinical regression.

Treatment

Lymphomatoid papulosis is seldom cured by therapy. The objective of treatment is to suppress the formation of new lesions and maintain the skin in an improved state. Various treatments with some effectiveness include antibiotics such as tetracycline, ultraviolet B light, PUVA, topical carmustine (BCNU) or mechlorethamine, and methotrexate.

It is important to avoid overtreatment of lymphomatoid papulosis with multiagent chemotherapy. A transient but only temporary remission of lesions is commonly observed during multiagent chemotherapy or ionizing radiation therapy for lymphoma in patients with lymphomatoid papulosis.

CUTANEOUS T-CELL LYMPHOMA

(CM&S Chapter 158)

Definition

Cutaneous T-cell lymphoma (CTCL) comprises a group of clinicopathologic entities that are neoplastic proliferations of T lymphocytes that home to the skin. Most of these begin as epidermotropic proliferations, but often eventually spread to the dermis, lymph nodes, blood, and viscera. Included in the spectrum of CTCL is mycosis fungoides and Sézary's syndrome.

Clinical Description

Lymphomas of cutaneous T cells produce a wide variety of clinical and pathologic changes. The following classification is based primarily on clinical morphology but also correlates with pathobiology, inasmuch as the progression from patches and plaques to tumors and erythroderma is associated with loss of epidermotropism, greater cytologic atypia, immunophenotypic alterations, and a poorer prognosis.

Patches and Plaques

CTCL in which lesions evolve from patches into plaques and ultimately into tumors is termed *mycosis fungoides.* Early lesions are typically dry, slightly scaly, pink lesions that can exhibit telangiectasia and atrophy. They tend to measure at least several centimeters across and are distributed asymmetrically. There is a predilection for areas of skin that are protected by two layers of clothing such as the buttocks and breasts, but lesions can occur anywhere. The eruption may be pruritic or asymptomatic and occasionally may be transitory. Often there is a preceding chronic, "resistant dermatitis" for 10 to 20 years. Some patients with patch-stage lesions have traditionally been said to have *large plaque parapsoriasis* or *parapsoriasis en plaques.* It is preferable to use the term CTCL where appropriate, and to simply express uncertainty as to the diagnosis if changes are not clear-cut.

The patch stage may last for months or years before progressing to the plaque stage, or plaques may appear to arise de novo. Plaques appear as elevated, scaly, indurated lesions that may be sharply demarcated and are often discoid in shape. The lesions tend to be of uniform color, ranging from an erythematous to a violaceous hue. Occasionally, the plaques simulate psoriasis, or are associated with crusts or papules. Plaques may spontaneously regress or may coalesce to form large plaques with annular, arcuate, or serpiginous borders, and may clear centrally with disease activity remaining at the periphery of the lesion, producing a geographic appearance.

Erythroderma

Sézary syndrome refers to patients with exfoliative erythroderma, leukocytosis, and Sézary cells (atypical circulating lymphocytes). Erythrodermic CTCL is a broader term that encompasses all stages of erythrodermic and leukemic disease, whether or not Sézary cells are identified in the blood.

Clinically, erythrodermic CTCL may start de novo, or appear after established plaque or tumor stage disease. The erythroderma is usually generalized, but isolated areas of normal skin may be present. Pruritus is often intense, resulting in excoriation and exudation. The patient may have fever, chills, weight loss, and malaise. There may be scaling and fissuring of palms and soles, alopecia, ectropion, nail dystrophy, and ankle edema. Such patients become severely debilitated by this fatal disease. Some patients with the erythrodermic form of CTCL develop tumors.

Tumors

Tumors are reddish-brown or purplish red and generally arise at sites of previous skin involvement by CTCL but may occur in clinically normal skin. They may become ulcerated and superinfected. Tumors have a predilection for the face and body folds—axillae, groin, antecubital fossae, neck, and the inframammary area. Spontaneous resolution of tumors is rare.

Variations

Poikiloderma vasculare atrophicans is a patch-stage form of CTCL dominated by a poikilodermatous appearance, in which there are atrophy and telangiectasis, often with hypo- or hyperpigmentation. Poikiloderma may also occur with dermatomyositis and radiation dermatitis.

Alopecia mucinosa (follicular mucinosis) refers to plaques that are clinically associated with alopecia and histologically associated with collections of mucin in follicular epithelium. Follicular mucinosis manifests clinically as solitary or multiple indurated plaques with superimposed follicular papules from which a gelatinous material can occasionally be expressed. Such lesions may occur before or after a diagnosis of CTCL is made. Follicular mucinosis also occurs as an idiopathic benign condition. The benign form clinically is indistinguishable from CTCL-associated follicular mucinosis and follow-up may be required to make this distinction. Childhood involvement, especially on the head and neck, favors the benign variety.

Pagetoid reticulosis or Woringer-Kolopp disease most often presents as a solitary verrucous plaque on acral skin. The long duration and slow growth of the disease are characteristic. The distinct histologic presentation is that of marked epidermotropism, similar to Paget's disease.

Granulomatous slack skin is a form of CTCL in which the lymphocytic infiltrate is associated with a granulomatous component and destruction of cutaneous elastic tissue. This presents clinically as large regions of lax skin, especially in the axillae and groins and breast destruction in women. Many with granulomatous slack skin are said to develop Hodgkin's disease.

Hypopigmented mycosis fungoides is a variant of patch or early plaque-stage mycosis fungoides that is seen in dark-skinned patients. Individual lesions clinically simulate vitiligo.

Some patients with CTCL have lesions resembling those of a pigmented purpuric eruption. Patients with such lesions tend to have their disease distributed in a fashion similar to other types of patch-stage CTCL.

Variations of CTCL have also been described as a result of immunophenotypic analysis. The vast majority of CTCLs are malignancies of cells with phenotypic characteristics of helper T cells (CD4+). Immunophenotypic variants include the CD8+(suppressor) and CD4+/CD2+/CD7− phenotypes and gamma-delta T-cell lymphoma. These phenotypic variants may have characteristic clinical presentations.

Pathology

There is a wide spectrum of histologic findings in cutaneous T-cell lymphoma, and the features are partially dependent on the type of lesion biopsied. Patches of CTCL show a sparse or moderately dense, perivascular or slightly lichenoid lymphocytic infiltrate with epidermotropism. The cells are slightly enlarged, hyperconvoluted, and hyperchromatic. Pautrier's microabscesses (epidermal clusters of lymphocytes) are a fairly specific finding, although not always present.

Plaques show similar changes, but the infiltrates are more lichenoid, denser, and containing eosinophils and/or plasma cells. The papillary dermis is expanded collagen bundles. Hyperkeratosis with subtle parakeratosis and psoriasiform epidermal hyperplasia may be present.

The histologic features of the erythrodermic stage vary and may resemble patch- or plaque-stage disease, but with less epidermotropism and, occasionally, with more spongiosis.

Tumors of CTCL feature dense diffuse or nodular infiltrates. Epidermotropism is seen less frequently. The lymphocytes are much more atypical, and immunophenotypic transformations may occur. In poikilodermatous CTCL, atrophy is associated with telangiectases, pigment incontinence, fibrosis, and sometimes subtle vacuolar alteration. Epidermotropism and cytologic atypia are subtle.

In follicular mucinosis, mucin and lymphocytes are present in follicular epithelium; associated features of CTCL may or may not be present.

Diagnosis and Differential Diagnosis

The differential diagnosis of CTCL depends on the clinical presentation. Patch-stage lesions can be difficult to distinguish from chronic allergic contact or nummular dermatitis, and rarely from drug eruptions. Erythrodermic CTCL needs to be distinguished from idiopathic erythroderma, and that due to pityriasis rubra pilaris, atopic dermatitis, psoriasis, and drug eruptions. Tumor-stage lesions can be confused with pseudolymphomas and with lymphomas of other types.

Skin Lesions

Diagnosis of CTCL in patients with patch/plaque-stage disease is usually accomplished by combining clinical features with findings in routine skin biopsy. A delay in the diagnosis early on (reported average of 6 years) is common and often due to the subtlety of the histology and similarities to other inflammatory dermatoses.

Immunohistochemical findings, such as a CD4+ phenotype or loss of CD7 antigen, can be supportive; however, one still needs to rely on clinical pathologic correlation. Evaluation of the T-cell receptor beta-chain variable region for clonality by Southern blot or PCR is currently being investigated and is a promising adjunct to routine histology in making the diagnosis of CTCL.

Lymph Nodes

A lymph node biopsy is usually not used for establishing an initial diagnosis of CTCL because in early stages of disease, when nodes are not clinically enlarged, the findings are noncontributory. Biopsy is usually recommended if lymph nodes are enlarged, especially for staging and prognosis.

Peripheral Blood

Morphology and enumeration of circulating CTCL cells by light microscopy alone are difficult unless there is marked lymphocytosis.

Flow cytometry has improved the reliability and reproducibility of detecting CTCL in the peripheral blood. An increased CD4/CD8 ratio is often seen. Values over 4 are very suggestive of CTCL.

Staging and Prognosis

Staging

Once the diagnosis of CTCL is established, an assessment should be made of the extent of cutaneous involvement and presence of extracutaneous involvement and its severity. The TNM scoring system (Table 10–8) is useful to assist staging but is in need of updating with current laboratory methods. Computerized axial tomography scan provides precise measurements of axillary and inguinal nodes along with surveillance pictures of viscera, pelvic, periaortic, and thoracic lymph nodes.

A practical approach for evaluating the peripheral blood includes checking a complete blood count for total lymphocyte count abnormalities, eosinophil count, and for overt lymphocyte nuclear abnormalities, flow cytometry panel to evaluate CD4, CD8, and CD45RO levels. Any elevation of the CD4/CD8 ratio or elevation of CD45RO, or any clinical suspicion of occult leukemia (widespread skin involvement) should be followed by gene rearrangement studies that could confirm leukemic disease.

Flow cytometry can also be used for monitoring the blood of patients with CTCL.

Prognosis

The outcome of CTCL is difficult to predict, but in general there is a worse prognosis for greater degrees of skin involvement, depth of infiltrate, blastic transformation, loss of normal T cells, leukemia, lymph node involvement, and visceral involvement. Involvement of

TABLE 10-8. TNM Classification of CTCL	
CLASSIFICATION	**DESCRIPTION**
T: skin	
T_0	Clinically and/or histopathologically suspicious lesions
T_1	Limited plaques, papules, or eczematoid patches covering 10% or more of the skin surface
T_2	Generalized plaques, papules, or erythematous patches covering 10% or more of the skin surface
T_3	Tumors, one or more
T_4	Generalized erythroderma
N: lymph nodes	
N_0	No clinically or palpably abnormal peripheral lymph nodes, pathology negative for CTCL
N_1	Clinically abnormal peripheral lymph nodes, pathology negative for CTCL
N_2	No clinically abnormal peripheral lymph nodes, pathology positive for CTCL
N_3	Clinically abnormal peripheral lymph nodes, pathology positive for CTCL
B: peripheral blood	
B_0	Atypical circulating cells not present or less than 5%
B_1	Atypical circulating cells present in 5% or more of total blood lymphocytes; record total white blood cell count and total lymphocyte counts and number of atypical cells/100 lymphocytes
M: visceral organs	
M_0	No involvement of visceral organs
M_1	Visceral involvement (must have confirmation of pathology and organ involved should be specified)

10% or less of the skin surface by patch-stage disease correlates with median survival of 12 years. Patients with patch-stage disease in general seem to have a median survival range of 7 to 12 years. Lymphadenopathy, whether due to dermatopathic change (N1) or infiltration by CTCL (N2, N3), is a sign of poor prognosis. The development of tumors, erythroderma, or node involvement signals a drop to 2 to 3 years' median survival. Patients with tumors or lymph node involvement have almost the same survival rate.

Matching the clinical activity of the disease with the appropriate treatment option is the science of CTCL management. Treatment options vary and may be dictated by the stage of the disease, familiarity of the physician with specific modalities, availability of modalities, geographic constraints, and personal patient factors such as compliance and commitment.

In early stages of CTCL (patch-plaque disease), photochemotherapy, topical chemotherapy, and electron beam radiotherapy usually induce remissions (rates of 80% to 90%) and often cures, if used early enough. Spot (localized) radiotherapy is more readily available and offers a shorter treatment course (five to ten sessions versus up to 3 months) versus electron beam radiotherapy. Its usefulness is limited to localized disease.

Topical nitrogen mustard (NM) and topical BCNU/carmustine are effective forms of therapy. Each are applied at home by the patient, which allows convenience. The main disadvantage is the frequent development of delayed hypersensitivity (greater with NM). This is decreased with the use of an ointment-based (instead of water-based) NM preparation, or with the induction of tolerance with PUVA. Secondary cutaneous malignancies and pigmentation variability are other potential undesirable complications of NM. Long-term maintenance is often required with NM. Topical BCNU has the advantage over NM of having an abbreviated treatment course; however, bone marrow depression and severe erythema can be limiting.

Photochemotherapy with PUVA (ingestion of 8-methoxypsoralen followed by ultraviolet A light exposure) or extracorporeal photochemotherapy (ECP) are effective forms of therapy in the appropriate patients. Both are limited in their availability and convenience. PUVA has the additional disadvantage of long-term cutaneous side effects, such as atrophy, dryness, and the development of secondary cutaneous malignancies. ECP is the first line of therapy for erythrodermic CTCL and, thus far, has a 15% to 30% complete response rate. Even partial responses can improve quality of life. ECP requires ingestion of 8-methoxypsoralen, followed by cycling of the patient's peripheral blood "extracorporeally" through a device that separates the leukocytes and preferentially exposes them to UVA irradiation, thus photoinactivating them. Side effects include fevers and exacerbation of erythroderma (both of which are transient).

Treatment options for more advanced or extracutaneous disease include systemic chemotherapy such as chlorambucil plus prednisone, fludarabine monophosphate, methotrexate, etoposide (VP 16), doxorubicin (Adriamycin), or combination chemotherapy. Other systemic treatment options include interferon (alpha, beta, or gamma) and diphtheria A toxin-interleukin-2 gene (DAB-IL2). Discussion of these options is beyond the scope of this text.

OTHER CUTANEOUS LYMPHOMAS: B-CELL LYMPHOMA, NON-MYCOSIS FUNGOIDES T-CELL LYMPHOMA, AND ADULT T-CELL LYMPHOMA/LEUKEMIA

(CM&S Chapter 159)

Non-mycosis fungoides (non-MF) lymphomas can be classified broadly into T- and B-cell subtypes. Almost 25% of cutaneous lymphomas are cutaneous B-cell lymphomas (CBCL), and 5% to 10% of cutaneous T-cell lymphomas (CTCL) are non–MF-CTCL.

Cutaneous B-Cell Lymphomas

Definition

CBCL are extranodal non-Hodgkin's lymphomas that occur primarily in the skin and are usually confined to the skin for many years. They can spread into extracutaneous sites, such as lymph nodes, peripheral blood, bone marrow, and viscera. The most frequent type of CBCL originates from follicular cells.

Clinical Description

Clinically, CBCL can usually be differentiated from CTCL, due to the monomorphous appearance of nodules and/or tumors, which may be solitary, grouped in a circumscribed area, or disseminated and which develop in a relatively short period of time from normal-looking skin.

The head and neck area appears to be preferentially involved. Diffuse infiltration may lead to leonine facies. The color of nodules and tumors of CBCL is deep red, and the surface is smooth without scaling or ulceration. The consistency of tumors is relatively firm compared with the soft consistency in CTCL.

As opposed to CTCL, the subtypes of CBCL cannot be differentiated on the basis of the clinical appearance of the skin lesions. The so-called reticulohistiocytosis of the back (Crosti's disease) is usually a follicular center cell lymphoma. Enlargement of peripheral lymph nodes, if at all, occurs early in the course of the disease and indicates neoplastic infiltration rather than dermatopathic lymphadenopathy as frequently seen in CTCL.

There is no current clinical staging classification for CBCL that can accurately predict the clinical course and prognosis of the disease.

The survival curve for cutaneous lymphoma flattens after about 7 years for CBCL. This indicates that there is a proportion of at least 50% of CBCL that has an exceptionally good prognosis. This is probably due to the special types, which are true clonal malignant B-cell lymphomas but that biologically show features of pseudo-lymphomas.

Pathology

Histologically, CBCL show a typical "B-cell pattern" that differs from the band-like infiltrate seen in CTCL. In CBCL, the infiltrate is characterized by a sharply demarcated nodular, mostly bottom-heavy infiltrate in the middle or deep dermis, sparing a subepidermal border zone. These features may be lost in large cell CBCL with high-grade malignancy.

Malignant B-Cell Lymphomas of Low-Grade Malignancy

Lymphocytic Lymphoma. Small lymphocytic lymphoma, B-cell type (SLL) differs from chronic lymphocytic leukemia (CLL) by the lack of a leukemic blood picture. Histologically, SLL displays the typical "B-cell pattern." The lymphocytes have a small, round, dark nucleus without visible cytoplasm. Germinal centers, eosinophils, and plasma cells are usually absent; κ and λ light chain, and B-cell differentiation antigens can be demonstrated.

Follicular Center Cell Lymphomas (Centroblastic [CB]/Centrocytic and Centrocytic Lymphoma [CC]). Reactive follicular centers mainly contain two types of B-lymphoid cells in addition to a network of dendritic cells and a few T lymphocytes. Centroblasts are medium-sized to large cells with a vesicular nucleus and basophillic cytoplasm. Centrocytes are small or medium-sized cells with irregular nuclei showing linear clefts.

Centroblastic/centrocytic (CBCC) lymphoma, also known as malignant lymphoma, intermediate grade, and mixed small and large cell, is the most frequent form, accounting for about 12% of cutaneous lymphomas and about 40% of CBCL. They are composed of centroblasts (at least 20%) and centrocytes and usually lack the sharp border between these two components, typically seen in follicular pseudolymphomas. In contrast to pseudolymphomas, in CBCL there are almost no tingible body macrophages and no eosinophils.

CC lymphoma (malignant lymphoma of small or large cleaved cells) comprises about 1% cutaneous lymphomas and about 4% CBCL. Due to the clefted nuclei and the lack of follicular structures, it may be misinterpreted as nonepidermotropic T-cell lymphoma. Therefore, immunophenotyping is mandatory in these cases.

Malignant B-Cell Lymphomas of High-Grade Malignancy

Centroblastic Lymphoma. CB lymphoma, formerly reticulum cell sarcoma, is referred to as malignant lymphoma, large cell, noncleaved. It comprises about 1.5% of cutaneous lymphomas and about 6% of CBCL and may arise secondary to CBCC lymphoma.

Histologically, typical features of B-cell or T-cell pattern are lacking. Epidermotropism and follicle-like structures may be present. The predominant proliferating cell type resembles the centroblast.

The differential diagnosis includes immunoblastic lymphoma, lymphoblastic lymphoma, and true histiocytic lymphoma.

Immunoblastic Lymphoma (IBL), B-Cell Type. This lymphoma, designated as malignant lymphoma, large-cell immunoblastic, was formerly referred to as reticulum cell sarcoma or histiocytic lymphoma and represents about 3% of cutaneous lymphoma and about 12% of CBCL.

Histologically, a diffuse pattern involving all levels of the dermis and subcutis is commonly found. Immunophenotyping is needed to differentiate B from T immunoblasts.

Lymphoblastic Lymphoma (LBL), Burkitt Type. Primary Burkitt-type lymphoma of the skin may occur that is rare. The categorization of this lymphoma is not yet completely clear. The histological hallmark is the starry-sky appearance due to large macrophages within a relatively monomorphous infiltrate of small to medium-sized lymphoid cells.

Non-Mycosis Fungoides Cutaneous T-Cell Lymphomas

Definition

Mycosis fungoides (MF) is the prototypical peripheral CTCL of small cerebriform cell type. One of the distinctive features is development of the disease from an "eczematous" stage to a tumor stage, whose diagnosis can be difficult. Non–MF-CTCL that display specific clinical, histologic, cytologic, or phenotypic features and therefore can be regarded as distinct nosologic subentities within the group of CTCL.

Clinical Description and Pathology

Pleomorphic and Large Cell Lymphomas

Pleomorphic T-cell lymphoma has an inconspicuous clinical appearance showing papules, plaques, tumors, or erythroderma with a male-to-female ratio of 5:1. The neoplastic cells, which may be small, medium sized, or large, are pleomorphic. Adult T-cell leukemia/lymphoma (ATL) is a human T-cell lymphotropic virus type I (HTLV-I)–positive variant of this subgroup. The clinical course of these lymphomas may be prolonged in the small cell variant or rapid in the medium and large cell variants.

Primary cutaneous CD30 (Ki-1)-positive anaplastic large cell lymphoma is a morphologic and phenotypic variant of large cell lymphomas, formerly referred to as histiocytic lymphoma or misdiagnosed as true malignant histiocytosis. Characteristic clinical features are solitary or localized skin lesions in almost 90% of the cases, frequent spontaneous remission of skin lesions, rare secondary involvement of extracutaneous sites (25%), and a good prognosis.

Histologically, there is a diffuse cohesive growth pattern with or without epidermotropism, often reaching into the subcutaneous tissue. The neoplastic cells are large with round or oval nuclei and abundant, often clear cytoplasm, simulating undifferentiated carcinoma, melanoma, or histiocytic disorders. Immunophenotypically, the hallmark is CD30 (Ki-1) positivity.

Immunoblastic lymphoma of T-cell type and multilobated T-cell lymphoma represent variants of large cell, non-MF peripheral T-cell lymphomas with high-grade malignancy showing distinct cytologic features.

Non–MF-CTCL Showing Features of Distinct Tissue Tropism

T-cell variants of angiotropic lymphomas (intravascular lymphomatosis), formerly referred to as systemic angioendotheliomatosis, exist. Clinically, multiple reddish-violet cutaneous patches, plaques, or nodules are seen. In the final stage of the usually treatment-refractory and rapidly fatal disease, extracutaneous involvement (lung, liver) occurs. Histologically, lymphoid cells are seen in the lumina of dermal vessels.

Subcutaneous ("lipotropic") lymphomas clinically often present as erythema nodosum or panniculitis. Histologically, they show dense infiltrates in the subcutaneous fat tissue. Rare variants may show clonal rearrangement of the δ chain of the T-cell receptor and produce high amounts of interferon gamma, resulting in progressing leukopenia and fever.

Epidermolytic (T8-positive) CTCL clinically appears with widespread erosions and ulcerations with rapid dissemination. Histologically, the epidermis is destroyed by a cytotoxic CD8-positive lymphoid infiltrate, which becomes tumorous in the final stage of the disease.

Granulomatous and Other Non-MF-CTCL

Granulomatous slack skin, originally described as progressive, atrophying, chronic granulomatous dermohypodermitis, represents a rare condition with plaque-like lesions showing a wrinkled surface and large pendulous folds of skin in the axillae and in the groins. Histologically, tuberculoid granulomas are found with almost complete loss of elastic fibers and remnants of elastic material in giant cells.

Angioimmunoblastic lymphadenopathy is a lymphoproliferative disorder that can give rise to T-cell lymphoma. Skin involvement is usually seen secondarily in 40% of the patients[7] after manifestations of the disease in the lung, brain, and other organs. Histology of skin lesions is not diagnostic.

Lymphomatoid granulomatosis is primarily an extracutaneous disease involving skin (plaques, papules, ulcers) in almost 50% of the cases. There are clinical similarities to Wegener's granulomatosis or to lethal midline granuloma. Histology shows characteristic angiocentric and angiodestructive infiltrates that range from cytologically bland to frankly malignant.

Diagnosis and Differential Diagnosis

Most CBCL can be diagnosed as such owing to their typical morphologic features of circumscribed, firm, dome-shaped nodules and tumors arising on normal-looking skin. In contrast to CTCL, differentiation of the various nosologic subtypes is not possible clinically. More information is provided by histomorphology showing a typical nodular B-cell pattern. In doubtful cases, confirmation of the B-cell nature of the infiltrate can be achieved by demonstration of κ or λ light chain restriction.

The differential diagnosis of CBCL primarily includes nodular pseudolymphomas and semimalignant (pseudolymphomatous) B-cell lymphomas of the skin with germinal center formation. Pseudolymphomas are reactive processes regressing either spontaneously or by nonaggressive treatment without recurrences. In some cases, the clinical course of the disease allows the conclusive diagnosis.

Adult T-Cell Lymphoma/Leukemia

Definition

Adult T-cell lymphoma/leukemia (ATL) is a lymphoproliferative disorder etiologically associated with HTLV-1 most frequently seen in endemic areas such as southern Japan and the Caribbean. The skin is involved in more than 50% of cases.

Clinical Description

The following subtypes of ATL have been differentiated: smoldering, chronic lymphoma, and acute. In general, the disease starts between the fourth to sixth decades and most commonly affects men. Generalized lymphadenopathy is the most consistent finding. However, hepatosplenomegaly, bone marrow involvement, and a leukemic blood picture are also present in more than 50% of the cases.

Skin involvement occurs almost regularly, presenting as papules, nodules, or tumors, as erythema, as lupus erythematosus-like lesions, or as erythroderma.

Typical laboratory findings are a leukemic blood picture, sometimes in conjunction with anemia, hypoalbuminemia, hypergammaglobulinemia, and hypercalcemia. A distinctive finding is the presence of peripheral blood lymphocytes with cloverleaf-shaped nuclei. The mean survival time is less than 3 years.

Pathology

The histopathologic findings are varied but include a diffuse infiltrate of medium-sized to large pleomorphic cells with or without epidermotropism. There is also pronounced heterogeneity of the immunophenotype of neoplastic cells from patients with ATL.

Pathogenesis and Etiology

In the endemic variants clonal integration (detected by Southern blot) of retroviral DNA into the host cell genome plays an important role in pathogenesis.

Diagnosis and Differential Diagnosis

The diagnosis is based on clinical findings described earlier and on the demonstration of HTLV-I antibodies in the serum.

The differential diagnosis, from a clinical point of view, includes the broad spectrum of peripheral CTCL and, from a pathologic point of view, other forms of HTLV-I–negative pleomorphic or anaplastic T-cell lymphomas.

Treatment

Like in other forms of noncurable T-cell lymphomas, the strategy of management of ATL should be control of the disease. Disease confined to a few skin sites is often amenable excision or local radiation therapy. For widespread lesions, the whole spectrum from watchful waiting to nonaggressive chemotherapy (e.g., low-dose chlorambucil) to highly aggressive polychemotherapy or electron beam radiation therapy may be considered. Recent studies have demonstrated effectiveness of the combination of zidovudine and interferon α in ATL, even in patients in whom prior cytotoxic therapy has failed.

LEUKEMIA CUTIS

(CM&S Chapter 160)

Definition

Cutaneous lesions in leukemias can be classified as either specific or nonspecific. Lesions resulting from the direct infiltration and proliferation of leukemic cells in the skin are ''specific lesions'' or ''leukemia cutis.'' This occurs in 3% to 11% of patients with adult leukemia. Nonspecific lesions (leukemids) occur in approximately 30% of patients with leukemia. They may be related to anemia, thrombocytopenia, infection, and drugs or result from immunologic responses to tumor antigens. Histologically, there is no leukemic infiltration.

Clinical Description of Specific Lesions

Lymphocytic Leukemia

In chronic lymphocytic leukemia (CLL), specific lesions occur in 4% to 45% of patients but are uncommon in lymphocytic leukemia of the acute type. Clinically, the patients present with papules, plaques, and nodules. Tumors and large nodules may be seen in 50% of patients. Although leukemic skin lesions can occur anywhere, the head, neck trunk, and especially the face appear to the most common locations.

Hairy-Cell Leukemia

Specific skin lesions in hairy cell leukemia (HCL) are uncommon. The few convincing cutaneous lesions reported were usually described as erythematous macules and papules.

Adult T-Cell Leukemia

Adult T-cell leukemia (ATL) is a disseminated malignancy of T lymphocytes infected by the human T-lymphotropic virus type I. The cutaneous manifestations, seen in 40% to 70% of cases, of ATL may vary from maculopapular rash, multiple nodular tumors, and bullous lesions to generalized erythroderma.

Granular Lymphocytic Leukemia

Lymphoproliferative disease of granular lymphocytes (LDGL) represents a heterogeneous family of diseases with an atypical lymphocytosis characterized by an expansion of lymphocytes (usually cytotoxic T cells or natural killer cells) with cytoplasmic azurophilic granules, usually referred to as ''granular lymphocytes.'' LDGL shows less predilection for skin involvement than other T-cell malignancies do, but when it occurs, it is a poor prognostic sign.

Myelogenous and Monocytic Leukemia

Involvement of the skin by acute myelogenous leukemia (AML) has been reported to occur in 13% of patients. Patients with acute monocytic leukemia (AMOL) and acute myelomonocytic leukemia (AMML) have the highest incidence of both specific and nonspecific skin lesions. The cutaneous manifestations are quite varied and consist of multiple papules, nodules, and infiltrative plaques ranging in size from a few millimeters to several centimeters. The most common areas of involvement are the scalp, face, trunk, and extremities. Congenital monoblastic leukemia with papular and nodular skin lesions or nodules with blueberry-muffin appearance has rarely been described.

Leukemic gingival infiltrations were present in 67% of patients with AMOL and in 18% of those with AMML. Hyperplasia, swelling, bleeding, and inflammation of the gingiva are characteristic findings. Usually skin involvement occurs during the course of disease or may be concomitant with or precede the diagnosis of systemic leukemia.

Cutaneous infiltration is rare with acute granulocytic leukemia (AGL). Skin lesions include papules, plaques, and nodules without any particular distribution. Chloroma (tumor of myeloblasts in the skin with a greenish color due to myeloperoxidase), or granulocytic sarcoma, is another rare condition that may occur in patients who have AGL or chronic granulocytic leukemia (CGL) in blast crisis. Granulocytic sarcomas develop in less than 3% of patients with AGL and may precede by months to years the development of systemic leukemia.

Specific skin lesions in CGL are uncommon. Skin involvement in chronic myelomonocytic leukemia (CMML), which almost exclusively affects elderly persons, is much less frequent, and only a few cases have been reported.

Pathology

Lymphocytic Leukemia

In most cases of B-cell CLL there is a perivascular and periadnexal infiltrate of dense small- to medium-sized lymphocytes. The infiltrate is usually present in the upper and lower dermis, with a grenz zone, but may extend to the subcutaneous tissue. The phenotype is heterogenous. Monoclonality of SIg (light-chain restriction) is pathognomonic of B-cell malignancy. The predominant heavy-chain type in typical CLL is IgM or IgM and IgD.

The distinctive pathologic feature of CLL is a dense, diffuse, or patchy infiltrate of small uniform tartrate-resistant acid phosphatase-positive mononuclear cells with indented nuclei in the dermis surrounding and invading the blood vessels and skin adnexa.

The histologic picture of ATL is that of a dense infiltrate of a variety of small, medium-sized, large, or pleomorphic lymphoid cells with convoluted nuclei that are perivascular or interstitial. Epidermotropism, Pautrier's microabscesses, and mitoses may be seen.

Myelogenous and Monocytic Leukemia

In AGL and CGL, dense infiltrates involve all levels of the dermis, leaving a distinct grenz zone. The cells spread contiguously destroying the blood vessels and adnexa, and infiltrating the collagen bundles and subcutaneous fibrous septa. AGL infiltrates are composed of large bizarre cells and immature atypical myeloid cells. Mitotic figures are common.

The infiltrates in AMOL composed of monomorphic cells with indented nuclei and basophilic or vacuolated cytoplasm. In AMML, the infiltrates contain a mixture of immature monocytes with irregular nuclei, atypical myeloblasts, myelocytes, and occasional neutrophils. Leukemic infiltrates are positive for lysozyme, CD43 (Leu 22), CD45 (LCA), and CD15 (Leu-M1) in almost all AMOL and in the majority of AMML cases. Chloroacetate esterase is detected in only a minority of the leukemic cells in AMML and is absent in AMOL.

Differential Diagnosis

The differential diagnosis of leukemia includes cutaneous lymphomas, Hodgkin's disease, histocytosis X, lymphomatoid papulosis, drug-induced pseudolymphoma, insect bite reactions, vasculitis, and mastocytosis.

Treatment

Treatment of leukemia cutis is the same as that of the underlying systemic leukemia and consists of local radiotherapy and chemotherapy.

Because systemic chemotherapy adequate to induce and to maintain bone marrow remission does not necessarily control specific skin lesions in AML, the optimal management of leukemia cutis should consist of electron-beam irradiation in conjunction with systemic chemotherapy. The skin lesions in HCL respond well to systemic interferon alpha therapy, which is the treatment of choice. Topical nitrogen mustard may also be helpful.

CUTANEOUS METASTASES

(CM&S Chapter 161)

Definition

Cutaneous metastases represent spread of a preexisting malignancy to the skin.

Clinical Description

Cutaneous metastases are relatively uncommon; they have been found in 2.7% and 10% of patients with internal cancer and metastatic cancer, respectively. The incidence of cutaneous metastasis depends on both the incidence and the site of the primary neoplasm. The incidence also varies by sex (Table 10–9).

The clinical appearance of skin metastases usually is not distinctive. They may resemble the primary tumor in color and consistency and vary in size up to several centimeters. Most skin metastases are

TABLE 10-9. Origins of Malignancies Most Commonly Metastatic to Skin

PRIMARY SITE IN MEN	RANGE OF PERCENTAGE OF CUTANEOUS METASTASES	PRIMARY SITE IN WOMEN	RANGE OF PERCENTAGE OF CUTANEOUS METASTASES
Melanoma	13-19	Breast	69-71
Lung	12-24	Melanoma	5-20
Colon	11-19	Ovary	3-4
Oral cavity	9-12	Lung	2-4
Kidney	5-6	Oral cavity	1-2
Stomach	1-6	Colon	1-9

*Data from Armed Forces Institute of Pathology.

freely movable cutaneous or subcutaneous nodules that may be discrete, firm, and indolent. Plaque-like lesions also occur. Lesions may appear skin colored, erythematous, violaceous, or pigmented.

Pathology

Metastases to skin generally show histologic features bearing some resemblance to those of the primary tumor. For example, metastatic adenocarcinoma from the gastrointestinal tract usually reveals glands with intracytoplasmic and luminal mucin. Although the histology of the metastasis may suggest the primary site of the tumor, not infrequently the cutaneous metastasis may be anaplastic or poorly differentiated and can be designated only as carcinoma, sarcoma, or undifferentiated malignant neoplasm.

Pathogenesis and Etiology

In general, the location of a cutaneous metastasis is related to the site of the primary neoplasm. Thus, head and neck cutaneous metastases are often associated with squamous cell carcinoma of the oral cavity or nasopharynx. Chest cutaneous metastases are most frequently associated with breast cancer in women and lung cancer in men. Gastrointestinal neoplasms usually metastasize to the anterior abdominal wall, while pelvic tumors tend to spread to the perineal region. Intra-abdominal malignancies, such as from the stomach, colon, and pancreas, will at times metastasize to the skin of the umbilicus, resulting in the so-called Sister Mary Joseph's nodule. Melanomas and neoplasms associated with vascular invasion, such as renal cell carcinoma, thyroid follicular carcinoma, and choriocarcinoma, show less tendency toward regional localization.

Diagnosis and Differential Diagnosis

Clinically, the differential diagnosis of neoplasms metastatic to skin is quite varied and is listed in Table 10-10.

TABLE 10-10. Differential Diagnosis of Neoplasms Metastatic to Skin
Epidermal/pilar cyst
Lipoma
Neurofibroma
Adnexal tumor
Fibroepithelial polyp
Pyogenic granuloma
Kaposi's sarcoma
Lymphoma
Morphea
Cicatricial alopecia

Treatment

The presence of cutaneous metastases in a patient with internal malignancy is usually a poor prognostic sign. The treatment of a specific cutaneous metastasis often depends on whether the lesion interferes with normal function of the body, is disfiguring, or is a source of great pain, frequent bleeding, or possible secondary infection.

chapter 11

What Diseases of the Skin Are Malformations or Are Predominantly Inherited?

THE ICHTHYOSES: DISORDERS OF CORNIFICATION

(CM&S Chapter 162)

The disorders of cornification constitute a diverse group characterized by focal or generalized scaling or hyperkeratosis. When generalized, these have been called *ichthyosis*, a term from the Greek root *ichthys* for "fish," to describe a similarity of appearance of the human scaling skin disorders to fish scales despite the facts that some forms show no resemblance to fish scales and that the term bears no relationship to disease pathogenesis.

Pityriasis Rotunda

Pityriasis rotunda, considered to be a localized form of acquired ichthyosis, occurs predominantly in South African blacks and Japanese and is clinically distinctive sharply circumscribed, strictly round, scaly patches, which may be slightly hyperpigmented but lack erythema or infiltration. Lesions are usually multiple, but countable, and vary in size from 0.5 to more than 25 cm. Pityriasis rotunda has been frequently linked to underlying disease, especially tuberculosis, malnutrition, malignant tumors, and hepatic disease. In whites, the disorder may not herald underlying disease and may be a familial trait.

Genetically Transmitted, Generalized Disorders of Cornification: Major Forms

Ichthyosis Vulgaris

Clinical Description

Ichthyosis vulgaris is a relatively common autosomal dominant trait. It commonly occurs in association with atopic dermatitis. Scaling is not usually evident at birth but appears during infancy and early childhood. In ichthyosis vulgaris, scales are fine and light colored and most prominent on the extremities, particularly the lower legs. The flexures are always spared. Involvement of the palms and soles is characteristic. Generally, involvement is mild and manifested by increased skin markings. In such cases, it may be difficult to distinguish from dry skin. The trunk is usually only mildly involved and scaling on the face, when present, is limited to the lateral margins.

Pathology

The most notable histopathologic feature in ichthyosis vulgaris is hyperkeratosis occurring above a thinned or absent granular layer. The hyperkeratosis of ichthyosis vulgaris is lamellar or compact and often plugs the orifices of hair follicles. Ultrastructural examination demonstrates few small, abnormal appearing keratohyaline granules.

Pathogenesis and Etiology

Ichthyosis vulgaris is a retention hyperkeratosis. The major protein of the keratohyaline granule, profilaggrin, and its proteolytic cleavage product, filaggrin, are decreased in involved epidermis.

Diagnosis and Differential Diagnosis

Ichthyosis vulgaris must be distinguished from excessively dry skin and from other cornification disorders, such as recessive X-linked ichthyosis (RXLI), which in certain cases can be differentiated only by a biochemical diagnosis of steroid sulfatase deficiency from nonbullous congenital ichthyosiform erythroderma (CIE) by its presence of flexural involvement and from acquired ichthyosis, which develops after childhood.

Treatment

Although a relatively mild form of ichthyosis, ichthyosis vulgaris can be difficult to treat effectively because of the coexistent atopic diathesis in most patients. The irritancy caused by keratolytic agents is not well tolerated by atopic patients and may cause their dermatitis to flare. Mild keratolytics, such as 10% urea creams or 5% to 10% lactic acid or glycolic acid in hydrophilic ointment (Aqua Glycolic or Lac-Hydrin), may be tolerated if the dermatitis is not active. Many patients prefer simple emollient therapy.

Recessive X-Linked Ichthyosis

Clinical Description

RXLI is a relatively common genetic trait that affects males only and is characterized by a nonerythrodermic, generalized hyperkeratosis of mild to moderate severity. Typically, the cutaneous disorder is not evident at birth and first manifests as a pronounced peeling or desquamation at 1 or 3 weeks of age. Thereafter, the characteristic pattern of a "dirty" brown scaling develops on the extremities and, to a lesser degree, on the trunk. During childhood, the scalp is often involved with a crusted hyperkeratosis, and involvement of the periauricular region and neck flexure is typical. In adults, the scalp usually is not clinically involved, but involvement of neck and axilla may persist. Typically, the popliteal and antecubital fossae are spared, as are palms and soles. Marked seasonal fluctuations in disease severity, with improvement in warm weather, are characteristic, but the disorder does not remit with age.

RXLI is due to deficiency of the enzyme steroid sulfatase. Extracutaneous manifestations of the enzyme deficiency are recognized and include corneal opacities, placental sulfatase deficiency syndrome, elevated serum steroid sulfate levels, cryptorchidism, and, perhaps, testicular cancer.

Pathology

The epidermis in RXLI shows slight hyperplasia with a normal, thickened, or slightly thinned granular layer. Compact and lamellar hyperkeratosis is present and can plug adnexal orifices.

Pathogenesis and Etiology

RXLI is due to deficiency of the microsomal enzyme steroid sulfatase, which is required to desulfate cholesterol sulfate. The steroid sulfatase gene is located on the X chromosome in a region that escapes X-inactivation. Hence, normal females have approximately twice the amount of active steroid sulfatase enzyme as do normal males. Steroid sulfatase activity in carrier females is similar to that of normal males, and activity in RXLI males is absent.

RXLI is a retention hyperkeratosis with normal epidermal proliferation rates but stratum corneum retention. As corneocytes and their membranes move outward toward the surface, the enzyme located in intercellular membranes hydrolyzes cholesterol sulfate to cholesterol. In some manner, this promotes dyshesion of corneocytes.

Diagnosis and Differential Diagnosis

RXLI should be considered in all males with a generalized, nonerythrodermic disorder of cornification. The diagnosis can be established either by direct enzymatic assay in skin, leukocytes, or cultured fibroblasts or by measurement of elevated stratum corneum or plasma cholesterol sulfate levels. The differential diagnosis includes ichthyosis vulgaris and CIE.

Treatment

The disorder responds well to topical therapies, including the α-hydroxy acids (e.g., Lac-Hydrin) or propylene glycol (60% in water) overnight under occlusion, and to exposure to a warm humid climate.

Lamellar Ichthyosis and Nonbullous Congenital Ichthyosiform Erythroderma

Clinical Description

The autosomal recessive group of primary disorders of cornification are characterized clinically by congenital onset, usually as a collodion baby, and later by a generalized uniform involvement of the skin surface with hyperkeratosis and erythroderma. All flexures are involved, as are palmoplantar surfaces. Facial involvement is characteristic, and in severely affected patients results in ectropion as well as underdevelopment of soft tissue portions of the nose and ear.

A wide range of clinical phenotypes is recognized within this group. A uniformly severe phenotype, designated classic lamellar ichthyosis, is characterized by very large, dark, plate-like scales and marked facial involvement with ectropion. Erythroderma is present in this phenotype, but it is much less striking at first inspection than the dense scaling. In contrast, the clinical spectrum of nonbullous CIE is broad and includes both patients with intense erythroderma and marked ectropion and patients with a very mild clinical phenotype. Scaling is uniform and generalized. As in other ichthyoses, scales on the lower legs may be large, dark, and plate-like; however, elsewhere, scales tend to be smaller, finer, and lighter. As in classic lamellar ichthyosis, facial involvement may result in severe ectropion as well as underdevelopment of soft tissue structures. In more mildly affected patients, erythroderma may be very subtle and ectropion absent. Here, the clinical clues to the correct diagnosis include generalized involvement without flexural sparing and facial tautness. History of congenital onset as a collodion baby may also suggest a diagnosis of CIE.

The skin of the ''collodion'' (collodion is a sticky substance that hardens in the air) baby at birth is thickened, taut, shiny, and inelastic, thus resembling a dried film of flexible collodion. The collodion baby is not a disease entity but represents a clinical phenotype that may have a variety of underlying causes, most commonly, lamellar ichthyosis and CIE. In the collodion baby, ectropion and eclabion are usually present. There is an increased incidence of premature births. In addition to the complications associated with prematurity, collodion babies are at risk for several complications arising from their abnormal skin, including skin infection and septicemia, hypernatremic dehydration, and temperature instability.

Pathology

Lamellar ichthyosis demonstrate striking hyperkeratosis. The granular layer is continuously present, and the epidermis often shows psoriasiform hyperplasia with broad rete ridges. In nonbullous CIE, there tends to be less marked hyperkeratosis, and even parakeratosis above a focally diminished granular layer can be present in biopsy specimens.

Pathogenesis and Etiology

For neither lamellar ichthyosis nor CIE has the underlying cause been defined.

Diagnosis and Differential Diagnosis

The severely affected child or adult with either the classic lamellar ichthyosis or CIE phenotype presents an unmistakable clinical picture. Patients who are more mildly affected with CIE must be differentiated from patients with the other ichthyoses.

A definitive diagnosis in a collodion baby may not be possible until the mature clinical pattern has evolved. Some collodion babies will resolve to normal skin or a very mild ichthyosis phenotype in *self-resolving collodion baby* or *lamellar exfoliation of the newborn.*

Treatment

Treatment is aimed at maintaining supple skin as well as improvement in appearance. Topical keratolytic agents, such as α-hydroxy acids and salicylic acid, are beneficial but often require highly motivated patients, due to the need for daily total-body applications. In addition, the stinging and irritancy from topical keratolytics are not well tolerated by young children. For these children, aggressive topical therapy usually is not indicated. Systemic absorption of topical medications is to be expected because the stratum corneum, although thickened, does not provide an effective barrier. Infants and young children are also at increased risk for systemic toxicity due to a higher surface area to volume ratio, as well as immaturity of detoxification and excretory mechanisms. More severely affected patients are candidates for treatment with oral retinoids; however, careful consideration of long-term risks is mandatory, particularly, bone toxicity (i.e., premature epiphyseal closure in children) and teratogenicity in women of childbearing age. Optimal management may require relatively high doses (e.g., isotretinoin, 1–2 mg/kg per day; etretinate, 1 mg/kg per day), increasing the risk of dose-dependent side effects. The disease can be expected to recur when treatment is interrupted.

Collodion babies should be kept in a humidified environment to minimize the formation of deep fissures as the membrane is shed. Serum electrolytes should be closely monitored because of the high risk for hypernatremic dehydration caused by the loss of free water across the skin. These infants are also at high risk for septicemia. Systemic antibiotic therapy should be initiated at the earliest sign of infection and should be directed against *Staphylococcus aureus*, in addition to the usual nursery pathogens. If a severe CIE or lamellar ichthyosis phenotype develops, the need for family support in adjusting to a child with potentially severe cosmetic impairment cannot be overemphasized. Parental counseling is essential. Because resolution to normal or near-normal skin may occur, undue pessimism should be avoided.

Families at risk for lamellar ichthyosis or CIE may be offered prenatal diagnosis by fetoscopy and fetal skin biopsy at about 22 weeks' gestation. Skin ultrastructure demonstrates premature and excessive keratinization in affected infants.

Bullous Ichthyosis (Epidermolytic Hyperkeratosis)

Clinical Description

Bullous ichthyosis (bullous CIE and epidermolytic hyperkeratosis) is a rare autosomal dominant trait characterized in the neonate with widespread blistering and denuded skin and thereafter by a generalized ichthyosiform erythroderma.

At birth, widespread denuded skin is precipitated by the trauma of passage through the birth canal. Hyperkeratosis may not be appreciated initially. Mechanically induced blistering is uncommon after the neonatal period; later on, blisters are usually focal and induced by secondary infection. Hyperkeratosis is usually generalized and in some patients includes the palm and soles. Flexures are characteristically involved with a peculiar ridging or exaggerated lichenification pattern. Scales in these areas often become macerated and secondarily colonized by bacteria, producing a foul odor. Another distinctive clinical feature is the tendency for stratum corneum to be shed in full-thickness sheets, often leaving a red, tender base. The face is involved, but ectropion does not develop. In some patients the involvement is predominantly focal and limited to extensor and flexure surfaces of elbows and knees and palms and soles. Erythroderma is prominent in some patients and minimal or absent in others.

Pathology

The epidermal reaction pattern, epidermolytic hyperkeratosis, which affects nearly the entire integument in bullous ichthyosis, is characterized by reticular alteration of the epidermis, produced by intracytoplasmic vacuolization of the spinous and granular layers. This is coupled with the occurrence of enlarged keratohyaline and trichohyaline–like granules in the upper half of the epidermis and hyperkeratosis and slightly papillated epidermal hyperplasia.

Pathogenesis and Etiology

Bullous ichthyosis is due to mutations, of either the keratin 1 gene on chromosome 12 or the keratin 10 gene on chromosome 17. These mutations presumably affect their ability to form a normal cytoskeleton, resulting in the abnormally aggregated tonofilaments that characterize the diagnostic ultrastructure of this disorder.

Diagnosis and Differential Diagnosis

In the absence of typical clinical features, a skin biopsy is usually diagnostic. The differential diagnosis includes neonatal blistering disorders and other ichthyosis.

Treatment

The neonate with bullous ichthyosis should be handled gently to minimize mechanical trauma and watched carefully for signs of sepsis and fluid and electrolyte imbalance. Management of the mature, hyperkeratotic phenotype is complicated by the tendency of scales to be shed as full-thickness stratum corneum, leaving a pink, tender base. For this reason, many patients do not tolerate the irritancy of topical keratolytic or synthetic retinoids, which may produce a similar tender base. Antibacterial soaps and topical and/or systemic antibiotics may be required to manage the problems of offensive body odor and secondary infections.

Harlequin Ichthyosis

Clinical Description

The infant at birth in this autosomal recessive disease of unknown etiology presents a grotesque appearance because of the massive, plate-like scales that distort facial features and restrict breathing and feeding. Severe ectropion and eclabion are present, and hands may be deformed by mitten-like skin encasements, although normal bone structures can be demonstrated radiographically. Many of these infants are stillborn, and others do not survive the neonatal period, explaining the previous term *harlequin fetus*.

Treatment

Treatment of the neonate with harlequin ichthyosis is similar to that of the collodion baby. In addition, retinoids may facilitate loosing and shedding of the abnormal scales.

Multisystem Disorders with Generalized Scaling

Netherton's Syndrome

Clinical Description

Netherton's syndrome is a rare, autosomal recessive trait characterized by the distinctive triad of ichthyosis, structural defects of the hair shaft, and atopic diathesis. *Ichthyosis linearis circumflexa* is the term used to describe the pattern of bizarre, migratory, polycyclic scaling with a characteristic double-edged scale, a pattern pathognomonic of Netherton's syndrome. The hair shaft defect diagnostic of Netherton's syndrome is trichorrhexis invaginata, a "ball and socket intussusception" of the distal into the proximal hair shaft. The atopic diathesis is manifested in approximately two thirds of patients by atopic dermatitis, allergic rhinitis, and/or an elevated serum IgE level.

Sjögren-Larsson Syndrome

Clinical Description

Sjögren-Larsson syndrome is an autosomal recessive trait due to deficiency of the enzyme fatty alcohol oxidoreductase. The syndrome is characterized by ichthyosis of moderate severity and tends to spare the face and palms and soles. Accentuation of flexures, forming a ridged, hyperkeratotic pattern, and accentuation of skin markings on the lower abdomen are typical. Other features include spastic diplegia or quadriplegia, mental retardation, and speech defects.

Treatment

Dietary restriction of long-chain fatty acids through the provision of fat in the form of medium-chain triglycerides has been associated with a marked improvement in ichthyosiform dermatosis, as well as some improvement in neurologic status, in some but not all patients.

Trichothiodystrophy

Trichothiodystrophy (i.e., sulfur-deficient brittle hair) is the common feature of a bewildering number of syndromes, most of which are inherited in an autosomal recessive pattern.

Erythroderma is usually not a striking feature. Other associated features include intellectual impairment, decreased fertility and short stature (BIDS), ichthyosis BIDS (IBIDS), photosensitivity plus IBIDS (PIBIDS), and osteosclerosis plus IBIDS (SIBIDS). Trichothiodystrophy should be excluded by hair mount and analysis of hair sulfur content in all children with scaling skin and brittle hair.

KID (Keratitis/Ichthyosis/Deafness) Syndrome

Clinical Description

The acronym KID syndrome denotes the triad of progressive corneal inflammatory disease (*k*eratitis), a distinctive and unusual ichthyosiform erythroderma (*i*chthyosis), and a congenital, usually profound neurosensory *d*eafness in an autosomal dominant inheritance.

The cutaneous phenotype is distinctive. In contrast to most other disorders of cornification, accentuated scaling is not seen. Instead, there is a generalized hyperkeratosis, producing a striking ridging or lichenification over acral surfaces, with markedly hyperkeratotic perioral plaques, and an underlying erythroderma. Palms and soles exhibit a distinctive, keratoderma that has been likened to the grained pattern of leather. Alopecia is often noted at birth; hair may subsequently grow, only to be later lost through a progressive alopecia. Eyebrows and eyelashes are sparse, and nails are often thickened and dystrophic. Impaired sweating and heat intolerance are frequent, presumably due to sweat duct obstruction rather than gland hypoplasia. Approximately half of patients suffer from recurrent skin infections. Cutaneous and mucocutaneous squamous cell carcinomas appear in early adulthood in as many as 15% of patients.

The keratitis usually begins in infancy and progresses with corneal opacities and ulcerations, neovascularization, and pannus formation. The deafness is congenital and nonprogressive.

Other Disorders or Cornification

Erythrokeratodermia Variabilis

Clinical Description

Erythrokeratodermia variabilis is a rare autosomal dominant trait characterized by fixed hyperkeratotic plaques and a changing configurate erythroderma. The onset is usually at birth, or within the first few months, but may be delayed until late childhood or early adulthood. The hyperkeratotic plaques are most frequently distributed on the face and extensor surfaces of the extremities. They are often dark red and densely hyperkeratotic. The number and extent of plaques are usually progressive until puberty and stable thereafter. There often is a dense palmoplantar keratoderma. The most striking clinical feature is the variable erythrodermic component in which geographic patterns of erythema induced by exposure to cold, heat, or wind or emotional stress are observed to shift and change within minutes, hours, or days.

Darier's Disease

Clinical Description

Darier's disease (Darier-White disease, keratosis follicularis) is an autosomal dominant trait in which approximately 75% of patients have the onset of their disease in the first or second decades. The disorder appears to be fully penetrant, with a wide range of expressivity. Keratotic papules in a seborrheic distribution are present in more than 90% of patients. Involvement of flexures, particularly axillae, groins, and inframammary folds, is seen in 80% of patients. In most patients, flexural involvement is mild, but some form extensive, macerated papillomatous plaques. Virtually all patients have hand involvement, which includes nail dystrophy, palmar pits, and acrokeratoses. Nail changes are highly characteristic and include short, broad nails, with longitudinal white and red streaks, nail fragility with V-shaped notches at the free edge, longitudinal ridges, and subungual hyperkeratoses. Oral manifestations are present in 15% to 50% of patients and include white papules on the hard palate and cobblestoning on the buccal mucosa and gingival margins.

Many patients note onset or flares of the disease after sun exposure. Heat and sweating may also trigger disease. Patients are at increased risk for widespread herpes simplex infections (eczema herpeticum), and one fourth of patients suffer from recurrent bacterial skin infections.

Pathology

Darier's disease is characterized by focal acantholytic dyskeratosis, in which suprabasal clefts lie beneath columns of acantholytic and dyskeratotic cells. The corps ronds of Darier's disease are simply acantholytic, dyskeratotic cells with prominent perinuclear vacuoles, and grains are their parakeratotic counterparts.

Diagnosis and Differential Diagnosis

The combination of the clinical picture and histopathology is distinctive and usually presents little diagnostic difficulty. The differential diagnosis includes Hailey-Hailey disease and seborrheic dermatitis.

Treatment

Once established, the disease tends to persist and gradually extend. The cutaneous lesions respond well to oral retinoids (e.g., etretinate, 0.5 mg/kg per day). To avoid long-term toxicities, patients should receive the lowest dose in intermittent courses that will suppress their disease. Sun protection is advised.

Hailey-Hailey Disease

Hailey-Hailey disease (benign familial pemphigus) is an autosomal dominant trait in which flexural involvement with moist vegetative plaques or scaly patches with vesiculopustules is the characteristic clinical sign. The disorder typically has onset in the second to fourth decade and may gradually improve with age. These lesions are similar to the flexural lesions of Darier's disease, but in Hailey-Hailey disease distinct keratotic papules are not seen. Extraflexural sites may be involved, with plaques on trunk, extremities, scalp, and face. The histopathology is distinctive, demonstrating suprabasilar acantholysis that may also affect the spinous layer. The epidermis is hyperplastic with slender, elongated dermal papillae lined by an intact basal layer that projects into the suprabasal cleft. Findings on direct immunofluorescence are nonspecific.

Lesions are provoked by a variety of traumatic stimuli. Avoidance of skin trauma, treatment with topical steroids, antibiotics, and antifungals are often beneficial. Rarely, surgical treatment by excision and grafting, CO_2 laser, and dermabrasion are indicated for resistant plaques.

Porokeratosis

Clinical Description

The porokeratoses are a group of disorders having in common a distinctive histopathologic structure—the cornoid lamella. At least four clinical forms can be delineated: (1) porokeratoses of Mibelli (including linear porokeratosis); (2) porokeratosis palmaris et plantaris disseminata; (3) punctate porokeratosis of palms and soles; and (4) disseminated superficial actinic porokeratosis. Most of these are inherited as autosomal dominant traits.

Porokeratosis of Mibelli is an autosomal dominant trait characterized by one or more well-demarcated erythematous, hyperkeratotic plaques outlined by a thickened, keratotic border often several millimeters in height. A furrow is evident running along the keratotic ridge. The inner portion of the lesion may be atrophic. Lesions are single or few in number, may be linear, and may occur anywhere, including mucous membranes. The initial lesion may be small (less than 1 cm) and slowly expands to exceed 10 cm in size. Most lesions have their onset in the first decade. In several instances, malignant degeneration to squamous cell carcinoma has been observed.

Porokeratosis palmaris et plantaris disseminata is a rare autosomal dominant form that differs from the Mibelli form in the multiplicity of lesions and onset in the second to third decade. Lesions too numerous to count develop over both sun-shielded and sun-exposed regions of the neck, trunk, and extremities.

Disseminated superficial actinic porokeratosis is common in whites and is more frequent in women. It has its onset in the third and fourth decades as multiple (usually more than 50), small erythematous or atrophic patches with a fine keratotic border, limited to the sun-exposed portions of the extremities. During the summer, the lesions may become more erythematous and keratotic. In addition to ultraviolet light, psoralens plus ultraviolet light A (PUVA) therapy may induce these lesions. Immunosuppression has also been associated with their appearance.

Pathology

Cornoid lamellation is the hallmark of the porokeratoses. In this reaction pattern, which defines the outer borders of lesions, narrow, sometimes slanting columns of parakeratotic cells are produced by an epidermis in which there are perinuclear vacuoles and individually dyskeratotic cells.

Treatment

Because of the risk of malignant degeneration, as well as the tendency to enlarge over time, treatment of porokeratosis of Mibelli is usually indicated. Topical 5-fluorouracil or ablation by surgery, dermabrasion, or CO_2 laser may be used. Recurrences are common. A number of therapies have been proposed for disseminated superficial actinic porokeratosis, including topical retinoids, cryosurgery, and topical 5-fluorouracil, as well as retinoids plus PUVA.

Palmoplantar Keratodermas

The palmoplantar keratodermas (PPKs) encompass numerous entities. The initial approach to the patient should focus on determining if the condition is part of a more generalized disorder of cornification (e.g., pityriasis rubra pilaris, psoriasis) or if it is predominantly localized to the palms and soles and whether it is acquired or genetically determined. The differential diagnosis of the genetic forms requires determination of the inheritance pattern and clinical evaluation of the pattern of involvement: focal versus diffuse, extension onto dorsal surfaces (transgrediens) or distant sites, and potential for constriction (pseudoainhum). As in the inherited generalized disorders of cornification (the ichthyoses), PPKs may also be part of a symptom-complex.

Acquired Palmoplantar Keratoderma

An acquired PPK should be considered in the patient with adult onset of disease and no known familial predisposition. Like acquired ichthyoses, it demands evaluation for an underlying cause. Calluses are a common form of focal acquired PPK that represent a response to chronic frictional injury. Removal of the hyperkeratosis by keratolytics or manual paring relieves the discomfort; however, the callus will recur unless the underlying stimulus is relieved. Diffuse palmoplantar hyperkeratosis may similarly develop on palms or soles in response to chronic mechanical trauma. These hyperkeratoses are usually functional. Painful callosities that sometimes develop in women after menopause (keratoderma climactericum) or bilateral oophorectomy, occasionally in association with hyperhidrosis, may respond to topical or systemic estrogen replacement therapy.

Like acquired ichthyosis, adult onset of palmoplantar hyperkeratosis may signify an underlying malignancy. An unusual pattern of hyperkeratosis characterized by a rugose or honeycombed morphology ("tripe palms") has been associated with a variety of internal malignancies. The Howel-Evans syndrome is the association of diffuse PPK with esophageal cancer and is inherited as an autosomal dominant trait. Cutaneous T-cell lymphoma may also present as an acquired PPK; here, the skin biopsy will reveal the correct diagnosis. Punctate palmar keratoses are also associated in some surveys with an increased risk of bladder and lung cancer; these lesions, however, are quite common in the population.

Inherited Palmoplantar Keratodermas: Diffuse Forms

Unna and Vörner Forms of PPK

The autosomal dominantly inherited form of diffuse PPK without transgrediens has been designated by two eponyms, the Unna-Thost form and the Vörner form, to denote histopathologic differences: the Unna-Thost form demonstrates orthohyperkeratosis, while the Vörner form shows epidermolytic hyperkeratosis. Mutations in the keratin 9 gene, a keratin species normally expressed only on palms and soles, have been described in the Vörner form. Clinically, the two forms are identical, with a sharply marginated, diffuse palmoplantar hyperkeratosis. A very dense keratoderma results in a yellow, waxy appearance, often rimmed with erythema. The onset is usually in infancy, but delay until childhood may occur. The initial involvement may be focal, over pressure points, and only later becoming diffuse. Hyperhidrosis is usually present. Mechanical debridement in conjunction with topical keratolytic therapy is the main line of therapy. Some patients may require oral retinoid therapy to maintain mechanical function.

Mutilating Forms of PPK

The mutilating keratoderma of Vohwinkel is inherited as an autosomal dominant trait and is characterized by infantile onset of keratoderma, often with a diffuse, honeycombed pattern. Star-shaped hyperkeratoses typically develop over the dorsa of the digits, elbows, and knees. The keratoderma is severely disabling and typically leads to the development of fibrous constrictions of the digits (pseudoainhum) and autoamputation. Retinoid therapy may prevent progression of the disease. Olmsted's syndrome is the association of massive, mutilating keratoderma with severe nail dystrophy and perioroficial sharply marginated, hyperkeratotic plaques.

PPK with Transgrediens

Mal de Meleda is a severe, autosomal recessive form of PPK with transgrediens originally described among inbred inhabitants of the Yugoslavian island of Meleda. The onset is at birth or shortly thereafter with erythema and hyperkeratosis of palms and soles spreading to the dorsa of the hands and feet in a stocking-and-glove pattern or forming focal, circumscribed hyperkeratotic plaques, often in association with plaques on elbows, knees, or angles of the mouth. Nails are dystrophic, and pseudoainhum may develop.

Papillon-Lefèvre syndrome is an autosomal recessive trait of diffuse PPK with transgrediens and focal keratotic plaques on elbows and knees, in association with severe periodontopathy, leading to premature loss of both primary and secondary teeth; onset is the first 3 years of life.

Kindreds are described with focal delayed-onset PPK and progressive sensorineural deafness. The association of PPK and deafness also occurs in pachyonychia congenita, Papillon-Lefèvre syndrome, Olmsted's syndrome, and the Vohwinkel form of PPK.

Inherited Palmoplantar Keratoderma: Focal Forms

Striate PPK is characterized by linear bands of hyperkeratosis that follow the midline of one or more digits, often continuing across the palm in a linear fashion. Plantar involvement may be nummular and centered over pressure points. The trait is inherited in an autosomal dominant manner and may not be expressed until late childhood or adulthood, when it is precipitated by mechanical stress. Painful hereditary callosities are also inherited as an autosomal dominant trait in which focal hyperkeratosis of one to several centimeters in diameter develops on palms and soles over pressure points. Palmoplantar hyperkeratosis is the most constant feature of the autosomal dominant pachyonychia congenita. Focal keratosis over pressure points develops with weight bearing, often accompanied by blistering and hyperhidrosis. Other common features include nail dystrophy with subungual hyperkeratosis, oral leukokeratosis, and follicular hyperkeratoses.

Small or punctate hyperkeratoses are also inherited as a dominant trait, but in most instances they occur sporadically and may be environmentally included. Two variants are recognized: punctate keratoses of the palms and soles and keratotic pits of the palmar creases. Both are quite common, occurring in 11% and 3% of dermatology patients, and both forms are more common in men and blacks. Punctate keratoses are 1- to 3-mm hyperkeratotic papules distributed over palms and soles. Lesions on the soles may be larger and symptomatic over pressure points and may be single or multiple. Keratotic pits of the palmar creases are discrete depressions in linear arrays. They can be painful and may require surgical intervention. Punctate keratoses are associated in some series with an increased incidence of smoking, as well as with bladder and lung cancer; both genetic and environmental factors may be involved in their formation. An association between punctate palmoplantar keratoses and gastrointestinal malignancy has also been reported. The differential diagnosis of punctate keratoses of the palms and soles is extensive and includes acquired causes (e.g., warts, arsenical keratoses, syphilis, and yaws) and other genetic traits (e.g., Darier's disease, basal cell nevus syndrome, and Cowden's disease).

In tyrosinemia type II (Richner-Hanhart syndrome), focal keratoses may develop over pressure points on the palms and soles. Dendritic corneal ulcerations and mental retardation are the other major clinical signs of this autosomal recessive disorder, which is caused by deficiency of the hepatic enzyme tyrosine aminotransferase. Serum tyrosine levels are markedly elevated, and normalization of tyrosine levels by dietary restriction may prevent full expression of the disease.

CONGENITAL ALOPECIAS AND DISORDERS OF MELANOSOME TRANSFER TO HAIR FOLLICLES

(CM&S Chapter 163)

Definition

Congenital alopecias represent a heterogeneous group of rare genetic and developmental disorders. Hair development requires the close coordination of multiple cell types of ectodermal and mesodermal origin, and thus hair development is susceptible to multiple forms of genetic insults. The genetic and developmental basis of few of these disorders is understood.

Metabolic Disorders

Menkes' Kinky Hair Syndrome

Menkes' kinky hair syndrome is a rare X-linked deficiency of copper metabolism. The deficiency of copper in certain tissues results in decreased activity of copper dependent enzymes, such as tyrosinase, dopamine hydroxylase, cytochrome oxidase, and lysyl oxidase. Diminished activity of these enzymes leads to the clinical stigmata of Menkes' syndrome, which include hypopigmentation of hair, mental retardation, degeneration of large vessel elastin, and bone abnormalities. No clinical treatment is effective in ameliorating the course of the disease. Prenatal diagnosis is available through copper measurements of fetal cells. Female carriers may have hypopigmentation following Blaschko's lines.

Disorders of Amino Acid Metabolism

Argininosuccinic aciduria is a deficiency of the urea cycle enzyme argininosuccinate lyase, which converts argininosuccinate to arginine. Clinical features of this disorder include mental retardation, hepatomegaly, dry and brittle hair with red fluorescence, trichorrhexis nodosa, monilethrix, and epilepsy. Clinical improvement has been noted by dietary supplementation with arginine. On polarizing microscopy, alternating light and dark bands are observed. Amino acid analysis of affected hair is essentially normal, but the polarized microscopic appearance can be reversed by placing these patients on a diet with low protein and with arginine supplementation. Serum levels of arginine are normal, but citrulline levels are elevated.

Homocystinuria, a deficiency of cystathionine beta synthase, is characterized by diluted hair pigmentation, ectopia lentis, marfanoid habitus, osteoporosis, and thrombotic tendency. A subset of patients respond to pyridoxine therapy. Homocysteine has been shown to be a growth factor for vascular smooth muscle.

Syndromes of Premature Aging

Hutchinson-Gilford progeria syndrome is an autosomal recessive disorder, which is characterized by onset during the first year of life, in contrast to Werner's syndrome, which is first noted toward the end of the first decade. Dermatologic findings in these disorders include alopecia and prominent scalp veins, loss of subcutaneous fat, dystrophic nails, scleredematous skin and yellowish discoloration of the skin, as well as hyperlipidemia. Alopecia develops at the age of a few months and is progressive. Alopecia is prominent in Werner's syndrome, but at a later age.

Congenital Triangular Alopecia

Congenital triangular alopecia is an uncommon developmental defect characterized by decreased hair mass, but not decreased hair number, on an isolated portion of the temporal scalp and is unilateral in 80% of cases. This defect may appear several years after birth. Scalp biopsy of these areas reveals increased numbers of vellus hair follicles and decreased terminal hairs. This defect is permanent but may be treated with scalp reduction.

Anhidrotic Ectodermal Dysplasia (Christ-Siemens-Touraine Syndrome)

Anhidrotic ectodermal dysplasia is an X-linked recessive disorder characterized by hypotrichosis, absence of sweat glands, and hypodontia in affected males. The earliest presentation may be extensive exfoliation of the skin as a newborn. Female carriers may show tooth malformations and slight abnormalities of breasts and sweat glands. Other clinical features include short stature, saddle-nose, periocular hyperpigmentation, and decreased mucous glands of the respiratory tract. Patients may have frequent respiratory infections, and care must be taken to avoid hyperthermia.

Hidrotic Ectodermal Dysplasia (Clouston's Syndrome)

Hidrotic ectodermal dysplasia is an autosomal dominant disorder that differs from anhidrotic ectodermal dysplasia in that sebaceous and eccrine function appear normal, but patients have nail dystrophy, hyperpigmentation of skin overlying joints, mental retardation, and alopecia. Analysis of hair from these patients has shown reduced birefringence with polarized light, and a disorganized fibrillar structure.

Keratosis Pilaris Atrophicans

Keratosis pilaris atrophicans describes a heterogeneous group of disorders of uncertain genetic transmission that are characterized by the triad of follicular hyperkeratosis, inflammation, and atrophic scarring. These disorders include keratosis pilaris atrophicans faciei (ulerythema ophryogenes), atrophoderma vermiculatum, and keratosis follicularis spinulosa decalvans. These disorders are characterized by follicular inflammation and scarring. Early pathologic changes include compact hyperkeratosis of the infundibulum and isthmus. Hair loss begins in early childhood, progresses to scarring alopecia at puberty, and may also involve eyebrows, trunk, and the extensor surfaces of the arms. This disorder may be associated with atopy, palmoplantar hyperkeratosis, and punctate corneal lesions. Retinoid, keratolytic, and topical corticosteroid therapy has been generally unsuccessful in treatment of these disorders.

Netherton's Syndrome

Netherton's syndrome is a disorder of uncertain genetic transmission characterized by hair shaft defects, especially trichorrhexis invaginata, atopy, and ichthyosis. This disorder has also been called ichthyosis linearis circumflexa. The differential diagnosis includes lamellar ichthyosis, Leiner's disease, and acrodermatitis enteropathica. These patients have recurrent bacterial infections of the skin and otitis, with organisms including *Staphylococcus aureus*, *Pseudomonas*, and streptococcal species. Hair defects noted in Netherton's syndrome include pili torti, monilethrix, and trichorrhexis nodosa. Aminoaciduria may be seen in these patients, but it may be secondary to long-term corticosteroid use. Multiple attempts at therapy have been tried, but with little success.

Loose Anagen Hair Syndrome

Loose anagen hair syndrome is a disorder characterized by the easy removal of anagen hairs from the scalp during a hair pull. Clinically, this is manifested as the painless loss of clumps of hair. Histologically, this disorder is characterized by distortion of the hair bulb and poor adhesion of the outer root sheath to the vitreous layer. Examination of plucked hairs by scanning electron microscopy reveals absence of the cuticle and root sheaths, as well as ridging and grooving of the shaft. This disorder often appears in lighter colored hair and tends to improve with age. Inheritance may be autosomal dominant.

Monilethrix

Monilethrix is an uncommon disorder of hair characterized by periodic constrictions that lead to hair shaft breakage and alopecia. Children are born with normal-appearing hair, which is lost within the first 4 months of life. Therapy is largely unsuccessful. Hair has been noted to improve during pregnancy.

Trichothiodystrophy

Trichothiodystrophy is a rare and heterogeneous disorder with the primary feature of brittle hair shafts. The hair protein has been found to contain an abnormally low sulfur content. Microscopic examination reveals a deficient cuticle. Other associated clinical features include photosensitivity, mental retardation, ichthyosis, nail dystrophy, dental anomalies, and decreased fertility.

Disorders of Melanin Transfer: Griscelli's Syndrome and Chédiak-Higashi Syndrome

Griscelli's syndrome is a rare autosomal recessive disorder. These patients usually present at 3 to 4 months of age with silver-tinged hair, neurologic abnormalities, and recurrent pyogenic infections. Leukocytes are normal in number upon initial presentation, but pancytopenia is a major cause of mortality after age 1. Lymphohistiocytic infiltration of liver, spleen, skin, and central nervous system are commonly observed, with prominent erythrophagocytosis.

Characteristic cutaneous findings include clumping of melanin within hair shafts and little transfer of melanin from melanocytes to keratinocytes. Electron microscopy reveals melanocytes containing stage 3 and 4 melanosomes, and keratinocytes that lack melanosomes.

Immunologically, patients may have normal levels of immunoglobulins but decreased T-cell response to mitogens. Chemotherapy with methotrexate, cytoxan, vincristine, VP-16, and steroids may be effective for ameliorating progression of this disorder, but bone marrow transplantation is the only effective therapy.

The differential diagnosis of this disorder includes Chédiak-Higashi disorder, a recessive disorder of melanocytes and granulocytes. Patients with Chédiak-Higashi syndrome do not have the prominent histiocytosis of Griscelli's syndrome and in general have a more indolent clinical course, with death in the teenage years. Recently, cyclosporine has been found to be useful in maintaining remissions in this disease.

The basic defect in Chédiak-Higashi appears to be in the lysosome and melanosome. The defect in the melanosome prevents transfer of melanosomes to keratinocytes, and the hair shaft reveals clumped melanin granules, which are diagnostic of this disorder. The failure in melanosome transfer results in pale blond hair, sometimes with a metallic sheen, and pale skin. Natural killer lymphocyte activity is deficient in this disorder.

Clinically, children with Chédiak-Higashi syndrome have recurrent bacterial infections, especially with *Staphylococcus aureus*. After the first decade of life, patients develop into an accelerated phase, characterized by lymphocytic infiltrates, pancytopenia, and hepatosplenomegaly. This accelerated phase is lethal unless treated with bone marrow transplantation. Death in the accelerated phase is usually secondary to hemorrhage or infection.

THE ECTODERMAL DYSPLASIAS

(CM&S Chapter 164)

Definition and Clinical Description

The ectodermal dysplasias are an extensive and diverse group of hereditary conditions that includes all conditions having a developmental defect that embryologically affects the ectoderm.

Although structures of ectodermal origin are most frequently involved in ectodermal dysplasias, a variety of nonectodermal structures may also be involved. Structures including the limbs, bones, palate, neurologic tissue, internal organs, and reproductive structures may be affected (Table 11–1). Hair is the most frequently altered tissue, with 90% of patients with ectodermal dysplasia showing changes in hair distribution, structure, quality, or composition. Often the hair will be twisted (pili torti) and small in diameter, have longitudinal grooves, and have an irregular cross-sectional shape and abnormal pattern of cuticulae. The other most common features in ectodermal dysplasia involve the skin (85%), teeth (80%), nails (75%), face (72%), psychomotor growth and development (61%), eyes (60%), limbs (48%), and hearing (24%).

TABLE 11–1. Tissues Involved in Ectodermal Dysplasias

TISSUE	CLINICAL AND STRUCTURAL CHARACTERISTICS
Hair	Sparse or absent, may be of small diameter, abnormal cross-sectional shape, longitudinal fissures, hypopigmentation, dystrophic bulb, abnormal slant
Teeth	Absent or reduced in number, peg-shaped, hypoplastic enamel, large pulp chambers, periodontal degeneration
Nails	Absent, thin, brittle, hyperconvex, conical, narrow, broad, thickened, hypopigmented, hyperpigmented, slow growing
Sweat glands	Regional absence, hypoplastic ducts and pores, functional alteration (decreased/increased sweat production)
Bones and limbs	Craniofacial deformities, cleft palate, syndactyly, ectrodactyly (split hands and feet), polydactyly, micromelia, generalized osteoporosis, osteosclerosis
Special senses	Microphthalmia, cataract formation, photophobia, frequent conjunctivitis, congenital deafness, conductive hearing loss
Glands	Decreased lacrimation, supernumerary nipples, mammary gland hypoplasia, decreased numbers of sebaceous and mucous glands, decreased saliva
Internal organs	Abnormal liver and kidney function, congenital heart disease
Reproductive organs	Hypospadias, hypogonadism, cryptorchidism, amenorrhea
Neurologic system	Mental retardation, hypotonia, seizures

Data from Holbrook KA. Structural abnormalities of the epidermally derived appendages in skin from patients with ectodermal dysplasia: Insight into developmental errors. In: Salinas CF, Opitz JM, Paul NW, eds. Recent Advances in Ectodermal Dysplasias. New York: Alan R Liss, 1988.

The skin of persons with ectodermal dysplasia is most commonly hyperplastic but may also be aplastic. Palmar-plantar hyperkeratosis and generalized ichthyosiform erythroderma are common. Increased or decreased pigmentation may also occur, depending on the tissue site and type of ectodermal dysplasia present. Abnormal sweat gland structure and/or function and altered dermatoglyphics are also common in the ectodermal dysplasia.

Diagnosis

The ectodermal dysplasias are inherited as autosomal dominant and recessive and X-linked dominant and recessive mendelian traits. Individuals with ectodermal dysplasia often have no prior family history, making determination of the mode of inheritance impossible in the absence of precise DNA probes. Careful analysis of the family history and evaluation of all at-risk individuals for subtle clinical features is, therefore, essential in obtaining an accurate diagnosis. Localization of the gene for X-linked recessive hypohidrotic ectodermal dysplasia to the Xq13.1 region now provides an accurate method for the diagnosis of cases both prenatally and postnatally in this specific type of ectodermal dysplasia. Further application of molecular biological techniques to the study of ectodermal dysplasia will lead to additional means for diagnosis and subclassification in the near future.

Treatment

Appropriate management of patients with ectodermal dysplasia often requires a team approach, due to the diverse spectrum of involvement. All interventions are preventive or palliative. Genetic evaluation and counseling should be provided to all families with ectodermal dysplasia. Individuals with severe hyperthermia may need to curtail activities causing exertion that could raise the body core temperature. Febrile seizures and even death have been reported in patients with ectodermal dysplasia having significant hypohidrosis and secondary hyperthermia.

Dermatologic therapy is rendered primarily in response to the xerosis, which may be striking in some patients. Individuals with severe hypotrichosis and hypodontia will benefit from hair and dental prostheses. These interventions are often best initiated before school age, thereby facilitating optimal socialization and peer interaction.

INCONTINENTIA PIGMENTI

(CM&S Chapter 165)

Definition and Clinical Description

Incontinentia pigmenti, also called Bloch-Sulzberger syndrome or Bloch-Siemens syndrome, is an X-linked, dominantly inherited disorder that affects, almost exclusively, females. The incontinence of pigment from which its name derives is the result of inflammation.

It is characterized by progression through three successive stages. In the first stage, a vesiculobullous eruption is present at birth or appears within 2 weeks in 90% of the patients. The vesicles are frequently in a linear arrangement, and the extremities are predominantly affected. Peripheral blood eosinophilia can occur.

The vesiculobullous stage is followed by a verrucous stage at 2 to 6 weeks of age. Rarely, the vesicular stage of incontinentia pigmenti occurs in utero and patients can be born with verrucous lesions. Linear verrucous and papillomatous lesions develop in previous vesicular areas.

In the third stage, the verrucous lesions give way to bizarre, whorled brown to slate-gray macular pigmentation that is most prominent on the trunk. This pigmentation gradually fades after 16 weeks of age. Occasionally, residual hypopigmentation remains for variable periods of time in the previously hyperpigmented areas.

Other cutaneous features include patchy cicatricial alopecia and dystrophic nails. Common extracutaneous anomalies include partial anodontia and/or conical teeth, seizures, mental retardation and/or spastic paresis, cataracts, papillitis, congenital retinal folds, and optical atrophy.

Incontinentia pigmenti may be associated with an increased frequency of childhood neoplasms. Retinoblastoma, Wilms' tumor, acute myelocytic leukemia, paratesticular rhabdomyosarcoma, and rhabdoid tumor of the kidney have been reported.

Pathology

Histologically, the vesicular lesions are characterized by eosinophilic spongiosis. In the dermis, there is a patchy infiltrate of mononuclear cells and many eosinophils. The verrucous lesions of the second stage show hyperkeratosis, papillomatosis, acanthosis, and scattered dyskeratotic cells within the epidermis. The pigmented whorls of the third stage display an accumulation of melanophages in the superficial dermis.

Differential Diagnosis

The differential diagnosis includes neonatal herpes simplex, infantile acropustulosis, epidermolysis bullosa, and neonatal herpes gestationis. Diseases that manifest with splashed pigmentation in older infants, such as the Franceschetti-Jadassohn syndrome and postinflammatory hyperpigmentation from atopic eczema or other causes, should also be considered in the differential diagnosis of incontinentia pigmenti in its third stage.

Treatment

No treatment is necessary except for control of secondary infection of the vesiculobullous lesions. Skilled dental intervention can minimize cosmetic disability related to the dental abnormalities. Neurologic and ophthalmologic consultation is advisable. Genetic counseling should be offered to all families with incontinentia pigmenti.

NEUROFIBROMATOSIS AND TUBEROUS SCLEROSIS

(CM&S Chapter 166)

Neurofibromatosis Type 1

Definition

The term *neurofibromatosis* implies neurofibromatosis type 1 (NF1), which formerly was known as as von Recklinghausen's disease. NF is no longer considered a single disease. NF1 is a multisystem disorder characterized by café-au-lait macules, neurofibromas, Lisch nodules, optic gliomas, bony dysplasias, intertriginous freckling, and autosomal dominant inheritance on the long arm of chromosome 17. The incidence of NF1 is approximately 1 in 3500; 50% of cases appear to be spontaneous mutations.

Clinical Description

Cutaneous Features

Neurofibromas. There are three types of neurofibromas: cutaneous, subcutaneous, and plexiform. The cutaneous type are pink, rubbery tumors that can be pedunculated or sessile, can number from just a few to over 1000, and vary in size from a few millimeters to more than 1 meter (average, 0.5 to 1.0 cm). All sites can be affected. Neurofibromas of the female areola and nipple are virtually pathognomonic for NF1. The lesions herniate easily or ''buttonhole'' through the dermis with gentle pressure. Subcutaneous neurofibromas may be firm, feeling like a pencil eraser. Cutaneous and subcutaneous neurofibromas appear initially in childhood, increase in number during puberty and pregnancy, and continue to appear at a slower rate throughout adulthood.

Plexiform neurofibromas are congenital and nearly pathognomonic for NF1. They are similar to a combination of cutaneous and subcutaneous types and feel like a ''bag of worms.'' They can be large but may be subtle at birth when the only sign of a plexiform neurofibroma may be a hair whorl or patch of hyperpigmentation.

Café-au-Lait Macules. The café-au-lait spot is a homogeneous tan-brown macule with smooth, sharp borders. It can vary in size from a few millimeters to many centimeters (average, 1–3 cm). Café-au-lait macules are found everywhere except the scalp, eyebrows, palms, and soles. They are congenital but may not be visible for the first few months of life.

Intertriginous Freckling. Intertriginous freckling, or Crowe's sign, consists of small 1- to 3-mm in diameter tan-brown macules. Freckling may be universal in NF1, but it is considered diagnostic of NF1 only when it is present in the axilla or groin.

Extracutaneous Features

Central Nervous System and Eye. Lisch nodules are the most common manifestation of NF1 but they are rarely seen in patients who do not have NF1. In one study, they were present in 100% of individuals with NF1. These melanocytic hamartomas of the iris that look like three-dimensional translucent brown spots do not interfere with vision and require a slit lamp to visualize in most cases.

Optic gliomas, the prototypical central nervous system (CNS) lesions of NF1, are present in approximately 15% of patients with NF1, but 80% of these may be asymptomatic. Both Lisch nodules and optic gliomas appear in childhood.

Orthopedic Features. Two lesions of the bone are considered specific for NF1: sphenoid wing dysplasia and pseudarthrosis of the tibia, although neither is frequently seen.

Course and Complications

NF1 is a progressive disease. It worsens with age; limited disease early in life is no guarantee of mild disease later. The lifetime risk for cancer in NF1 patients is approximately 5% above the lifetime risk of the general population. The prototypical adult NF1-specific cancer is neurofibrosarcoma, which can develop within plexiform neurofibroma or within large nerves but rarely with typical cutaneous or subcutaneous neurofibromas. Pheochromocytomas, malignant melanoma, and embryonal tumors such as Wilms' tumor and rhabdomyosarcoma and childhood leukemia are also more common in NF1.

Cosmetic disfigurement is a complication of NF1. Two thirds of patients with NF1 have mild disease, one half of whom consider cutaneous neurofibromas to represent their major concern. Of the remaining third, one half have severe but correctable problems and one half have persistent, severe difficulties.

Pathology

Neurofibromas are characterized by replacement of the dermis with a blue-gray gelatinous-appearing, nonencapsulated collection of palisading, loosely arranged, endoneurial fibroblasts and Schwann cells.

Diagnosis

Diagnostic criteria are provided in Table 11–2.

Differential Diagnosis

The differential diagnosis includes McCune-Albright syndrome (polyostotic fibrous dysplasia, irregular skin pigmentation, and sexual precocity); Watson syndrome (café-au-lait macules, dull intelligence, and pulmonary stenosis); and Proteus syndrome (mesodermal malformations, hemihypertrophy, scoliosis, cerebriform masses of palms and soles, and subcutaneous masses that can be mistaken for neurofibromas).

Neurofibromatosis type 2 (NF2), the only other type of NF having its own universally accepted criteria, inherited on chromosome 22, is characterized by bilateral acoustic neuromas. The characteristic cutaneous features include neurofibromas and schwannomas but not café-au-lait macules or freckling.

TABLE 11-2. Criteria for Neurofibromatosis Type I

Two of seven criteria are required for a definitive diagnosis:
1. Six or more café-au-lait macules over 5 mm in greatest diameter in prepubertal individuals and over 15 mm in greatest diameter in postpubertal individuals.
2. Freckling in the axillary or inguinal regions.
3. Two or more neurofibromas of any type or one plexiform neurofibroma.
4. Two or more Lisch nodules.
5. Optic glioma.
6. A distinctive osseous lesion such as sphenoid wing dysplasia or thinning of the long bone cortex with or without pseudarthrosis.
7. First-degree relative with neurofibromatosis type 1 by these criteria.

From Mulvihill JJ (moderator). Neurofibromatosis 1 (Recklinghausen's disease) and neurofibromatosis 2 (bilateral acoustic neurofibromatosis): An update. Ann Intern Med 1990;113:39–52.

Treatment

Management is based on genetic counseling and monitoring for and treatment of complications. Identification of children at risk is important because early intervention in children with learning disabilities due to neurofibromatosis is extremely valuable. For all subjects with NF1 routine age-specific cancer screening examinations are indicated. The development of focal neurologic complaints, especially referred pain, or a history of a rapidly enlarging mass, suggests neurofibrosarcoma in a patient with NF1.

A variety of surgical techniques can be used to treat neurofibromas. Café-au-lait macules respond variably to short pulsed lasers, such as the Q-switched ruby, Q-switched NdYAG, and Q-switched alexandrite lasers.

Tuberous Sclerosis

Definition

Tuberous sclerosis, Bourneville's disease, or tuberous sclerosis complex (TSC), is an autosomal dominant disorder characterized by seizures, mental retardation, and a variety of skin lesions such as "ash leaf" macules, facial angiofibromas, ungual fibromas, and shagreen patches. It can affect almost every organ but the most frequently involved are brain, eye, skin, kidneys, heart, and lung. Almost three fourths of cases may be spontaneous mutations and the phenotype varies from family to family and even within families. The birth incidence could be as high as 1 in 10,000.

Clinical Description

Cutaneous Features

Ninety-six percent of patients with TSC and their affected relatives have one or more of the five typical skin signs, of which maybe three are pathognomonic. In order of decreasing frequency they are

1. Hypomelanotic macules
2. Multiple facial angiofibromas
3. Periungual fibromas
4. Shagreen patches
5. Fibrous plaques

Hypomelanotic Macules. Hypomelanotic or "ash leaf" macules are found in 90% of affected individuals. Affected individuals usually have more than four white spots. The macules are often present at birth but may not be recognized until the skin has been exposed to ultraviolet light. The hypopigmented macules are off-white, not snow-white like those of vitiligo. The three types of spots are polygonal (like a thumbprint), lance-ovate (ash leaf), and confetti-like.

Identification is aided with Wood's light examination. Although common, hypomelanotic macules are not specific: 0.8% of neonates normally have white spots; the prevalence is 0.4% for white children and 2.4% for black children. The hypomelanotic macules must be differentiated from vitiligo, nevus anemicus, nevus depigmentosus, and piebaldism.

Multiple Facial Angiofibromas. Most patients have at least one of three different connective tissue hamartomas: (1) facial angiofibromas, (2) ungual fibromas, and (3) shagreen patches. When present in the typical bilateral and symmetrical distribution, multiple facial angiofibromas are pathognomonic for TSC. Originally considered necessary to make the diagnosis of TSC, the prevalence of angiofibromas was 100%. Fewer than half of patients with TSC, however, have angiofibromas.

Angiofibromas are usually symmetrically found over the cheeks, nasolabial folds, and chin; they cross the midline over the nasal bridge and chin. They are rarely seen on the upper lip. The original name, adenoma sebaceum, arises from the fact that these locations have abundance of normal sebaceous glands. Angiofibromas first appear as small red spots and are usually present by age 5. In adolescents, they can be mistaken for acne vulgaris. They are histologically similar to sporadic angiofibromas or fibrous papules.

Periungual Fibromas. Periungual fibromas, pathognomonic of TSC, first appear in the second decade and present in 20% of patients. They are visible as a fibrous growth at the nail edge or may present as a longitudinal groove in the nail plate.

Shagreen Patch. The shagreen patch presents as a skin-colored or yellow-brown plaque that can resemble the skin of an orange, and is usually located on the lumbosacral area. Shagreen patches are found in one fifth of all patients with TSC, usually appearing after puberty. Found alone, they are not diagnostic.

Fibrous Plaques. Fibrous plaques are skin-colored to yellow-brown, smooth elevations of the skin of the forehead and scalp with a rubbery consistency with a histologic similarity to angiofibromas. The plaques usually present in the first 2 to 3 years of life. They are likely pathognomonic of TSC, but their frequency is unknown.

Extracutaneous Features

Central Nervous System. There are two nontumorous features —seizures, the most common presenting feature of TSC, and mental retardation, which correlates with the occurrence of seizures early in life, and has been reported in over 40% of individuals with TSC. Both findings correlate with the size and number of tubers. There are three characteristic tumors—cortical tubers, subependymal nodules, and subependymal giant cell tumors.

Nodules. Tubers are hamartomatous proliferations of glial and neuronal tissues and can give rise to gliomas. There may be as many as 40 lesions per patient, and the distribution is random but symmetrical. The size varies from a few millimeters to a few centimeters.

Subependymal nodules are firm, pea-sized and larger excrescences on the ventricular wall, similar in composition to tubers. They give rise to gliomas termed giant cell subependymomas.

Other Organs. Tumors seen in other affected organs include retinal hamartomas, renal cysts and angiomyolipomas, cardiac rhabdomyomas, and in the lung, cystic disease and lymphangiomyomatosis.

Course and Complications

The prognosis of TSC depends on what organs are involved and to what degree these organs are compromised. Brain abnormalities are associated with almost half of the deaths in TSC. Renal involvement is second most common cause of death.

Diagnosis and Differential Diagnosis

Because there are no markers or blood tests, diagnostic clinical criteria have been developed in an effort to more accurately make a TSC diagnosis. They have been ranked in order of significance to distinguish between common but nonspecific features such as hypomelanotic macules and apparently pathognomonic features such as facial angiofibromas (Table 11–3).

Treatment

Management of TSC consists of monitoring for and treatment of complications. Genetic counseling is extremely important for families of persons with TSC. Since it is an autosomal dominant disorder with suspected complete penetrance, 50% of children of an affected parent are at risk. For families with an affected child in whom no evidence of TSC can be detected in either parent there is still a finite risk for transmission to future children. Since gonadal mosaicism and nonpenetrance can never be completely ruled out, the risk for having future children with TSC is probably 2% to 5%, rather than the 1 in 10,000 risk that would be expected if the event were unrelated.

Management of facial angiofibromas with a variety of treatments from surgical excision to dermabrasion to laser abrasion with either the CO_2 or argon laser can substantially improve the quality of life.

Surgical treatment of periungual fibromas may be indicated if the tumors are painful or disfiguring. Partial or complete nail avulsion may be required in some cases to access the base of the tumor, which usually arises under the proximal or lateral nail fold. This can be accomplished using an electrosurgical device or preferably the more precise CO_2 laser.

TABLE 11-3. Abbreviated Diagnostic Criteria* for Tuberous Sclerosis

PRIMARY FEATURES

Facial angiofibromas†
Multiple ungual fibromas†
Cortical tubers
Subependymal nodule or giant cell astrocytoma‡
Multiple calcified subependymal nodules§
Multiple retinal astrocytomas†

SECONDARY FEATURES

Affected first-degree relative
Cardiac rhabdomyoma‡§
Other retinal hamartoma or achromic patch†
Cerebral tubers§
Noncalcified subependymal nodules§
Shagreen patch† or forehead plaque†
Pulmonary lymphangiomyomatosis‡
Renal cysts‡

TERTIARY FEATURES

Hypomelanotic macules† or "confetti" skin lesions†
Renal cysts§
Randomly distributed enamel pits in teeth
Hamartomatous rectal polyps‡
Bone cysts§
Pulmonary lymphangiomyomatosis§
Cerebral white matter "migration tracts" or heterotopias§
Gingival fibromas†
Hamartoma of other organs‡

*Definite: either one primary feature, two secondary features, or one secondary plus two tertiary features; Probable: either one secondary plus one tertiary feature or three tertiary features; and Suspect: either one secondary feature or two tertiary features.

†Histologic confirmation not required *if* lesions clinically obvious.

‡Histologically confirmed.

§Radiographic evidence.

Data from Roach ES, Smith, M, Huttenlocher P, et al. Report of the Diagnostic Criteria Committee of the National Tuberous Sclerosis Association. J Child Neurol 1992:7:221–224.

BASAL CELL NEVUS SYNDROME

(CM&S Chapter 167)

Definition and Clinical Description

The basal cell nevus syndrome (BCNS) (nevoid basal cell carcinoma syndrome) is a rare autosomal dominantly inherited disorder characterized by one or more of a large number of abnormalities, most often, cutaneous basal cell carcinomas, pits of the palms and soles, cysts of the jaws, and ectopic calcification of cranial membranes.

Basal cell carcinomas are the hallmark of the syndrome, and patients may have several dozen or hundreds. They typically begin around puberty, but the initial lesion may develop only in adulthood, and new tumors usually continue to appear even in later years. The tumors occur more commonly on sun-exposed areas; however, a greater percentage of basal cell carcinomas occur on the trunk in patients with BCNS than in patients with sporadic basal cell carcinomas. Many of the basal cell carcinomas have an appearance no different from that of sporadic basal cell carcinomas, and their biologic behavior is similar: they metastasize only very rarely and are occasionally locally aggressive, especially around the eyes and ears. Other lesions, especially on the trunk, may be more nonspecific, appearing as tiny nontranslucent papules that the unwary may misdiagnose as "tags" or nevi.

The second cutaneous abnormality characteristic of BCNS is the presence of pits of the palms and soles. These 1- to 3-mm in diameter, asymptomatic, ice pick–like defects in the stratum corneum demonstrating crowding of basaloid cells at the bases of rete ridges, but fully developed basal cell carcinomas are rarely present.

Superficial milia and deeper cysts are also frequently seen. There are three skeletal abnormalities seen frequently in BCNS. Jaw cysts (odontogenic keratocysts) are often the presenting sign of BCNS, beginning typically at the end of the first decade. These are usually asymptomatic but may present as jaw pain and swelling and may cause dysfunction, such as by causing loss of teeth or by eroding into a sinus. Usually more than one cyst is present.

Calcification of the dural membranes separating the lobes of the brain, particularly of the falx cerebri, is frequent. Abnormalities of bony outline are also seen. Bifid ribs and changes in skull shape are common. Also occasionally reported are marfanoid habitus, scoliosis, and shortened fourth metacarpals. Skull abnormalities that are usually considered characteristic of BCNS are a large head with bulging ("bossing") of the frontal and temporal bones, which gives the eyes a sunken appearance, and a protruding jaw.

A variety of tumors is seen in the BCNS. Brain tumors are probably the most common fatal "complication" of BCNS. Meningiomas probably occur more often in patients with BCNS than in the general population. The more common tumors are medulloblastomas, which occur typically at age 2, considerably earlier than the age of development in patients with sporadic tumors.

Ovarian fibromas, cysts of the mesentery, and cardiac fibromas are also manifestations of the syndrome. Ovarian fibromas also occur commonly. They do not inhibit fertility; they often calcify and so present on radiographic examination of the abdomen and pelvis with an unusual appearance that may be confused with calcified uterine leiomyomas; and they can become symptomatic if they twist on their pedicle, a complication requiring prompt surgical intervention to prevent destruction of the ovary. Although more commonly developing after adolescence, they have been reported rarely in young children.

Cysts of the mesentery (lymphomesenteric cysts) may be large enough to be apparent on abdominal palpation. Calcification of the cyst walls can cause a balloon-like appearance on radiographic examinations.

Cardiac fibromas have been reported in young children with BCNS, as have fetal rhabdomyomas.

Diagnosis and Differential Diagnosis

In most instances, the combination of several basal cell carcinomas at a young age, jaw cysts, and palmoplantar pits allows for a

TABLE 11–4. Treatment of Basal Cell Nevus Syndrome

1. Regular follow-up with complete cutaneous examination for early detection of lesions
2. Sun protection
3. Genetic counseling
4. Dental examination with surgical treatment of jaw cysts
5. Topical 5-fluorouracil to reduce formation of new lesions
6. Systemic etretinate to prevent new tumor formation may be effective for short periods (1 mg/kg)

ready diagnosis. However, since no single pathognomonic abnormality occurs solely in patients with BCNS and not in otherwise normal individuals, since abnormalities develop in some persons only well into adult life, and since extensive clinical data on the age at onset of different manifestations are not available, diagnosis is often uncertain, especially if no family members have more typical abnormalities.

The dermatologic differential diagnosis includes patients who develop multiple basal cell carcinomas but have no other phenotypic abnormalities of the BCNS, and patients with arsenic-induced skin cancers.

Treatment

Individual basal cell carcinomas can be treated with a variety of modalities, including excisional surgery, electrodesiccation and curettage, cryotherapy, and Mohs micrographic surgery. Radiation therapy is contraindicated. For the general management of patients with BCNS, see Table 11–4.

XERODERMA PIGMENTOSUM

(CM&S Chapter 168)

Definition and Clinical Description

Xeroderma pigmentosum and the related diseases Cockayne syndrome and trichothiodystrophy are rare genetic diseases inherited as autosomal recessive traits.

Xeroderma pigmentosum is characterized by an inordinate susceptibility to develop photodamage and sun-induced skin cancers due, apparently, to ultraviolet (UV) radiation. The skin is normal at birth, and changes are usually first noted between 6 months and 3 years of age. Initial skin changes consist of freckling and dryness of sun-exposed skin. With progression, telangiectasia, angiomas, then depigmented atrophic macules, crusts, ulcers, warty growths, actinic keratoses, and vesiculobullous lesions occur. The skin develops the poikilodermatous appearance of chronic, severe actinic damage, leading to skin cancers of all types, especially squamous cell carcinoma and melanoma.

Cutaneous Changes

Basal cell carcinomas and squamous cell carcinomas are the most common cancers in the general population and in patients with xeroderma pigmentosum. In patients with xeroderma pigmentosum, these malignancies occur at a much higher rate and a much earlier age. Keratoacanthomas, angiomas, and fibrosarcomas also occur in patients with xeroderma pigmentosum.

Malignant melanoma is the third most common skin cancer in patients with xeroderma pigmentosum, as it is in the general U.S. population. A 10- to 20-fold increase in internal malignancies over age-matched controls has been reported.

Ocular Changes

Sunlight-induced changes appear primarily on the eyelids, the conjunctivae, and the cornea. Photophobia may be one of the earliest symptoms of the disease. Blepharospasm and conjunctivitis without infection are common. Macular pigmentation, symblepharon, telangiectasia, pinguecula, and pterygium formation of the conjunctivae occur. Corneal vascularization, clouding, keratitis, and ulcers may be seen, with the subsequent development of corneal opacities. The eyelids show the same changes as the adjacent skin. Atrophy of the eyelids, loss of lashes, ectropion, and entropion have also been noted. Squamous cell carcinoma, basal cell carcinoma, and melanomas of the ocular tissues and limbus are almost exclusive to these sun-exposed structures.

Neurologic Abnormalities

Neurologic changes can be important associated symptoms in xeroderma pigmentosum involving up to 18% of patients.

Oral Changes

Severe atrophy and cancers of the oral structures appear to be due to sun exposure. In the oral cavity, the tip of the tongue may show telangiectasias and other changes, including squamous cell carcinoma.

Photosensitivity

The earliest skin abnormalities in patients with xeroderma pigmentosum include exaggerated sunburn reaction, delayed appearance of and/or the peak of erythema, excessive persistence of the erythema, telangiectasia and pigmentation persisting for several months, and light and electron microscopic evidence of chronic sun damage following a single UV exposure. The clinical action spectrum appears to fall primarily in the UVB range (290–320 nm). The minimal erythema dose to UVB radiation is usually normal in patients with xeroderma pigmentosum, and certainly some patients tan without an acute photosensitivity reaction. Some evidence also exists for impaired immune function.

Course and Prognosis

In the largest review of patients with xeroderma pigmentosum, only 5% were older than 45 years of age. The average age of death at that time (1975) was 30 years younger than that of the general U.S. population. The most common causes of death are melanoma and squamous cell carcinoma.

Pathogenesis and Etiology

Xeroderma pigmentosum is due to a genetic defect in the biochemical pathways by which damage caused by sunlight (UVB) to DNA is processed to eliminate its carcinogenic potential. Ezymatic DNA repair defects prevent proper DNA repair after UV-induced damage. The two major photoproducts induced are the cyclobutane pyrimidine dimer and, at about one fourth the frequency, the pyrimidine-pyrimidone (6-4) photoproduct. These photoproducts may play a major role in UVB (solar) mutagenesis.

Treatment

The cutaneous malignancies of patients with xeroderma pigmentosum are treated in a similar manner as those occurring in the general population. It is important for these patients to have regularly scheduled full skin exams to afford the earliest possible education regarding prevention of sun exposure, genetic counseling, and detection and treatment of cutaneous malignancies.

THE PORPHYRIAS

(CM&S Chapter 169)

Definition

Porphyrias are a group of inherited or acquired disorders that result from partial deficiency in activities of the enzymes of the heme biosynthetic pathway. Each porphyria is associated with a specific defective enzyme (Table 11–5), the reduced activity of which results in accumulation of intermediaries or by-products of the pathway in a characteristic pattern.

Clinical Description

Porphyrias are divisible into hepatic or erythropoietic types according to the site in which the heme synthetic defect is predominantly expressed. Porphyrias can also be divided into those manifesting cutaneous photosensitivity, neurovisceral symptomatology, or both. Among porphyrias with photocutaneous manifestations, division is possible between those exhibiting immediate or delayed phototoxicity. Porphyrin-sensitized immediate phototoxicity occurs during or shortly after sunlight exposure and is typified by stinging or burning pain followed by erythema, edema, and purpura. Immediate phototoxicity is induced by protoporphyrin, a hydrophobic

TABLE 11-5. Enzyme Defects Associated with Porphyrias	
DEFECT	**AFFECTED ENZYME**
Aminolevulinic acid dehydratase porphyria	Aminolevulinic acid dehydratase (porphobilinogen synthase)
Acute intermittent porphyria	Porphobilinogen deaminase (formerly uroporphyrinogen I synthase)
Congenital erythropoietic porphyria	Uroporphyrinogen III synthase (formerly uroporphyrinogen cosynthase)
Porphyria cutanea tarda	Uroporphyrinogen decarboxylase
Hepatoerythropoietic porphyria	Uroporphyrinogen decarboxylase
Hereditary coproporphyria	Coproporphyrinogen oxidase
Variegate porphyria	Protoporphyrinogen oxidase
Erythropoietic protoporphyria	Ferrochelatase (heme synthase)

molecule. Delayed porphyrin-sensitized photocutaneous lesions are induced by the more hydrophilic porphyrins and are indistinguishable among the several forms of porphyrias in which hydrophilic porphyrins accumulate: mechanical fragility, subepidermal blistering with subsequent milia formation and scarring, scarring alopecia, hypertrichosis, pigmentary changes, sclerodermoid lesions that may become calcified, and photo-onycholysis.

The Heme Biosynthetic Pathway

The heme biosynthetic pathway is shown in Figure 11–1. Reduced activity of any of its enzymes results in accumulation of its substrates. Large amounts of accumulated substrates escape conversion into pathway intermediaries and enter the blood circulation, either unchanged or as oxidized by-products of the pathway.

Porphyrins are red-brown crystalline pigments that are photoactive and cause photosensitivity; porphyrinogens and the porphyrin precursors are colorless and not photoactive. Porphyrins and precursors vary greatly in water solubility; molecules with greater hydrophilicity occur earlier in the pathway.

Accumulation of porphyrins and porphyrin precursors leads to an array of signs and symptoms that typify each clinical syndrome. Characteristic patterns of these metabolites in blood, urine, and feces distinguish porphyrias biochemically and are the usual means of confirming clinical diagnostic suspicions in the laboratory.

Photochemistry and Photobiology of Porphyrins and Porphyrias

The electronic configuration of porphyrin molecules permits their absorption of light radiation, with major absorption peaks in the

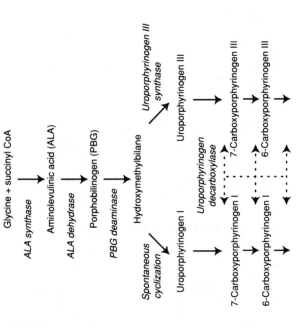

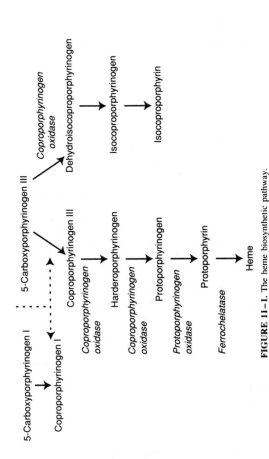

FIGURE 11-1. The heme biosynthetic pathway.

visible violet spectral range (400–410 nm). Long ultraviolet and longer visible light wavelengths can also photoexcite porphyrin molecules, but less strongly. The absorbed energy creates electronically excited-state molecules that can emit light energy (fluorescence), react directly with other biomolecules, or transfer excitation energy to oxygen, creating highly reactive oxygen species.

The Erythropoietic Porphyrias

Congenital Erythropoietic Porphyria

Congenital erythropoietic porphyria (CEP) is an autosomal recessive disorder in which defective activity of uroporphyrinogen III synthase leads to accumulation of the isomer I series of porphyrins (uroporphyrin I to coproporphyrin I) in erythroid cells. These porphyrins are released into plasma by hemolysis or diffusion; are deposited in tissues, bones, and teeth; and are excreted in urine and feces. The diagnosis is often manifested in the neonatal period by pink staining of diapers by porphyrin pigment in urine. Adult-onset cases have also been observed.

CEP is typified by marked cutaneous photosensitivity of the delayed type. Urine, bones, and teeth are stained red-brown. Hemolytic anemia with splenomegaly is common; bony fragility has been observed. Some patients are far less severely affected than others.

Laboratory diagnosis is based on demonstration of increased levels of the isomer I porphyrins in blood and urine. The differential diagnosis includes disorders that may present in childhood with porphyrinuria and bullous cutaneous photosensitivity:hepatoerythropoietic porphyria, childhood-onset porphyria cutanea tarda, or rare cases of homozygous inheritance of hepatic porphyrias typically transmitted as autosomal dominant traits.

Treatment of the cutaneous photosensitivity begins with sunlight avoidance; topical sunscreens are not useful unless formulated to block long ultraviolet and visible light wavelengths. Oral beta-carotene for photoprotection typically offers only limited benefit. Circulating porphyrin levels can be lowered by inhibiting erythropoiesis: hypertransfusion regimens and chemically induced bone marrow suppression have been effective in reducing clinical and biochemical disease expression. Splenectomy may decrease the rate of erythrocyte destruction but is not invariably associated with lasting biochemical or clinical benefit. The risks of therapies must be carefully weighed against the severity of the disorder in each individual case.

Erythropoietic Protoporphyria

Typically presenting in childhood as immediate phototoxicity with stinging, burning, erythema, and edema of skin developing within minutes to 1 hour or so of sunlight exposure, followed by a painful purpura, erythropoietic protoporphyria (EPP) occurs far more frequently than CEP. Vesiculation or hypertrichosis is infrequent. Exposed skin, especially of the dorsum of the hands and occasionally of the face, may become thickened, waxy, leathery, or hyperkeratotic. Facial skin may bear scattered shallow elliptical or linear scars and linear perioral furrowing. Anemia, if present, is typically mild. There is an increased incidence of cholelithiasis at unusually early ages in both males and females. Life-threatening hepatic dysfunction may develop at any age.

Laboratory diagnosis is based on demonstration of increased protoporphyrin in erythrocytes, plasma, and feces, all of which are normal in cases of solar urticaria, the major differential diagnosis for EPP. Urinary porphyrins are normal in EPP unless hepatic failure occurs, producing coproporphyrinuria.

Immediate porphyrin-induced phototoxicity produces acute cutaneous signs and symptoms. Biopsy specimens from the acute wheal-like lesions of EPP demonstrate sparse perivascular and interstitial neutrophilic infiltrates. Specimens of long-standing lesions of EPP examined by light microscopy most often reflect effects of chronic damage: markedly thickened papillary dermal capillary walls and an amorphous, hyaline material deposited perivascularly and scattered throughout the dermis.

Treatment of EPP begins with avoidance of sun exposure. Topical sunscreens must block long ultraviolet and visible light wavelengths to be effective. Preparations containing titanium dioxide or zinc oxide offer the protection of physical barriers; those with agents absorbing well into the ultraviolet A spectrum afford some benefit. Many individuals with EPP can increase their solar tolerance with oral beta-carotene in amounts sufficient to produce carotenodermia. Typical adult doses are 120 to 180 mg per day, increasing to 300 mg per day if efficacy is inadequate at lower doses. Children's doses range from 30 to 120 mg per day. Solar tolerance increases slowly; 3 to 4 weeks of treatment may be necessary to reach full benefit. In many latitudes, treatment is needed only in spring and summer months.

The dire prognosis of protoporphyrin-induced hepatic dysfunction warrants vigorous medical intervention. Oral cholestyramine resin has been used to sequester protoporphyrin in the enteric tract, thus protecting the liver from the toxic effects of its enterohepatic recirculation. Vitamin E has been given concomitantly in the hope of regulating hyperactive porphyrin synthesis. Administration of iron has been followed by clinical improvement in a few cases but has been linked to exacerbation of photosensitivity in others. Infusion of heme analogues, agents apparently effective in "acute attack" porphyrias by reducing hepatic heme synthesis by negative feedback repression of the rate-limiting enzyme ALA synthase, may affect erythropoietic heme synthesis as well but is not suited to long-term treatment. Liver transplantation is indicated as a last resort.

The Hepatic Porphyrias

Porphyria Cutanea Tarda

Porphyria cutanea tarda (PCT) is the only porphyria with both familial and acquired forms. Heterozygous inheritance of a gene mutation encoding partial deficiency of the activity of the enzyme uroporphyrinogen decarboxylase results in a disorder that presents typically in adults but occasionally in children. Childhood PCT is usually of the familial type. Homozygous inheritance of mutant genes results in a PCT-like disorder in childhood termed *hepatoerythropoietic porphyria* (HEP). Children with HEP can be differentiated from those with heterozygous PCT by demonstration of increased levels of zinc photoporphyrin in erythrocytes of those with HEP but not PCT. Measurement of residual erythrocyte uroporphyrinogen decarboxylase activity also permits differentiation.

Clinical signs of PCT and HEP include darkening of the urine and cutaneous photosensitivity of the delayed type, most often manifested by blistering, milia, scarring, and hypertrichosis of sun-exposed skin. Other cutaneous signs (pigmentary changes, sclerodermoid lesions, dystrophic calcification, alopecia, photo-onycholysis) are variably present; occasionally sclerodermoid changes occur alone. PCT (and HEP) is confirmed in the laboratory by demonstration of the excess porphyrin by-products resulting from the enzyme defect: chiefly uroporphyrin and heptacarboxylic porphyrins in urine and plasma or serum and isocoproporphyrin in feces. In most familial cases of PCT, deficient activity of uroporphyrinogen decarboxylase can be detected in erythrocytes as well as in liver cells, whereas in acquired or sporadic cases the erythrocyte enzyme activity is normal. In some families, PCT occurs with normal erythrocyte enzyme activity.

In sporadic or acquired PCT, and in many familial cases, disease expression requires exposure to additional factors or circumstances: ethanol intake, estrogenic hormone therapies, certain aromatic hydrocarbon hepatotoxins, causes of increased iron stores, or dialysis treatment of chronic renal disease. Serologic evidence of exposure to hepatitis B or C viruses or human immunodeficiency virus is increasingly recognized. Increased incidences of abnormal glucose tolerance and antinuclear antibody tests and of hepatocellular carcinoma are linked to PCT.

In PCT (and in all other porphyrias manifesting delayed-type phototoxicity), bullae form subepidermally and are characterized by "festooning," or upward protrusion of dermal papillae into the blister cavity and little or no dermal inflammatory infiltrate. Immunohistochemical studies demonstrate that the plane of separation in bullae due to porphyria is in the lamina lucida.

Therapeutic interventions can lead to biochemical and clinical remission of PCT but have not been successful in HEP. Avoidance of exogenous agents known to exacerbate the disease should be advised. If there are no contraindications, serial phlebotomy or low-dose chloroquine regimens or a combination of the two are the most frequently used therapies. The success of serial phlebotomy protocols appears related to removal of excess hepatic iron stores, which can be monitored by progressive diminution of serum ferritin levels. In practice, this can be accomplished by removal of approximately 500 mL of whole blood at weekly or biweekly intervals, while monitoring the hemoglobin level to limit symptoms of iatrogenic anemia.

Oral chloroquine or hydroxychloroquine regimens offer another approach suitable for patients in whom phlebotomy may be contraindicated or technically difficult. Given in low doses, these agents appear to facilitate liberation of porphyrins accumulated in hepatocytes, which are then excreted, accompanied by an increase in urinary iron excretion. Doses of 125 mg twice weekly of chloroquine or 100 mg thrice weekly of hydroxychloroquine appear to be appropriate levels for initiation of treatment. Liver function tests are recommended before treatment and at biweekly intervals thereafter.

Glucose-6-phosphate dehydrogenase testing before treatment and interval ophthalmologic evaluations are recommended.

The differential diagnosis of PCT and HEP includes all of the other porphyrias that may present with similar skin lesions (CEP, variegate porphyria, hereditary coproporphyria), all being distinguishable by their different porphyrin laboratory profiles. A wide array of drugs, exposure to tanning beds, and maintenance hemodialysis treatment are linked to occurrence of photocutaneous bullae that are clinically and histologically similar to those of PCT. Such occurrences have been termed *pseudoporphyria*. Absence of abnormal porphyrin laboratory profiles allows differentiation of these from true PCT. Epidermolysis bullosa acquisita and bullous lupus erythematosus, which may also resemble PCT clinically, are similarly differentiated.

Acute Intermittent Porphyria

Acute intermittent porphyria (AIP) is not manifested by cutaneous photosensitivity but rather by a wide array of episodic or chronic neurologic dysfunctions that may affect peripheral, autonomic, or central nervous systems. These neurovisceral symptoms occur most often after puberty, vary in frequency and severity, and can be precipitated by many drugs, infections, carbohydrate restriction, or endogenous or exogenous hormonal fluctuations. Similar attacks of potentially life-threatening severity also characterize aminolevulinic acid dehydratase porphyria, variegate porphyria, and hereditary coproporphyria.

During such episodes, urinary ALA and PBG are excreted copiously in all of the "acute attack" porphyrias and typically remain abnormal even in quiescent periods in AIP. AIP can be confirmed by demonstration of deficient activity of erythrocyte PBG deaminase at about 50% of normal values.

Treatment of AIP (and of the other acute attack porphyrias) is primarily preventive: patients must avoid drugs and factors that induce heme biosynthesis. Once an attack has begun, intensive care may be required. Oral or intravenous loading with glucose may repress the induced heme biosynthetic pathway, as may intravenously administered heme analogues.

Hereditary Coproporphyria

Photosensitivity resembling that of PCT occurs in about 30% of cases of hereditary coproporphyria (HCP). Neurovisceral problems are more frequently manifested. Many heterozygotes remain biochemically and clinically silent. As in AIP and variegate porphyria, onset of symptoms in heterozygotes is rare until after puberty. Although laboratory diagnosis of HCP is based on demonstration of increased excretion of coproporphyrin III in both urine and feces as a result of deficient activity of coproporphyrinogen oxidase, levels of ALA and PBG in urine become elevated during "attack" episodes.

Variegate Porphyria

Individuals with variegate porphyria (VP) may exhibit either cutaneous or systemic manifestations or both and can be shown to have approximately 50% reduction in protoporphyrinogen oxidase activity.

The diagnostic porphyrin profile includes elevated levels of both protoporphyrin and coproporphyrin in feces, with protoporphyrin usually in greater proportion. Abnormal porphyrinuria is variably present, with coproporphyrin generally in excess of uroporphyrin when observed. Plasma or serum porphyrin levels are elevated when the disease is active and exhibit a distinctive fluorescence emission spectrum peak that is diagnostic.

The differential diagnosis and approaches to treatment are as noted for the other ''acute attack'' porphyrias. In the absence of neurovisceral symptoms, misdiagnosis of individuals with VP as having PCT is not uncommon. Treatments effective in PCT are not beneficial and are inappropriate in VP.

ACRODERMATITIS ENTEROPATHICA

(CM&S Chapter 170)

Definition and Clinical Description

Acrodermatitis enteropathica is a rare autosomal recessive disorder characterized by acral and periorificial dermatitis, alopecia, and diarrhea. The disease results from an inability to absorb sufficient amounts of zinc from the diet and generally affects infants and young children. Premature infants are especially at risk because the full complement of neonatal gene is not received until the late third trimester.

Acquired forms of acrodermatitis enteropathica occur in patients with malabsorption or abnormal excretion of zinc or with malnutrition and in patients receiving inadequate hyperalimentation.

The disease is usually not present at birth but typically develops either after weaning from breast milk or during the first few weeks or months of life. The clinical syndrome of acrodermatitis enteropathica is characterized by dermatologic, gastrointestinal, and psychological abnormalities.

Affected individuals develop a symmetrical acral (extensor surfaces of the major joints, fingers, and toes) and periorificial (mouth, nose, eyes, ears, and perineum) vesiculobullous dermatitis that becomes crusted and psoriasiform. Involvement of the digits is manifested by an erythematous dermatitis, paronychial tissue swelling, and nail dystrophy. Perlèche is a common early sign. The tongue and buccal mucosa may either develop superficial aphthous-like lesions or be secondarily infected with *Candida albicans*. Alopecia results when the scalp is involved. In addition, conjunctivitis, blepharitis, and photophobia may be present.

The gastrointestinal disturbance is primarily diarrhea with irregular exacerbations and remissions. Psychological symptoms include mental depression, irritability, and loss of appetite.

Pathology

Histopathologically, the psoriasiform plaques of acrodermatitis enteropathica are characterized by diffuse parakeratosis and psori-

asiform epidermal hyperplasia with characteristic large pale keratinocytes in the upper spinous layers and dyskeratotic cells.

Differential Diagnosis

The differential diagnosis of acrodermatitis enteropathica includes candidiasis, pustular psoriasis, epidermolysis bullosa, porphyria, and other deficiency states such as pellagra and necrolytic
migratory erythema.

Treatment

The clinical findings of acrodermatitis enteropathica are rapidly
and dramatically reversed by dietary supplementation with zinc sulfate in a daily dose of 1 to 2 mg/kg in children or 220 mg three times
daily in adults. Supplemental zinc should probably be maintained
indefinitely and be monitored twice a year, particularly in women of
childbearing age who either may become pregnant or want to take
oral contraceptives.

INHERITED ENZYME DISEASES

(CM&S Chapter 171)

Gaucher's Disease

All of the inherited disorders of glucosylceramide catabolism are
collectively known as Gaucher's disease. Each of the three subtypes
of Gaucher's disease is inherited as an autosomal recessive trait.
The gene for glucocerebrosidase has been cloned and mapped to
chromosome 1q21.

The three types of Gaucher's disease are related biochemically in
that all accumulate the lipid glucosylceramide and all types are deficient in lysosomal glucocerebrosidase (also called acid β-glucosi-
dase). Each subtype represents a grouping of similar phenotypes
rather than a single genotype that may or may not be representative
of different mutations.

Type 1 (nonneuronopathic) encompasses 99% of the cases of
Gaucher's disease evaluated. This form has a chronic time course
and manifests with hepatosplenomegaly, thrombocytopenia, anemia, bleeding diathesis, and bone disease. Although the severity and
onset of symptoms may vary widely, type 1 disease is distinguished
by the lack of neuropathology. This disorder may become manifest
at any age and is panethnic, but it occurs more frequently in Eastern
European (Ashkenazi) Jews. This group tends to have less severe
disease than the general population, with more severe disease being
evident in affected blacks.

Type 2 Gaucher's disease (acute neuronopathic) is clinically a
stereotypic, rapidly progressive neurovisceral storage disease that is
usually fatal within the first 2 years of life. Hepatosplenomegaly is
common to this as well as all subtypes of this disorder.

Type 3 (subacute neuronopathic) varies in severity but is usually less rapidly progressive than types 1 or 2. Afflicted children develop ataxia, myoclonus, seizures, and dementia. The degree of hepato-splenomegaly and skeletal involvement is variable, but death occurs in early childhood. All ethnic groups may be affected, but this form of Gaucher's disease is rare.

Patients with Gaucher's disease are deficient in glucocerebrosi-dase, which is a specialized lysosomal acid β-glucosidase. The glu-cosylceramide accumulates primarily in the lysosomes of the reticu-loendothelial cells.

The skin in adult patients with Gaucher's disease may have an abnormal diffuse yellow-brown skin pigmentation. This may be most evident on the face and legs. Gaucher's cells are not found in the skin, but afflicted patients may have increased deposition of hemosiderin and melanin is present in increased amounts in the basal layer of the epidermis.

Therapy

Enzyme replacement therapy that is macrophage targeted has been developed and tested in patients with Gaucher's disease. This macrophage-targeted human placental glucocerebrosidase (alglu-cerase) is administered intravenously and has resulted in objective clinical improvement in patients with type 1 Gaucher's disease.

Hartnup's Disorder

Hartnup's disorder is an impairment of neutral amino acid trans-port that involves the kidneys, the intestine, or both. The diagnosis is based on biochemical rather than clinical abnormalities. Affected individuals show a characteristic urinary pattern of monoamino-monocarboxylic amino acids (alanine, serine, threonine, valine, leu-cine, isoleucine, phenylalanine, tyrosine, tryptophan, and histidine) and monoaminodicarboxylic amides (glutamine and asparagine), which are excreted in amounts 5 to 20 times normal. Blood amino acids are either low or normal in amount in these patients. Hartnup's disorder is an autosomal recessive trait.

The most frequent clinical abnormality seen in Hartnup's patients is an unusual ''pellagra-like'' skin rash. Affected individuals can have onset from as early as 10 days to as late as 13 years. The rash appears on uncovered areas of the body after sunlight exposure. Histopathologic examination shows changes similar to those in pel-lagra, acrodermatitis enteropathica, and other conditions in which there are deficiencies of amino acids. Other clinical manifestations that are sometimes seen are primarily neurologic and include ataxia, mental retardation, increased muscle tone, and increased deep ten-don reflexes. Ataxia is the most commonly reported neurologic symptom, and it is intermittent in nature. Somatic abnormalities occasionally seen in some Hartnup's patients that are thought to be related to the disease include atrophic glossitis and small stature.

Therapy

Due to the similarities to pellagra, nicotinic acid and nicotinamide have been used as therapies in patients with signs suggesting a defi-ciency of this vitamin. Amounts from 50 to 300 mg daily given orally have been tried. The rash, ataxia, and psychotic behavior have been reported responsive; however, neither the hyperaminoaciduria nor the intestinal transport defect responds to this therapy.

INHERITED ELASTIC TISSUE MALFORMATIONS

(CM&S Chapter 172)

Pseudoxanthoma Elasticum

Definition

Pseudoxanthoma elasticum is an inherited disorder of connective tissue of unknown cause in which the elastic fibers of the skin, retinae, and cardiovascular system become slowly calcified. Both autosomal recessive and autosomal dominant inheritance patterns occur in affected kindreds, with approximately 90% showing an autosomal recessive pattern.

Clinical Description

The estimated prevalence of pseudoxanthoma elasticum in the population is 1 in 100,000. There is a 2 to 1 female predominance. There is a tight clustering of new cases starting in the 10- to 15-year age group and a broad age range of 2 years to 50 years. Overall longevity is believed to be normal.

Cutaneous Manifestations

There are two major diagnostic features: (1) characteristic yellow-orange, plucked chicken skin, linear papules that coalesce to form larger plaques; and (2) a unique localization to flexural sites —predominantly lateral neck, antecubital fossae, axillae, groin, and popliteal space—with almost perfect symmetry. The initial diagnostic manifestation of pseudoxanthoma elasticum is almost always lateral neck skin lesions. Gradual centripetal extension beyond the primary flexural neck lesions may occur.

Ocular Manifestations

Calcification of the elastic fibers in Bruch's membrane layer of the retina allows for cracking of this layer, producing angioid streaks most commonly appearing several years after the first skin lesions. Angioid streaks are a hallmark, but not specific or pathognomonic of pseudoxanthoma elasticum and eventuate in nearly 100% of patients.

Retinal hemorrhages occur with increasing frequency in the fifth decade, and by the seventh decade, about 90% of persons with pseudoxanthoma elasticum will have experienced at least one retinal hemorrhage and will have varying degrees of loss of central vision.

Cardiovascular Manifestations

The cardiovascular manifestations of pseudoxanthoma elasticum develop later; the first sign is often symptomatic calcification of the elastic media and intima of arteries. The most significant vascular complication is gastrointestinal (primarily gastric) hemorrhage, which may come without warning, usually in the 2nd or 4th decade, and be severe enough to warrant hospitalization, blood transfusion, and occasionally surgery with a partial gastrectomy. It affects approximately 10% of patients with pseudoxanthoma elasticum.

Pathology

The three known pathophysiologic events in pseudoxanthoma elasticum include (1) mineralization of elastic fibers; (2) increased concentrations of glycosaminoglycans in the affected dermis; and (3) an increase in elastic fibers in the dermis. The principal finding in the lesional skin of patients with pseudoxanthoma elasticum is an accumulation of fragmented elastic fibers in the mid and deep reticular dermis.

Differential Diagnosis

Long-term penicillamine therapy produces clinical changes that resemble pseudoxanthoma elasticum, but they are not usually flexural and they are histologically dissimilar.

Treatment

Despite the incurable nature of pseudoxanthoma elasticum, there are numerous measures that can alter the course of the disease and prevent or minimize risk factors. The earlier in life prophylactic measures are instituted, the more effective most will be (Table 11–6).

Ehlers-Danlos Syndrome

Definition and Clinical Description

Ehlers-Danlos syndrome is a clinically heterogeneous syndrome made up of nine (possibly ten) types of all three major inheritance patterns—autosomal dominant, autosomal recessive, and X-linked. Except for one of the types (type V), the skin is light in color, thin,

---

TABLE 11–6. Treatment of Pseudoxanthoma Elasticum

Maintenance of a low calcium diet
Avoidance of head-contact sports
Control of serum lipids
Exercise and weight control
Detect and treat retinal changes early
Limitation of the number of pregnancies
Control of hypertension
Avoidance of tobacco
Awareness of possible gastrointestinal hemorrhage
Avoidance of aspirin and nonsteroidal anti-inflammatory drugs
Genetic counseling

---

smooth with a velvety feel, and extremely hyperelastic such that when pulled it rapidly retracts when released.

Cutaneous fragility (dermatorrhexis) is markedly increased and is particularly troublesome over bony pressure points (knees, elbows, forehead, shins) where mild trauma causes gaping "fish mouth" wounds that are difficult to close because the skin does not hold sutures well. Healing is slow, leaving a thin, shiny, cigarette paper—like scar. Such lacerations are common during childhood when minor trauma is common. After multiple traumatic episodes with scarring and cutaneous hemorrhages, soft, heaped-up pseudotumors develop.

Another feature of Ehlers-Danlos syndrome skin is easy bruisability and hemorrhage believed due to the poor connective tissue support of the vasculature and direct involvement of the vessel wall. Gingival bleeding after brushing is a common experience, as is excessive hemorrhage after surgical procedures. Life-threatening cerebral and coronary aneurysms may occur, especially in type IV.

The other major characteristic of Ehlers-Danlos syndrome is variable and sometimes dramatic hyperextensibility of the joints with marked laxity of the joint capsules, ligaments, and tendons.

Hernias are common. Pregnancy is often complicated by premature rupture of the membranes and premature delivery with severe postpartum hemorrhage in all types, but especially in type IV. Ocular complications including retinal detachment and retinal hemorrhages are frequent.

There are probably multiple genetic defects to account for the clinical heterogeneity seen in this disorder. The most common recognized types of Ehlers-Danlos syndrome are summarized in Table 11–7.

Differential Diagnosis

Several heritable syndromes have features of hyperelastic skin or joint hyperextensibility similar to those of Ehlers-Danlos syndrome; however, they are seldom combined. Some of the disorders include Marfan's syndrome, osteogenesis imperfecta, and cutis laxa.

Treatment

Genetic counseling is essential. Some of the more important prophylactic and therapeutic measures include physical therapy; protective garments worn over bony prominences to pad fragile skin and reduce tears; extra suturing to close torn wounds; avoiding vigorous contact sports; counseling regarding increased risks for sudden arterial hemorrhages and bowel perforation; and taking antibiotics before surgery and dental procedures in individuals with mitral valve prolapse.

Acrokeratoelastoidosis

Clinical Description

In acrokeratoelastoidosis 2- to 4-mm shiny hyperkeratotic papules appear during childhood or adolescence, occurring on the dorsal hands, usually over the knuckles and often in groups. The lateral margins of the palms and soles may also be involved.

690

TABLE 11-7. Types of Ehlers-Danlos Syndrome

TYPE	SKIN SIGNS Elasticity	Fragility	Bruising	JOINT LAXITY	COMPLICATIONS	INHERITANCE	PRIMARY DEFECT
I (gravis)	(+++)	(+++)	(++)	(+++)	Bowel, aorta rupture	AD	Unknown
II (mitis)	(++)	(++)	(+)	(++)	Few complications (often undiagnosed)	AD	Unknown
III (hypermobile)	(+)	(+)	(+)	(+++)	Arthritis muscle pain	AD	Unknown
IV	(−)	(+++)	(+++)	(+)	Aneurysms with rupture; severe obstetric hemorrhage; pneumothorax	AD	Type III collagen deficiency
V	(+++)	(+)	(+)	(+)	Same as I, II, and III but less severe	Probably XL	
VI	(+++)	(++)	(++)	(+++)	Muscle hypotonia; kyphoscoliosis; osteoporosis; eye globe rupture	AR	Lysyl hydroxylase deficiency in most cases
VII	(++)	(+)	(+)	(++++)	Severe ligament and joint laxity; congenital hip arthritis	AD	Missing N-telopeptid of α_1(I) or α_2(I) chains of collagen type I (three possible subtypes)

680

Pathology

Fibers in the reticular dermis are fragmented and diminished in number.

Treatment

Essentially no treatment is needed. Shave excision or electro-desiccation may be tried but may leave scars.

FOCAL DERMAL HYPOPLASIA AND APLASIA CUTIS CONGENITA

(CM&S Chapter 173)

Focal Dermal Hypoplasia

Definition and Clinical Description

Focal dermal hypoplasia (Goltz syndrome; Goltz-Gorlin syndrome) is an X-linked recessive disorder characterized by ectodermal and mesodermal abnormalities. The skin, bones, and teeth are the most common sites of involvement, but multiple other organ systems can be affected.

Several diverse skin lesions have been noted, primarily in linear patterns corresponding to the lines of Blashko. These include pink or reddish-brown atrophic-appearing macules in a cribriform pattern; poikiloderma; scar-like areas; soft, yellow-brown fat "herniation"; macular hyper- and hypopigmentation; and papillomatous areas, particularly around the mucous membranes and periorificial areas. At birth, areas of aplasia cutis may be noted. An inflammatory or desquamative phase and even blistering or crusting may be present, occasionally preceding the development of other skin findings. Other less common cutaneous manifestations include hyper- and hypohidrosis, lichenoid follicular papules, urtication or intense erythema upon stroking the skin, radial folds around the mouth, and keratotic lesions of the palms and soles. The hair may be brittle or sparse, contain areas of localized poliosis, and be totally missing with areas of scarring noted. The nails may also be absent, poorly developed, dystrophic, spooned, grooved, or hypopigmented. In addition to the diverse array of skin lesions, the severity of skin and systemic manifestations may vary considerably; in mild cases, only faint reddish-brown linear atrophic areas may be present, making diagnosis elusive, until a more severely affected offspring is born.

Skeletal abnormalities are very common, especially syndactyly, often of the third and fourth fingers or of the second and third toes. Other reported skeletal abnormalities include short stature; hemiatrophy; microcephaly; complete hypoplasia, absence or fusion of digits; camptodactyly; clinodactyly; kyphosis; scoliosis; fusion of vertebrae; rib anomalies; and multiple giant cell tumors of the bone.

Oral and dental abnormalities are also relatively common, occurring in approximately one half of affected patients. These include missing teeth, enamel defects, irregular spacing, malocclusion, notching of incisors, extra teeth, mandibular hypoplasia, prognathism, papillomatous lip and gingival lesions.

The wide variety of other described manifestations include eye abnormalities, facial asymmetry, mental deficiency, renal and ureteral anomalies, and cardiac anomalies.

Pathology

Areas of aplasia cutis congenita demonstrate absence of appendages and a thinner than normal dermis, either covered by an epidermis or devoid of one. The atrophic areas, whether irregular in shape or linear, have clusters of adipocytes that are abnormally situated in the mid or upper reticular dermis or in the papillary dermis.

Diagnosis and Differential Diagnosis

Diagnosis is made based on the clinical findings, correlated with the skin histopathology of affected skin. Long-bone films looking for osteopathia striata may be helpful. Differential diagnosis includes incontinentia pigmenti, the epidermal nevus syndrome, linear porokeratosis, and the ectodermal dysplasia ectrodactyly clefting syndrome.

Treatment

There is no specific treatment of focal dermal hypoplasia. Papillomatous lesions may be excised if they become cosmetically or functionally bothersome. Orthopedic surgery may help some limb abnormalities. All affected individuals should have dental and ophthalmologic evaluations and be carefully monitored for musculoskeletal, genitourinary, and developmental problems. Other family members should be examined for abnormalities. Genetic counseling should be given to the affected individual and family. Even in the absence of a precise genetic marker, prenatal diagnosis may be helpful in identifying a female infant at greater risk by using ultrasound to search for severe skeletal anomalies.

Aplasia Cutis Congenita

Definition

Aplasia cutis congenita, *congenital localized absence of skin*, is characterized by localized area(s) of absent skin at birth. This clinical finding is caused by a heterogeneous group of diseases including autosomal dominant and recessive genetic disorders, chromosomal abnormalities, teratogens, intrauterine infections, and intrauterine vascular accidents. Many cases are of unknown etiology.

Clinical Description

The clinical findings of aplasia cutis congenita depend at least in part on the cause and location of the defect. The condition is by definition present at birth, but small lesions may occasionally be overlooked during the newborn period, particularly in an infant with thick hair. Lesions may also appear as scars, rather than skin defects, presumably due to in utero healing.

The scalp is the most common site of involvement, occurring in approximately 80% of cases. The size of the defect varies from a few millimeters to as large as 100 cm. Larger defects are often deeper and may extend to the dura or meninges. Seventy-five per cent of scalp lesions are solitary. The lesions may have a variable appearance, with a raw friable surface, crusted, blister-like with a thin or thick membrane covering the defect or with a mature atrophic scar at the time of birth.

Pathology

Affected skin in aplasia cutis congenita shows a range of findings from complete absence of the epidermis and dermis, with a thin or thick band of scar in their place, either covered by a re-epithelialized epidermis or bare of one.

Differential Diagnosis

The differential diagnosis includes obstetrical trauma, bullous diseases, and congenital alopecia.

Treatment

Virtually all lesions of aplasia cutis congenita will heal with resultant scarring, but the extent of scarring and need for medical and/or surgical intervention are directly related to the size and extent of lesions. Small lesions heal by secondary intention without significant complications. Larger lesions, especially those more than 3 to 4 cm in diameter, are more susceptible to secondary infection and hemorrhage and may require skin grafting. In deep lesions, full-thickness skin flaps or bone grafting may be necessary.

NEVOID CONDITIONS OF EPIDERMIS, DERMIS, AND SUBCUTANEOUS TISSUE

(CM&S Chapter 174)

In its broadest and original sense, the term *nevus* refers to abnormalities of either structure (malformations) or cellular composition (hamartomas) of the skin. These conditions, which can be classified according to the malformed tissue or cell of origin (Table 11–8), are usually congenital, but sometimes their appearance is delayed into childhood or even young adult life.

Epidermal Nevi

Definition and Clinical Features

Epidermal nevi are inborn abnormalities of the epidermis and often also of the papillary dermis. The term *epidermal nevus syndrome* refers to a heterogeneous group of disorders in which there is an association of epidermal nevi with abnormalities in other organ systems. Epidermal nevi of the keratinocytic type come in an array of sizes and shapes, ranging from trivial lesions of a few centimeters to catastrophic ones covering much of the trunk, limbs, and head

---

TABLE 11-8. Classification of Nevoid Conditions of the Skin

Nevoid conditions of the epidermis and appendages
  Epidermal nevus, keratinocytic type
  Sebaceous nevus
  Follicuar nevus—nevus comedonicus
  Sweat gland nevus (see Chapter 10 in this text or Chapter 145 in CM&S)
    Apocrine
    Eccrine
  Becker's nevus (see Chapter 7 in this text or Chapter 132 in CM&S)
  Vascular nevi and malformations (see Chapter 10 in this text or Chapter 146 in CM&S)
Melanocytic nevi

Dermal and subcutaneous nevi
  Collagen and elastic tissue nevi—collagenoma
  Elastic tissue nevus
  Fat nevi
    Nevus lipomatosus
  Muscular nevi
    Congenital smooth muscle hamartoma

---

that disfigure a child and can be associated with important extracutaneous abnormalities. They may involve any area of skin and even extend into the oral cavity. They may be congenital or appear in the first months or years of life. Almost all nevi on the head and neck present at birth and enlarge in proportion to the patient's growth. Delayed-onset lesions may extend far beyond their original distribution.

Epidermal nevi may have a flat surface or one that is papillated, or they may be very raised and warty. The color varies from black through brown to pale gray. Single or multiple plaques or lines are seen, often arranged in a streaky, swirled, or segmental distribution. Inflammatory epidermal nevus appears as a linear array of pink to red papules, usually on the lower limb and/or adjacent buttock and hip area, clinically resembling psoriasis or eczematous dermatitis. Epithelial neoplasms rarely develop in epidermal nevi, usually in adult life.

Pathology, Pathogenesis, and Etiology

In the most common form of epidermal nevus (nevus verrucosus), the epidermis is papillated and there is compact hyperkeratosis. Abnormalities of keratinocytic maturation are present in other types of epidermal nevi, such as focal acantholytic dyskeratosis (as occurs in Darier's disease), suprabasilar acantholysis without dyskeratosis (the pattern evident in Hailey-Hailey disease), and cornoid lamellation (the hallmark of porokeratosis). These findings may reflect mosaicism for genes that would ordinarily produce the corresponding diseases in a widespread distribution.

Epidermal nevi arise from the embryonic ectoderm, which gives rise to keratinocytes and also to the cells of epithelial appendages. The mesoderm may also be affected, as the papillary dermis in nevus verrucosus is also abnormal and therapies that do not ablate it are often unsuccessful. Each type of epidermal nevus may represent the cutaneous manifestation of a different mosaic phenotype. In favor of the mosaic hypothesis is the fact that most epidermal nevi follow the lines of Blaschko, which do not correspond to any known neural or vascular structures but probably represent the migration tracks of clones of genetically identical cells.

There are probably many epidermal nevus syndromes, each representing a particular mosaic phenotype. Most reported associations have been ocular, neurologic, and skeletal. In general, nevi of the head and neck are associated with ocular and neurologic abnormalities and those on the trunk and limbs with skeletal anomalies. Several entities are well defined. There is a subgroup of patients with nevi of the sebaceous type (see below) on the head and neck who demonstrate ipsilateral hemimegalencephaly and gyral malformations, mental retardation, seizures, and contralateral hemiparesis. In the Proteus syndrome, a folded type of epidermal and dermal nevus is associated with hemihypertrophy, partial gigantism of hands and feet, and a variety of vascular and connective tissue hamartomas. In the CHILD syndrome, congenital hemidysplasia and an ichthyosiform verrucous epidermal nevus occurs with limb defects. Significant developmental abnormalities occur in about 1.7% of all neonates.

Differential Diagnosis

Verrucous epidermal nevi are sometimes confused with seborrheic keratoses and with nevus sebaceus.

Treatment

Therapy of epidermal nevi is difficult. Recurrence is almost invariable with destructive modalities unless the dermis underlying the nevus is also destroyed. Excision is appropriate for small lesions and narrow linear lesions and for cosmetically troublesome or irritating areas of some widespread nevi. Topical retinoic acid or lactic acid may temporarily flatten very thick areas.

Nevus Sebaceus

Definition

Nevus sebaceus (of Jadassohn) is a circumscribed abnormality of the skin that includes many of the findings of a verrucous epidermal nevus but also is accompanied by malformations of the dermis, including most prominently abnormal positioning and hypertrophy of sebaceous epithelium. Mesenchymal elements can also be abnormal; hence the name *organoid nevus*.

Clinical Features

Nevus sebaceus occurs almost always on the scalp and face, areas rich in sebaceous glands. They are characteristically yellow or occasionally pink in color and are present at birth as fairly flat, hairless plaques, with a smooth waxy surface, linear or oval in shape. They have a tendency to become raised and warty and are often irritable at puberty. The development of a variety of benign and malignant secondary neoplasms in nevus sebaceus at or after puberty, such as syringocystadenoma papilliferum, leiomyoma, keratoacanthoma, and basal cell, squamous cell, sebaceous, and apocrine carcinoma, is much more common than in epidermal nevi of the keratinocytic type.

Differential Diagnosis

The differential diagnosis of nevus sebaceus is essentially the same as that of epidermal nevi.

Treatment

Complete excision with conservative margins is the best approach when feasible.

Nevus Comedonicus

The typical nevus comedonicus is composed of dilated follicular openings filled with comedo-like keratin plugs. Groups of these structures occur in a linear or swirled configuration sometimes covering large areas of face, trunk, or limbs. Particularly after puberty, inflamed acne-like cysts and deep scars can develop within the lesion.

Dermal and Subcutaneous Nevi

Cutaneous Collagenoma

Collagenomas are uncommon connective tissue nevi composed of dense dermal collagen, often with a reduction in elastic fibers. Occasionally they occur as solitary lesions, but most commonly they present as multiple asymptomatic, firm, flesh-colored dermal nodules symmetrically distributed on the upper trunk and arms. They vary in size from a few millimeters to several centimeters. They may be slightly elevated, flat, or indented producing a peau d'orange appearance. The usual time of onset is in adolescence. The condition may be autosomal dominant or sporadic, and it may occur in several syndromes, including tuberous sclerosis, in which the collagenoma presents as the ''shagreen patch,'' a firm dermal plaque with a pebbly surface, usually in the lumbosacral area. Excision is curative but may not be practical in patients with many lesions.

Elastic Tissue Nevus and the Buschke-Ollendorff Syndrome

Elastic tissue nevi are dermal papules within which there are increased numbers of elastic fibers. They can occur as yellow or flesh-colored solitary or multiple lesions. When dominantly inherited, they are termed the Buschke-Ollendorff syndrome. Multiple connective tissue nevi, usually of the elastic tissue type, but occasionally collagenomas, are associated with osteopoikilosis, or focal thickening of the long bones.

Nevoid Conditions of Adipose Tissue —Superficial Lipomatous Nevus

This rare hamartoma, also termed *nevus lipomatosus superficialis,* consists of soft, clustered yellow to skin-colored nodules caused by the abnormal presence of adipose tissue within the dermis, which are usually present at birth or in the early years of life. Nevus lipomatosus can be removed by shave excision.

Muscular Nevi

Congenital Smooth Muscle Hamartoma

Smooth muscle hamartomas are uncommon lesions that may be congenital or arise in childhood or adolescence. The typical appearance is of a solitary, slightly hyperpigmented plaque or patch, usually located on the trunk, buttocks, or proximal limbs with associated hypertrichosis. The lesion may become raised on firm stroking as a result of the contraction of large arrector pili muscles. The condition is not associated with any systemic abnormalities or malformations.

chapter 12

What Are the Disorders of Deposition and Cellular Secretion?

XANTHOMAS

(CM&S Chapter 176)

Definition

Xanthomas, which are localized infiltrates of lipid containing foamy macrophages in either the dermis or tendons, are important clinical clues to underlying systemic disturbances in lipoprotein metabolism that subsequently lead to the development of two life-threatening conditions: atherosclerotic cardiovascular disease and pancreatitis. The lipids that accumulate in xanthomas and in the intima of blood vessels are derived from lipids carried in lipoproteins (1) when the lipoproteins are found in high plasma concentrations or (2) when the lipoprotein levels are normal but their biochemical structure is altered.

Clinical Description

Xanthomas usually appear in one of four general forms, occurring either in the skin or in tendons or tendon sheaths: tendinous, planar, tuberous, and eruptive. The form of the xanthomas helps to identify the lipoprotein abnormality.

Tendinous xanthomas arise in tendons, ligaments, and fascia and are noted initially as deeply situated, smooth, firm nodules of various sizes covered by normal-appearing, freely movable skin. They occur most frequently in extensor tendons of the hands, knees, elbows, and Achilles tendons.

The finding of tendinous xanthomas almost always indicates an underlying disturbance in cholesterol and in low-density and intermediate-density lipoprotein metabolism. Coronary atherosclerosis is also a frequent finding. Rarely, tendinous xanthomas are found in the presence of normal plasma cholesterol.

Planar xanthomas appear as yellow, soft, and either macular or slightly elevated smooth-surfaced plaques. The most common planar xanthoma is xanthelasma palpebrarum, which occurs on the eyelids. Although such xanthomas suggest the presence of underlying hypercholesterolemia, when these are seen in patients younger than 40 to 50 years of age only about half will have plasma lipid elevations. A frequent accompanying clinical finding in patients with tendinous xanthomas, xanthelasmas, and hypercholesterolemia is corneal arcus, consisting of whitish yellow infiltrates of cholesterol, triglyceride, and phospholipid in the peripheral corneal limbus.

A second type of planar xanthoma has been termed *xanthoma striatum palmare* and appears as flat, yellow to orange, linear lesions in the creases of the palms and fingers. Conditions causing elevated plasma cholesterol and triglycerides (increases in very-low-density and intermediate-density lipoproteins) are usually associated with this form of xanthomas.

A third form of planar xanthomatosis is extensive, yellow-orange infiltrative, soft plaques that diffusely involve the face, neck, and even upper portions of the trunk and arms observed in association with paraproteinemias or various causes of cholestatic liver disease. Increases in blood cholesterol levels are usually found.

Tuberous xanthomas appear as yellow to red papules that evolve into larger firm nodules, usually over extensor surfaces of the body (elbows, knees, buttocks) as well as the palms. Such xanthomas indicate a systemic alteration in lipid metabolism when cholesterol and/or triglyceride amounts are increased. Increases in intermediate-density lipoproteins (as occurs in type III, dysbetalipoproteinemia) are most frequent, but they can also occur with increases in low-density lipoproteins (LDL).

Eruptive xanthomas are characterized by small, yellow, cutaneous papules, 1 to 4 mm in diameter, with an erythematous halo around the base. They erupt suddenly in crops over the extensor surfaces of the arms, legs, and buttocks. These forms of xanthomas develop almost exclusively in the presence of hyperlipemic plasma due to elevated serum levels of triglycerides (i.e., increased chylomicrons, very-low-density lipoproteins [VLDL], and intermediate-density lipoproteins [IDL]). Pancreatitis is frequently associated.

Lipoproteins Atherogenicity and Propensity to Form Xanthomas

In general, chylomicrons and VLDL when found in high concentrations predispose to eruptive xanthomas; elevated levels of LDL are associated with tendinous and planar xanthomas (xanthelasma and intertriginous xanthomas); while IDL, when increased, can cause tuberous xanthomas and xanthoma striatum palmare.

Pathology

The various forms of cutaneous xanthomas due to altered lipid metabolism have in common the accumulation of macrophages with foamy cytoplasm but differ in respect to their location and the degree of fibrosis that accompanies them.

Pathogenesis

Disorders of Lipoprotein Metabolism

Abnormal accumulation of lipoprotein in the plasma results from (1) excessive production, (2) defective removal or decreased catabolism, or (3) a combination of both mechanisms. Defective removal of lipoprotein has been shown to be due to several processes, including enzyme deficiencies, defective formation of certain apoproteins that serve as ligands for cellular receptors, and deficiencies in cellular receptors.

These metabolic aberrations in lipoprotein metabolism may be seen either as a primary manifestation of specific genetic disorders (primary hyperlipoproteinemia) or as an associated phenomenon secondary to specific underlying disease (e.g., diabetes, hypothyroidism, pancreatitis, from drugs causing or accentuating hyperlipoproteinemias, cholestatic liver disease, and dysgammaglobulinemias and paraproteinemia)—so-called secondary hyperlipoproteinemia.

Normolipidemic Xanthomatosis

Xanthomas can arise in the absence of elevated blood lipids (or at least in the absence of hypercholesterolemia or hypertriglyceridemia) or lipoproteins. At least three general mechanisms can be identified in playing a role in the evolution of xanthomatous infiltrates.

1. Alterations in lipoprotein content or structure in which normal amounts of lipoproteins are found but there is an accumulation of unusual lipids within the lipoproteins that predispose to their accumulations in skin and other tissues.
2. Lymphoproliferative changes in the skin with secondary accumulation of lipids in macrophages.
3. Local tissue abnormalities such as inflammatory reactions in the skin increase vascular permeability to otherwise normal levels of lipoproteins in the circulation.

Diagnosis

Finding xanthomas mandates a careful history and physical examination, with attention directed to the familial incidence of xanthomas or premature atherosclerotic disease, as well as to lipemia retinalis, arcus senilis, hepatosplenomegaly, and abdominal pain. Biopsy may be necessary to rule out other conditions.

Quantitative measurement of fasting plasma cholesterol and triglyceride levels is followed by lipoprotein measurements if the initial tests are abnormal. If lipoprotein levels are elevated, every effort must be made to determine if the alterations are a primary genetic defect or due to a secondary underlying disease.

Differential Diagnosis

Tendinous xanthomas are nearly pathognomonic clinically when multiple. Giant cell tumor of tendon sheath or pigmented villonodular tenosynovitis is usually solitary. Xanthelasmas are pathognomonic when multiple small plaques are present on the eyelids, but early, small lesions can be confused with sebaceous hyperplasia, syringoma, or milia. Diffuse or generalized planar xanthomas do not have the flexural distribution seen in xanthoma disseminatum, and are yellow, not orange, in color. Tuberous xanthomas can be confused with nodular lesions of erythema elevatum diutinum and with rheumatoid nodules. Eruptive xanthomas can be confused clinically and histologically with generalized granuloma annulare.

Treatment

The choice of treatment to resolve xanthomas (and, it is hoped, atheromatous infiltrates) depends on the underlying lipoprotein abnormality. In secondary hyperlipoproteinemia, the condition should be specifically treated. If no secondary disease is found, then two major approaches to therapy are available for treating primary hyperlipoproteinemias: (1) diet and (2) antihyperlipidemic drugs.

Diet

Dietary manipulation, by reducing caloric intake, altering cholesterol and triglyceride intake, altering carbohydrate intake, or altering the type of triglyceride in the diet, alone is often effective in lowering lipoproteins in most primary hyperlipoproteinemias except in familial hypercholesterolemia.

Antilipid Pharmacologic Agents

When dietary restrictions, alterations, and weight reduction are ineffective a number of drugs may be added to the regimen. Three types of drugs affect lipoprotein metabolism:

1. Drugs altering cholesterol and bile salt absorption (anion exchange resins).
2. Drugs altering lipoprotein synthesis and catabolism, including nicotinic acid, clofibrate, gemfibrozil, dextrothyroxine, probucol, and nicotinic acid.
3. Drugs altering endogenous cholesterol synthesis such as lovastatin.

Prognosis

Diet and drugs are often effective in clearing eruptive xanthomas. Tuberous xanthomas, found in broad beta disease, resolve with weight reduction, diet (restricted carbohydrates), and drug therapy. Tendinous and tuberous xanthomas and xanthelasma seen in familial hypercholesterolemia, although difficult to resolve, have been reported to regress with strict dietary restriction of cholesterol and a combination of drugs, especially lovastatin and cholestyramine.

AMYLOIDOSIS

(CM&S Chapter 177)

Amyloid is a filamentous substance of uniform diameter (6 to 10 nm) with fibrils that are straight and neither branch nor anastomose. Varying amounts of amorphous materials are embedded on these filaments. Amyloid stains metachromatically with basic aniline dyes, such as crystal violet, and orthochromatically with dyes used to stain cotton, such as Congo red and Dylon, which exhibit green-ish birefringence under polarized light. Thioflavin-T binds amyloid and exhibits fluorescence under an appropriate filter combination. These tinctorial characteristics of amyloid filaments are related to their β-pleated antiparallel sheet configuration. Chemically, amyloids are diverse; keratin, immunoglobulins, insulin, and other substances are known to be amyloidogenic, and each amyloid produced from these building materials satisfies the criteria mentioned earlier.

Amyloidoses are classified mainly according to their chemical origins. Other considerations include whether the condition is systemic or localized and isolated or familial and its etiologic factors and clinical appearance.

Systemic Amyloidosis

Clinical Description

In this category of amyloidoses, skin involvement accompanies or may precede more serious systemic disease. Systemic amyloidosis derived from altered light chains (AL) can be associated with multiple myeloma or other gammopathies. Those patients with myeloma are designated as having myeloma-associated amyloidosis, and those without gammopathy, who are more numerous, have primary systemic amyloidosis. Some cases seem to begin without an immunocyte dyscrasia, which develops later, or a dyscrasia is discovered after repeated examinations with more sensitive methods.

Clinical findings in AL amyloidosis are most often (1) macroglossia with or without hardening of oral mucous membrane, (2) periorbital waxy papules and plaques with ecchymosis, and (3) pinch hemorrhages. Less commonly, amyloid deposition becomes more generalized and causes purpuric or ecchymotic lesions on folded areas such as the retroauricular and nasolabial folds, neck, umbilicus, and anogenital area. Waxy, shiny, and frequently semi-translucent papulonodules may also be found in flexural areas. Massive amyloid deposition can result in leonine facies, condyloma latum–like growths in the genital skin, and xanthomatous lesions in other sites. Postpurpuric hemosiderin pigmentation and jaundice due to hepatic involvement may occur. Perivascular deposition of amyloid may produce cord-like blood vessel thickening. Diffuse dermal infiltration can cause induration, and when the fragile amyloid in the lesion is split it may produce hemorrhagic bulla. Alopecia and nail dystrophy can occur. Typically, elderly patients begin to complain of fatigue and weight loss. Carpal tunnel syndrome is common.

Pathology

The primary sites of amyloid deposition in the skin in systemic AL amyloidosis are around small vessels, sweat glands, and lipocytes. In more advanced lesions, amyloid is found diffusely in the dermis and subcutis. Masses of amyloid are often fissured forming small islands. Inflammatory cells are absent or few.

Pathogenesis and Etiology

The amyloid substance is derived from monoclonal expansion of plasma cells. These cells produce either λ or κ light chain of immunoglobulin, which then produce amyloid light-chain proteins. The final AL amyloid is conjugated with neutral polysaccharides and therefore is often periodic acid–Schiff (PAS) positive and diastase resistant.

Diagnosis and Differential Diagnosis

The differential diagnosis of systemic AL amyloidosis includes nodular amyloidosis, hyalinosis cutis et mucosae, and colloid milium.

Treatment

There is no effective therapy for AL amyloidosis. Chemotherapy for multiple myeloma with melphalan-prednisone or colchicine(1 to 2 mg daily), which is effective for secondary amyloidosis due to familial Mediterranean fever, has been used with variable results. Amyloid is insoluble, and once deposited in the tissue, it is difficult to remove with ordinary tissue proteases. Temporary relief of gastrointestinal symptoms may be obtained with systemic antibiotics, but no change is seen in the skin lesions.

Systemic AA Amyloidosis

Clinical Description

Systemic AA amyloidosis is also referred to as secondary systemic amyloidosis because there are preceding chronic inflammatory diseases such as rheumatoid arthritis and familial Mediterranean fever or chronic infectious diseases such as osteomyelitis, bronchiectasis, and lepromatous leprosy. Skin lesions are rare, but the subcutaneous fat of the lower abdomen or rectal mucosa contains AA amyloid. Predilection sites of AA amyloid deposition are parenchymatous organs such as kidney (nephrosis, uremia), liver, and spleen.

Pathology

As in AL amyloidosis, amyloid deposition in AA amyloidosis is seen surrounding blood vessels, lipocytes (amyloid rings), and eccrine glands. As more amyloid accumulates in the skin, it can be found diffusely in the dermis.

Pathogenesis

AA amyloid is not immunoglobulin but is instead derived from the amino-terminal portion of serum amyloid A (SAA)–related protein. SAA is an α-globulin and is apparently present in normal sera in association with high-density lipoproteins, but its cleavage into AA amyloid may be stimulated in chronic inflammation or infections.

Diagnosis and Differential Diagnosis

Aspiration needle biopsy of the subcutaneous fat tissue of the lower abdomen is more sensitive than rectal biopsy. AA amyloid in tissue sections becomes alkaline Congo red negative after it is treated with potassium permanganate. This oxidation method is useful to differentiate AA amyloid from AL or keratin amyloids, which are alkaline Congo red positive after permanganate treatment.

Treatment

Correction of an underlying disease may not alleviate secondary AA amyloidosis, because once deposited in the tissue, amyloid is difficult to remove. However, colchicine is significantly effective for AA amyloidosis secondary to familial Mediterranean fever.

Familial Mediterranean Fever
Clinical Description

As sporadic attacks of fever are repeated, amyloidosis develops with clinical evidence of peritonitis, pleuritis, and synovitis. Skin lesions may develop in the form of erysipelas-like erythema of legs and feet and of Henoch-Schönlein purpura. Inheritance is autosomal recessive.

Pathology

Parenchymatous organs such as spleen (lardaceous spleen), kidneys, adrenals, and pulmonary alveolar septa are involved. Hepatic sinusoids are spared. The amyloid is the permanganate-sensitive AA type. Skin lesions have not been studied.

Skin-Limited Keratin Amyloidoses

Idiopathic Keratin Amyloidoses
Clinical Description

Lichen amyloidosus, macular amyloidosis, and biphasic amyloidosis (a combination of both) are related and most often affect dark-skinned races such as Asians, Latinos, and those of Middle Eastern extraction. Typically, lichen amyloidosus affects the extensor surfaces of the extremities, such as the shins and outer arms. Lesions on the upper back are relatively common. The condition is more frequent in males, occurring most often between 50 and 60 years of age. Small pruritic papules become larger and confluent as the patient constantly scratches because of intense pruritus. Well-developed lesions are hyperpigmented, lichenified, and hyperkeratotic. Papules and small nodules similar to prurigo nodularis are strewn over a grater-like rough skin surface. Excoriations and hemorrhagic crusts are common.

Macular amyloidosis is more common in women. Frequent sites are areas subject to friction such as the upper back, neck, shin, thigh, and buttocks. In contrast to the lichenoid variety, pruritus is not usually noted. Typically, a middle-aged woman seeks medical attention when neck lesions creep up to the face and cannot be concealed with high-necked clothing. Macular lesions consist of hyperpigmentation with a characteristically rippled pattern (i.e., parallel waves of hyperpigmentation). Constant friction with nylon brush or towel may cause macular amyloidosis (i.e., friction or irritant amyloidosis).

Biphasic amyloidosis shows both lichenoid and macular amyloidoses in the same location or at separate sites. Lichenoid lesions are pruritic. The peak incidence of the biphasic type is between 50 and 60 years of age.

Pathology

The epidermis is acanthotic and hyperkeratotic in lichenoid lesions. There may be eosinophilic cytoid bodies in the epidermis, which are rich in disulfide bonds and are Congo red positive. Amyloid deposition principally expands dermal papillae and presses rete ridges into thin septa. Amyloid globules can be scattered in the upper reticular dermis, but perivascular deposition as seen in systemic amyloidoses is not prominent. In macular amyloidosis, the lesional epidermis is often atrophic and the amount of amyloid deposition may be very small.

Pathogenesis and Etiology

Trauma, insect bites, mild chronic infection, and other injurious factors may be involved in the initial damage to the epidermal keratinocytes. No matter what the cause of keratinocyte damage might be, the first step in keratinocyte-derived amyloidosis appears to be apoptosis (i.e., nuclear pyknosis and fragmentation followed by cytoplasmic disruption). Tonofilaments become thicker and bundled into a wavy mass that occupies the whole cytoplasm (filamentous degeneration) and can be seen on light microscopy as cytoid bodies or hyaline bodies. During filamentous degeneration and after dropping into the dermis there must be certain modifications, and sulfhydryl linkages, rich in lower epidermal keratinocytes, may be reduced to disulfide bonds.

Differential Diagnosis

Atopic dermatitis with prurigo nodularis should be differentiated from lichen amyloidosus. For macular amyloidosis, the differential diagnosis is often poikilodermas of various etiologies (Civatte type, mycosis fungoides, dermatomyosis, scleroderma), postinflammatory hyperpigmentation, erythema dyschromicum perstans, dyskeratosis congenita, and, if on the face, melasma.

Treatment

Etretinate therapy for 10 to 20 weeks has been shown to be effective in some cases of lichen amyloidosus. Topical dimethyl sulfoxide, retinoic acid, fluorinated corticosteroids, and mercaptoethanolurea solution give some relief. Dermabrasion removes the source of amyloid keratin and is reportedly very effective with long-term remission.

Actinic Amyloidosis

Both ultraviolet A and B light cause keratinocyte degeneration. Chronic exposure to actinic rays produces a large number of damaged keratinocytes in which filamentous degeneration of tonofilaments occurs. These keratinocytes are observed as cytoid bodies on light microscopy and eventually drop into the dermis to form keratin amyloid. The most common example is the keratin amyloid found in actinic keratosis. The colloid substance in juvenile colloid milium is actually keratin amyloid despite its clinical resemblance to colloid milium of the adult face. Chronic psoralens and ultraviolet A light therapy frequently produces keratin amyloid in the upper dermis. No clinical symptoms are elicited.

Epithelioma Keratin Amyloidosis

Epithelial tumors derived from the epidermis contain keratin species, which become amyloid in lichenoid, macular, and biphasic amyloidoses. Basal cell carcinoma, Bowen's disease, and seborrheic keratoses are commonly laden with stromal and sometimes parenchymal amyloid. Neoplastic cells undergo apoptosis and accumulate in the stroma, where they become keratin amyloid.

Nodular Amyloidosis

Clinical Description

Single or multiple lesions can occur anywhere, but the face, scalp, and leg are common sites. Middle-aged women are most often affected with this relatively rare amyloidosis. Individual lesions are waxy, yellowish tumor-like nodules or atrophic plaques. Some nodules are semi-transparent and appear like bulla, while others are covered with telangiectases or hemorrhagic skin. Nodular amyloidosis may be associated with Sjögren's syndrome.

Pathology

There is massive infiltration of the entire dermis and often the subcutis by amyloid. Perivascular and periappendageal deposition may be particularly heavy. Immunoglobulin κ or λ light chains or both are demonstrable in this amyloid. Epitopes of keratins, type IV collagen, and laminin are absent, suggesting that this amyloid is of immunoglobulin origin.

Diagnosis and Differential Diagnosis

The clinical differential diagnosis includes cutaneous lymphoma, pseudolymphoma, sarcoidosis, Sweet's syndrome, colloid milium, and hyalinosis cutis et mucosae. Nodular lesions of AL amyloidosis are usually a part of more generalized cutaneous manifestations.

Treatment

Small numbers of nodular amyloidosis lesions are best treated by surgical removal. Intralesional corticosteroid injections, if repeated, reduce the size of the nodule.

CUTANEOUS OSSIFICATION AND CALCIFICATION

(CM&S Chapter 178)

New bone formation or calcium deposition in the skin may be present in a variety of clinical settings, both inherited and acquired (Table 12–1). Osteoma cutis, formation of new bone in the skin, may be primary or secondary. Primary cutaneous ossification frequently occurs in Albright's hereditary osteodystrophy and as idiopathic osteoma cutis. In secondary cases of cutaneous ossification, bone formation occurs within a preexisting lesion, usually a tumor. Calcinosis cutis is the deposition of calcium in the skin and subcutaneous tissues. Four principal forms of calcinosis cutis are recognized: metastatic calcinosis, dystrophic calcinosis, idiopathic calcinosis, and subepidermal calcified nodule.

Pathology

The pathologic appearance of cutaneous ossification is that of spicules of bone of varying size within the dermis or in the subcutaneous tissue. Osteocytes, cement lines, and haversian canals are seen along with osteoblasts. The x-ray appearance is that of true bone.

Treatment

A variety of treatments have been attempted for osteoma cutis and cutaneous calcification. Treatments include 0.05% tretinoin cream, surgical excision, and treatment of the underlying condition.

TABLE 12–1. Differential Diagnosis and Evaluation of Cutaneous Ossification and Calcification

CONDITION	CLINICAL EXAMPLES	CALCIUM PHOSPHORUS
Osteoma Cutis		
Primary osteoma cutis		
Localized	Isolated nodule, multiple papules	Normal
Generalized	Albright's hereditary osteodystrophy	Normal, hypocalcemia
Secondary osteoma cutis		
Neoplasms	Pilomatricoma, others	Normal
Inflammatory processes	Morphea, myositis ossificans progressiva	Normal
Calcinosis Cutis		
Metastatic calcification	Renal failure patients with firm nodules around large joints, white papules/plaques, calciphylaxis	Hypercalcemia/hyperphosphatemia
Dystrophic calcification		
Universalis	Dermatomyositis	Normal
Circumscripta	Scleroderma, subcutaneous fat necrosis of the newborn	Normal
Neoplasms	Pilomatricoma, others	Normal
Other	Local infiltration, traumatic implantation	Normal
Idiopathic calcification		
Tumoral calcinosis	Subcutaneous masses	Hyperphosphatemia
Scrotal calcinosis	Nodules on scrotum	Normal
Cutaneous calculi	Fascial or mucosal nodules	Normal

THE CUTANEOUS MUCINOSES

(CM&S Chapter 179)

The cutaneous mucinoses are a heterogeneous group of disorders in which mucin accumulates in the skin either diffusely or focally. Mucin is a jelly-like amorphous mixture of glycosaminoglycans (GAGS)—mainly hyaluronic acid and dermatan sulfate bound to small amounts of chondroitin sulfate and heparin sulfate. All types of GAGS can be demonstrated in tissue sections by the Alcian-blue at pH 2.5 stain or the colloidal iron stain. The causes of these conditions are unknown. Mucinoses can be divided into those in which mucin deposition results in clinically distinctive lesions (Table 12–2) and diseases in which mucin deposition is an epiphenomenon (Table 12–3).

Dermal Mucinoses with Distinctive Features

Lichen Myxedematosus

Definition and Clinical Description

Lichen myxedematosus is a localized or generalized papular eruption due to dermal deposition of mucin without thyroid disease and has three forms—a localized type affecting a single site, a

---

TABLE 12-2.   Cutaneous Mucinoses with Distinctive Features

A. Dermal
  1. Lichen myxedematosus
  2. Acral persistent papular mucinosis
  3. Reticular erythematous mucinosis
  4. Scleredema
  5. Dysthyroidotic mucinoses
      a. Localized (pretibial) myxedema
      b. Generalized myxedema
      c. Papular mucinosis associated with thyroid disease
  6. Papular and nodular mucinosis associated with lupus erythematosus
  7. Self-healing juvenile cutaneous mucinosis
  8. Cutaneous mucinosis of infancy
  9. Cutaneous toxic mucinoses
      a. Papular mucinosis of the toxic oil syndrome
      b. Papular mucinosis of the eosinophilia-myalgia syndrome
  10. Cutaneous focal mucinosis
  11. Mucous cyst
      a. Digital
      b. Of the oral mucosa (mucocele)
  12. Miscellaneous mucinoses
B. Follicular
  1. Follicular mucinosis (alopecia mucinosa)
  2. Urticaria-like follicular mucinosis

From Rongioletti F, Rebora A: Les mucinoses cutanées. Ann Dermatol Venereol 1993;120;75–87.

TABLE 12-3. Disorders Associated with Histologic Deposition of Mucin

A. Epithelial Mucinosis
1. Mycosis fungoides
2. Spongiotic dermatitis
3. Basal cell carcinoma
4. Warts
5. Keratocanthoma
6. Squamous cell carcinoma
B. Dermal Mucinosis
1. Lupus erythematosus
2. Dermatomyositis
3. Scleroderma
4. Degos' disease
5. Granuloma annulare
6. UV radiation and PUVA
7. Actinic elastosis
8. Hereditary progressive mucinous histiocytosis
9. Epithelial tumors (basal cell carcinoma, eccrine tumors)
10. Mesenchymal tumors (fibroma, lipoma)
11. Neural tumors (neurofibroma, neurilemoma)
C. Follicular Mucinosis
1. Lymphoma/Pseudolymphoma
2. Cutaneous leukemia
3. Spongiotic dermatitis
4. Lupus erythematosus
5. Hypertrophic lichen planus
6. Insect bites
7. Angiolymphoid hyperplasia with eosinophilia
8. Hodgkin's disease
9. Photo-induced eruptions
10. Familial reticuloendotheliosis

UV, ultraviolet; PUVA, psoralen plus ultraviolet A.
From Rongioletti F, Rebora A: The new cutaneous mucinoses. A review with an up-to-date classification of cutaneous mucinoses. J Am Acad Dermatol 1991;24:265–70.

disseminated type involving more than one site, and a generalized type, termed *scleromyxedema* affecting large portions of the skin or even the entire body.

Lichen myxedematosus is most commonly seen in patients 30 to 50 years old and affects both sexes equally. It features multiple, waxy, flat-topped papules that remain isolated or coalesce into plaques. Linear and annular, nodular, urticarial, or cyst-like lesions may also be seen. In scleromyxedema, a sclerodermatous induration affects the mouth and fingers. Vertical furrows on the glabella give some patients a leonine appearance. The elbows, forearms, upper trunk, and neck are also involved.

A serum paraprotein, usually 7S-IgG with lambda light chains, is present in most cases of lichen myxedematosus. Unpredictably, a small number of patients with lichen myxedematosus develop myeloma or Waldenström's macroglobulinemia. Other laboratory tests are usually normal. Scleromyxedema has a number of internal manifestations, including neurologic, cardiovascular, renal, and rheumatologic disorders as well as necrotizing myopathy, dermatomyositis, esophageal aperistalsis, and laryngeal involvement.

The localized and disseminated types of lichen myxedematosus may clear spontaneously. Scleromyxedema is often progressive, with death usually resulting from pneumonia or thrombosis.

Differential Diagnosis

The differential diagnosis of localized forms include granuloma annulare, lichen amyloidosus, lichen planus, and eruptive collagenoma. Scleromyxedema can be distinguished from systemic scleroderma and scleredema in which papules do not occur.

Treatment

No therapy is curative. Electron-beam and radiotherapy, extracorporeal photochemotherapy, PUVA, retinoids, dermabrasion, plasmapheresis, melphalan, cyclophosphamide, methotrexate, local steroids, and dimethyl sulfoxide have been useful. Potentially toxic drugs should be limited to patients who are disfigured, disabled, or very ill.

Acral Persistent Papular Mucinosis

Acral persistent papular mucinosis affects mostly women with multiple, symmetrical, ivory- or flesh-colored, 2- to 5-mm-wide papules located on the back of the hands and wrists. Acral persistent papular mucinosis may be a variant of lichen myxedematosus.

Reticular Erythematous Mucinosis (Plaque-like Cutaneous Mucinosis)

Definition and Clinical Description

Reticular erythematous mucinosis (REM) is a persistent photoaggravated erythematous reticular or plaque-like eruption in the midline of the back or chest. REM occurs most often in middle-aged women.

Reddish macules and papules merge into reticulate annular or plaque-like, slightly pruritic lesions in the midback or chest, at times spreading to the abdomen. Sun exposure worsens the eruption, but it has even been beneficial. Phototesting may reproduce REM lesions. Usually, REM is not associated with systemic diseases and altered laboratory tests. Oral contraceptives, menses, and pregnancy may promote or exacerbate REM. REM may clear spontaneously.

Differential Diagnosis

The differential diagnosis includes lupus erythematosus, Jessner's lymphocytic infiltration, and polymorphic light eruption.

Treatment

Antimalarials are usually effective in 2 to 4 weeks.

Scleredema

Definition

This disorder is a symmetrical diffuse induration of the upper part of the body due to thickening of the dermis and deposition of mucin.

Clinical Description

There are three types of scleredema, although a simpler division into patients with and without diabetes has been suggested. The first type affects mostly middle-aged women but also children. It is preceded by fever, malaise, and infection, usually streptococcal, of the upper and lower respiratory tracts. The skin of the cervicofacial region, then of the trunk and proximal upper limbs, suddenly hardens. The face is expressionless, and opening the mouth and swallowing are difficult because of involvement of the tongue and pharynx. This type usually resolves in a few months.

The second type shares the same clinical features but has a subtle onset without preceding illness and persists for years.

The third type occurs mainly in obese middle-aged men with insulin-dependent diabetes (scleredema diabeticorum). The onset is subtle and the disorder persistent. Erythema and induration of the back are common, irrespective of whether hyperglycemia is corrected.

Serositis, dysarthria and dysphagia, myositis, ocular and cardiac abnormalities, parotiditis, monoclonal gammopathy, and myeloma may occur in all forms. There may be also hyperparathyroidism, rheumatoid arthritis, Sjögren's syndrome, and malignant insulinoma. Scleredema causes little morbidity besides the limitation of movement. Type I may clear in 1 to 2 years, whereas the other types last longer. Type III scleredema is occasionally fatal.

Differential Diagnosis

The differential diagnosis includes systemic scleroderma and scleromyxedema.

Treatment

There is no reproducibly effective treatment.

Dysthyroidotic Mucinosis Associated with Altered Thyroid Function

Localized (Pretibial) Myxedema

Definition. Localized or pretibial myxedema is a cutaneous induration of the shins due to mucin deposition, associated with hyperthyroidism, or occurring after thyroidectomy.

Clinical Description. Localized myxedema develops as erythematous to skin-colored, sometimes purple-brown or yellowish, waxy, indurated peau d'orange nodules or plaques. Usually, they are located on the anterolateral aspect of the legs or feet.

Differential Diagnosis. Lichen simplex chronicus, lymphedema, elephantiasis, and hypertrophic lichen planus lack mucin deposition and are generally not seen in the setting of thyroid disease.

Treatment. Therapy of hyperthyroidism does not improve the cutaneous lesions and, often, localized myxedema develops after it. Steroids administered under occlusive dressings or delivered by intralesional injection may help.

Generalized Myxedema

Definition and Clinical Description. Generalized myxedema is a manifestation of severe hypothyroidism in which mucin is stored in the dermis leading to induration of the skin. In adult hypothyroidism, the most common form, initial symptoms are subtle, including mental and physical sluggishness, weight gain, constipation, leg cramps, loss of appetite, and cold intolerance. As the disease progresses, the face has a dull expression; eyelids, lips, tongue, and hands become puffy; the nose becomes broad; and the speech becomes hoarse and slurred. The skin is pale, cool, waxy, and dry for the absence of sweating with ichthyosis or eczema craquelé. Hair and nails are dry and brittle. A diffuse nonscarring alopecia is common. Purpura on the limbs, blue telangiectatic fingertips, delayed wound healing, and xanthomas are present.

Diagnosis and Differential Diagnosis. The diagnosis is made clinically. Low levels of T_3 and T_4 confirm the diagnosis. The thyroid-stimulating hormone level is high in primary hypothyroidism and low in secondary hypothyroidism, in which myxedema does not occur.

Treatment. Early treatment is crucial for proper mental development of neonates with hypothyroidism. Usually, symptoms subside with thyroxin treatment and recur if it is stopped.

Papular and Nodular Mucinosis in Lupus Erythematosus

Papular and nodular mucinosis (PNM) occurs in 1.5% of lupus erythematosus cases as symptomless skin-colored, at times reddish, 0.5- to 2-cm-wide papules and nodules that rarely merge into plaques. The back and V of the neck are mostly involved. Usually, patients with lupus erythematosus who develop PNM have systemic disease. Only a few patients respond to antimalarials; the remainder require systemic steroids.

Cutaneous Focal Mucinosis

The lesion, a symptomless, skin-colored papule or nodule, less than 1 cm wide, on the face, trunk, or limbs of adults. Rarely is it linked to a thyroid disorder or to scleromyxedema. Lesions of cutaneous focal mucinosis can be surgically excised. Relapses are uncommon.

Mucous Cysts

Mucous Digital Cyst (Myxoid Cyst, Synovial Cyst)

Mucous digital cyst occurs at any age, mostly in women, as a raised, cystic nodule, almost translucent, and seldom wider than 2 cm. Usually, it is located on the fingers (rarely on the toes) at the nail base. Clear viscous material comes out, but older cysts may be solid. The adjacent nail may show a longitudinal furrow and a Heberden's (osteophytic) nodule.

Mucous digital cyst is neither a cyst nor a tumor but rather the result of connective tissue degeneration. Trauma is a promoting factor.

Excision, incision and drainage, electrodesiccation, CO_2 laser, vaporization, aspiration of the content, and intralesional injections of triamcinolone or sclerosant agents are used, but relapses are frequent.

Mucous Cyst of the Oral Mucosa (Mucocele)

Mucoceles are single, symptomless, dome-shaped, translucent, blue-whitish cysts that contain a clear, viscous fluid. They are usually located on the inner surface of the lower lip or on the floor of the mouth. Most are smaller than 1 cm in diameter and wax and wane over several months. Rarely, multiple mucoceles arise in the superficial labial epithelium, and they can resemble a blistering disease. Mucoceles result either from a ruptured mucous salivary gland duct or from retention of mucus due to obstruction of a duct.

They occasionally disappear spontaneously but can be excised or treated with cryotherapy, electrodesiccated, or vaporized with a CO_2 laser.

Distinctive Follicular Mucinoses

Mucin accumulates in follicular epithelium in two distinctive clinical conditions—alopecia mucinosa and urticaria-like follicular mucinosis. Otherwise, follicular mucinosis is a histologic epiphenomenon most often seen in cutaneous T-cell lymphomas and other skin disorders (see Table 12–3).

chapter 13

What Are the Dermatologic Manifestations of Internal Disease? What Are the Dermatologic Disorders Commonly Found in Neonates?

PARANEOPLASTIC SYNDROMES

(CM&S Chapter 180)

Definition

There are two essential criteria to a paraneoplastic syndrome: (1) the dermatosis must develop only after the genesis of the malignant tumor, and (2) the dermatosis and the malignant tumor should follow a parallel course.

Only diseases not described elsewhere in the text are discussed here. For Sweet's syndrome, see Chapter 38 (Chapter 2 in this text); subcutaneous fat necrosis, see Chapter 71 (Chapter 2 in this text); pruritus, see Chapter 8 (Chapter 2 in this text); dermatomyositis, see Chapter 25 (Chapter 2 in this text); erythroderma, see Chapter 31 (Chapter 2 in this text); pemphigus, see Chapter 74 (Chapter 3 in this text); flushing, see Chapter 6 (Chapter 2 in this text); and xanthomas, see Chapter 176 (Chapter 12 in this text).

Necrolytic Migratory Erythema

Necrolytic migratory erythema (the glucagonoma syndrome) is a marker for a glucagon-producing tumor of the pancreas. Necrolytic migratory erythema is manifested by erythema, vesicles, pustules, bullae, and erosions that typically involve the face and the intertriginous areas, particularly the groin, but they can occur in acral sites as well. It is often initially mistaken for an intertriginous candidal infection. The vesicles are often very superficial, tend to become confluent, and rupture easily. Brownish-red papules are often scattered over much of the skin surface. Peripheral expansion of the lesions results in an arcuate or gyrate morphology. Associated abnormalities include glossitis, stomatitis, dystrophic nails, alopecia, weight loss, anemia, and diabetes.

In most patients resection of the pancreatic islet cell tumor of the glucagon-producing type, that results in high serum glucagon levels and mild diabetes mellitus, clears the eruption, sometimes within 48 hours. The cutaneous eruption is most likely due to the toxic effect of amino acids or keratinocytes, which are in excess because of their enhanced hepatic uptake.

While the diagnosis can be suspected on biopsy, which demonstrates psoriasiform epidermal hyperplasia with pallor, ballooning, and necrosis of the upper spinous layer of the epidermis, confirmation may require serum glucagon levels.

Hypertrichosis Lanuginosa Acquisita

In hypertrichosis lanuginosa acquisita, there is excessive growth of lanugo (vellus) hairs. These long, soft, downy hairs initially cover the face and ears, but eventually all hair-bearing skin may be involved. Associated abnormalities include glossitis, which is often painful, and red papules occurring extensively on the tongue. Fully expressed hypertrichosis lanuginosa acquisita, usually secondary to malignant tumors of a variety of sites, appears suddenly and is rapidly progressive. Excessive lanugo hair growth can also be caused by anorexia nervosa or drugs such as steroids, phenytoin, and minoxidil.

Erythema Gyratum Repens

Erythema gyratum repens is a cutaneous eruption consisting of concentric, raised, erythematous bands migrating in waves over the body surface and resulting in a wood-grain pattern. These bands move quickly—up to 1 cm per day.

Only rare cases of erythema gyratum repens have been reported in the absence of an underlying tumor. Carcinoma of the breast, lung, bladder, prostate, cervix, stomach, and esophagus and with multiple myeloma are most common.

Multiple Eruptive Seborrheic Keratoses

Multiple eruptive seborrheic keratoses, also known as the sign of Leser-Trélat, have been mentioned in association with many internal malignancies, including tumors of the stomach, breast, prostate, lung, and colon; malignant melanoma; as well as lymphoma, primary lymphoma of the brain, and mycosis fungoides.

Evidence to support the presumed relationship of seborrheic keratoses to malignant disease is meager. Most of the cancers so described are common. Seborrheic keratoses are ubiquitous in the elderly, who are also at greatest risk for developing cancer. Pseudoeruptive seborrheic keratoses can occur secondary to any inflammatory skin eruption, especially widespread dermatitis.

Paraneoplastic Acrokeratosis of Bazex

Paraneoplastic acrokeratosis of Bazex is a symmetrical dermatosis that most commonly affects acral sites including the digits, nails, feet, ears, and nose with an erythematous to violaceous, scaling eruption that, except for a bluer hue, resembles psoriasis. There is gradual progression of the eruption to include involvement of the cheeks, elbows, knees, and central trunk. Nail changes include subungual hyperkeratosis, onychomadesis (shedding), flaky white surface changes to the nail plate, and periungual fissuring and suppuration.

Bazex's syndrome is almost always associated with cancer, usually of the upper respiratory system, which includes cancer of the tongue, pharynx, esophagus, and lung. The eruption frequently predates evidence of the cancer.

Acquired Ichthyosis

Paraneoplastic ichthyosis is a true hyperkeratosis and can be differentiated clinically and histologically from simple dry skin (xerosis). While the ichthyosis usually occurs as a late manifestation of a lymphoma, it may precede the diagnosis by several years. Acquired ichthyosis has also been associated with a variety of other cancer types.

Acanthosis Nigricans

Unlike the benign form, malignant acanthosis nigricans is usually of sudden onset, is rapidly progressive, and is often pruritic. Diffuse keratoderma involving the palms and soles is also common in the malignant form. Otherwise, acanthosis nigricans is clinically indistinguishable from benign acanthosis nigricans, which is manifested as a gray-brown, symmetrical, velvety thickening of skin with increased skin fold markings. The appearance of acanthosis nigricans can precede other evidence of the internal malignant disease. There may be an association with eruptive seborrheic keratoses.

Malignant acanthosis nigricans is usually due to an intra-abdominal tumor, with gastric adenocarcinoma being the most common.

Thrombophlebitis

Peripheral thrombophlebitis is typically associated with gastric carcinoma, although other associated cancers include tumors of pancreas, prostate, lung, liver, bowel, gallbladder, and ovary, as well as lymphoma and leukemia. The sometimes "migratory" nature of the thrombophlebitis probably relates to a generalized hypercoagulable state.

Mondor's disease, usually benign but sometimes associated with breast cancer, is thrombophlebitis of the anterior chest wall presenting as a tender or nontender cord.

Patients younger than 50 years with deep venous thrombosis appear to have a very significant risk of occult cancer.

HIRSUTISM AND ITS RELATED ENDOCRINE DISORDERS

(CM&S Chapter 181)

Definition

Hirsutism is the abnormal growth of terminal hair in androgen-sensitive areas such as the moustache and beard regions. The presence of terminal hair in these regions is not necessarily abnormal for some women, and the determination of whether a patient has hirsutism must take into consideration the normal hair pattern for the genetic makeup of the individual.

Excess hair may also be present in *hypertrichosis*, in which uniformly long, smooth, silky hair is distributed over the entire body rather than just the androgen-sensitive areas. Hypertrichosis is a common result of certain medications (e.g., cyclosporin), certain malignancies (e.g., hypertrichosis lanuginosa), and accompanying metabolic disorders, including hypothyroidism, porphyria, anorexia nervosa, and starvation.

In hirsutism, a woman has terminal hair in the characteristic male distribution of androgen-responsive areas, including the moustache and beard regions, pubic escutcheon, trunk, and thighs. The upper lip, chin, lower abdomen, and thighs are the most sensitive areas to evaluate.

Clinical Presentation

Polycystic Ovarian Syndrome

In the majority of hirsute women, *polycystic ovarian syndrome,* a group of related disorders that culminate in the development of chronic anovulation (usually perimenarchal), hyperandrogenism, relative insulin resistance, and acanthosis nigricans, is considered. Obesity is common, but further signs of virilization, such as hypertrophy of the clitoris or husky voice, are rare. Enlarged cystic ovaries are decisive for diagnosis.

Laboratory evaluation indicates a high serum luteinizing hormone (LH) level and normal or low follicle-stimulating hormone (FSH) concentrations (i.e., increased ratio of LH to FSH). Testosterone concentrations in patients with polycystic ovarian syndrome are usually mildly elevated (not more than 200 ng/dl).

Ovarian Tumors

A variety of neoplasms of the ovary may be responsible for excess ovarian androgen production, either by direct secretion of testosterone or by stimulation of adjacent ovarian stroma and thecal tissue to secrete this hormone. Serum free testosterone levels may be only slightly elevated but are generally more than 200 ng/dl. Patients who present with virilization (acne and hirsutism) should be evaluated for one of these tumors by ultrasonography.

Cushing's Disease and Syndrome

Cushing's disease (excess pituitary adrenocorticotropic hormone [ACTH] secretion) and syndrome (pituitary independent) are conditions of hypercortisolism that may be accompanied by hirsutism. The clinical diagnosis is usually made on the presence of common physical signs such as moon facies and buffalo hump. Hirsutism is a secondary consideration. The traditional tests are a 24-hour urinary cortisol (normal levels, less than 100 ng/24 hr) or low-dose dexamethasone suppression testing. The corticotropin-releasing hormone and overnight high-dose dexamethasone are followed by plasma ACTH measurements by radioimmunoassay and alternative tests.

Hyperprolactinemia

Prolactin-secreting pituitary tumors may induce hirsutism.

Congenital Adrenal Hyperplasia

Congenital adrenal hyperplasia occurs when there is a partial blockage of the synthesis of cortisol caused by a variety of enzyme deficiencies. This form of adrenal hyperandrogenism results from excess corticotropin levels and, thus, increased androgen secretion. These enzyme deficiencies usually manifest early in life, with the patient developing ambiguous genitalia. However, a subset of these deficiencies is considered to be late onset or attenuated, in which the clinical manifestations are hirsutism or anovulation. A substantial proportion of women with hirsutism have mild defects in adrenal steroidogenesis, revealed by an ACTH stimulation test, that are indicative of late-onset (nonclassic) congenital adrenal hyperplasia.

The most common enzyme causing adrenal hyperplasia is 21-hydroxylase deficiency. The diagnosis is usually made by demonstration of an increased concentration of 17-hydroxyprogesterone, the substrate for the deficient enzyme.

In 11β-hydroxylase deficiency, a much less common condition, the 17-hydroxyprogesterone levels are usually midrange. Diagnosis is made by measuring 11-deoxycortisol after adrenal stimulation with ACTH.

Adrenal Neoplasms

Adenoma and carcinoma of the adrenal gland may cause hirsutism associated with very high dehydroepiandrosterone sulfase (DHEA-S) or testosterone levels.

Idiopathic Hirsutism

Many patients have hirsutism in the face of normal adrenal and ovarian function, including normal levels of bound and free serum testosterone. Although this subset of patients has been hypothesized to have an increased metabolism of testosterone within the target tissue, characterized by increased 5α-reductase activity resulting in increased conversion of testosterone to dihydrotestosterone, tests have not substantiated this theory.

Pathogenesis and Etiology

In women, there are three sources of circulating androgens: ovarian, adrenal, and peripheral tissue conversion of precursors. The ovaries and adrenal glands produce testosterone, androstenedione, and dehydroepiandrosterone (DHEA). The adrenal cortex also produces DHEA-S. Of these compounds, testosterone is the physiologically active compound. One third of testosterone production comes from ovarian production, and the remainder comes from ovarian and adrenal precursors metabolized to testosterone by peripheral tissue. Ovarian, and perhaps adrenal testosterone, production is normally regulated by the pituitary via LH.

Androstenedione, DHEA, and DHEA-S, although designated as weak androgens, are best thought of as androgen precursors because they can be converted to testosterone in peripheral tissues. Their production appears to be gonadotropin independent and ACTH responsive. Peripheral conversion of androgen precursors is likely the major source of circulating androgen.

Diagnosis and Differential Diagnosis

A screening work-up should be done on all patients with hirsutism. This should include a serum free testosterone, LH, FSH, DHEA, and DHEA-S, 17α-hydroxyprogesterone, and an ultrasound examination (for polycystic ovaries).

For patients with virilism, as demonstrated by concurrent acne, deepening of the voice, amenorrhea, increased muscle mass, and clitoral hypertrophy, the investigation involves imaging, selective venous sampling, or laparotomy.

Treatment

General Considerations

Before initiating therapy for patients with hirsutism, there should be an accurate identification of any underlying abnormalities in androgen production or metabolism. History should be taken to ensure that the hirsutism is not due to medications such as androgens, anabolic steroids, danazol, and progestational compounds.

Medical treatment usually manages to decrease the rate of hair growth but may not eliminate the need for physical removal of undesired hair. Areas of the body that appear to respond to medical therapy include the hair on the face, chest, abdomen, and upper thighs. In contrast, hair around the nipples and on the arms, back, and lower legs responds less well.

In the presence of elevated levels of 17α-hydroxyprogesterone and DHEA-S, the presumptive diagnosis is adrenal source of androgens. The treatment of choice then is glucocorticoid suppression.

When there is hirsutism in the setting of normal menses and normal serum testosterone and DHEA-S, the diagnosis is usually considered to be idiopathic hirsutism, and the antiandrogens are usually the drug of choice.

The anti-androgens are usually effective and are first-line agents for most causes of hirsutism. The combination of spironolactone and oral contraceptive is excellent for treating this condition. Oral contraceptives serve to prevent a contraindicated pregnancy as well as to control dysfunctional bleeding caused by the spironolactone. Patients with adrenal hyperplasia are usually treated with dexamethasone or anti-androgens. Spironolactone may also be given in combination with dexamethasone.

Specific Agents

Oral Contraceptives

The most commonly used agents for the treatment of hirsutism, oral contraceptives, suppress the secretion of LH, increase sex hormone–binding globulin concentrations, and decrease testosterone and DHEA-S concentrations. Recommended oral contraceptives for this treatment are estrogen dominant and contain progestin with minimal androgenic activity, such as ethynodiol diacetate. Once inproved, bimonthly treatment may be effective maintenance.

Synthetic Progestins

Synthetic progestins such as medroxyprogesterone acetate and megestrol, which suppress gonadotropin secretion and testosterone production, may be effective alone at 20 to 40 mg per day orally or 150 mg intramuscularly every 6 weeks for 3 months.

Dexamethasone

Dexamethasone is often successful in treatment of hirsutism of ovarian or adrenal origin, given orally in doses as low as 0.25 mg every other day. In treatment of congenital adrenal hyperplasia, dosages up to 1.0 mg per day may be needed to suppress corticotropin secretion.

Gonadotropin-releasing Hormone Agonists

These drugs, which work by desensitization of gonadotropin-releasing hormone receptors on the gonadotropes, result in decreased gonadotropin secretion and appear to be effective in polycystic ovarian disease.

Ketoconazole

The oral antifungal drug ketoconazole inhibits cytochrome P-450–dependent enzymes involved in adrenal and gonadal steroid synthesis. It may be useful in a number of instances, including polycystic ovarian disease, adrenal adenoma or carcinoma, Cushing's disease, and idiopathic hirsutism, at a dosage of 400 to 1200 mg per day. However, it should be reserved for patients with hyperandrogenism unresponsive to other medical therapy.

Spironolactone

This potassium-sparing diuretic inhibits 5α-reductase activity, interferes with binding of dihydrotestosterone to its receptor, and inhibits testosterone synthesis. A dosage of 50 to 200 mg per day is the recommended anti-androgen dosage. Larger doses appear to be more efficacious.

Cyproterone Acetate

This anti-androgen compound is not available in the United States but is widely used in Europe for the treatment of hirsutism. This synthetic progestin works as a competitive inhibitor of testosterone and dihydrotestosterone to androgen receptors, inhibits gonadotropin secretion, and increases the metabolic clearance of testosterone. It is administered in a dosage of 50 to 200 mg per day on days 5 to 14 of the menstrual cycle or as a monthly 300-mg intramuscular injection.

Flutamide

Unavailable in the United States, this nonsteroidal anti-androgen appears to act solely through the blockade of the androgen receptor. Administered in conjunction with oral contraceptives to inhibit gonadotropin rise (and to prevent pregnancy), the recommended dosage is 250 mg twice a day. Favorable effects may be noted within 3 months.

NUTRITIONAL ABNORMALITIES

(CM&S Chapter 182)

Skin lesions are often a critical clinical feature of some inborn errors of metabolism. The cutaneous manifestations may be characteristic of a specific disorder.

Inborn errors of amino acid metabolism that have prominent cutaneous features and may be treated with appropriate nutritional intervention are reviewed in Table 13–1. Some defects of amino acid metabolism are covered elsewhere in this text. Other inborn errors of metabolism, such as zinc deficiency, Menkes' disease (copper transport), and glycogen storage diseases, are covered elsewhere in the text.

NEONATAL DERMATOLOGY

(CM&S Chapter 184)

Neonatal Dermatoses

Transient Vascular Phenomena

During the first few weeks of life, cold stress may be associated with a number of transient vascular phenomena. Acrocyanosis, in which the hands and feet become variably and symmetrically blue, disappears quickly when the child is bundled or warmed. Central cyanosis of the lips or face may be a marker for underlying cardiac or pulmonary disease. Cutis marmorata or livedo reticularis also develops with cold exposure. Diffuse marbling or mottling appears on the trunk and extremities for seconds to minutes intermittently up to 1 month of age. If cutis marmorata persists beyond the neonatal period, associated disorders including Down syndrome, trisomy 18, hypothyroidism, and Cornelia de Lange's syndrome should be considered. Congenital phlebectasia (cutis marmorata telangiectatica

TABLE 13-1. Dermatologic Signs of Disorders of Amino Acid Metabolism

DISEASE	METABOLIC DEFECT	MAJOR CLINICAL FEATURES	DERMATOLOGIC SIGNS	EFFECT OF TREATMENT ON SKIN INVOLVEMENT
Phenylketonuria (PKU)	Phenylalanine hydroxylase deficiency	Developmental delay Mental retardation	Flexural eczema Scleroderma-like changes • proximal • childhood onset Pigment dilution	Dietary phenylalanine restriction improves skin; skin may darken with diet
Tyrosinemia, type II (Richner-Hanhart syndrome)	Hepatic tyrosine aminotransferase deficiency	Photophobia Corneal scarring Developmental delay Mental retardation	Hyperkeratosis • hands and feet • painful, focal Leukokeratosis of tongue	Dietary phenylalanine and tyrosine restriction improves skin
Albinism Oculocutaneous • classic • other (see Chapter 7 in this text or Chapter 131 in CM&S)	Absence of tyrosinase Tyrosinase positive	Decreased pigment Decreased visual acuity, photophobia	Decreased pigmentation of skin, hair, eyes	No repigmentation (photoprotection is essential)
Prolidase deficiency	Reduced activity of prolidase	Mental retardation Splenomegaly Recurrent infections	Skin ulcers • legs	Manganese supplementation (prolidase cofactor) may help

Continued

713

TABLE 13-1. Dermatologic Signs of Disorders of Amino Acid Metabolism *(Continued)*

DISEASE	METABOLIC DEFECT	MAJOR CLINICAL FEATURES	DERMATOLOGIC SIGNS	EFFECT OF TREATMENT ON SKIN INVOLVEMENT
Argininosuccinicaciduria	Deficiency of argininosuccinate lyase		Trichorrhexis nodosa Dry, brittle hair	Hair may improve spontaneously with age
Multiple biotin-dependent carboxylase deficiency	Holocarboxylase Synthetase deficiency (early onset) Biotinidase deficiency (later onset)	Seizures, ataxia Failure to thrive Hypotonia Keratoconjunctivitis Metabolic acidosis	Seborrheic-like dermatitis Refractory candida intertrigo Pigment dilution Diffuse alopecia	Biotin treatment improves skin
Homocystinuria	Cystathionine synthase deficiency (pyridoxine-dependent)	Lens dislocation Other eye abnormalities Osteoporosis—spine Developmental delay Vascular occlusion	Pigment dilution Brittle hair Malar flushing Livedo reticularis	Methionine-restricted diet and pyridoxine supplementation may improve skin

Hartnup disease	Defective intestinal transport of tryptophan	Occasional ataxia Retardation	Pellagra-like rash Photosensitivity	Oral nicotinamide improves skin
Maple syrup urine disease	Branched-chain amino acids accumulate	Hypoglycemia seizures, acidosis Growth retardation Urine odor	Exfoliative erythroderma associated with inadequate dietary intake of branched-chain amino acids	Skin improves with less restriction of diet
Alkaptonuria	Homogentisic acid Oxidase deficiency	Dark urine Discoloration and degeneration of cartilage	Dark cerumen Cutaneous ochronosis	

congenita) may mimic persistent cutis marmorata. Although this permanent vascular anomaly may be generalized, lesions are usually localized to a small part of the skin surface. Infants with congenital phlebectasia deserve a careful medical evaluation for other mesodermal and neuroectodermal anomalies.

The harlequin color change is noted when the infant is placed in the lateral decubitus position. The dependent half of the body turns deep red in contrast to the pale upper half. The color reverses when the infant is rocked from side to side. Although this phenomenon may develop in up to 10% of infants, the color change usually lasts for under a minute. Recurrences are common during the first month of life. The cause is unknown, and it has not been associated with serious underlying disease.

Minor Anomalies

Minor congenital anomalies, such as skin tags of the auricle, epicanthal folds, simian creases, and café-au-lait spots, are of little or no physiologic consequence and occur in up to half of newborns. Nearly 10% of newborns have three or more minor anomalies, many of which are inherited in a multifactorial familial pattern. Although the risk of an associated syndrome with multiple major anomalies is low, the presence of multiple minor anomalies should prompt a thorough pediatric evaluation to exclude occult major defects, such as structural congenital heart disease, congenital cataracts, cleft palate, and choanal atresia.

Benign Pustular Dermatoses

Several innocent pustular eruptions that occur commonly in neonates must be distinguished from potentially serious infections.

Erythema toxicum neonatorum develops in up to 70% of healthy full-term infants typically on the second or third day of life. Erythematous macules and papules evolve over hours into 2- to 3-mm yellow papules and pustules on a broad urticarial base, giving a "flea-bitten" appearance. Although any part of the skin surface may be involved, lesions tend to cluster on the trunk, face and proximal extremities. Cultures of material obtained from pustules are sterile, and smears usually reveal sheets of neutrophils and eosinophils. Although biopsy is not needed for diagnosis, specimens taken to rule out other vesiculopustular conditions show that erythema toxicum neonatorum is a pustular folliculitis in which neutrophils and eosinophils predominate.

Transient neonatal pustular melanosis commonly develops in utero or during the first day of life. Macules or pustules on the sacrum or buttock may be the only cutaneous finding. However, pustules can spread over much of the skin surface. Pustules tend to aggregate on the chin, neck, upper chest, sacrum, abdomen, and thighs. Lesions typically arise on a noninflammatory base, and over a period of several days develop a central crust, then dry, leaving a collarette of scale, and finally heal with postinflammatory hyperpigmentation that resolves over 4 to 6 weeks. The pustules are subcorneal collections of neutrophils with few eosinophils. Pigment in basal keratinocytes, rather than an accumulation of melanophages, accounts for the hyperpigmentation of resolving macules. Unlike erythema toxicum neonatorum, scrapings from pustules of transient neonatal pustular melanosis show mostly neutrophils. This dermatosis occurs in only 4% of newborns, primarily in black males.

Both erythema toxicum neonatorum and transient neonatal pustular necrosis must be distinguished from *staphylococcal pustulosis*. Pustules in staphylococcal infection tend to be relatively large compared with the surrounding erythema. They often cluster in the diaper area, around the umbilical stump, or intertriginous areas. Gram's stain of purulent exudate reveals gram-positive cocci, and cultures are positive for *Staphylococcus aureus*. Prompt local care with compresses and topical antibiotics may result in rapid clearing. Widespread lesions require oral antibiotics. If the infant is febrile or appears ill in any way, a thorough evaluation for possible sepsis, hospital admission, and parenteral antibiotics are usually warranted. These benign pustular dermatoses should also be distinguished from candidiasis, *Herpes simplex* infection, and scabies.

Neonatal acne develops in at least 20% of newborns at birth or within the first few weeks of life (see Chapter 2 in this text or Chapter 49 in CM&S). Closed comedones predominate on the face. However, extensive eruptions over the trunk and occasionally the extremities may also include inflammatory papules and pustules. Lesions resolve without treatment within 1 to 3 months. The risk of severe acne in adolescence does not seem to be increased in these children.

Scaly Dermatoses

At 7 to 10 days of life, physiologic desquamation peaks, with large sheets of scale peeling from the extremities, leaving normal skin beneath. Deep cracking and fissuring of the skin the first day of life should alert the practitioner to the risk of postmaturity syndrome. In these infants, peeling may be noted in the delivery room. Other cutaneous markers include decreased subcutaneous fat and meconium staining. These children require close monitoring during the first few days of life for increased risk of temperature instability, hypoglycemia, hypocalcemia, poor feeding, and sepsis.

Ichthyosis refers to a heterogeneous group of genodermatoses, some of which present in the newborn period (see Chapter 11 in this text or Chapter 162 in CM&S). In the newborn, the first clues of disease include generalized scaling and erythema typical of an erythroderma (congenital ichthyosiform erythroderma) or a thick cellophane-like collodion membrane (lamellar ichthyosis).

Diaper dermatitis includes a number of acute and chronic disorders that present with rash primarily or initially in the diaper area (see Chapter 2 in this text).

Vesiculobullous Eruptions

Blistering eruptions in the newborn may present a confusing clinical picture. Once common bacterial, viral, and fungal infections have been excluded, only a limited number of disorders remain.

Several conditions, which do not commonly blister, may present with vesiculation in infancy because of decreased efficacy of intraepidermal attachments and dermal-epidermal adhesion. In rare cases of *bullous mastocytosis*, recurrent blistering may be so severe that fluid and electrolyte balance is disrupted and the risk of infection is high (see Chapter 10 in this text or Chapter 152 in CM&S).

More commonly, children with solitary mastocytomas or urticaria pigmentosa occasionally develop localized areas of blistering that are often mistaken for bullous impetigo. In both settings, blistering decreases with increasing age.

Localized or widespread blistering on a noninflammatory base, especially over bony prominences and areas of mechanical trauma, should suggest the diagnosis of *epidermolysis bullosa* (see Chapter 3 in this text or Chapter 73 in CM&S). These disorders can be characterized by histopathologic and clinical findings, inheritance patterns, and biochemical and molecular markers. Epidermolytic hyperkeratosis and pachyonychia congenita are both commonly associated with blistering in infants and should be considered in the differential diagnosis of epidermolysis bullosa.

Lumps and Bumps

Although cutaneous malignancies are rare, two forms of panniculitis cause self-limited disease regularly in otherwise healthy infants.

In *subcutaneous fat necrosis* of the newborn, red or hemorrhagic nodules and plaques up to 3 cm in diameter appear most commonly on areas exposed to trauma and cold stress, such as the cheeks, back, buttocks, arms, and thighs, during the first few days of life. Although the cause is unknown, complicated deliveries, hypothermia, perinatal asphyxia, and maternal diabetes predispose to the development of fat necrosis. In most cases the general health of the child is unaffected. However, recalcitrant life-threatening hypercalcemia has been rarely reported. Skin biopsies characteristically demonstrate fat necrosis, foreign body giant cells, and residual lipocytes with needle-shaped clefts in a radial arrangement. Most lesions resolve without scarring in 1 to 2 months. However, some nodules become fluctuant, ulcerate, and heal with atrophy.

Cold panniculitis appears as red indurated nodules and plaques on the cheeks of infants exposed to cold weather (see Chapter 2 in this text or Chapter 70 in CM&S).

Index

Note: Page numbers in *italics* indicate figures; those followed by t indicate tables.